BACKCOUNTRY TRIPS IN CALIFORNIA'S SIERRA NEVADA

SIERRA SOUTH

9TH Edition

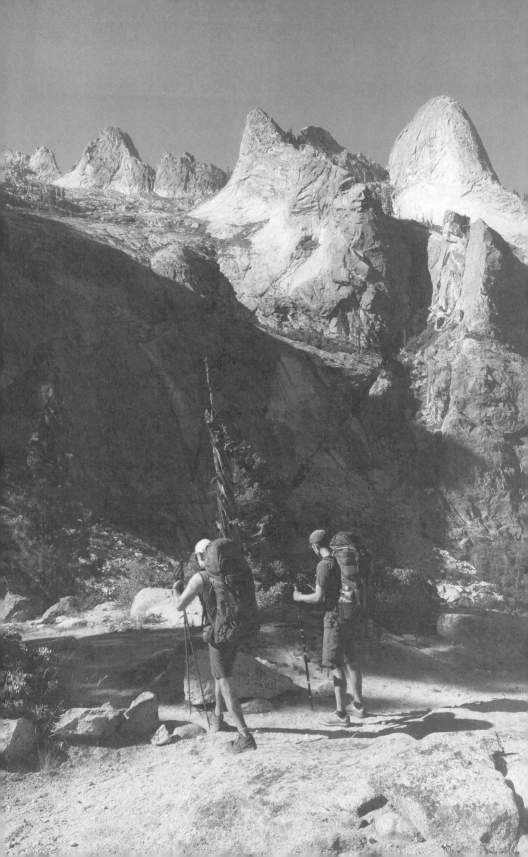

BACKCOUNTRY TRIPS IN CALIFORNIA'S SIERRA NEVADA

SIERRA SOUTH

9TH Edition

ELIZABETH WENK
and MIKE WHITE

WILDERNESS PRESS . . . *on the trail since 1967*

SierraSouth: Backcountry Trips in California's Sierra Nevada

1st edition, 1968; 2nd edition, 1975; 3rd edition, 1980; 4th edition, 1986; 5th edition, 1990; 6th edition, 1993; 7th edition, 2001; 8th edition, 2006; 9th edition, 2021
   2nd printing 2022

Cover design: Scott McGrew
Text design: Andreas Schüller, with updates by Annie Long
Cartography: Scott McGrew, Elizabeth Wenk, and Mike White
Cover photo: © Videowokart/Shutterstock
Frontispiece: Hamilton Towers (Trip 25, page 149); © Elizabeth Wenk
Project editor: Holly Cross
Copy editor: Kerry Smith
Proofreaders: Emily Beaumont and Ritchey Halphen
Indexer: Potomac Indexing LLC

ISBN 978-0-89997-884-0 (pbk.); ISBN 978-0-89997-885-7 (ebook)

Library of Congress Control Number: 2020947927

Published by: 🏃 **WILDERNESS PRESS**
         An imprint of AdventureKEEN
         2204 First Ave. S., Ste. 102
         Birmingham, AL 35233
         800-678-7006, fax 877-374-9016

Manufactured in the United States of America
Distributed by Publishers Group West

Visit wildernesspress.com for a complete listing of our books and for ordering information. Contact us at our website, at facebook.com/wildernesspress1967, or at twitter.com/wilderness1967 with questions or comments. To find out more about who we are and what we're doing, visit blog.wildernesspress.com.

Safety Notice Although Wilderness Press and the authors have made every attempt to ensure that the information in this book is accurate at press time, they are not responsible for any loss, damage, injury, or inconvenience that may occur to anyone while using this book. You are responsible for your own safety and health while in the wilderness. The fact that a trail is described in this book does not mean that it will be safe for you. Be aware that trail conditions can change from day to day. Always check local conditions and know your own limitations.

Acknowledgments

I have thoroughly enjoyed the opportunity to be a part of the 9th edition of *Sierra South*. Hiking 54 trips for this book required a bit of a time commitment, and I always appreciate my family's enthusiasm for book-driven Sierra adventures, as well as my husband's willingness to be a single parent for a month each summer while I continue exploring the mountains on my own.

Thank you as well to the many friends who have joined me on trips, especially the Rengers, who are my companions each summer. A number of friends have read segments of this book, confirming that my writing matches their memory of trips: thank you, Inga Aksamit, John Ladd, Ethan Gallogy, and Peter Hirst.

As my coauthor, Mike White, will attest, updating this book did not go quite as smoothly as either of us had planned, with record snowpacks in 2017 and 2019 and fires in the region in 2017 and 2018 repeatedly interrupting hiking schedules; I felt unusually relieved when I finished mapping the trails.

I hope that you have the chance to experience many of the trips described—and that you consider the landscape as beguiling as I do.

—*Elizabeth Wenk*

I am always indebted to the ongoing support of my wife, Robin, for the opportunity to be in the wilderness and to write about its wonders. Companionship on the trail is usually desirable, and many have walked along with me on this project, including Dal and Candy Hunter, Keith Catlin, and Joe and Chris Tavares. The folks at Wilderness Press certainly deserve kudos for guiding this project to completion, especially with the delays caused by forest fires and a pandemic. Thanks also to my coauthor, Lizzy Wenk, for all of her support and help in making this new edition a reality.

—*Mike White*

We jointly wish to acknowledge the Indigenous tribes who have been the custodians of the southern Sierra's lands for millennia and who continue to maintain a close cultural connection to these lands and waters.

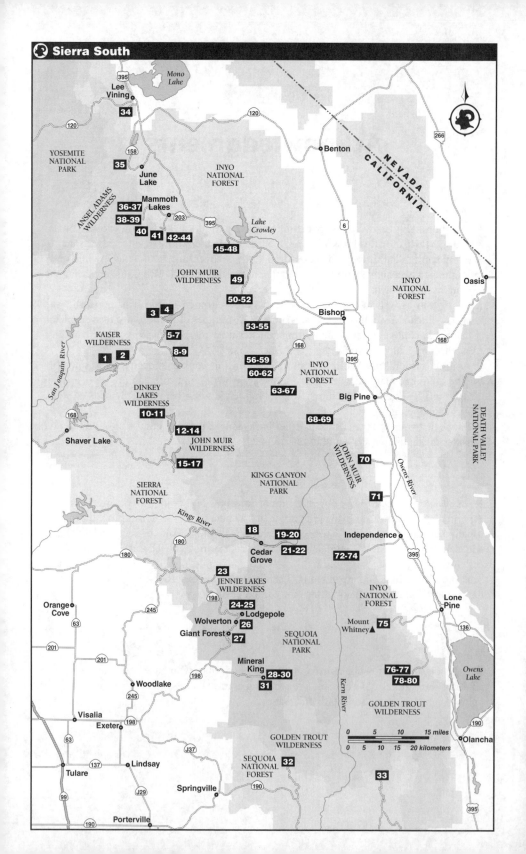

Contents

Climbing above Deer Lakes toward Deer Lakes Pass (Trip 41, page 249)   Photo by Elizabeth Wenk

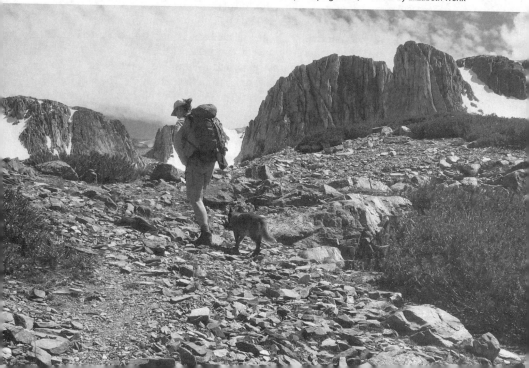

Going High to Get High

Note for the 9th Edition

This is the first edition of Sierra South *that Wilderness Press's founder, Tom Winnett, will not see go to press. We hope he would be pleased with the latest edition. The authors have tried to merge in modern guidebook expectations, including GPS coordinates, while keeping true to Tom's pledge to make this a series that accurately portrayed the trail, campsites, landscape, and natural history, providing readers with enticing trips. About 15 years ago Tom wrote:*

By Thomas Winnett (1922–2011), Wilderness Press Founder

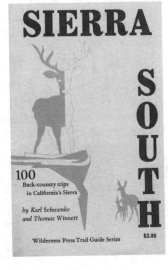

As I write this, it is nearly 40 years since we at Wilderness Press held a celebration to promote the first edition of *Sierra North* and the upcoming *Sierra South*, one-of-a-kind books Karl Schwenke and I wrote to recommend 100 of the best backpacking trips into the northern Sierra and 100 into the southern Sierra.

It was the summer of 1967, and we celebrated in the backcountry with a high-altitude cocktail party. We invited everyone we thought would help get the word out about the book: people from the Sierra Club, outdoor writers, and friends. We held the celebration in August, in Dusy Basin, in the eastern Sierra, 8 miles from the nearest car. The hike went over a 12,000-foot pass, so we were delighted when 15 people showed up. It was a real party. We used snow to make our martinis, ate hors d'oeuvres, and spent the night. In a mention of the event, *San Francisco Chronicle* columnist Herb Caen wondered, "How high can you get to get high?"

It was a spectacular occasion, not only because we were launching the book but also because we were starting a new company, Wilderness Press. Karl and I had been complaining about how hard it was to get accurate information about the out-of-doors. At the time, there were only one or two guidebooks to the Sierra—our favorite place—so we decided to write our own. We planned to create prepackaged trips that specified which trails to take and where to stop each night. We would do a series of small books, each covering a 15-minute quadrangle, and they would be called the Knapsacker/Packer Guide Series.

In the summer of 1966, we started doing the field research. Our approach was simple: we wanted to accurately describe where the trails led and what was there. On my scouting trips, I carried more than your average backpacker. In addition to all the standard gear, I packed two cameras, two natural history books to help me identify flowers and birds, and my Telmar tape recorder. The tape recorder ran about half the speed of the recording devices that are available today, and I'd walk along, dictating into the microphone everything I thought our customers would be interested in reading. So in addition to the basics—how to get to where you start walking, where to go, the best campsites—we also described what we saw: the animals, flowers, birds, and trees.

By the end of the summer, we had enough material to cover most of the trails in the northern Sierra, so we published a book of 100 trails and called it *Sierra North*. Next, we set about work on *Sierra South,* which we published in 1968.

The first edition of *Sierra South* sold like the proverbial hotcakes; we sold out our entire print run of 3,000 books. Since then, this book has sold more than 140,000 copies, and it gives me great joy to see it in its eighth edition.

As I think back to that high-altitude cocktail party in 1967, I wonder how many people have used this book to "go high to get high" in the Sierra. I have personally walked more than 2,000 miles in this most beautiful of mountain ranges, and although I can't do that anymore, I am still hooked on the experience—the splendid isolation, the scenery that really lights up your eyeballs, the strength you feel climbing with the weight of your pack on your back, the myriad trout. I hope this guidebook hooks you too.

Isoceles Peak and Columbine Peak rise above Dusy Basin (Trip 65, page 341). Photo by Elizabeth Wenk

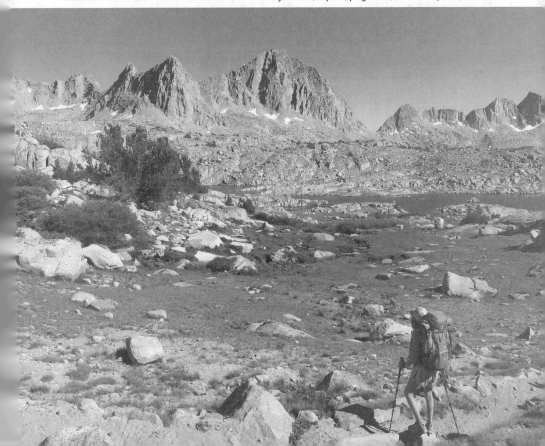

TRIP CROSS-REFERENCE TABLE

TRIP NO.	PAGE NO.	TRIP TYPE				BEST SEASON			HIKING DAYS	MILEAGE	GOOD FOR BEGINNERS
		OUT & BACK	LOOP	SEMILOOP	SHUTTLE	EARLY	MID	LATE			
1	23		•			•	•	•	2	18.7	
2	29	•				•	•	•	2	9.6	•
3	35			•			•	•	4	29.1	
4	41	•					•	•	3	15.0	•
5	45			•			•	•	5	37.2	
6	55			•			•	•	4	32.8	
7	59				•		•	•	4	35.0/31.0	
8	64	•					•	•	6	39.4/47.4	
9	69	•					•	•	6	44.4/52.4	
10	73	•					•	•	2	10.6	•
11	77			•			•	•	3	21.1	
12	82	•					•	•	2	14.2	•
13	86	•					•	•	6	33.0	
14	89			•			•		6	32.1	
15	91	•				•	•	•	2	19.6	
16	96	•					•	•	5	42.8	
17	99			•		•	•	•	4	29.3	
18	105				•		•	•	5	30.0	
19	114	•				•	•	•	3	21.8	
20	119		•				•	•	9	78.7	
21	131	•					•	•	4	29.6	
22	135			•			•	•	6	40.7	
23	141			•		•	•		3	18.6	•
24	144	•					•	•	2	20.0	
25	149			•			•	•	11	113.4	
26	163	•					•	•	2	11.8	•
27	166				•		•	•	9	68.0	
28	178	•					•	•	2	16.4	
29	182	•					•	•	6	39.0	
30	184		•				•	•	6	38.7	
31	189	•				•	•	•	4	23.6	
32	195	•				•	•	•	3	19.0	
33	198			•		•	•	•	3	18.8	
34	208	•					•	•	2	5.2	
35	211			•			•	•	3	20.1	•
36	220		•				•	•	2	18.9	
37	225	•					•	•	2	13.8	•
38	229	•					•	•	2	14.4	•
39	232		•				•	•	3	14.6	•
40	238			•			•	•	6	46.6	

TRIP CROSS-REFERENCE TABLE

TRIP NO.	PAGE NO.	TRIP TYPE			SHUTTLE	BEST SEASON			HIKING DAYS	MILEAGE	GOOD FOR BEGINNERS
		OUT & BACK	LOOP	SEMILOOP		EARLY	MID	LATE			
41	249		•				•	•	2	13.1	
42	251				•		•	•	3	17.1	•
43	257				•	•	•	•	4	28.2	
44	263			•			•	•	4	24.8	
45	267	•					•	•	2	11.6	•
46	271			•				•	5	27.0	
47	276	•					•	•	2	15.0	•
48	278				•		•	•	5	31.7	
49	285	•				•	•	•	3	13.8	
50	292	•					•	•	2	7.2	•
51	293				•		•	•	3	24.6/19.7	
52	298	•					•	•	4	18.0	
53	302	•					•	•	2	10.4	
54	305			•			•	•	4	19.0	
55	308			•			•	•	3	21.3	
56	314	•					•	•	2	14.4	
57	316	•					•	•	2	5.0	•
58	318	•					•	•	3	14.0	
59	320		•				•	•	6	39.0	
60	324				•		•	•	2	8.1	
61	328	•					•	•	2	11.8	•
62	330	•					•	•	2	9.4	
63	337	•					•	•	2	5.8	•
64	339			•			•	•	2	6.8	•
65	341	•					•	•	2	14.0	
66	344			•			•	•	6	37.4	
67	350				•		•	•	8	55.0	
68	360			•			•	•	3	12.2	•
69	366	•					•	•	2	9.2	
70	370				•		•	•	5	33.4	
71	381	•				•	•	•	2	15.6	
72	385	•				•	•	•	2	5.0	•
73	388			•			•	•	5	27.4	
74	392			•			•	•	4	34.5	
75	400	•					•	•	4	20.8	
76	407			•		•	•	•	2	12.6	•
77	412		•				•	•	4	23.4	
78	420				•		•	•	6	39.5	
79	427				•		•	•	7	55.6	
80	435	•					•	•	4	26.8	

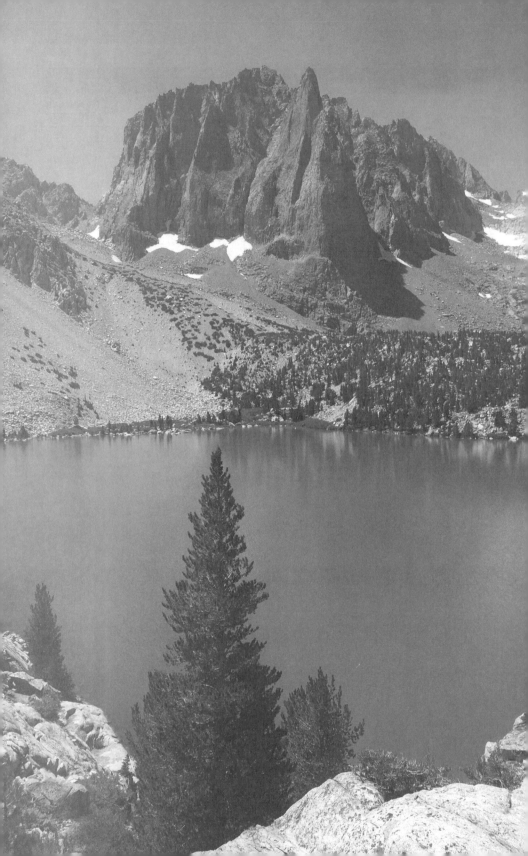

Introduction

Welcome to what we think is just about the most spectacular mountain range in the contiguous 48 states. The Sierra Nevada is a hiker's paradise filled with huge wilderness areas; thousands of miles of trails; countless lakes, rugged peaks, and canyons; vast forests; giant sequoias; and terrain ranging from deep, forested river valleys to sublime, rugged alpine country.

Updates for the 9th Edition

Welcome, too, to the 9th edition of Wilderness Press's second book, *Sierra South*. The original edition of *Sierra South* was published in 1968, a year after its first book, *Sierra North*, became an instant bestseller—among Sierra hikers at least. *Sierra South* has proved to be equally popular for the past half century. As always, the authors involved in the update have rotated, and the updates this time have been led by Elizabeth Wenk and Mike White.

In the 15 years since the eighth edition was published, GPS units have become commonplace additions to hikers' gear lists, and the waypoints and trail distances included in this book have (nearly) all been verified by electronic devices. While most of the trips remain the same, there were regions where the hikes included had been unchanged for 52 years but trail networks and use patterns have evolved. Hence, some hike routes have been altered, while a few have been removed and replaced with new hikes. We've strived to include the vast majority of the southern Sierra's trails, as we expect readers want to explore widely. In addition, all-new elevation profiles clearly show junctions and waypoints described in the text.

For this edition, coordinates for waypoints are given as latitude and longitude in decimal degrees, a relatively simple format to enter into digital devices. If you'd like to upload the waypoints embedded in the text directly to a GPS device, visit tinyurl.com/sierrasouthgps to download a file that you can view online or on your device. *Note:* This file does not contain all trail junctions—just trailheads, notable campsites, ranger stations, and the occasional cryptic junction where having a coordinate is particularly useful.

The maps provided in the book are nearly identical to those in previous editions; that is, they are simple sketch maps of the hikes, including prominent nearby place-names. The only notable change is that, where relevant, we reference nearby or overlapping trips, by number, to make it easier for users to merge segments of different described hikes into a unique route of their choosing. Similarly, in the text, at junctions we reference how different trips link together.

As in the eighth edition, *Sierra South* spans wilderness areas from a little south of Yosemite National Park on the west and from Yosemite's eastern boundary south of CA 120 (Tioga Road) on the east to the Sherman Pass area to the south. The previous edition included a

Temple Crag stands proudly behind Second Lake (Trip 68, page 360).   Photo by Elizabeth Wenk

cluster of hikes beginning in the Clover Meadow area of Ansel Adams Wilderness; these are now covered in *Sierra North*. The wilderness areas and national parks covered include most of Ansel Adams Wilderness and all of John Muir Wilderness, Kings Canyon National Park, Sequoia National Park, Kaiser Wilderness, Dinkey Lakes Wilderness, Monarch Wilderness, Jennie Lakes Wilderness, and Golden Trout Wilderness. (*Sierra North* then covers the Sierra from a little south of Yosemite north through the Tahoe area to I-80 and to the Castle Peak Wilderness Study Area, including the northwestern corner of Ansel Adams Wilderness, Yosemite National Park, Hoover Wilderness, Emigrant Wilderness, Carson-Iceberg Wilderness, Desolation Wilderness, Granite Chief Wilderness, and the National Forest lands connecting these regions.)

Unlike the region covered by *Sierra North,* in the territory this book covers, no roads cross the range, a distance of some 140 air miles between CA 120 to the north and Sherman Pass to the south. Instead, in this region many spur roads lead from corridors to the west, east, and south into the range, accessing countless trailheads. The book's first major trip section covers the region's west side and presents roads into the west side from north to south. The second major trip section covers the Sierra's east side and, also from north to south, the roads into the range from the east.

Measuring distances in the backcountry used to be more art than science, but modern GPS units make it possible to accurately determine trail distances. Your authors each have their own methods to measure trail distance, but Lizzy Wenk measures all tracks she walks with a pair of GPS units, verifies the tracks in Google Earth, and generally trusts the resultant distances to within 2%. With a few exceptions, trail distances are still rounded to the closest 0.1 mile.

It's our hope that this new edition will help you enjoy our magnificent southern Sierra as well as give you an incentive to work to preserve it.

We appreciate hearing from our readers. Many of the changes and updates for this edition are a direct result of readers' requests and comments. Please let us know what did and didn't work for you in this new edition, and about any errors you find. You can email us at info@wildernesspress.com or leave comments at our website: go to wildernesspress.com and click "Contact Us" at the top of the page.

Care and Enjoyment of the Mountains

Be a Good Guest: Wilderness and Leave No Trace

The Sierra is home—the only home—to a spectacular array of plants and animals. We humans are merely guests—uninvited ones at that. Be a careful, considerate guest in this grandest of nature's homes. Indeed, the vast majority of hikes included in this guide lie within one of the Sierra's many wilderness areas, lands designated by the 1964 Wilderness Act to remain *untrammeled,* defined in the *Oxford English Dictionary* as "not deprived of freedom of action or expression; not restricted or hampered." Moreover, *wilderness* is defined as areas where humans and their works do not dominate the landscape and indeed where humans are visitors who do not remain.

Several hundred thousand people camp in the southern Sierra's wilderness areas each year. The vast majority care about the wilderness and try to protect it, but it is threatened by those who still need to learn the art of living lightly on the land. The solution depends on each of us. We can minimize our impact. The saying "Take only memories (or photos), leave only footprints" sums it up. Hikers or equestrians entering the Sierra's many wilderness areas must accept that, in order to preserve the wilderness in its natural form, perhaps they cannot enter the trailhead they want because the quota is filled or they might be slightly inconvenienced by packing out toilet paper or not lighting a campfire.

Following the seven Leave No Trace principles is an easy way to ensure you are minimizing your impact when camping in (and out of) wilderness areas. Indeed, if you look carefully at the regulations on your backpacking permit, you will realize that the specific requirements—from human-waste management to campfire regulations to campsite selection and food storage—are all necessary if visitors are going to "leave no trace," as embodied by these principles:

- Plan ahead and prepare.
- Travel and camp on durable surfaces.
- Dispose of waste properly.
- Leave what you find.
- Minimize campfire impacts.
- Respect wildlife.
- Be considerate of other visitors.

© 1999 by the Leave No Trace Center for Outdoor Ethics: lnt.org.

The information below applies Leave No Trace principles to on-the-ground guidelines for hikers. More than anything else, learn to go light. John Muir, traveling along the crest of the Sierra in the 1870s with little more that his overcoat and his pockets full of biscuits, was the archetype. Muir's example may be too extreme for many (and he did stay warm by building campfires in locations now deemed unacceptable), but the concept that you should strive to get by with less, not more, is a powerful starting point. A lot of the stuff people take into the mountains is burdensome, harmful to the wilderness, or just plain annoying to other people seeking peace and solitude.

Carry Out Your Trash

- Pack out all trash—do not attempt to burn plastic, foil packaging, or toilet paper. The remnants of foil-lined hot-chocolate packets linger indefinitely in fire pits to the ire of rangers and backpackers alike.
- Anglers, take all your lures, bait, and monofilament out with you. Don't leave fishing line tangled over trees, shrubs, or logs or floating in the lake.
- Prepare only as much food as you think you will eat in a sitting. Discarded leftovers are likely to attract bears and other wildlife (see page 5).

Protect the Water

Keeping the Sierra's water sources pristine is as important for wilderness users as for nature itself. Humans (and stock) can damage Sierra water sources by introducing disease agents through poor sanitation practices, by adding nutrients to the Sierra's naturally low-nutrient waters, or by increasing streambank erosion. Notably, augmenting nutrient concentrations in the water leads to algal blooms that, in turn, provide habitat for waterborne parasites such as *Giardia* (see page 7).

- Wash and rinse dishes, clothes, and yourself a minimum of 100 feet away from water sources; never wash in lakes or streams. Even though a soap may be marketed as biodegradable, it still isn't OK to put it in the water. A good, lightweight solution is to carry a large zip-top bag for washing clothes and then carry the water away from the creek or lake.

- Do not put any soap in water—even biodegradable soap.
- Follow the sanitation practices described in the next section.

Practice Good Sanitation

- Bury waste 6 inches deep, a minimum of 100 feet from trails, and 200 feet from water sources. Intestinal bacteria can survive for years in feces when they're buried, but burial reduces the chances that critters will come in contact with them and carry pathogens into the water, or that these pathogens will wash into the water following snowmelt or a thunderstorm.
- Pack out toilet paper. This is now a requirement throughout the Sierra, but one that is poorly complied with by many hikers. Burying your toilet paper does not work—animals rapidly dig it up, and tissue "flowers" are a blossoming problem in popular areas. Also pack out facial tissues, wet wipes, tampons, and sanitary pads.

  Place used toilet paper and sanitary products in a heavy-duty zip-top bag. Add a little baking soda to the bag to minimize odors, and/or place the plastic bag in an opaque ditty bag to keep it out of sight.
- Consider using a bidet instead of toilet paper. A growing contingent of Sierra hikers has ditched (or mostly ditched) toilet paper in favor of portable bidets. In addition, many women now carry a "pee cloth" to greatly reduce their backcountry use of toilet paper. You can use a standard cotton bandanna or purchase a dedicated cloth.

Practice Good Campsite Selection

- Whenever possible, camp in an established campsite.
- Otherwise, pick a campsite on a durable surface, such as sand, a polished granite slab, or the forest floor.
- Camp at least 100 feet from water (in some wilderness areas you can camp closer than 100 feet *if* you are using an established site).
- Never camp in meadows, on lakeshores, or on streamsides. The fragile sod is easily compacted and, once the soil is hardened, meadow grasses are replaced by shrubs and trees.
- Don't make campsite "improvements" like rock walls or tent ditches. These are illegal.
- For your safety, don't camp beneath a dead tree or large dead branch. So-called widowmakers are a particular danger in forests hard hit by recent droughts and bark-beetle and leaf-miner infestations.
- Also take care with the vegetation beside your tent—walking back and forth to a water source can also damage riparian vegetation, and moving rocks exposes the roots of nearby plants, possibly killing them.

Avoid Campfires

- Use a modern, lightweight backpacking stove. Campfires waste a precious resource: wood that would otherwise shelter animals and, upon decaying, return vital nutrients to the soil. Campfires can also start—and have started—forest fires. As detailed on your wilderness permit, campfires are prohibited in many areas, especially at high elevations and at lower elevations during the hot midsummer months.
- Each year, campfires are prohibited in ever more popular areas—because some wilderness visitors use the available wood resources irresponsibly. If having a *small* campfire is an

important part of your backcountry experience, take care to build only legal and responsible fires, so that you will have this option on future trips.

- Build a small fire.
- Only build a fire in an existing campfire ring.
- Never leave the fire unattended.
- Make sure your fire is out and cold before leaving your campsite (or retiring to your tent).
- *Always* obey campfire bans when they are in effect.
- Likewise, *do not* build a campfire in areas where they are prohibited. This increasingly includes popular subalpine lake basins where previous campers have scoured the landscape for every piece of dead wood, leaving nothing to decompose or as shelter for the animal residents.
- Make sure to pick up a California Campfire Permit at a ranger station (or online) if you don't need a wilderness permit or if your wilderness permit doesn't double as a campfire permit.

Protect Your Food from Wildlife

Remember, the wilderness is wildlife's home, not yours, and you must always respect the wildlife. Avoid trampling on nests, burrows, or other homes of animals. Observe all fishing limits. If you come across an animal, just quietly observe it. Don't go near any nesting animals and their young. Get "close" with binoculars or telephoto lenses. And most importantly, make sure only you eat your food—letting animals eat your food not only cuts short your trip, but is bad for the animals. They may become too aggressive toward humans, dependent on human food, or sick from eating processed food (and wrappers).

Bears are the animals most likely to attempt to eat your food, but marmots, ravens, and even deer will grab a snack if your food is accessible to them. While most animals can easily be thwarted by hanging your food sloppily in a tree or off a rock, bears are very clever and innovative: mothers give their cubs a piggyback to reach a low-lying bag. Mothers encourage their cubs to climb out on the branch, too flimsy to hold an adult bear's weight, but perfect for a cub. And even a perfectly hung pair of counterbalanced food bags can be foiled if a bear shakes a tree until one bag drops down.

Marmots love people food, so take precautions to make sure they don't steal yours.

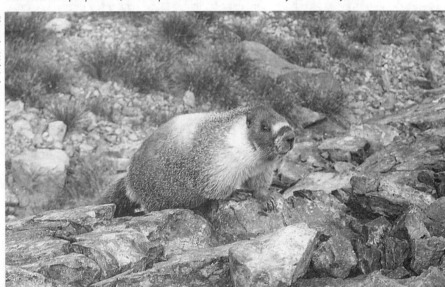

Photo by Walt Lehmann

Bear canisters—plastic, carbon fiber, or metal containers, generally in a cylindrical shape—first appeared on the market in the early 1990s and are now considered the *only* acceptable way to store your food in some of the Sierra's wilderness areas (including parts of Sequoia and Kings Canyon National Parks and parts of John Muir Wilderness). The remaining areas covered in this book still allow hikers to hang their food using the counterbalance method but strongly recommend the use of canisters. Another alternative, prohibited in Sequoia and Kings Canyon National Parks but currently allowed in all national-forest wilderness areas described in this book, is the Ursack, a Kevlar bag in which you can store your food. Most ranger stations rent bear canisters for a modest fee, so if you don't own one, you can pick one up together with your wilderness permit.

In addition, in Sequoia and Kings Canyon National Parks quite a few established camping areas have food-storage lockers—colloquially known as bear boxes. See nps.gov/seki /planyourvisit/bear_box.htm for a current list of their bear box locations. Food-storage lockers are also located at many Sierra trailheads to store your extra food before a trip. Everyone shares the bear box; you may not put your own locks on one. Never leave a bear box unlatched or open, even when people are around.

Overall:

- Store all food in your bear canister (or hung or in an Ursack, where legal) anytime you leave it unattended.
- All toiletries and fragrant items from your first aid kit must be stored with your food.
- After cooking, clean up food residue and leave your pots out.
- Don't leave any food in your backpack when you aren't wearing it.
- Don't store any food in your tent.
- Do not leave any food in your car at the trailhead. Many trailheads have animal-proof food storage lockers in which to store your extra supplies.
- Never use a backcountry bear box as a food drop; its capacity is needed for people actually camping in its vicinity.

Safety and Well-Being

Hiking in the high country is far safer than driving to the mountains, and a few precautions can shield you from the discomforts and dangers that do threaten you in the backcountry.

Health Hazards

ALTITUDE SICKNESS If you normally live at sea level and you come to the Sierra Nevada to hike, it will take your body several days to adjust. Headaches and a sense of nausea are the most common symptoms of acute mountain sickness (AMS), the least severe and by far most common type of altitude sickness in the Sierra Nevada. Though most cases of altitude sickness occur above 10,000 feet in elevation, 20%–25% of people experience some degree of altitude sickness already at 8,200 feet (2,500 meters). For unknown reasons, some people are much more prone to altitude sickness than others—if you hike often at higher elevations, you will know how susceptible you are and how hard you can plan to push yourself at altitude. While going slowly, staying hydrated, and regularly eating some food are important to reduce the chance you will experience nausea or headache, they aren't explicitly reducing your AMS symptoms—the only way you can actually reduce the likelihood of altitude sickness is to acclimate. Afterall, acclimation refers to the multiday physiological adjustments to altitude that your body can make only through exposure to high elevation.

One of the best things you can do is to stay in a trailhead campground the night before your trip to begin the acclimization process, especially one above 6,000 feet. If you are particularly susceptible to altitude sickness, either avoid the hikes in this guide that suggest a campsite above 9,000 feet for the first night, or spend several nights car camping and day hiking before you begin your backpacking trip.

An Unofficial Acclimatization Guideline: Your High-Altitude Guideline for the John Muir Trail is a handy, inexpensive reference you can read in advance and load onto your mobile device to read on the trail. It covers the symptoms associated with different types of altitude sickness, prophylactic medications, and treatment options. Free copies of this guide are also available in the archives of the Altitude Acclimatization Facebook group: facebook.com /groups/altitudeacclimatization.

WATERBORNE ILLNESS For many decades, hikers in the Sierra Nevada have been advised to filter their water due to the risk of contamination by *Giardia lamblia,* a waterborne protozoan, and other waterborne pests that cause severe diarrhea and abdominal pain. Aside from areas with cattle grazing and very high stock use, the risk of waterborne illness is actually quite low, but most hikers treat all their drinking water as a precaution. *Giardia* populations are generally only high in water bodies where algae provide habitat for the cysts. In the Sierra, algal blooms are generally associated with cattle grazing and high stock use, but in the future poor human sanitation or camp practices (see pages 3–4) or warming water temperatures could increase algal prevalence and in turn *Giardia* risk.

Some hikers are likely asymptomatic *Giardia* carriers, and their sloppiness in burying waste or cooking for a group can contaminate water sources and infect others, so always assume you're contagious and sanitize your hands before sharing food. Note that with *Giardia,* symptoms appear two to three weeks after exposure.

There are additional disease agents that could be present in Sierran lakes and rivers. *Cryptosporidium* is another, smaller, very hardy pest that causes a disease similar to giardiasis. A recent study has found the feces of the resident yellow-bellied marmots contains

This may look cool and refreshing, but it's advisable to chemically treat, filter, or boil water before drinking it.

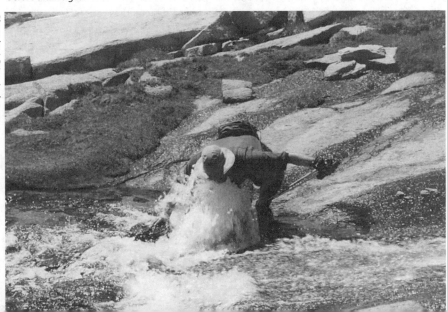

Photo by J. Brian Anderson

strains of *Cryptosporidium* that could infect humans, although no one has collected evidence that it regularly contaminates water sources.

Viruses do not survive long in the cold, harsh conditions of the alpine environment and are unlikely to infect water in the Sierra. *E. coli* is uncommon but could be present in lower-elevation Sierra water bodies.

Hikers have myriad water-treatment options. Keep in mind that different treatments kill or remove different microbes:

- **Chemical purification** *(for example, iodine or chlorine)*: This is the easiest method of treating water—simply add drops or a tablet—but you have to wait about 20 minutes to drink your water. Some chemical purification methods leave a distinct chemical flavor, while others do not. In addition, *Cryptosporidium* is resistant to chlorine, so if this microbe becomes more common in the Sierra, this method will no longer be practical.

- **Water filters:** Water filters should remove all bacteria and protozoa, but the pores of many filters are too large to remove viruses. The advantages of filtering are removal of all microorganisms of concern (in the Sierra Nevada) and not leaving a flavor in your water. There are both pump filter and gravity filter setups. The prior requires you to actively pump your water through the filter, while with the latter, filtering is a passive process; you fill a bag with water and return 5 minutes later to find a gallon of freshly filtered water. Another variant of water filters are squeeze filters (for example, Sawyer Mini) that screw straight onto your water bottle. You effectively purify the water as you drink. They are lightweight and allow each person to easily carry his or her own filter, but some brands clog easily and have quite low flow.

- **Ultraviolet light purifier** *(such as SteriPen)*: Ultraviolet light damages the DNA of all microorganisms, rendering them harmless. Water must be clear for the ultraviolet light to function, so water with silt must settle or be filtered through a cloth or equivalent. And make sure you have spare batteries with you. (As an aside, a clear, still alpine lake, devoid of algae, is the best place from which to drink if you aren't purifying your water. The top 6 inches of an alpine lake have been irradiated by the sun to a similar extent as a UV purifier performs.)

- **Boiling:** This kills all microorganisms but is very time-consuming and uses considerable fuel.

HYPOTHERMIA Hypothermia refers to subnormal body temperature. Caused by exposure to cold, often intensified by wet, wind, and weariness, the first symptoms of hypothermia are uncontrollable shivering and imperfect motor coordination. These are rapidly followed by loss of judgment, so that you yourself cannot make the decisions to protect your own life. "Death by exposure" is death by hypothermia.

To prevent hypothermia, stay warm: carry wind- and rain-protective clothing, and put it on as soon as you feel chilly. Stay dry: carry or wear wool or a suitable synthetic (not cotton), and bring raingear even for a hike with an apparently sunny forecast.

Treat shivering at once: get the victim out of the wind and wet, replace all wet clothes with dry ones, put him or her in a prewarmed sleeping bag with hot water bottles, and give him or her warm drinks.

LIGHTNING Although the odds of being struck are small, almost everyone who goes to the mountains thinks about it. If a thunderstorm comes upon you, avoid exposed places—mountain peaks, passes, open fields, a boat on a lake—and avoid small caves and rock overhangs. The safest place is an area where you are less than 50 feet from, but not directly next to, a much taller object such as a tree.

If you are stuck in flattish terrain above treeline, crouch on top of a rock (but not the highest one, of course) that is somewhat elevated or otherwise detached from the rocks underneath it to protect yourself from any current flowing through the ground. Make sure to get all metal—such as frame packs, hiking poles, tent poles, and so on—away from you. The best body stance is one that minimizes the area where your body touches the ground. The National Outdoor Leadership School recommends squatting on the balls of your feet as low as possible and wrapping your arms around your legs. This position minimizes your body's surface area, so there's less chance for a ground current to flow through you, reducing the seriousness of injuries should you be struck. Close your eyes, cover your ears, hold your breath, and keep your feet together to prevent the current from flowing in one foot and out the other. Once a storm is upon you, getting in this position is more important than trying to seek more sheltered ground.

If you get struck by lightning, hope that someone in your party is adept at CPR—or at least artificial respiration if your breathing has stopped but not your heart. Eighty percent of lightning victims are not killed, but it can take hours for a victim to resume breathing on his or her own. As soon as possible, a victim should be evacuated to a hospital; other problems often develop in lightning victims.

SUNBURN Sunburns can be particularly bad at high elevations, where the ultraviolet radiation is greater. You can even get burned on cloudy days because the radiation penetrates clouds. Therefore, always wear a wide-brimmed hat and apply strong sunscreen to all exposed skin. The best sun protection is, of course, long sleeves and long pants—even if you've been resistant to long clothing in the past, try some of the new fabrics on the market. Some of them are—finally—true to their advertisement of keeping you pleasantly cool on a hot day.

Wildlife Hazards

RATTLESNAKES Rattlesnakes mainly occur below 7,000 feet but have been seen up to 9,000 feet. They live in a range of habitats but most commonly along canyon bottoms. Watch where you place your hands and feet; listen for the rattle. If you hear a snake rattle, stand still long enough to determine where it is, then leave in the opposite direction. They are frequently curled up alongside a rock or beneath a fallen log—look carefully before stepping across a fallen log or sitting atop a log or rock for a break.

Rattlesnake bites are rarely fatal to an adult, but a bite that carries venom may still cause extensive tissue damage. If you are bitten, get to a hospital as soon as possible. There is no substitute for proper medical treatment.

MOSQUITOES Mosquitoes in the Sierra fall more in the nuisance category than the danger category, but as they may (at lower elevations) carry diseases, it is best to avoid being bitten. That is easier said than done, for mosquitoes are common near stagnant water sources (including many Sierra lakes and slow-flowing rivers) and in moist forest terrain until mid-July. In some years they are only pesky near dusk and other years are an all-day nuisance. Camping in windier, drier, higher-elevation locations is one good way to avoid them—but such campsites don't appeal to everyone.

The best way to avoid being bitten by mosquitoes is to cover your skin by wearing long sleeves, long pants, and a wide-brim hat, possibly topped by a head net. There are a number of topical solutions hikers carry to thwart mosquitoes on exposed skin. N,N-diethyl-meta-toluamide, known commercially as DEET, is the most common, and products with at least 20% DEET do a very good job of keeping mosquitoes off of you, but also can etch plastics and must be kept far from your mouth, eyes, and so on. You must also never wash yourself in streams or lakes with DEET on your skin—it is toxic to many animals, including frogs. Other products, such as picaridin and lemon eucalyptus, do as well as DEET in trials (commercial trials and your authors') but must be reapplied more frequently. An alternative (or additional) approach is to, before your hike, spray or soak your clothes in permethrin. Permethrin can be purchased in ready-to-spray formulations or as a concentrate. There are also companies that commercially apply permethrin—and a growing contingent of outdoor clothing retailers that sell pretreated clothing.

Of course, the best method of mosquito prevention is to plan your trips from late July to September.

BLACK BEARS The bears of the Sierra are American black bears; their coats range from black to light brown. American black bears are fast, immensely strong, and very intelligent. They're not usually aggressive, however, unless they're provoked, and their normal diet consists largely of plants. In California's mountains they pose no danger to you, just to your food; some of the black bears in Canada and Alaska are more aggressive. Long ago black bears learned to associate humans with easy sources of food, leading to incessant human–bear conflicts, especially broken-into cars and stolen food. Over past decades steady progress has been made in outsmarting the bears—or, more specifically, educating humans about the need to store food in bear canisters and not leave food in unattended cars (see pages 5–6). Sadly, a food-habituated bear is usually soon a dead bear.

Don't let the possibility of meeting a bear keep you out of the Sierra. Respect these magnificent creatures. Just remember, if a bear does get your food, it now belongs to the bear, not you; don't attempt to get it back, but do realize it is your responsibility to pick up the wrappers that get scattered around.

Terrain Hazards

SNOW BRIDGES AND CORNICES Stay off of these.

STREAMS Stream flows can be dangerous during peak snowmelt or following a severe thunderstorm. When stream flows are high, drowning is the greatest danger facing a backpacker. Peak snowmelt usually occurs in June, but it can extend into July in high snow years. Stream flows can also rise (and drop) rapidly following a summer thunderstorm. If a river is running high, you should not cross it solo, and you should spend considerable effort looking for an alternative (for example, a log or a broader, shallower, less turbulent ford) before starting across. And if a stream is dauntingly high or swift, forget it; the best option is to retreat or wait until the water level subsides. Snowmelt flows are much higher in the evening than the following morning, and thunderstorm flows usually subside within 12 hours.

Here are some suggestions for stream crossing:

- Wear closed-toe shoes, which will protect your feet from injury and give them more secure placement. If you don't have good water shoes—not flip-flops—wear your hiking boots or shoes.
- Cross in a stance in which you're angled upstream. If you face downstream, the water pushing against the back of your knees could cause them to buckle. Or, following the other school of thought, face slightly downstream, where you're not battling against the current.
- Move one foot only when the other is firmly placed.
- Keep your legs apart for a more stable stance. You'll find a cross-footed stance unstable even in your own living room, much less in a Sierra torrent.
- One or two hiking sticks will help keep you stable while crossing. You can also use a stick to probe ahead for holes and other obstacles that may be difficult to see and judge under running water.

- One piece of advice used to be that you should unfasten your pack's hip belt in case you fell in and had to jettison the pack. However, modern quick-release buckles probably make this precaution unnecessary. Keeping the hip belt fastened will keep the pack more stable, and this will in turn help *your* stability. You may wish, however, to unfasten the sternum strap so that you have only one buckle to worry about.

Maps and Profiles

Today's Sierra traveler is confronted by a bewildering array of maps, and it doesn't take much experience to learn that no single map fulfills all needs. Three main categories of maps are described below: government-issued topographic maps, trail maps, and online maps. While the book includes grayscale maps for each hike, these do not suffice for on-the-trail navigation; they are included only to provide an overview of the regions through which the trip wanders.

USGS Topographic Maps

Topographic maps of various scales exist for all areas covered in this guidebook. The most detailed maps are those produced by the U.S. Geological Survey (USGS), generally referred to as the 7.5-minute (abbreviated henceforth as 7.5′) topo series. These have become increasingly hard to purchase except directly from the USGS, but if you plan to explore off-trail, they are still the gold standard. The data from these maps is available to the public, and you can download the maps to print yourself directly from the USGS: visit the **National Map Viewer** at usgs.gov/core-science-systems/national-geospatial-program/national-map. The trail locations depicted on the National Map Viewer are more current than those on the print maps.

While some visitor centers still stock USGS 7.5′ (1:24,000-scale) maps for the local area, they are increasingly difficult to find in outdoor-equipment stores. For an off-trail trip when you truly need the detail only provided by USGS maps, plan ahead and order them directly through the USGS website.

Since USGS maps are public domain, they are also used as the base maps by other online services, such as the free **CalTopo.com,** where you can easily print the pieces of map required for your trip. The USGS maps required for each hike are indicated in the introductory material for that hike. If the hike traverses more than one USGS map, they are listed in the order they are encountered on the walk.

Trail Maps

While USGS topo maps provide the best detail for landscape features, they do not include trail distances, trail names, or similar annotations. The U.S. Forest Service publishes a series of "inch to the mile"–scale (1:63,360-scale) maps for many wilderness areas and national forests. These are excellent resources for driving to trailheads because they include all U.S. Forest Service road names (and numbers) and provide a good overview of the local trail network. However, they lack trail distances, often fail to acknowledge which trails haven't been maintained in a generation, and are a bit bulky for backpacking. These maps are generally available at ranger stations or can be ordered through store.usgs.gov. The content from these maps can also be purchased as georeferenced PDFs from **Avenza** (avenza.com) for use on digital devices.

In addition, a number of other cartography companies produce topo maps annotated with trail distances. These vary in accuracy, but the two brands most commonly used for Sierra trails are **Tom Harrison Maps** and **National Geographic Trails Illustrated maps,** which cover nearly every hike in this book.

Map Apps

The past decade has brought a change in how people navigate in the wilderness. A growing number of people no longer carry paper maps, instead using an app to preload topo maps onto their phones, GPS units, or other digital devices. Of these, the **Gaia GPS** app is the most widely used and allows you to upload both waypoints (that is, those provided in this book) and USGS 7.5′ topo maps. CalTopo.com offers a similar service.

The benefits of these apps are obvious:

- You're already carrying a phone, so you now have maps at no additional weight.
- You always know where you are; your location is identified by a little dot on your screen.
- These apps are an easy way to plot waypoints onto a map.

The downsides of these apps *should* also be obvious—and scare your authors into *always* carrying a paper map as well:

- Digital devices eventually run out of battery power—and map apps are notorious battery sinks.
- Digital devices can break, get wet, and so on.
- You have a very limited understanding of the broader landscape because you see only a tiny piece of the map at once.
- It is very easy to have the maps for some segment of your trip not download properly—and you won't realize it until you're on your trip.

One of your authors (Lizzy) has, over the past five years, transitioned to doing a fair bit of navigating using Gaia GPS. She finds it incredibly convenient for trying to follow a trail across snow and making sure she is aiming for the correct cross-country location. However, she also still carries USGS 7.5′ topo maps when hiking off-trail and either a trail or topo map when hiking on trail because she has (1) had her phone's battery run out faster than expected, (2) been frustrated with herself for forgetting to look at the big picture and made poor big-picture navigation decisions off-trail, and (3) realized the maps downloaded at the wrong scale and were useless for cross-country navigation.

But really, the biggest problem is that people no longer have that wonderful sense of connectedness to the entire landscape that you have if you stare at your entire trip on a giant mosaic of maps.

How to Use This Book

Terms This Book Uses

DESTINATION/COORDINATES In this edition, coordinates are provided in latitude and longitude, in decimal degrees. If you prefer UTM coordinates (which are easier to plot on a paper map), download a copy in that format from tinyurl.com/sierrasouthgps or use a GPS coordinate conversion program (many are available online). All the coordinates provided by your authors have been field-checked or checked on a mapping program like Google Earth. The coordinates use the WGS 84 horizontal datum (equivalent to the NAD83 for UTM coordinates).

TRIP TYPE This book classifies a trip as one of four types. An **out-and-back** trip goes out to a destination and returns the way it came. A **loop** trip goes out by one route and returns by another with relatively little or no retracing of the same trail. A **semiloop** trip has an out-and-back part and a loop part; the loop part may occur anywhere along the way. A **shuttle** trip starts at one trailhead and ends at another; usually, the trailheads are too far apart for you to walk between them, so you will need to leave a car at the ending trailhead, have someone pick you up there, or rely on public transportation to get back to your starting trailhead. The shuttle information indicates whenever public transportation is an option.

BEST SEASON Deciding when in the year is the best time for a particular trip is a difficult task because of California's enormous year-to-year variation in snowpack and melt-off times. In one year the subalpine and alpine lands are mostly snow free by Memorial Day (late May) and another year you must wait until mid-July to cross the higher passes—and even then you will encounter considerable snow, which may require the use of an ice axe and crampons. On the other end of the season, some years receive their first winter storm in mid-September, and in others you can traverse the high country until late October. Therefore, describing hiking season by month is problematic; if you aren't sure how the current year tracks the long-term average, visit cdec.water.ca.gov/snowapp/swcchart.action to get a sense.

Hence, instead of describing hikes by month or descriptors like "early summer," this book uses the terms **early, mid,** and **late season.** In an average year, early season is mid-May–June, midseason is July and August, and late season is September–mid-October. Low-country hikes, which are almost always listed as early season, are perfect as warm-up excursions for the itchy hiker who may be stiff from a winter's inactivity.

And if a hike lists a variety of hiking seasons, in addition to snow pack consider the following to help you decide when to go:

- Mosquitoes can be bad through mid-July.
- June–mid-July is the peak wildflower bloom.
- Day length starts to shorten noticeably starting in August, with days becoming quite short by September.
- Temperatures are warmest in mid- to late July.
- Thunderstorms can occur anytime but are most prevalent in July and August, corresponding with monsoon moisture coming north from the Gulf of Mexico and Gulf of California.
- Wildfires become increasingly likely as the summer progresses; these rarely pose a danger to hikers, but they can ruin the views with hazy air or make the air unhealthy to breathe.

PACE For each trip, we give a suggested number of days to spend completing the trip as well as the number of layover days (see below) you might want to take. Galen Clark, Yosemite's beloved "Old Man of the Valley," was once asked how he "got about" the park. Clark scratched his beard and then replied, "Slowly!" And that is the philosophy we have adopted in this book. Most trips are divided across enough days to be either **leisurely** or **moderate** in pace, depending on where the best overnight camping places are along the route. We also call a few trips **strenuous,** usually because the terrain requires significant elevation gain on one or more days. In today's era of lightweight backpacking gear and short vacations, hiking longer days is in vogue—your authors are also guilty of this—but, with extra time, a leisurely pace lets hikers absorb more of the sights, smells, and "feel" of the country they have come to see. If you do choose to hike two of the described days in a single day or come up with your own itinerary, make use of some of the other campsites described in the text. Pace may not be everything, but Old Man Clark lived to the ripe old age of 96, and it behooves us to follow in his footsteps.

LAYOVER DAYS Also called "zero days" by long-distance thru-hikers, these are days when you'll remain camped at a particular site. You can spend your layover day on a day hike to see other beautiful places around the area, enjoy some adventures like peak bagging, or spend a quiet day fishing or reading in camp. The number of layover days you take will most likely be dictated by how many days you have off work and how much food you can fit in your bear canister. In the text, we often provide suggestions for activities on your layover day, usually an easy peak to ascend or a spur trail that is good to explore.

TOTAL MILEAGE The trips in this book range in length between 5.0 miles and 113.4 miles, and many trips can be shortened or extended, based on your interest and time.

CAMPSITES The trips are divided to spend each night in a location with a decent campsite and, whenever possible, one that can accommodate several groups and that is ecologically robust enough to host campers most nights throughout the summer. Scattered throughout the daily hike descriptions are mentions of other established campsites if you wish to make your day shorter or longer. If you establish your own campsite, make sure you follow both the regulations detailed on your wilderness permit and follow good campsite-selection practices, outlined on page 4. Occasionally we reference "packer campsites"; these are generally larger, long-established sites favored by large stock groups, often with log furniture. Some are, to many backpackers, objectionably overused, dusty, and accompanied with piles of dung, but others are very pleasant stopping points and are usually in ecologically appropriate areas. Using this descriptor is not meant to be an explicit slight—it's simply a description.

FISHING Angling, for many, is a prime consideration when planning a trip. As background, within the scope of Sierra South, all mountainous areas above the first significant topographic barrier (waterfall or high cascades) were fishless before the arrival of white emigrants; glaciers had scoured all the high country lakes and the fish could not recolonize upstream of the barriers. Many of these lakes were stocked beginning in the 1870s, and although stocking has ceased in the wilderness areas covered in this book, many High Sierra lakes still hold healthy fish populations. In the Kern River drainage in the far southern Sierra is the native range of three subspecies of golden trout: the California golden trout (Kern Plateau); Kern River rainbow trout (main Kern River, below barriers); and the Little Kern rainbow trout (Little Kern River). Conservation efforts are underway to protect these populations, so be sure you know local fishing regulations if you visit these areas.

Stocking in naturally fishless lakes has stopped to protect native mountain yellow-legged and Sierra Nevada yellow-legged frog populations. Most lakes that were once stocked still have self-sustaining fish populations, but fish have vanished from some lakes (usually at

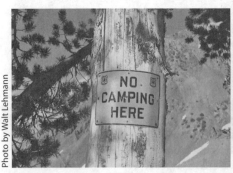
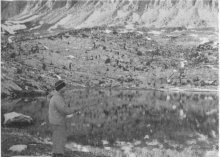

Be careful to observe all camping and fishing regulations.

Photo by Walt Lehmann

Photo by Bryan Rodgers

high elevations, without good spawning habitat), and fish have been explicitly removed from a few other lakes to provide frog habitat (almost always off-trail). While we note the most recent information on which lakes have which fish species, accept that this is a bit of a moving target. For the eastern Sierra, visit fs.usda.gov/activity/inyo/recreation/fishing to download a pamphlet detailing which fish are currently in each water body. And, of course, that indefinable something known as "fisherman's luck" plays a big role in what you'll catch. Generally speaking, the old "early and late" adage holds: fishing is better early and late in the day, and early and late in the season.

STREAM CROSSINGS We mention man-made bridges and other means of crossing streams. We also include descriptions of currently available naturally fallen logs, as these may last for decades or—like some bridges—be washed out during high flows. Asking the rangers about stream-crossing conditions when you pick up your permit is always a good idea. (See page 10 for stream-crossing tips.)

TRAIL TYPE AND SURFACE Most of the trails described here are well maintained (the exceptions are noted) and are properly signed. If the trail becomes indistinct, look for blazes (peeled bark at eye level on trees) or cairns (two or more rocks piled one atop another; also called *ducks*). Trails may fade out in wet areas like meadows, and you may have to scout around to find where they resume. Continuing in the direction you were going when the trail faded out is often, but not always, a good bet.

Two other significant trail conditions are also described in the text: the degree of openness (type and degree of forest cover, if any, or else *meadow, brush,* or whatever) and underfooting (talus, scree, pumice, sand, duff—a deep ground cover of humus, or rotting vegetation—or other material).

A *use trail* is an unmaintained, unofficial trail that is more or less easy to follow because it is well worn by use. For example, nearly every Sierra lakeshore has a use trail worn around it by anglers in search of their catch.

LANDMARKS The text contains occasional references to points, peaks, and other landmarks. These places are shown on the appropriate topographic maps cited at the beginning of the trip. For example, "Point 9,426" in the text would refer to a point designated as simply "9426" on the map itself. The actual numbers are an eclectic mix of feet and meters because USGS topo maps vary in the units they use.

FIRE DAMAGE Fire creates a mosaic of habitats throughout the Sierra Nevada. Historically, ground fires were common throughout the Sierra's montane forests and an essential ecological disturbance. In the process of clearing the ground and understory of thick brush, fire significantly altered the populations of ground-dwelling plants and animals. These fires would rarely have killed most of the canopy trees, allowing the landscape to rapidly recover from the fire. Then, from the late 1800s until the 1970s (or later), fire suppression was a general policy; every fire was extinguished immediately. This led to the accumulation of thick litter, dense brush, and overmature trees—all prime fuel for a hot, destructive blaze when a fire inevitably sparked to life. Foresters now know that natural fires should not be prevented but only regulated.

In recent decades, a combination of controlled burns (mostly alongside road corridors) and large wildfires (started by a combination of lightning strikes, careless campers, and arson) have passed through many of the Sierra's low- and midelevation forests. The years of fuel accumulation mean many of these fires become behemoths, often decimating the entire forest and killing the vast majority of trees, a very different process to what ecologists hypothesize occurred previously. If most of the trees in a region are killed, there is no longer a seed source, and it can be decades before seedlings establish, dependent on the rare seeds that arrive from afar. A second problem is that the hottest fires burn organic material within the soil and sterilize it, such that even wildflowers and shrubs struggle to establish.

Nonetheless, you should not consider fire as a negative force. Without fires, a plant community evolves toward a climax, an end stage, of plant succession, and only the plant and animal species that thrive in this climax community remain common. The mosaic of burned and unburned patches allows such a diversity of plant and animal species to thrive in the Sierra. For instance, species of the genus *Ceanothus* rapidly colonize the burned landscape, only to be shaded out by young lodgepoles and Jeffrey pines a few decades later. They are in turn replaced by red and white firs, the main species in the characteristic climax communities of the Sierra's midelevations.

From a practical hiker's standpoint, fire-ravished landscapes offer less shade but an abundance of spring wildflowers. Less-traveled trails often become yet more difficult to navigate as mountain whitethorn, a particularly fast-growing, dense, prickly shrub, consumes the trail. In the text we note where fire has recently passed across patches of landscape and how much forest remains. We recommend visiting charred landscapes in spring and early summer, when vibrant blooms make up for the lack of shade.

As a final note, as this book goes to press in late 2020, the Creek and Castle Fires are both raging in the western Sierra, changing the character of quite a few of the trips in this book and *Sierra North*. The Creek Fire is already the Sierra's largest fire, burning across the San Joaquin River drainage and into the North Fork Kings. Abundant dead trees from drought and beetle kill are providing ample fuel—the fire is likely to continue burning eastward (away from populated areas) until it reaches rockier terrain or winter rains extinguish it. Sierra backpackers will increasingly need to accept that the lower elevation trails will be more open, while the subalpine (and alpine) lake basins will be fairly untouched.

How This Book Is Organized

In this region, roads penetrate the range from the west and from the east without crossing the range. Therefore, *Sierra South* is organized first by which side of the Sierra you must start on (west or east) and then, in north to south order, by the roads you must take into the range to get to the trailheads. The two hikes in the far southern Sierra, Maggie Lakes (Trip 32) and Redrock Meadows and Jordan Hot Springs (Trip 33) are both listed as western hikes because the trailheads lie west of the Sierra Crest. With the western and eastern sections, the trailheads and hikes are listed in a north-to-south sequence.

TRAILHEAD AND TRIP ORGANIZATION As previously noted, each trip is located within trailhead sections in the book. These sections begin with a summary table, such as the example on the facing page, that uses the trailhead's name, elevation, and latitude–longitude coordinates as its title. If relevant, the table also includes the names of shuttle trips that start at a different trailhead but end at this trailhead; these are included should you want to walk a described trip in reverse—for example, because you are unable to obtain a permit for the direction as described.

Following the table are details about information and permits, along with driving directions to the trailhead.

Next comes the first trip from this trailhead; see example also on the facing page. The trip data—GPS coordinates, total mileage, and hiking/layover days—is included with each trip entry. All trips include an elevation profile, a list of maps, and highlights. Some include Heads Up!, or special considerations for that trip; shuttle trips include directions to the ending trailhead.

Bishop Pass Trailhead (at South Lake)
9,825'; 37.16934°N, 118.56580°W

Destination/ GPS Coordinates	Trip Type	Best Season	Pace & Hiking/ Layover Days	Total Mileage	Permit Required
63 Treasure Lakes 37.14522°N 118.57544°W	Out-and-back	Mid to late	Leisurely 2/1	5.8	Treasure Lakes
64 Chocolate Lakes 37.14841°N 118.54932°W	Semiloop	Mid to late	Leisurely 2/0	6.8	Bishop Pass– South Lake
65 Dusy Basin 37.10369°N 118.55158°W (Lake 11,347)	Out-and-back	Mid to late	Moderate 2/1	14.0	Bishop Pass– South Lake
66 Palisade Basin 37.08201°N 118.50601°W (Glacier Creek Lake 11,673)	Semiloop	Mid to late	Strenuous 6/2	37.4	Bishop Pass– South Lake
67 South Lake to North Lake 37.11205°N 118.67093°W (Muir Pass)	Shuttle (public transport option)	Mid to late	Moderate 8/1	55.0	Bishop Pass– South Lake (Piute Pass in reverse)

trip 63 Treasure Lakes

Trip Data: 37.14522°N, 118.57544°W (lowest Treasure Lake); 5.8 miles; 2/1 Days
Topos: *Mount Thompson*

HIGHLIGHTS: Few trips offer so much High Sierra beauty for so little effort. Not only is there a wealth of dramatic scenery, there's also good camping and fishing. This trip also makes a good day hike.

DAY 1 (Bishop Pass Trailhead at South Lake to lowest Treasure Lake, 2.9 miles): Starting just left of the information sign, the trail crosses an unmapped creeklet and meets the trail climbing from the pack station; turn right here, heading south. The trail descends slightly toward South Lake and then immediately begins a steady climb up the sandy slope rising from the shore with splendid views across the lake. Soon out of sight of the lake, you wind upward, through pocket meadows and conifer stands . . . This lake, the largest in the Treasure Lakes basin (12 acres), affords fair-to-good fishing for golden-rainbow hybrids. There are additional campsites at fishless Lake 11,159 (Lake 3); see the sidebar below. The listed mileage ends where you ford the lowest lake's inlet stream—usually a wade.

DAY 2 (lowest Treasure Lake to Bishop Pass Trailhead at South Lake, 2.9 miles): Retrace your steps.

After this comes the next trip, if any, from this same trailhead. Trips in the same general area, especially multiple trips from the same trailhead, often share the same first day's hiking. For example, the first trip from a trailhead is usually the shortest—one day out to a destination, the next day back to the trailhead. The second trip will build on—extend—the first trip by following the first trip's first day and then continuing on a second and subsequent days to more-distant destinations. Rather than repeat the full, detailed description for the first trip's first day, we simply reference the first day's description from the first hike.

TRAILHEAD MAPS A simple sketch map is included for each trailhead. It shows the location of roads, trailheads, and trails. It shows the route of each described trail and the names of key landmarks, but it is not meant to be a comprehensive hiking map of the area. The goal of these maps is for you to easily be able to find the described route on a larger topographic map or trail map. Gray numbers indicate trips departing from other trailheads that share a trail segment or traverse adjacent trail segments, should you wish to piece together your own route, combining pieces of multiple trail descriptions. Nearby trailheads are also marked and named, again in gray, so you can easily find adjacent trailhead maps. The map legend on the facing page details the symbols you'll find on the trailhead maps.

East Lake (Trip 21, page 131)   Photo by Elizabeth Wenk

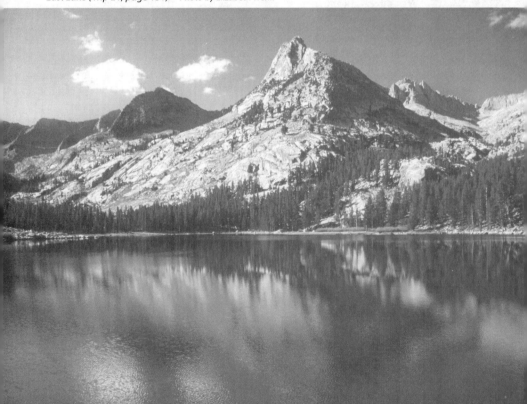

Map Legend

▪▪▪▪▪▪▪▪▪	Main trail	
▬ ▬ ▬ ▬ ▬ ▬	Other trail	
•••••••••••	Cross-country route	
- - - - - - - -	Use-trail	
▬ ▬ ▬ ▬ ▬	4WD road	
═══════	Freeway	
═══════	Major road	
──────	Minor road	
═ ═ ═ ═ ═ ═	Unpaved road	

28 **56**	Trip Number/linked
T **T**	Trailhead/linked
P **P**	Parking/linked
⌂	Ranger station
?	Information
⛺	Campground
⊞	Picnic area
⌒	Dam
▲	Peak/summit
■	General point of interest

▨	National Park
▨	Wilderness
▨	National Forest
▪▪▪▪▪▪▪	Adjacent boundary

◌	Glacier
◌	Lakes
～	Rivers/creeks

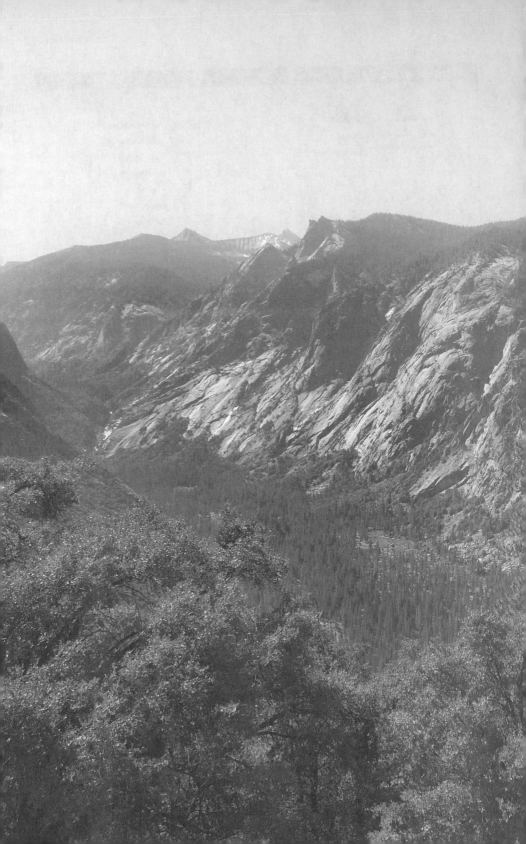

West Side

Getting to the starting trailheads on the west side of the Sierra south of Yosemite means long, gradual, winding, scenic drives on mountain roads and highways from some major road in the western foothills or the Central Valley, like CA 49 or CA 99. Be sure to allow plenty of time to enjoy these beautiful drives. A few shuttle trips will end at roads not listed below. Along the way, small towns, tiny villages, and rustic resorts provide lodging and some supplies. For supplies, there are more choices in the larger towns nearer the roads' west ends than closer to the trailheads.

On the west side, you'll enter the Sierra on these roads and highways:

- **CA 168 West Side to Kaiser Pass Road** *(yes, there is an east side, too, but 168 doesn't cross the range)*

- **CA 168 West Side to Dinkey Creek Road**

- **CA 180** *(into Kings Canyon proper)*

- **CA 198** *(Generals Highway, runs along the far western edge of Kings Canyon and then Sequoia National Parks, passing through part of Sequoia National Forest)*

- **CA 198 to Mineral King Road**

- **CA 190** *(into the southern Sierra's Golden Trout Wilderness)*

Take in the beautiful views to the South Fork Kings and the Sphinx near the base of the Copper Creek Trail (Trip 19, page 114).   Photo by Elizabeth Wenk

CA 168 WEST SIDE TO KAISER PASS ROAD TRIPS

Kaiser Pass Road leads deep into the Sierra, accessing trails near Lake Edison and Florence Lake that head up the major forks of the South Fork San Joaquin River, Mono Creek, Bear Creek, and the South Fork San Joaquin itself, each with enticing glacial lake basins at their heads. Less convenient is the long, slow, winding drive, but it's well worth it once you experience the diverse trips on offer.

The first pair of trailheads, Deer Creek and Potter Pass, lead into Kaiser Wilderness from near the start of Kaiser Pass Road, a small wilderness area centered on view-rich Kaiser Peak. The other trailheads lie farther east in the South Fork San Joaquin drainage. From north to south, they are Mono Creek Trailhead (at Lake Edison), Bear Diversion Trailhead (along Lake Edison Road), and Florence Lake Trailhead (at Florence Lake). A cluster of trails departs from the Mono Creek Trailhead. Mono Creek Trail leads up the drainage, intersecting the John Muir Trail (JMT) and numerous spurs, while other trails access the lake basins surrounding the Silver Divide, including the Margaret Lakes Trail and Goodale Pass Trail (with a spur to Graveyard Lakes). The Bear Creek Trail, departing from the Bear Diversion Trailhead, intersects the JMT (from which spurs provide the easiest access to the Hilgard Branch and East Fork Bear Creek) and leads to the renowned Bear Lakes Basin. Finally, the Florence Lake Trailhead ascends the main South Fork San Joaquin Valley, leading to the JMT corridor, and up to remote lake basins tucked beneath monumental ridges, the Goddard Divide, White Divide, and Le Conte Divide. Trips along two other forks of the South Fork San Joaquin, Piute Creek and Evolution Creek, are included in the east side portion of this book.

Trailheads: **Deer Creek**

Potter Pass

Mono Creek

Bear Diversion

Florence Lake

Deer Creek Trailhead (Huntington Lake)
7,224'; 37.25958°N, 119.17225°W

Destination/ GPS Coordinates	Trip Type	Best Season	Pace & Hiking/ Layover Days	Total Mileage	Permit Required
1 Kaiser Loop Trail 37.29428°N 119.18556°W (Kaiser Peak)	Loop	Early to late	Strenuous 2/0	18.7	Deer Creek (Billy Creek for alternative route)

INFORMATION AND PERMITS: This trailhead is in Sierra National Forest. Permits are required for overnight stays and quotas apply. Details on how to reserve permits are available at fs.usda.gov/detail/sierra/passes-permits. For advance reservations (60% of quota; reservable starting in January each year), there is a $5-per-person reservation fee, while walk-up permits (40% of quota) are free. Permits can be picked up at 29688 Auberry Road, Prather, CA 93651; if you call 559-855-5355 in advance they will leave your permit in a dropbox. Permits can also be picked up in person at the Eastwood Forest Service Office at the corner of Kaiser Pass Road and CA 168, at Huntington Lake. If you plan to use a stove or have a campfire, you must also have a California campfire permit, available from a forest service office or online at preventwildfireca.org/campfire-permit. Campfires are prohibited above 10,000 feet. Bear canisters are not required but are strongly encouraged.

DRIVING DIRECTIONS: From the intersection of CA 168 and CA 180, just east of Fresno, take CA 168 northeast through Clovis and up into the foothills, to the community of Shaver Lake. Here, continue straight along CA 168 to Huntington Lake (versus right to Courtright Reservoir along Dinkey Lakes Road), and reach a T-junction near the community of Lakeshore, 67.5 miles from CA 180, where the Kaiser Pass Road branches right. Continue left on the Huntington Lake Road for 0.9 mile, past the College Campground and Lakeshore Resort, turning right (north) onto Upper Deer Creek Lane. Over the coming 0.6 mile, you pass several spurs left to vacation houses and each time stay right; there is no mention of a trailhead. Just before the road bends right (east) to the D&F Pack Station, there is a pullout on the left side of the road. Park here and continue on foot to the trailhead, located at the back of the pack station and marked by an information sign.

trip 1   Kaiser Loop Trail

see map on p. 24

Trip Data: 37.29428°N, 119.18556°W (Kaiser Peak);
18.7 miles; 2/0 days

Topos: *Kaiser Peak*

HIGHLIGHTS: This demanding trip's highlight is the ascent of Kaiser Peak, with its spectacular views that encompass the central Sierra Nevada's San Joaquin River's watershed. The lack of permanent water sources makes this a difficult trip. Delightful Nellie Lake is the only site with big campsites and guaranteed water, which necessitates a 10-mile day with more than 2,000 feet of elevation gain and 3,000 feet of loss on Day 2. A small party can break the second day with a stop at Line Creek Lake (if there is good weather) or, in early summer, a camp alongside a seasonal creek. Note the shuttle alternative given on page 25, which unfortunately only shortens Day 1.

HEADS UP! *Take plenty of water, for long stretches of this strenuous trip are usually dry by mid-July; the watercourses are seasonal.*

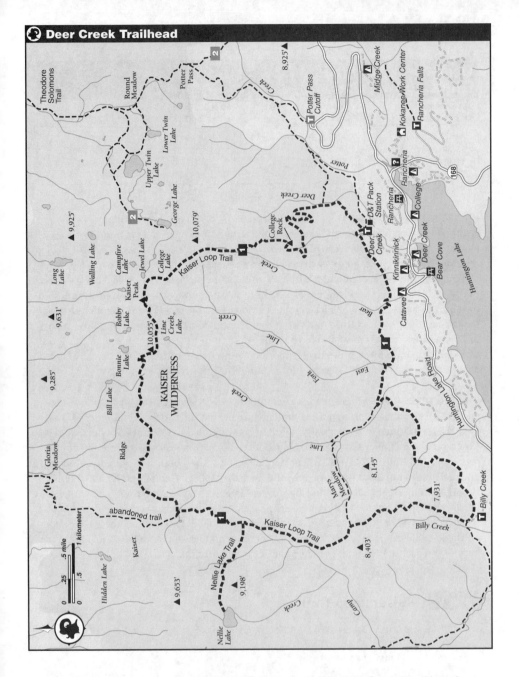

HEADS UP! *If you just want to day hike Kaiser Peak, follow the first 5.25 miles in the opposite direction, completing a 10.5-mile out-and-back hike.*

HEADS UP! *The landscape along the Kaiser Loop Trail was severely burned in the 2020 Creek Fire and will bear little resemblance to the text in this book. Fire passed through all forested sections between the trailhead and the Nellie Lake basin. The upper ridge is untouched by fire, but campsites along this stretch are sparse. Contemplate an out-and-back day hike to Kaiser Peak for the coming few years.*

DAY 1 (Deer Creek Trailhead to Nellie Lake, 8.5 miles): From the trailhead parking area, you follow the dirt road across a gully toward the D&F Pack Station and then walk left (north) to the back of the pack station. Here a standard national forest placard marks the Deer Creek Trailhead. Just 180 feet later, a somewhat indistinct junction is signposted left (west) to Billy Creek and you follow it, looping back above the road and parking area, past a large water tank. For the first 4.6 miles the trail makes a long, undulating traverse above the vacation homes lining Huntington Lake. It is not a showy hike, offering few views, but is certainly pleasant forest walking. Maybe you'll be as lucky as your author was last time and spend 30 minutes watching a spotted owl, perched in his favorite, white-splattered tree beside the trail.

There are a few waypoints that require your attention along these miles: first, a little over a mile from the trailhead, the trail drops to ford Bear Creek and then switchbacks up to a closed road (at 1.2 miles). You must turn right onto the road and jog 100 feet north to find the continuing trail; then turn left (west) back onto the trail. At the 2.5-mile mark you reach a junction where the Kaiser Loop Trail continues left, while right leads to Marys Meadow. Heading to Marys Meadow shaves 1.9 miles off your distance to Nellie Lake—it is a pleasant walk, first alongside mostly bedrock-lined Line Creek and later through verdant Marys Meadow, but since this trip description is for the official Kaiser Loop Trail, the description stays left; in addition, the Marys Meadow connector is less maintained at times.

Beyond the Marys Meadow junction, you cross alder-lined Line Creek and admire its beautiful slab bed. You then round a dry slope and drop into an unmapped creek drainage, thick with early-season flowers. Just before crossing the creeklet, a quite prominent use-trail-to-nowhere departs south, straight down the slope. Do not take it—it drops to forest service buildings. The proper route—at times less distinct—crosses the creeklet and then climbs gently, soon crossing a mapped but unnamed creek, next turning more southwest to skirt a rounded spur, then dropping toward a junction with the Billy Creek Trailhead. See the sidebar "Shuttle Alternative" below if your group has two cars and you'd like to start your hike at the Billy Creek Trailhead, lying just 350 feet south of this junction.

SHUTTLE ALTERNATIVE
If you have two cars, a possible alternative is to leave one car at the Deer Creek Trailhead and the other at the Upper Billy Creek Trailhead, lying just 350 feet off the Kaiser Loop Trail (7,230'; 37.24213°N, 119.22730°W). If you choose this alternative, you will bypass the first 4.6 miles, turning this loop into a 14.2-mile shuttle trip. The spur road to Upper Billy Creek Trailhead lies within Lower Billy Creek Campground. *Note:* If you start here, you need a wilderness permit for the Billy Creek Trailhead.

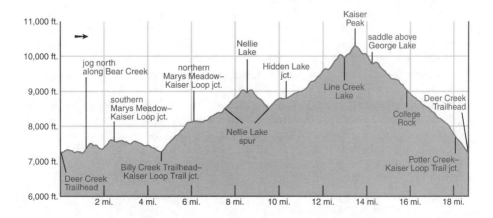

Continuing on the Kaiser Loop Trail, at the Billy Creek Trailhead junction, you turn right (north) and begin ascending the Billy Creek drainage, through a mix of red fir and white fir. The meadowed creek corridor is just visible to the west as you climb onward, passing a few open, sandy patches and then diving back into lush red fir forest as you approach the northwestern junction with the Marys Meadow connector. Onward, a few granite outcrops break the forest cover and splendid swathes of lupine color sandy openings. You sidle into a tributary of the Home Camp Creek drainage and follow it north to the Nellie Lake junction, the first lodgepole pine now mixed with the still-dominant red fir. At the Nellie Lake junction, straight ahead (north), is the continuing Kaiser Loop Trail to Kaiser Peak, tomorrow's route, while now you turn left (west) toward Nellie Lake.

Following a narrower trail, you angle across a slope, drop into a seasonally lush drainage with a usually robust flow, and climb up a shallow draw to a broad forested saddle, set beneath the Kaiser Ridge's escarpment. A brief descent leads to lovely, deep Nellie Lake, ringed by a mature mixed-conifer forest (lodgepole, red fir, and the occasional airy western white pine and droopy-topped mountain hemlock) and steep ridges. There are a few campsites along the northern shores (for example, 8,934'; 37.28204°N, 119.24592°W), although respect NO CAMPING signs at this popular destination, where current regulations require you to be 200 feet from the shoreline. Heading clockwise around the lake leads to additional campsites on the southern shores.

DAY 2 (Nellie Lake to Deer Creek Trailhead, 10.2 miles): In the morning, fill all your water bottles, especially by August, when this is likely to be the last available water on the hike. Then reverse the 1.0 mile walk east to the Kaiser Loop Trail and turn left (north). A steady ascent leads past some giant red firs, through wet glades of early-summer flowers, and across some drier, sandier slopes. After about 0.75 mile you step across a seasonal Line Creek tributary and reach a junction, where left (north) is signposted for the abandoned trail to Hidden Lake. You continue straight ahead (right; east).

The forest cover is notably thinner as you ascend toward the crest of Kaiser Ridge. By late summer the next miles will be dry and dusty, but in June and early July the powdery soils are a riot of color—vibrant pink from pussypaws, a sustained yellow from frosted wild buckwheat, and the purple carpeting of Brewer's lupine, each forming dense near-monocultures in their preferred patches. Meanwhile, your views are broadening and you stare north to the Ritter Range, southern Yosemite border country, and Balloon Dome, a prominent, granite knob jutting nearly 3,000 feet above the banks of the San Joaquin River. To the south you look toward the neighboring Dinkey Lakes Wilderness. These expansive views are yours to enjoy all the way to the summit of Kaiser Peak.

The trail now winds approximately along the crest, gaining elevation in spurts and occasionally dropping just a little. The southern slopes are reasonably gentle, while to the north is a vertical escarpment, at the base of which lie a trio of fairly inaccessible lakes: Bill, Bonnie, and Bobby Lakes. At 9,750 feet you curve into a flat, a lovely hemlock glade that lies just north of the crest; here you'll find, in early summer, a shallow tarn with translucent water and later a dry talus flat, for the water has percolated down through the porous soils. A steeper ascent leads you back to the crest through many-stemmed whitebark pine krummholz. Then as you turn east (left) again, you'll spy Line Creek Lake in the broad tundra to the south. There are some flat, open sites near the southeast corner of the lake where you could camp—but it will be windy and is inadvisable if there are thunderstorms about. The underlying rock is now metamorphic, decomposing to fine, powdery, nutrient-rich soils, which allows the unusually thick ground cover of plants. But the diminutive flowers are only noticed if you stare at your feet—and it is probably the views to the San Joaquin drainage that are more enticing.

Crossing the minor saddle above Line Creek Lake, you begin your final ascent toward Kaiser Peak, continuing across pleasant alpine tundra to a signed spur trail. Turn left (north) and you quickly gain the summit (10,293'; 37.29428°N, 119.18556°W).

VIEWS FROM KAISER PEAK

The ridge culminating in 10,310-foot-high Kaiser Peak sits alone in the vast western San Joaquin River catchment, offering outstanding views of the drainage's highest peaks. Gaze around you at this great river's watershed. If you have cell coverage—many carriers do on this summit—load peakfinder.org to identify your surroundings. In the north, you look deep into the San Joaquin River canyon, above which rise the peaks on the southern Yosemite boundary. Balloon Dome is the steep knob standing like a lone thumb rising straight above the river. Swiveling a little to the right, you look up the North Fork San Joaquin River with the dark, serrated Ritter Range rising to the east, Mount Ritter and Banner Peak the two tallest summits. The Middle Fork San Joaquin flows down the east side of the Ritter Range and is hidden from view, with the quite staid San Joaquin Ridge visible to its east. To the northeast is the Silver Divide, crowned by large, gray Silver Peak. Red Slate Peak, a little farther east, is the first prominent peak on the Sierra Crest, a massive red pyramid rising north of McGee Pass. The reservoir you see is Lake Edison. Nearly due east is Seven Gables, a large, steep-sided, buttressed summit looming over the Bear Lakes. On the southeastern boundary of the San Joaquin watershed, most of the Evolution Peaks are visible, including steep-sided, flat-topped Mount Darwin. Mount Goddard is the massive black pyramid to the southeast. On a brilliantly clear day you can ostensibly see all the way to Mount Whitney and the Kaweah Peaks in southern Sequoia National Park. What a brilliant treat!

Line Creek near the Marys Meadow Trail junction   Photo by Elizabeth Wenk

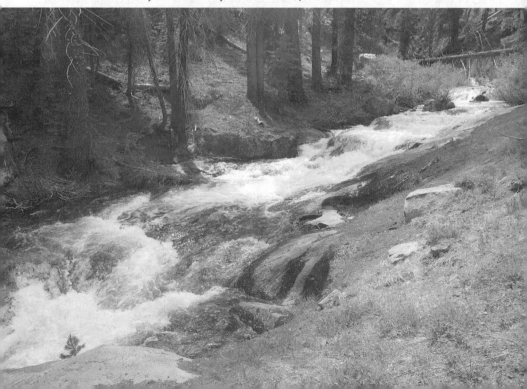

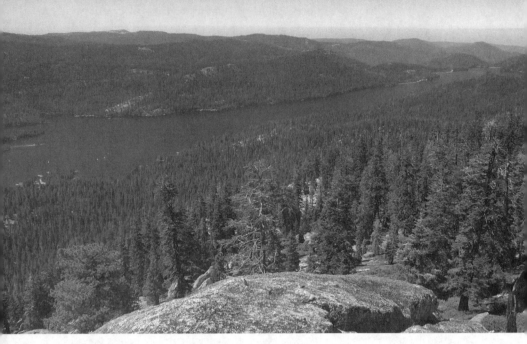

View of Huntington Lake from College Rock   Photo by Elizabeth Wenk

You now have 5.25 miles to the trailhead, much of it a steep downhill. The trail continues nearly on the ridge, soon turning to the south and dropping down some rockier terrain via a few switchbacks. Looking east over the escarpment you'll spy Campfire and Jewel Lakes nearly 400 feet below. A long traversing descent across a slope peppered with spreading phlox and Brewer's lupine leads to a saddle with a faint use trail that drops to College and George Lakes (Trip 2). Nearby are some plausible campsites among stunted whitebark pine—although no water source. Beyond, you sidle around the western side of Peak 10,079, climbing just slightly to surmount a saddle that drops you to the headwaters of Bear Creek.

Now begins the serious downhill, as you wind steeply down coarse, sandy slopes between slabs. The path meanders toward and away from seasonal Bear Creek, through lodgepole and western white pine. At 9,340 feet the trail cuts across the head of a seasonally marshy meadow—if there is still water, there are campsites here—and continues east to a spur. Switchbacks lead down it, first through more western white pine and then through more bouldery terrain (a moraine) covered with pinemat manzanita, the trail efficiently dropping to a sandy flat just north of College Rock. If you're keen for a detour, a use trail leads south to the summit, the final rocks requiring some third-class scrambling. The views are nothing compared to those from Kaiser Peak, but College Rock provides a nice panorama south to the Huntington Lake environs and beyond to the Three Sisters and Dogtooth Peak in Dinkey Lakes Wilderness.

After a short westward traverse, switchbacks lead south down an open rib, alternating between red fir shade and open shrubby slopes where slabs are just below the surface. At 8,700 feet you have a final view over Huntington Lake from atop steep slabs decorated with mountain pride penstemon. Continuing down through open red fir forest and past blocky, rounded outcrops where Jeffrey pines grow, switchbacks lead south and east into the Deer Creek drainage. Finally, you follow the creek corridor south, passing a faint trail that leads east to Potter Creek, and soon reach the Deer Creek Trailhead.

Potter Pass Trailhead (Huntington Lake)
8,313'; 37.26956°N, 119.12136°W

Destination/ GPS Coordinates	Trip Type	Best Season	Pace & Hiking/ Layover Days	Total Mileage	Permit Required
2 George Lake 37.29239°N 119.17042°W	Out-and-back	Early to late	Moderate 2/1	9.6	Potter Pass *(Potter Cutoff for alternative route)*

INFORMATION AND PERMITS: This trailhead is in Sierra National Forest. Permits are required for overnight stays and quotas apply. Details on how to reserve permits are available at fs.usda.gov/detail/sierra/passes-permits. For advance reservations (60% of quota; reservable starting in January each year), there is a $5-per-person reservation fee, while walk-up permits (40% of quota) are free. Permits can be picked up at 29688 Auberry Road, Prather, CA 93651; if you call 559-855-5355 in advance, they will leave your permit in a dropbox. Permits can also be picked up in person at the Eastwood Forest Service Office at the corner of Kaiser Pass Road and CA 168, at Huntington Lake. If you plan to use a stove or have a campfire, you must also have a California campfire permit, available from a forest service office or online at preventwildfireca.org/campfire-permit. Campfires are prohibited above 10,000 feet. Bear canisters are not required but are strongly encouraged.

DRIVING DIRECTIONS: From the intersection of CA 168 and CA 180, just east of Fresno, take CA 168 northeast through Clovis and up into the foothills, to the community of Shaver Lake. Here, continue straight along CA 168 to Huntington Lake (versus right along Dinkey Lakes Road to Courtright Reservoir), and reach a T-junction near the community of Lakeshore, 67.5 miles from CA 180. Here CA 168 ends, and Huntington Lake Road leads left around the lake's north shore, while Kaiser Pass Road/FS 80 branches right. Turn right onto Kaiser Pass Road and go 4.8 more miles to a large parking area on the right, with vault toilets and bear boxes; the trailhead is across the street.

Note: If you are starting from the alternate Potter Cutoff Trailhead, turn left onto a dirt road 2.7 miles up the Kaiser Pass Road and follow the road 0.2 mile to its end.

see map on p. 30

trip 2 ## George Lake

Trip Data: 37.29239°N, 119.17042°W; 9.6 miles; 2/1 days
Topos: *Kaiser Peak*

HIGHLIGHTS: In the heart of the Sierra National Forest, little Kaiser Wilderness boasts 35 square miles of pristine forests, emerald lakes, and rugged alpine terrain. This trip visits three delightful lakes, with others nearby for off-trail explorers. An added bonus is an impressive marble sinkhole through which Upper Twin Lake's water vanishes. This region has become popular with day hikers and backpackers alike, but George Lake still offers decent solitude.

HEADS UP! *There are two Potter trailheads, the lower Potter Cutoff Trailhead, 2.7 miles from the start of Kaiser Pass Road, and the higher Potter Pass Trailhead that is a much larger pullout with toilets 4.8 miles up Kaiser Pass Road, a locale also termed Badger Flat. Separate permits are required for these two trailheads, although they both access the same*

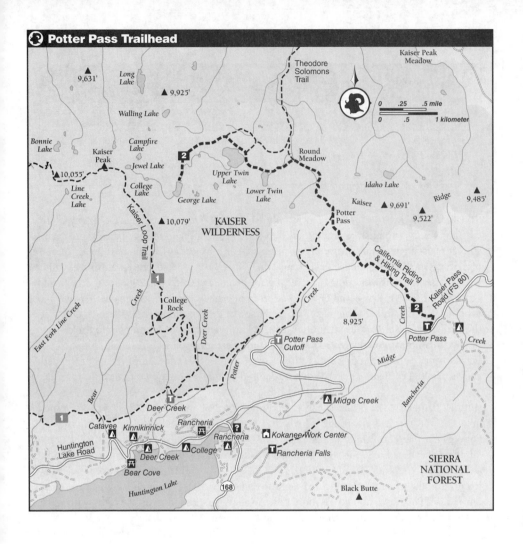

Kaiser Peak Meadow

9,631'

Long Lake

9,925'

Walling Lake

Theodore Solomons Trail

0 .25 .5 mile
0 .5 1 kilometer

Bonnie Lake

Campfire Lake

Round Meadow

Kaiser Peak

10,055'

Line Creek Lake

Jewel Lake

College Lake

Upper Twin Lake

Lower Twin Lake

George Lake

Idaho Lake

Kaiser Ridge

9,691'

9,485'

9,522'

10,079'

KAISER WILDERNESS

Potter Pass

California Riding & Hiking Trail

College Rock

Deer Creek

Creek

8,925'

Kaiser Pass Road (FS 80)

Potter Pass

Potter Pass Cutoff

Creek

Midge

Potter

Rancheria

Deer Creek

Midge Creek

Catavee

Kinnikinnick

Rancheria

Rancheria

Kokanee Work Center

Huntington Lake Road

Deer Creek

College

Rancheria Falls

SIERRA NATIONAL FOREST

Bear Cove

Huntington Lake

168

Black Butte

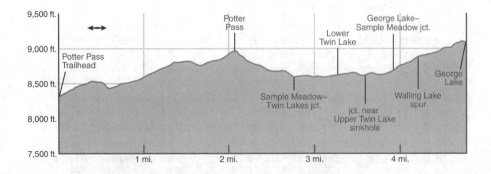

9,500 ft.

Potter Pass

George Lake–Sample Meadow jct.

9,000 ft.

Lower Twin Lake

Potter Pass Trailhead

8,500 ft.

Sample Meadow–Twin Lakes jct.

George Lake

Walling Lake spur

8,000 ft.

jct. near Upper Twin Lake sinkhole

7,500 ft.

1 mi.   2 mi.   3 mi.   4 mi.

area. The Potter Cutoff Trailhead is actually 0.15 mile shorter, but requires nearly 500 feet extra elevation gain, so the route starting at the Potter Pass Trailhead is written up here.

HEADS UP! *The hike to George Lake is one of the few trips in the area not burned in the 2020 Creek Fire.*

DAY 1 (Potter Pass Trailhead to George Lake, 4.8 miles): Across the street from the parking area, the Potter Pass Trail heads up through open lodgepole pine and red fir forest to scrubbier slopes, and soon back to dense red fir forest. It sees heavy use, and is notably dusty by midseason, but simultaneously soft underfoot as it works its way diligently but gently upward. The trailside flowers can be delightful—violets and spotted coralroot in deep shade and corn lilies, shooting stars, and crimson columbines in wet meadow strips along seasonal drainages. Cresting a ridge after 1.4 miles, the trail traverses a more open slope, again a delightful wildflower garden in season, with scarlet gilia, mountain mule ears, and Leichtlin's mariposa lilies staring up at you. This pleasant route leads to Potter Pass (8,974'), from which you are treated to far-ranging views north to the Ritter Range and into southern Yosemite. To the southeast you stare at the highest peaks of neighboring Dinkey Lakes Wilderness—10,000-plus-foot Three Sisters (seen as a series of rounded granite studs) and barren, serrated, 10,302-foot Dogtooth Peak (Trips 10 and 11). At the pass, the Potter Pass Cutoff Trail merges from the left (west), signposted for Huntington Lake.

VIEWS FROM POTTER PASS

Epic views await at the pass! In the north, Balloon Dome stands alone as a prominent granite knob jutting from the enormous San Joaquin River valley. Farther north, the dark, jagged Minarets of the Ritter Range are easily identified. These peaks are comprised of metavolcanic rock derived from volcanoes that erupted some 100 million years ago. To the northeast, the Middle Fork San Joaquin River curves north below the distant Mammoth Crest. East-southeast, the South Fork San Joaquin River drains the mountains of northern Kings Canyon National Park.

The merged trails continue ahead (north), winding down a delightfully red fir-shaded draw and crossing to the east side of the drainage near the bottom. Passing a flat, strikingly dense with flowers, you reach a junction where straight ahead (right, northwest) leads to Sample Meadow, while you turn left (west) toward Twin Lakes. Stepping across a minor drainage, the trail trends west across an open rocky slope, verdant Round Meadow visible below. The aspens ringing the meadow provide a burst of yellow and orange color for the autumn hiker. The rough rock outcrops above and below the trail are limestone, a rarity in the Sierra, and the soils here host some unusual plant species, including periwinkle-colored western blue flax. Cresting a minor lump, the trail soon drops to the Lower Twin Lake basin, the lake backdropped by steep, 800-foot-tall granite cliffs. There is a large campsite along the western lakeshore beneath mixed-conifer canopy. Lower Twin Lake (8,627') has a gentle, mature feel, with large trees and smooth, lichen-covered cliffs. Small brook trout are plentiful. Continuing, the trail skirts a diminutive seasonal pond and traverses an easy half mile to exquisite Upper Twin Lake's east shore (8,606' by current USGS calculations, meaning Upper Twin Lake has the nominally lower elevation of the twin lakes.) The lake's sparkling blue waters are interrupted by smooth granite-slab islands that host surprisingly large Jeffrey pine, red fir, and lodgepole pine. But the lake's most peculiar feature is that it has no outflow. A few steps north of where the trail intersects the shore, a conspicuous outcrop marks a rocky limestone pit—a sinkhole—through which the water exits the lake underground.

Some of the flow reemerges at a spring in the valley to the northwest and more probably irrigates Round Meadow. During snowmelt, the pit can be blocked (and hidden), causing the lake's water level to rise dramatically above its shores. There are campsites on the ridge to the east of the lake and near its southeastern corner; respect the NO CAMPING signs placed near the shores of this popular destination.

Not far from Upper Twin Lake's southeastern corner, you reach a signed junction, where left (north) leads to George Lake and right (northeast) to Sample Meadow (8,622'; 37.29626°N, 119.15742°W). Turning left, you continue along the northeastern shore of Upper Twin Lake under a canopy that is a delightful mix of western white pine, lodgepole pine, Jeffrey pine, and junipers, passing a selection of view-rich campsites. As the slope steepens you reach another junction, where right (east) leads back in the direction of Sample Meadow, while your route turns left (west) toward George Lake; at this junction, your route transitions back onto granite. You ascend a dry, mat manzanita–covered slope above Upper Twin Lake, slowly transitioning to a red fir forest. At a conspicuous turn in the trail, 0.3 mile above the last junction, a use trail trends north (right) toward Walling Lake, while the main trail continues west (left), skirting beneath bluffs through some magnificent western white pine. For the final stretch, the trail winds to and fro beside the creek draining George Lake, eventually crossing the creek, and 70 feet later arriving at a large flat near the lake's outlet. Here it reaches the first of several campsites along George Lake (9,100'; 37.29239°N, 119.17042°W). The most scenic sites are located along the western shore between the inlet from College Lake and the large granite wall that rims the northwest shore, although the biggest are closer to the northeastern corner where the trail terminates.

George Lake on an early-season hike   Photo by Elizabeth Wenk

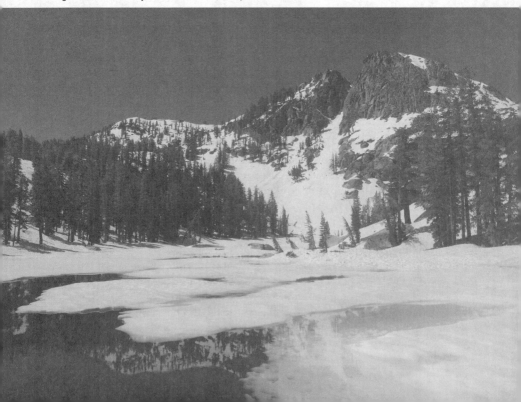

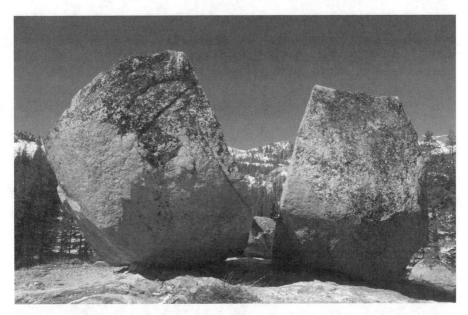

A giant boulder at Upper Twin Lake   Photo by Elizabeth Wenk

SIDE TRIP: CROSS-COUNTRY DAY HIKE TO COLLEGE LAKE AND THE KAISER LOOP TRAIL
From George Lake, an adventurous cross-country route leads to College Lake and, with a bit of scrambling suitable for a day pack but not a full backpack, to a saddle where you meet the Kaiser Loop Trail (Trip 1) to Kaiser Peak. From George Lake's outlet, follow a use trail counter-clockwise around George Lake and ascend approximately west-northwest up slabs and across shelves to the east of the creek connecting College Lake to George Lake. From College Lake, follow the western edge of a broad meadowed shelf nearly due south for about 0.25 mile to its end. Near here (9,610'; 37.28850°N, 119.17692°W), you should pick up a use trail—if you haven't already stumbled upon it—that climbs another approximately 0.2 mile to the saddle; this is a loose, rocky scramble that zigzags west, then north, and finally southwest to avoid a late-lasting, very steep snowfield. Right at the saddle, this route joins the Kaiser Loop Trail (9,765'; 37.28773°N, 119.17811°W). If you are venturing for a grander tour of the wilderness, turn right (north and then west) at this unmarked and unofficial junction and continue an additional 0.8 mile to 10,310-foot Kaiser Peak.

DAY 2 (George Lake to Potter Pass Trailhead, 4.8 miles): Retrace your steps. At each junction, your route is labeled BADGER FLAT.

Mono Creek Trailhead
(at Lake Thomas A. Edison)
7,800'; 37.38122°N, 119.01034°W

Destination/ GPS Coordinates	Trip Type	Best Season	Pace & Hiking/ Layover Days	Total Mileage	Permit Required
3 Arch Rock and Margaret Lakes 37.46151°N 119.03849°W (Big Margaret Lake)	Semiloop	Mid to late	Moderate 4/1	29.1	Margaret Lakes
4 Graveyard Lakes 37.44524°N 118.96882°W (lower Graveyard Lake)	Out-and-back	Mid to late	Leisurely 3/1	15.0	Devils/ Graveyard
51 Mono Creek (in reverse of description; see page 293)	Shuttle	Mid to late	Leisurely 3/2	24.6	Mono Creek (Mono Pass as described)

INFORMATION AND PERMITS: This trailhead is in Sierra National Forest. Permits are required for overnight stays and quotas apply. Details on how to reserve permits are available at fs.usda.gov/detail/sierra/passes-permits. For advance reservations (60% of quota; reservable starting in January each year), there is a $5-per-person reservation fee, while walk-up permits (40% of quota) are free. Permits can be picked up at 29688 Auberry Road, Prather, CA 93651; if you call 559-855-5355 in advance, they will leave your permit in a dropbox. Permits can also be picked up in person at the Eastwood Forest Service Office at the corner of Kaiser Pass Road and CA 168, at Huntington Lake or at the High Sierra Visitor Information Station, 15.7 miles along Kaiser Pass Road (shortly before the Lake Edison–Florence Lake split). If you plan to use a stove or have a campfire, you must also have a California campfire permit, available from a forest service office or online at preventwildfireca.org/campfire-permit. Campfires are prohibited above 9,600 feet in the Margaret Lakes Basin and within 0.25 mile of Lower Graveyard Lake. Bear canisters are not required but are strongly encouraged.

DRIVING DIRECTIONS: From the intersection of CA 168 and CA 180, just east of Fresno, take CA 168 northeast through Clovis and up into the foothills, to the community of Shaver Lake. Here, continue straight along CA 168 to Huntington Lake (versus right along Dinkey Lakes Road to Courtright Reservoir), and reach a T-junction near the community of Lakeshore, 67.5 miles from CA 180. Here CA 168 ends, and Huntington Lake Road leads left around the lake's north shore, while Kaiser Pass Road branches right. Turn right onto Kaiser Pass Road and drive 16.7 miles over Kaiser Pass to a fork, where left leads to Lake Edison and Mono Hot Springs and right to Florence Lake. Turn left onto the Lake Edison Road (Forest Service Road 5S80) and continue 8.5 miles, driving past Mono Hot Springs, across the base of the Lake Edison Dam, past Vermilion Valley Resort to a junction with FS 6S78. Here, left leads to the pack station (Trip 3) and right to the Mono Creek Trailhead (Trip 4). For Trip 3, turn left and continue 0.5 mile, until just past the pack station; then park in any of the roadside pullouts. For Trip 4, turn right and drive 0.3 mile to the road-end parking lot and hiker campground. Note that once you are 5.5 miles past Huntington Lake, both Kaiser Pass Road and Lake Edison Road are very slow, often single lane, and very exposed in places; expect to drive much of it at just 10 miles per hour.

VERMILION VALLEY RESORT (VVR)

This resort, powered by its own generators, is on the west shore of Lake Edison. It is well known for its hospitality, especially among John Muir Trail and Pacific Crest Trail thru-hikers who flock to its rooms, tent cabins, store, and restaurant. Traditionally, the resort buys the thru-hiker's first beverage and offers a free stay in the (shared) hikers' camping area. It's a good opportunity to share information about trail conditions and exchange trail tips.

Thru-hiking or not, VVR is a nice stop on an extended trip, and daily ferry service from June to October makes for easy access to the resort from main trails across the lake (for instance, Trip 51). The ferry (fee) leaves the resort at 9 a.m. and 4 p.m. and departs the Mono Creek landing at 9:45 a.m. and 4:45 p.m. Call the resort for updated information or to make reservations in a room or tent cabin: 559-259-4000. The resort website has good hiking links, food drop details, and driving directions: edisonlake.com.

trip 3   Arch Rock and Margaret Lakes

see maps on p. 36–37

Trip Data: 37.46151°N, 119.03849°W (Big Margaret Lake);
29.1 miles; 4/1 days

Topos: *Sharktooth Peak*

HIGHLIGHTS: A private lakes basin nestled beneath precipitous walls and one of the Sierra's largest granite arches are the reward for hikers drawn to this out-of-the-way trailhead. A 4.6-mile walk along a jeep road to reach the true trailhead is probably what keeps most visitors away, but as you set up your tent, you'll be pleased you chose Rainbow and Margaret Lakes, tucked against the Silver Divide, as your destination.

HEADS UP! *The first 4.6 miles are along the Onion Springs OHV Route. A high-clearance four-wheel drive can navigate this road, saving you nearly half your distance on the first (and last) days.*

HEADS UP! *Campfires are prohibited above 9,600' in the Margaret Lakes Basin, meaning fires are prohibited at the suggested campsites at Frog Lake, Coyote Lake, and Big Margaret Lake.*

HEADS UP! *The 2020 Creek Fire burned stretches along and above the Onion Valley OHV Route, but the fire stopped a short distance up the climb to Arch Rock Pass.*

DAY 1 (Onion Springs OHV Route to Frog Lake, 10.75 miles): Just to the north of the High Sierra Pack Station is the start of the Onion Springs OHV Route. If you lack a vehicle that can navigate this road, there are pullouts near the start where you can park. Don't try and continue with a standard SUV—the road almost immediately crosses bedrock slabs that require high clearance and not long afterward is one of the steeper, more eroded road sections.

Assuming you're walking, you climb alongside an unnamed creek, pass popular car-camping sites, and soon cross an unnamed creek. After climbing quite steeply through white fir forest along a rough stretch of road, you turn west (about 1.0 mile from the start of the Onion Springs OHV Route) and the ascent moderates. For the coming 1.8 miles you are following the crest of a moraine, dropping a gentle 240 feet along the way. Here you have excellent views south to Kaiser Ridge and to Lake Edison, already far below you. Ahead, the road turns north, crossing a broad saddle and dropping to Onion Spring Meadow, where you'll find an ancient campsite, now 4.1 miles from the start. Climbing steadily again, you

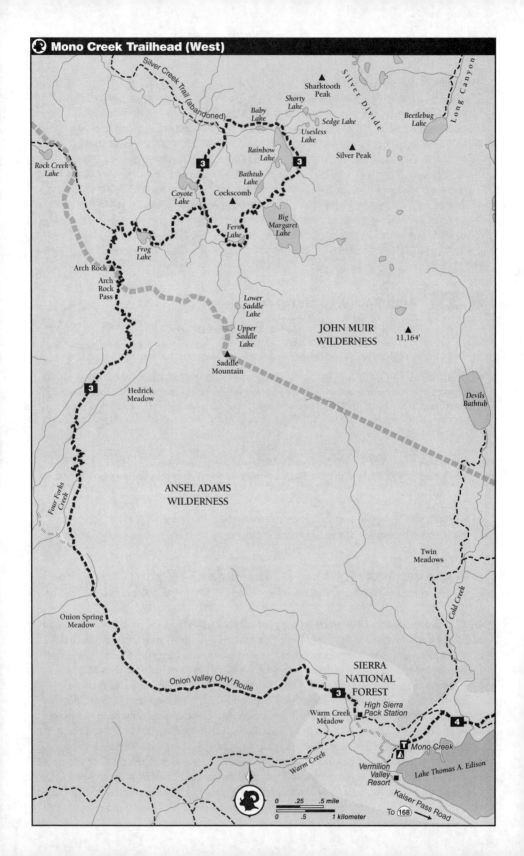

Silver Creek Trail (abandoned)

Long Canyon

Silver Divide

Sharktooth Peak ▲

Shorty Lake

Baby Lake

Sedge Lake

Beetlebug Lake

Usesless Lake

Rock Creek Lake

3

Rainbow Lake

3

Silver Peak ▲

Bathtub Lake

Coyote Lake

Cockscomb ▲

Big Margaret Lake

Fern Lake

Frog Lake

Arch Rock ▲

Arch Rock Pass

Lower Saddle Lake

JOHN MUIR WILDERNESS

11,164' ▲

Upper Saddle Lake

Devils Bathtub

Saddle Mountain ▲

3

Hedrick Meadow

ANSEL ADAMS WILDERNESS

Four Forks Creek

Twin Meadows

Cold Creek

Onion Spring Meadow

SIERRA NATIONAL FOREST

Onion Valley OHV Route

3

High Sierra Pack Station

Warm Creek Meadow

4

T

Mono Creek

Warm Creek

Vermilion Valley Resort

Lake Thomas A. Edison

Kaiser Pass Road

To (168) →

0   .25   .5 mile

0   .5   1 kilometer

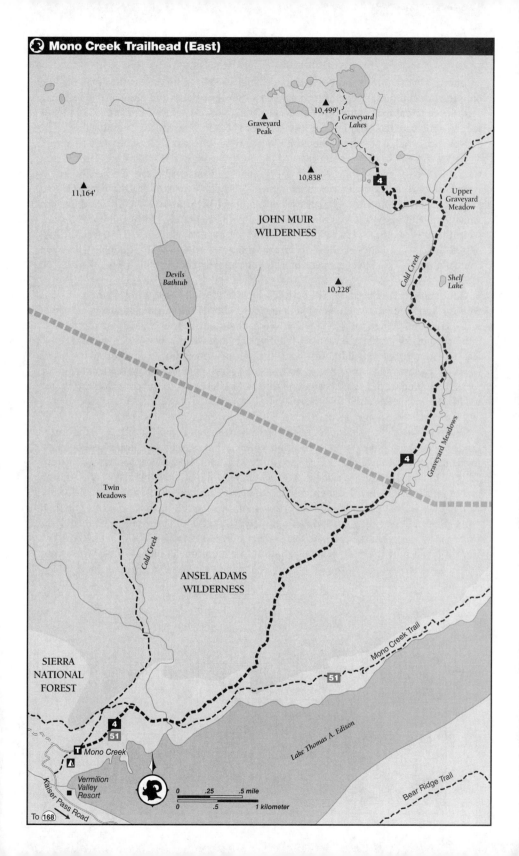

Graveyard Peak

10,499'

Graveyard Lakes

4

11,164'

10,838'

Upper Graveyard Meadow

JOHN MUIR WILDERNESS

Devils Bathtub

Cold Creek

Shelf Lake

10,228'

Graveyard Meadows

4

Twin Meadows

Cold Creek

ANSEL ADAMS WILDERNESS

Mono Creek Trail

SIERRA NATIONAL FOREST

51

4

51

T Mono Creek

Lake Thomas A. Edison

Bear Ridge Trail

Vermilion Valley Resort

Kaiser Pass Road

To 168

0   .25   .5 mile

0   .5   1 kilometer

are alternately in white fir forest and along slabbier stretches with more Jeffrey pine. Rolling onto the broad top of a ridge, you come across four bear boxes and a small sign declaring TRAIL, the actual start of the Margaret Lakes Trail (8,081'; 37.40986°N, 119.07459°W); it is wise to anticipate this junction, for it would be easy to march past the cryptic sign.

Now on a trail, a steeper climb ensues, leading up through a pleasant white fir forest. There are some gigantic trees and century-old mulching logs, indicating a fire hasn't passed through here in a long time. Crossing one small seasonal tributary, the headwaters of Four Forks Creek, the trail switchbacks upward through a splendid mixed-conifer forest; lodgepole pines dominate, yet your eyes will probably be drawn to the towering western white pines and marvelous red firs, for the lodgepole pines tend to form a uniform "forest" while the trees of other species more often stand out as "individuals." At 8,950 feet, the trail passes pleasant campsites beside a stream that will *usually* hold water; through late July you could dependably plan to camp here, breaking the long first day in half (8,894'; 37.42782°N, 119.07454°W).

Continuing briefly west, the trail crosses a sandy moraine crest and follows it upward, with just scattered Jeffrey pines and junipers rising above the endless chinquapin and pine-mat manzanita. Where the moraine crest ends, the trail traverses a little east and resolves into switchbacks beside a seasonal tributary. This stretch of trail is steep, gaining 1,000 feet over a mile. Spring wildflowers color the ground—spreading phlox, coyote mint, and ivesia—while by midsummer it is a parched slope of whitebark pine and scattered volcanic rocks. Emerging from forest cover along the final switchbacks to the crest, you are treated to far-reaching views south: Seven Gables rises prominently above the Bear Creek drainage, and Florence Lake, along the main South Fork San Joaquin River, lies farther south.

When you reach the pass, colloquially referred to as Arch Rock Pass (10,535'), the northern San Joaquin drainage is laid before you, with views both into the lower river gorge and to the dark Ritter Range, flanked by the North Fork and Middle Fork San Joaquin Rivers. To your immediate east is a ridge of 3.5-million-year-old basalt, while the pass itself is on granite. (Printed USGS 7.5' topo maps place the label "Arch Rock" on a ridge to the southwest of the pass, but the arch is to the northwest of the pass; this has been corrected on their online maps.) Descending north down sandy switchbacks (with late snow some years), the trail soon swings west onto a broad, flat, sandy saddle (10,369'; 37.45204°N, 119.06628°W). Here you will note use trails heading south into picturesque boulder stacks. Weave your

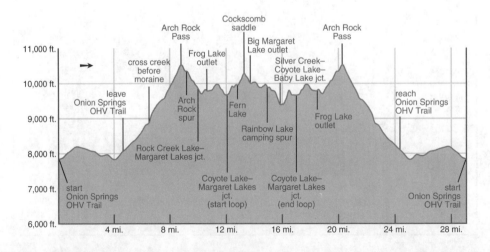

way through these and you're soon treated to a view of Arch Rock—a granite arch that rivals Indian Rock Arch in Yosemite.

Continuing, the trail completes tight switchbacks, routed just east of another slope of volcanic rock. The view north continues to impress: the lower San Joaquin drainage toward Balloon Dome, the Ritter Range and all of southern Yosemite laid out before you. Slowly the hemlocks and whitebark pine increase in stature and the trail reaches a junction, where right (east) leads to the Margaret Lakes, your route, and left (west) leads to Rock Creek Lake. Turning right, the trail continues down a rocky rib, then cuts north into a draw with a seasonal stream (and campsites while water persists) and then loops north again, climbing atop the next bedrock ridge. Descending again, you cross Frog Lake's outlet creek and find pleasant campsites about halfway along its north shore (9,785'; 37.45762°N, 119.06060°W; no campfires).

DAY 2 (Frog Lake to Big Margaret Lake, 3.2 miles): From Frog Lake, the trail continues snaking eastward, but actually traveling mostly north or south as it winds between a succession of granite ribs. Throughout this basin, the granite is broken by broad-scale, near-parallel joints. As the glaciers flowed downhill approximately parallel to the fracture planes, they created a landscape of smoothed granite ribs alternating with linear valleys, gulches, and draws. You are mostly cutting across these ribs and so the trail must either climb up and over each crest or sidle around them—it does a lot of both.

Leaving Frog Lake, the trail follows a meadowed corridor over a taller ridge and then drops south into the basin holding Coyote Lake, zigzagging on its descent to the broad lakeside meadow. Cockscomb dominates the view to the east—an imposing fin of fractured granite that you will loop around. Coyote Lake offers campsites on its southern peninsula or along its eastern border. At the southeast corner of the meadow, you ford the lake's inlet creek and just beyond reach a junction, where the loop part of this hike begins. For now, stay right (southeast), signposted for Fern Lake.

The trail continues up, climbing between and then across polished slabs between stands of lodgepole pine. Soon you are alongside Fern Lake's outlet stream, splayed delightfully across the bedrock. From Fern Lake you have, perhaps, the best views of the Cockscomb. Looping through the meadow turf surrounding Fern Lake (and past small campsites on knobs), tight, steep switchbacks lead up a broad sandy gully just north of the Cockscomb, the summit itself soon blocked from view. The east side of the ridge leads down similarly sandy passageways between rocky ribs, depositing you near the outlet of Big Margaret Lake. Big Margaret Lake offers all the features you seek in a Sierran lake: large, island dotted, slab ringed, backdropped by a rugged crest, endless options for exploring, and of course plenty of campsites. You will quickly find a tent site in sandy flats between slabs along the lake's northern shores (10,015'; 37.46275°N, 119.03501°W; no campfires). From Margaret Lake, peak baggers can scramble up Silver Peak, heading first east and then north to the summit.

DAY 3 (Big Margaret Lake to Frog Lake via Rainbow Lake, 4.4 miles): From Big Margaret Lake your loop continues north to Rainbow Lake. Many hikers will choose to explore the Rainbow Lake environs without a pack and then return the way they came—it makes for less hiking with a pack, but once you're at Rainbow it is actually faster to complete the loop. The lumpy topography continues, as you climb briefly and then descend a gully toward Rainbow Lake and continue around its eastern shores on a deteriorating trail. Cockscomb becomes less prominent, but the Silver Divide remains a spectacularly steep backdrop, its angular ungla-ciated profile contrasting with the rounded, polished granite ribs ringing the lake. There are beautiful campsites halfway along Rainbow Lake, where a bulbous peninsula juts out.

Continuing across rivulets descending from Useless, Sedge, and Shorty Lakes, the trail turns west to skirt Baby Lake (grassier, lodgepole pine–ringed, with less-enticing camping), and then descends steeply down broken slabs to a deep-set lodgepole pine flat with a just-visible junction that declares stock aren't recommended down Silver Creek (9,400'; 37.47268°N, 119.04563°W). Indeed, the right-hand branch, the abandoned Silver Creek Trail, that leads down Silver Creek to Fish Creek is not recommended for pack animals, but it does traverse some phenomenal slab country along the eponymous creek; if you have time for a detour, you can gaze upon the upper slab basin just 1.0 mile from this junction. To continue the loop, however, turn left (south) to return to Coyote Lake.

For the first 0.2 mile the trail has mostly vanished as it, in theory, skirts the eastern edge of the marshy-meadow-and-lodgepole-pine forest environment, endless deadfall hastening its disappearance. But at the southern end of the flat it reappears intact, leading southwest up a hemlock and western white pine–clad gully. Sinuous switchbacks lead up the passageway, located, once again, between two steep-sided bedrock ribs. A short, easier descent then leads back to the Coyote Lake basin. Now enjoying excellent views to Cockscomb again, you head south along the lake's eastern shores, passing possible campsites as you cross sandy flats and pass the expansive meadow at Coyote Lake's head to reach the trail junction where you close the loop part of this trip. Turning right (west) you now retrace your steps to Frog Lake for the night—or maybe camp at Coyote Lake's peninsula campsites (9,750', 37.46252°N, 119.05273°W; no campfires), if you're willing to have a longer final day.

DAY 4 (Frog Lake to start of Onion Springs OHV Route, 10.75 miles): Retrace your steps from Day 1.

Arch Rock is a highlight of this trip.   Photo by Elizabeth Wenk

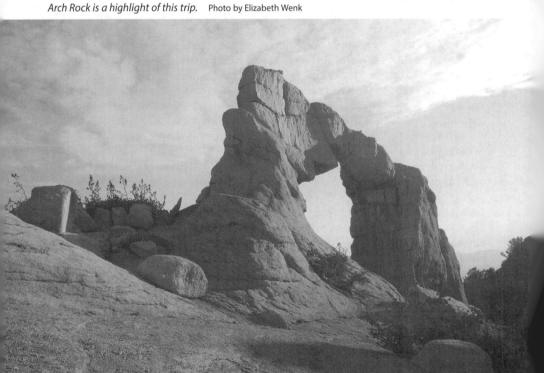

see
maps on
p. 36–37

trip 4 ## Graveyard Lakes

Trip Data: 37.44524°N, 118.96882°W (lower Graveyard Lake);
15.0 miles; 3/1 days
Topos: *Sharktooth Peak, Graveyard Peak*

HIGHLIGHTS: Phantom, Murder, Headstone, and Ghost Lakes: don't let the ominous names fool you—the granite-covered Graveyard Lakes basin is one of the loveliest and most regal in the Silver Divide country. The walk to these lakes can easily be completed in a single day, but here it is split over two for a very relaxing pace. Don't forget to budget a layover day to explore the upper lakes, a divine alpine basin that is part of the excuse for this hike.

HEADS UP! *Campfires are prohibited within 0.25 mile of Lower Graveyard Lake, including at the suggested campsite.*

HEADS UP! *The 2020 Creek Fire passed through the first 3 miles of this hike, but the rest of the forests are still intact.*

DAY 1 (Mono Creek Trailhead to Graveyard Meadows, 3.8 miles): Two trails depart from the trailhead, the more northern one ascending to Devils Bathtub and the slightly more easterly-trending (right-hand one) continues along Lake Edison's shore; head right. After 0.6 mile, a sandy trail merges from the left, signposted to the pack station; again you stay right (east). The trail now loops into the Cold Creek drainage, crossing the creek on a bridge, and then jogging back to the southeast. Just beyond, now 1.0 mile from the trailhead, you reach another junction, where left (northeast) leads to Goodale Pass, your route, while right (east), signposted for Mono Creek, continues around Lake Edison (Trip 51).

Diverging just slowly from Lake Edison, the trail toward Goodale Pass makes a gradual forested climb, reaching a marshy meadow after 0.8 mile. As the trail cuts across the meadow, you can, in early summer, admire fields of shooting stars and western bistort. Ascending briefly up the seasonal drainage, the trail then diverges north and begins a steadier climb. In part you are in a beautiful open forest of Jeffrey pine and juniper and elsewhere under less varied lodgepole pine cover. You are ascending a giant lateral moraine left by the glacier that once spilled down Mono Creek. From the top of the ridge, the moraine crest, around 8,800 feet, there are good views of Lake Edison and the peaks of the Mono Divide. After crossing the dry, sandy flat among scattered lodgepole pine, the trail turns east to descend the back side of the moraine into the Cold Creek drainage. The creek is soon just below, and you follow up its southern bank, passing a selection of mostly shadeless, but popular, campsites.

Crossing Cold Creek on logs, you reach a junction where left (west) is an alternate route to Devils Bathtub, while you stay right (northeast) to continue up Cold Creek's valley through open lodgepole pine forest with a grassy understory. You soon spy a sea of grass to the right, magnificent Graveyard Meadows. The long, oval-shaped meadow sits trapped between two moraine crests, the moraine deposits likely the "dam" that raises the water table here, preventing trees from establishing. You could camp in the fringing lodgepole pine forest anywhere along its length, but the creek is difficult to access across the fragile meadow grasses. It is best to select a campsite where you can collect water from the stream as it exits the meadow, but stare across the meadow for views (for example, 8,859'; 37.40838°N, 118.96660°W).

DAY 2 (Graveyard Meadows to Lower Graveyard Lake, 3.7 miles): Continuing north, the trail skirts the edge of the Graveyard Meadows under a dense cover of lodgepole and red fir—a wonderful bird habitat and a pleasant, easy way to start the day. A mile later, at the north end of the meadows, the trail passes a few more campsites and begins climbing moderately on slabs and broken cobble. It soon fords Cold Creek, a broad cobbly wade or rock hop that can be difficult in early season. After a brief respite in a lodgepole pine flat, you climb again across slab and then the trail turns north. Suddenly the slabs are less broken by forest and the terrain has a more subalpine feel; you pass tiny streamside pocket meadows with straggly lodgepole pine and dwarf bilberry cover. At the end of one such meadow, you find a junction signed for the Graveyard Lakes (9,388'; 37.44029°N, 118.95938°W).

Turning left (west) and climbing just briefly up this spur trail leads to Upper Graveyard Meadow. Here you must ford Cold Creek again—only the longest-legged hikers will be able to leap its meandering channel in the middle of the meadow; others have an easy wade. Beyond the meadow, in the fringing forest there are small campsites, but much better ones lie ahead—and up. The trail now enters lodgepole and hemlock cover and begins a steep, rocky climb to the basin above. The switchbacking trail is steep and the slope it climbs steeper; you are relieved when the gradient lessens and you spill onto sumptuous meadows ringing the lowest lake. You pass an unmarked Y-junction, where you stay right (north) to reach the lake's northeastern shore. Here in the fringing lodgepole pine forest you'll find especially appealing campsites (9,961'; 37.44524°N, 118.96882°W; no campfires).

From the shores of Lower Graveyard Lake, there are marvelous views of Graveyard Peak and the tumbled granite cirque wall that surrounds the entire Graveyard Lakes basin. Graveyard Peak may be reminiscent of a tombstone with its salt-and-pepper granite, but its name memorializes the unfortunate resolution of a shepherd's dispute at Graveyard Meadows long ago. William A. Dill, with the California Department of Fish and Game, added the names Ghost, Headstone, Murder, Phantom, Pumice, Spook, and Vengeance to the small lakes in the basin (in addition to the larger two, known as the Lower and Upper Graveyard Lakes), but fortunately these ominous names for a decidedly heavenly basin were never added to the topo maps.

Lower Graveyard Lake makes an excellent, sheltered base camp from which to fish (for brook trout) and explore the remaining lakes in the basin. However, additional gorgeous campsites for a small group are found at the next two lakes upstream and at Upper Graveyard Lake. To reach them—and the upper basin in general—follow the trail around to the head of Lower Graveyard Lake, cross the outlet from Upper Graveyard Lake, and then climb over a small saddle to reach a pair of lovely deep lakes. Beyond the second lake, where you encounter a major headwall with a waterfall, turn to the right (northeast) to

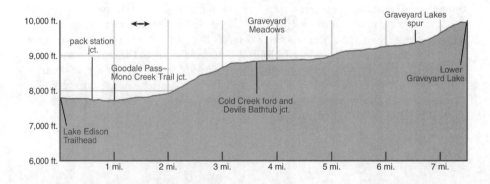

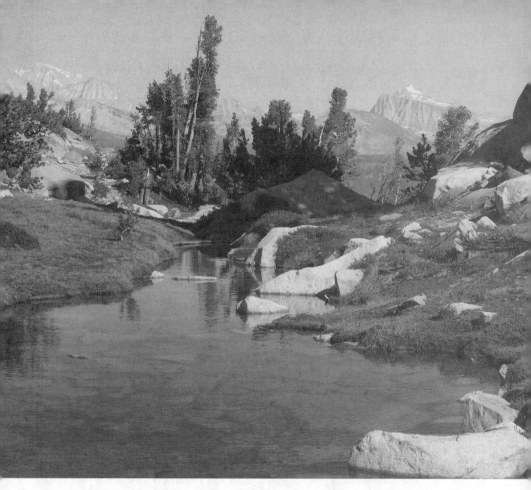

Lovely view to Seven Gables from high up in the Graveyard Lakes basin   Photo by Elizabeth Wenk

ascend a broad swale to Upper Graveyard Lake, possibly still following the dwindling use trail. Campsites are generally absent at the uppermost lakes, but a visit is worthwhile. The view from atop the knob in the center of the basin (10,499'; 37.45110°N, 118.97600°W) is stupendous and is easily reached from its northwestern side.

DAY 3 (Graveyard Lakes to Lake Edison Trailhead, 7.5 miles): Retrace your steps for Days 1 and 2.

Bear Diversion Trailhead			7,011'; 37.33823°N, 119.00438°W		
Destination/ GPS Coordinates	**Trip Type**	**Best Season**	**Pace & Hiking/ Layover Days**	**Total Mileage**	**Permit Required**
5 Bear Lakes Basin 37.32367°N 118.81049°W (Vee Lake)	Semiloop	Mid to late	Strenuous 5/1	37.2	Bear Diversion
6 Medley Lake 37.30666°N 118.85469°W	Semiloop	Mid to late	Moderate 4/1	32.8	Bear Diversion
7 Bear Creek to Florence Lake 37.30666°N 118.85469°W (Medley Lake)	Shuttle	Mid to late	Moderate 4/1	35.0/ 31.0	Bear Diversion *(Florence Lake in reverse)*

INFORMATION AND PERMITS: This trailhead is in Sierra National Forest. Permits are required for overnight stays and quotas apply. Details on how to reserve permits are available at fs.usda.gov/detail/sierra/passes-permits. For advance reservations (60% of quota; reservable starting in January each year), there is a $5-per-person reservation fee, while walk-up permits (40% of quota) are free. Permits can be picked up at 29688 Auberry Road, Prather, CA 93651; if you call 559-855-5355 in advance, they will leave your permit in a dropbox. Permits can also be picked up in person at the Eastwood Forest Service Office at the corner of Kaiser Pass Road and CA 168, at Huntington Lake or at the High Sierra Visitor Information Station, 15.7 miles along Kaiser Pass Road (shortly before the Lake Edison–Florence Lake split). If you plan to use a stove or have a campfire, you must also have a California campfire permit, available from a forest service office or online at preventwildfireca.org/campfire-permit. Campfires are prohibited above 10,000 feet. Bear canisters are not required but are strongly encouraged.

DRIVING DIRECTIONS: From the intersection of CA 168 and CA 180, just east of Fresno, take CA 168 northeast through Clovis and up into the foothills, to the community of Shaver Lake. Here, continue straight along CA 168 to Huntington Lake (versus right along Dinkey Lakes Road to Courtright Reservoir), and reach a T-junction near the community of Lakeshore, 67.5 miles from CA 180. Here CA 168 ends, and Huntington Lake Road leads left around the lake's north shore, while Kaiser Pass Road branches right. Turn right onto Kaiser Pass Road and drive 16.7 miles over Kaiser Pass to a fork, where left leads to Lake Edison and Mono Hot Springs and right to Florence Lake. Turn left onto Lake Edison Road (Forest Service Road 5S80) and continue 2.7 miles to the Bear Diversion Dam Road/FS 6S83. A high-clearance, four-wheel-drive vehicle, not the average, urban SUV, can travel this road another 2.25 miles to the true trailhead above the reservoir. Note that once you are 5.5 miles past Huntington Lake, both the Kaiser Pass Road and the Lake Edison Road are very slow and often single lane; expect to drive much of it at just 10 miles per hour.

trip 5   Bear Lakes Basin

see maps on p. 46–47

Trip Data: 37.32367°N, 118.81049°W (at Vee Lake);
37.2 miles, part cross-country; 5/1 days
Topos: *Mount Givens, Florence Lake, Mount Hilgard*

HIGHLIGHTS: This spectacular hike tours one of the western Sierra's most stunning basins. Starting from the forested depths of Bear Creek Canyon, this trip climbs to the picturesque and secluded Bear Lakes through glacially carved valleys, across polished slabs, and past lush meadows. Although several parts of the terrain are strenuous, the cross-country route-finding is not difficult, and solitude and breathtaking beauty richly reward the determined hiker.

HEADS UP! *This trip is for experienced hikers only. The route involves some cross-country travel as well as stretches of poorly maintained trail.*

HEADS UP! *The first mile of the four-wheel-drive road to Bear Diversion Dam was burned in the 2020 Creek Fire, but the landscape upstream was spared.*

HEADS UP! *The route around Lake Italy can be covered all summer by a steep snowfield that plummets straight into the lake. If you're planning this route in early season or in a high-snowfall year, be prepared for this snowbank.*

DAY 1 (Bear Dam Junction to John Muir Trail junction, 9.1 miles): The trail description begins along the Lake Edison Road at the junction with the road to the Bear Diversion Dam, Forest Service Road 6S83, for this rugged four-wheel-drive route can only be navigated by jeeps—not any four-wheel drive will do. If you can drive to the true trailhead, you'll have 2.25 miles less walking each direction. These first miles are, fortunately, relatively fast, pleasant walking, nearly continually traversing broken slabs high above the South Fork San Joaquin with views of seemingly infinite granite bedrock, although the river itself remains hidden. You loop southeast and then northeast around the base of Dome 8,533, looking down toward the incised course of Bear Creek after 1.4 miles. The road then follows a bench about 200 feet above the river course across slabs, interrupted by brief forest stands. At the west end of the Bear Diversion Dam, you reach the end of the road and the true Bear Creek Trailhead (7,435′; 37.33617°N, 118.97652°W).

You continue around the Bear Diversion Dam reservoir on slab slopes, then cross dry flats of mountain mule ears, before entering stands of white fir. Traversing broken orange granite with scattered Jeffrey pine, you come to an often-indistinct junction with the northbound (left-bearing) Bear Creek Cutoff Trail that leads to a separate trailhead closer to Lake Edison; this trail is actually slightly shorter than your route, but it has more elevation gain. It is used predominately by Pacific Crest Trail (PCT) and John Muir Trail (JMT) hikers cutting north from the Bear Creek Trail toward Lake Edison.

Entering an aspen glade, the trail parallels the course of Bear Creek upstream. The creek runs over short, rocky falls and swift rapids and then collects in long, quiet pools shaded by aspens, lodgepole pine, and white fir. Occasional switchbacks help the trail maintain a mostly even gradient, as it climbs across sandy slopes and up exposed broken slabs with scattered Jeffrey pine and junipers. With upward progress, there are ever briefer interludes beneath a shaded conifer canopy. The creek's profile continues repeating the cascades-pools-cascades-pools mantra, but the cascades become ever more impressive. Their locations are delineated by broad-scale bedrock fractures, along which disproportionate erosion occurs.

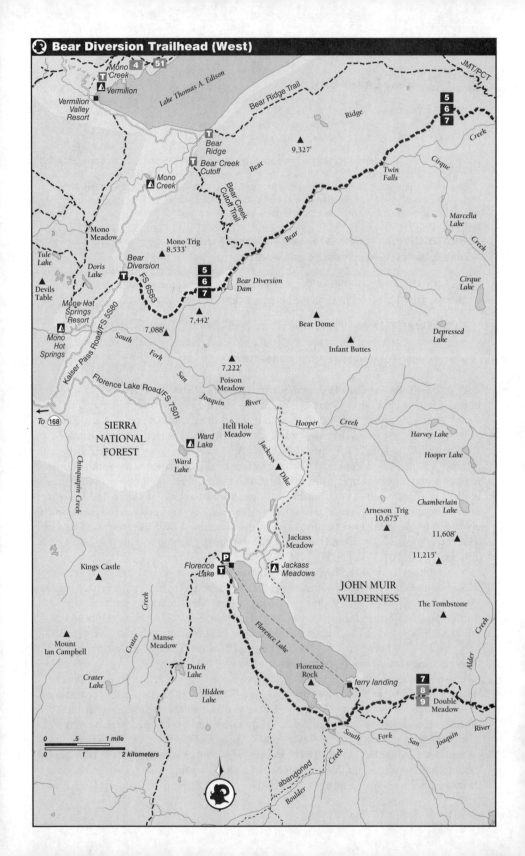

Mono Creek 4 51

T Mono Creek

▲ Vermilion

Vermilion Valley Resort

Lake Thomas A. Edison

Bear Ridge Trail

Ridge

JMT/PCT

Creek

5 6 7

T Bear Ridge

T Bear Creek Cutoff

▲ Mono Creek

Bear Creek Cutoff Trail

Bear

9,327' ▲

Twin Falls

Cirque

Marcella Lake

Creek

Mono Meadow

Mono Trig 8,533' ▲

Bear

Cirque Lake

Tule Lake ▲

Doris Lake

Bear Diversion

5 6 7

Bear Diversion Dam

Devils Table ▲

FS 6S83

Mono Hot Springs Resort

7,088' ▲

7,442' ▲

Depressed Lake

Mono Hot Springs ▲

Kaiser Pass Road/FS 5S80

South

7,222' ▲

Bear Dome ▲

Infant Buttes ▲

To (168) ←

Florence Lake Road/FS 7S01

Fork

San

Poison Meadow

Joaquin

River

Hooper

Creek

Harvey Lake

SIERRA NATIONAL FOREST

Hell Hole Meadow

Jackass

Hooper Lake

Chinquapin Creek

▲ Ward Lake

Ward Lake

Dike

▲

Arneson Trig 10,675' ▲

Chamberlain Lake

11,608' ▲

Jackass Meadow

11,215' ▲

Kings Castle ▲

Florence Lake

P

T

▲ Jackass Meadows

JOHN MUIR WILDERNESS

The Tombstone ▲

Mount Ian Campbell ▲

Crater

Creek

Manse Meadow

Dutch Lake

Florence Lake

Alder

Creek

Crater Lake ▲

Hidden Lake

Florence Rock

ferry landing ■

7 8 9

Double Meadow

South

Fork

San

Joaquin

River

0   .5   1 mile

0   1   2 kilometers

abandoned

Boulder

Creek

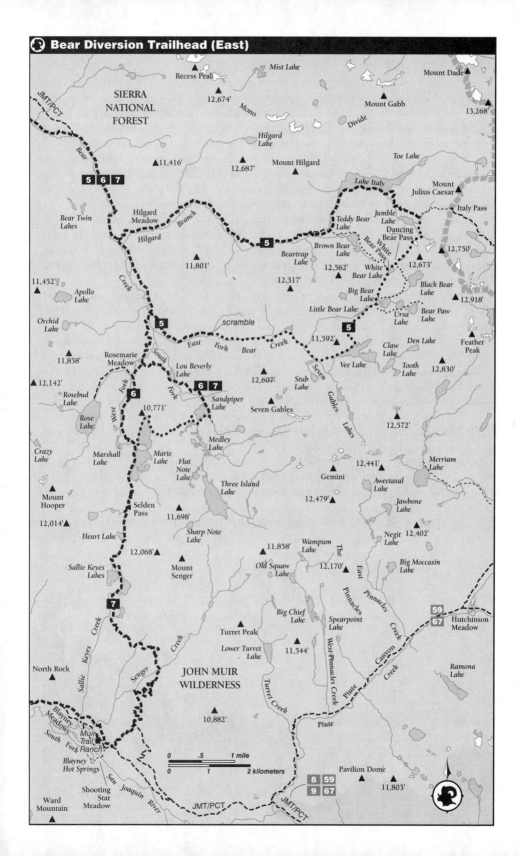

There are a few falls you should particularly take time to admire. The first truly dazzling set of trailside cascades begins just below 8,000 feet: you pass a spectacular swimming hole and ahead watch the creek's slalom course chute from cascade to cascade with barely a pause. Partway through this segment, there are some campsites on juniper-and-Jeffrey-pine-shaded benches above the creek. Half a mile later are Bear Creek's showiest falls, Twin Falls (8,119'; 37.36253°N, 118.93179°W), where a pair of parallel cascades drop into a giant, inviting swimming hole—and there are ample campsites on the slopes to the northeast. You have covered just 5.9 miles (of the recommended 9.1 miles), but if you're game for a long day tomorrow, you may be tempted to while away your afternoon here.

Upstream, the river is no less showy, but the trail now diverges north around a granite dome and away from its course and you'll sadly miss a trio of spectacular pothole-pools and the river's continually chuting, cascading, bubbling flow. But the streamside terrain becomes rougher and the trail follows an easier route high above the creek, only dropping back to the banks of Bear Creek after 2.5 miles.

Climbing south alongside a seasonal tributary, you soon bend east along a creeklet beside which the landscape is marshy in early summer and brightly colored with water-loving flowers through most of August. The ensuing miles are hard, hot walking on a sunny afternoon. The trail continues up nominally forested passageways between bluffs and slabs, but the soils are thin and the sparse tree cover provides little shade. The tree cover further lessens until suddenly, around 8,900 feet, you emerge into a fabulous landscape of bare slabs decorated by weathered junipers. You climb to the shoulder of a ridge and then turn to the northeast to follow a trough between two rounded ribs. (*Note:* For the previous 0.75 mile, the trail trends well north of the route plotted on the USGS 7.5' topo maps.) Beyond, the trail descends an unwelcome 200 feet into a verdant lodgepole-pine-and-aspen forest, crosses a robust tributary, and soon reaches the banks of Bear Creek.

As soon as you approach the riverbank, campsites appear on benches and in lodgepole pine flats overlooking the vivacious river. If you'd like solitude for the night, stop here, about 0.6 mile before the JMT junction (8,837'; 37.36988°N; 118.89784°W). Beyond the campsites, continue through an often-boggy stretch of trail, past wet meadows, and soon reach large campsites, Old Kit Camp (8,912'; 37.36829°N, 118.88992°W), under lodgepole pine cover; these are the final campsites for 2 miles. The junction with the JMT is just around the corner.

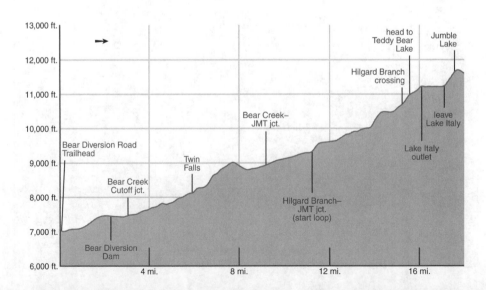

DAY 2 (John Muir Trail junction to Teddy Bear Lake, 6.4 miles): Turn right (south) from the Bear Creek Trail onto the JMT (and PCT), paralleling the banks of Bear Creek southbound. The gradient of rollicking Bear Creek is lower here and the trail much less rocky—the coming 2.0 miles to the Hilgard Branch are delightfully easy walking, mostly beneath lodgepole pine cover. Note that along this stretch, camping is currently prohibited between the trail and the river. Bear Creek, in stretches lined by granite slabs, contains enticing swimming holes when the water is low and striking cascades when the water level is high. Eventually, the lodgepole forest gives way to broken slabs with dry sedge patches and you round a small knob to reach a sign for LAKE ITALY. Here you turn left (east) onto the rarely maintained trail up the Hilgard Branch (9,333'; 37.34565°N, 118.87621°W), beginning the loop part of this trip, while the JMT continues straight ahead (right; south), the continuing routes of Trips 6 and 7.

For the first miles, the trail is in decent shape, leaving the forested valley bottom and wiggling up broken slabs beneath juniper-decorated bluffs to reach flatter terrain in Hilgard Meadow. You pass some good campsites beneath forest cover and later ones on open slabs bordering the northwest side of this subalpine meadow. Mount Hilgard looms almost 4,000 feet above, and the meadow underfoot is adorned with thousands of purple Lemmon's paintbrush and tundra aster flowers in midseason.

Climbing again, the trail crosses the outlet of Hilgard Lake and continues across broken slab to reach the foot of massive Mount Hilgard about 1.5 miles past the JMT. The trail now turns right (southeast), following the foot of the steep bluffs and cliffs. The face is cut by numerous creeks, rolling down aspen-and-willow clogged corridors, or initiating as springs at the base. Winter avalanches and rockfall also tumble down these chutes, creating huge talus fans and preventing the establishment of forest. Along much of this stretch, the landscape is too sloping and wet to permit camping, with the next good choice around the 10,000-foot mark in a lodgepole pine flat.

Channeled by walls to either side, the creek soon assumes a due-easterly bearing. You initially switchback up through lush lodgepole pine forest with abundant red mountain heather and western Labrador tea underfoot, and then cut right (south) onto open slabs, where the trail is marked by cairns. The trail is leading you to a fortuitously located shelf just above the river's entrenched course, providing easy passage through otherwise steep terrain. Along this fantastic meandering path you are sandwiched between bluffs below

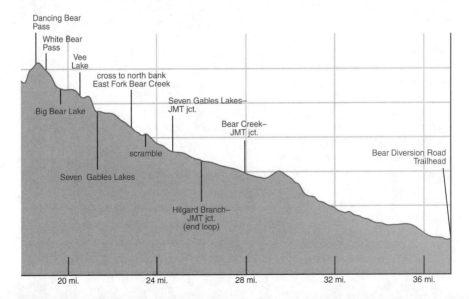

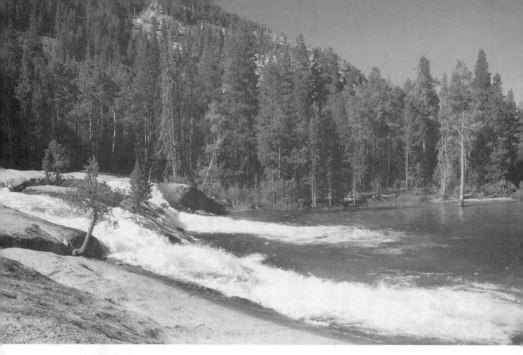

Twin Falls along Bear Creek   Photo by Elizabeth Wenk

and above and are relieved that the passageway continues until the terrain broadens again upstream. The variation in the width of the canyon, from a narrow gorge to a wide, gently sloping meadow, is due to differences in the structure of the bedrock.

EFFECTS OF GLACIAL EROSION

Although stream erosion began the difficult work of carving this canyon, glaciers continued the effort and modified the canyon's shape. Before glaciers reshape them, stream canyons usually have a V-shaped cross section, for most of their erosive power is focused at the very base of the canyon. Glaciers create a more U-shaped cross section, plucking loose rock from the valley walls. The efforts of both erosion agents are apparent in most Sierra canyons.

As you walk up the Hilgard Branch you pass through both broad, flat U-shaped stretches, such as near Hilgard Meadow, and narrow more V-shaped sections like the narrow gorge. This juxtaposition is initially puzzling as the same river and glaciers flowed through both sections. Here, the variations in the canyon width and steepness of its walls likely reflect variation in the prevalence and spacing of joints—fractures in the bedrock. Neither glaciers nor rivers are very effective at eroding unfractured bedrock or bedrock with very widely spaced fractures.

The orientation of fractures also influences canyon shape. Where joints are mostly oriented vertically, glaciers break off columnlike pieces from the valley sides, thereby undermining the canyon walls above. Where jointing is primarily horizontal, the glaciers, of course, flow parallel to the joints. In such a place, glaciers tend to just slide along the surface, eroding less and leaving more of the original V-shaped profile. This is the process that shaped the narrow, steep sections of Hilgard Branch's canyon.

Exiting the narrow gorge you emerge in a small creekside meadow and walk through it, cutting across avalanche debris and open slabs. Where the terrain next steepens, your final step up before Teddy Bear Lake and Lake Italy, you may lose the trail. With ever more slabs, repeat avalanche chutes (and resultant messes of downed trees), and marshy corridors, the sparse foot traffic fans out and there is no single established path. Simply head upstream—slabs generally make for the best travel unless they are covered with water. Avoid the marshier ground where you compact and damage the fragile soils. Not only is the trail indistinct, but the foot traffic forks near where the Teddy Bear Lake outlet creek flows into the Hilgard Branch. To most efficiently reach Teddy Bear Lake (which offers better campsites than does Lake Italy), cross the Hilgard Branch just 40 feet upstream of the Teddy Bear Lake outlet confluence. Here, where the Hilgard Branch is entrenched in a little gorge, is a safe crossing point (10,705'; 37.34687°N, 118.82223°W). Climbing up talus blocks to exit the chasm, you emerge on open slab that you follow upstream until it is easy to cut over to Teddy Bear Lake (at about 10,985'; 37.34798°N, 118.81746°W). You'll find sandy sites among slabs on the ridge overlooking the lake (11,027'; 37.34726°N, 118.81664°W; no campfires).

(If you wanted to continue up to Lake Italy for the night, most people stay on the northern bank, walking up steeper slabs and crossing the creek where it becomes wider and shallower, about 0.25 mile upstream of Teddy Bear Lake. I'd only recommend this route if you're worried about high water at the crossing because the walking is easier by cutting to the southern side sooner.)

DAY 3 (Teddy Bear Lake to Vee Lake via Lake Italy and Jumble Lake, 5.0 miles, part cross-country): From Teddy Bear Lake it is possible to continue upcanyon to Brown Bear Lake and then over White Bear Pass to White Bear Lake, the route followed by the High Sierra Route as described by Steve Roper. It is only 1.1 miles to White Bear Lake, versus 3.5 miles via the described route, but you miss Lake Italy. Also, it is a steeper route, with the headwall beneath White Bear Pass requiring careful route-finding. However, this is the safer alternative if there is an icy snowbank along Lake Italy.

Returning to the Hilgard Branch Trail from Teddy Bear Lake, the route continues across slabs, trending north and then northeast to arrive at the outlet of large Lake Italy (11,220'). Here you'll enjoy great vistas of Mount Gabb, the tip of Mount Abbot, Mount Dade, Bear Creek Spire, and Mount Julius Caesar. Lake Italy gets its name from its similarity in shape to the European peninsula; consider this west end of it to be the "boot top." This is a spectacular 124-acre lake and a sublime basin, but with very limited campsite options, except along the northern shore—far out of your way. There are a few established campsites near the outlet and others along the first 0.4 mile around the shore, but none is the requisite 100 feet from water. Slightly larger (and legal) campsites are just east of where the creek from Jumble Lake spills into the lake.

Onward, you continue along Lake Italy's southern shore, initially on a faint trail through flat meadow patches and sand quite close to the lake's edge. This fast, pleasant walking continues for just under a mile, until you round a slight promontory and turn into a bay. Here the steep slabs that have been looming to the south (right) suddenly extend to the lakeshore and are often snow covered through July. Your skill set and the snow's condition will determine your preferred route—if the snow isn't icy, you can traverse it, but there is the potential to slide straight into the lake. When the snow is reduced to a short, very icy patch in late season, it can be easier (and safer) to wade briefly through the lake's knee-deep water. Beyond, there are no obstacles, but the use trail becomes fainter as you continue along the lakeshore and across the inlet from Jumble Lake, flowing through a small meadow; this is considered Lake Italy's "heel." You want to continue about 0.1 mile beyond the creek crossing before beginning your ascent; there are sandy campsites nearby.

For the first stretch of your climb, there is no use trail, so where you head up is a little arbitrary, but make sure you are east of (beyond) an expanse of low-angle broken rock—one decent option is to start climbing at 37.35618°N, 118.80029°W (11,233'). Your winding route climbs east of Jumble Lake's outlet creek, staying outside of the bouldery creek corridor until about 11,430 feet. Here you'll pick up a use trail that quickly climbs northeast up a narrow corridor between bluffs (to the north) and the top of the moraine that dams Jumble Lake (to the south). If you don't find the use trail, aim for 37.35230°N, 118.79792°W (11,646'), where you'll find yourself on a remarkably sandy slope above Jumble Lake's jumbled shores and can traverse southeast above the lake. At the far end of Jumble Lake, where there is a more vegetated strip with rills, you are beyond the cumbersome moraine deposits and can drop toward the lake's shore (11,700'; 37.35061°N, 118.79286°W). This is also the point where the use trail bound for Italy Pass turns northeast to climb alongside an inlet stream (Trip 54, Royce Lakes).

The high point of this trip, informally named Dancing Bear Pass, can be seen to the south, a long, narrow, flat-bottomed valley bracketed by two nondescript peaks. There are various ways to reach this pass—one possibility is to drop to the shores of the tarn at the head of Jumble Lake (and part of Jumble Lake just after the snow melts) and follow around its eastern side until you've skirted a blocky talus field and can begin ascending. You ascend less than 100 feet, jog 150 feet right on a shelf, and then resume your ascent southeast up a steep, sand-and-boulder drainage. Once the terrain "flattens" (around 11,850'), you head south, southeast, and then south again toward the pass. Late-lasting snow is found here; it is not particularly steep or dangerous—as alpine snowfields go—but, of course, exercise caution. Soon you crest the nearly imperceptible Dancing Bear Pass (12,158'; 37.34375°N, 118.79546°W) and beyond spy a long linear tarn (or a dry flat where you can imagine a tarn) and continue gently downhill until you are staring at rock-entombed, deep White Bear Lake, perched on a saddle. White Bear Pass, the route from Teddy Bear Lake, is just on its right side. This is an awe-inspiring location in which to rest and drink in the view.

GLACIAL SCENERY

The lip of East Fork Bear Creek's basin marks the upper limit of glaciers that flowed over the top of the dome to the south and then through White Bear Pass toward Brown Bear Lake. Most of this basin was under ice many times during the Pleistocene Epoch, 2 million to 10,000 years ago. However, where you are standing always remained above the glaciers.

To tell which areas remained above the ice, note the jagged or pointed peaks and ridges and high elevation, sloping plateaus of sand and boulders. These high points protruded above the glaciers, which eroded them from several sides, leaving them steep sided, but not smoothed over.

The domelike peaks and ridges formed where the land was completely covered by the glaciers. The sandy, bouldery area where you are standing was never glaciated (or at least, not recently), and it shows no clean or fresh bedrock, as emerges after glaciers scrape away surface debris. In unglaciated locations, over hundreds of thousands or even millions of years, the rock cracks into angular boulders, which, in turn, weather into gravel and sand.

From this majestic vantage point, look beyond the outlet of White Bear Lake (the narrow end) down the linear valley to the southwest. This valley is your route to Vee Lake. The descent to White Bear Lake follows the steep, sandy slope below. The path skirts White Bear Lake's west shore, past White Bear Pass, and follows the west side of the outlet to Big Bear Lake.

URSA, BEARPAW, AND BLACK BEAR LAKES
Ursa and Bearpaw Lakes are an easy detour east from Big Bear Lake. Big Bear Lake can be circumnavigated on either side, but Ursa Lake is best bypassed on its south side and Bearpaw Lake along its north shore. Black Bear Lake is also beautiful (and harbors campsites near its outlet) and you could alternatively head from Dancing Bear Pass east to Black Bear Lake before descending to Big Bear Lake. Continuing updrainage from Bearpaw Lake leads to Feather Pass and down to Merriam Lake and onward to French Canyon.

Once at the outlet of Big Bear Lake, the best path follows the outlet's south side west-southwest through a gorge to Little Bear Lake's inlet. Continue along the south shore of Little Bear Lake, diverging slightly south of the shore to follow a grassy passageway. This leads to a marshy meadow, and then a meadow-and-sand corridor appears that you follow southwest past an elongate tarn to a broader meadowy shelf overlooking Vee Lake. Here are some splendid sandy campsites with wonderful views. Continue south and even slightly southeast to the lip of the shelf, before dropping toward Vee Lake. You want to intersect the north shore of Vee Lake about two-thirds of the way east, right where a pair of bedrock peninsulas jut into the water (11,193'; 37.32367°N, 118.81049°W; no campfires). Here you will find spectacular campsites on benches above the lake and in sandy flats. The views down the length of Vee Lake to the face of Seven Gables couldn't be better, while the pinnacled skyline leading to Feather Peak dominates the eastern vista. This is a perfect place to spend a well-deserved rest day—you could return to explore the uppermost Bear Lakes Basin; hike above Vee Lake to the broad open basin holding Claw, Tooth, and Gruff Lakes; or simply search for your own special places in this secluded glacial wonderland. Part of what makes the Bear Lakes Basin so enticing to explore are the endless narrow grassy passageways that have formed along joints, making for (relatively) easy, but secretive, travel that forever leads to another lake filling a tiny glacier-carved basin. You could easily follow one such ramp from Vee Lake to Bearpaw Lake.

DAY 4 (Vee Lake to JMT at Bear Creek junction, 7.6 miles): An unmapped trail traverses Vee Lake's north shore west-southwest to its bedrock-dammed outlet (there is one small campsite here). Then head west across a small grassy flat and down an unlikely route, a narrow slot. (The top of this slot may be snow covered in early summer. If it is too steep or icy, instead descend down slabs just west of the Vee Lake outlet. This alternative requires a little scrambling at the very bottom. It then requires you to cross the Seven Gables Lakes outlet creek, rejoining with the described route at the inlet to the lowest Seven Gables Lake—or possibly even the outlet of the lowest Seven Gables Lake.) The slot has a use trail for parts and offers a steep but mostly talus-free sandy descent route. At the bottom of the chute (10,775'; 37.31990°N, 118.82093°W) you hug the base of steep bluffs along the north side of the lowest Seven Gables Lake. Along a very short stretch a snowfield may block your way; if icy, sloping snow extends right to the water's edge, you may have to loop around the lake on the south side—a long detour.

Once past the lowest Seven Gables Lake, a squiggly use trail follows the northern bank of the creek. You ford a creek—the outlet of the main Bear Lakes (wet feet if the hop-across rocks are submerged)—and just beyond cross to the south bank of East Fork Bear Creek, right before it descends into a small gorge. You are still following a use trail, but it is now mostly quite distinct; just pay attention each time you cross slabs to ensure you pick it up again. Pleasant walking leads past a last lake and then around the base of Peak 11,151. The rock here is superbly exfoliated—notice the thin slabs of granite that flake off—and be careful, for sometimes these dinner-plate slabs decide they'd rather be flying saucers.

Down and down, across slabs and through pocket meadows you continue, hopefully impressed by the imposing northern ramparts of Seven Gables, for these are some of the author's favorite avalanche-polished chutes in the entire Sierra. Eventually, the trail crosses onto a small talus field and you'll notice a second talus field on the north side of the stream. Where the northside talus slope ends, you need to cross to the northern bank, an indistinct crossing through a thicket of willows (10,267'; 37.32423°N, 118.84282°W). The trail reappears after you cross, its downward course now alternating between lodgepole pine cover, across spectacularly polished slabs, and through a few cumbersome stretches of avalanche debris. These lead to a very short, easy scramble that must be surmounted—climbing uphill, it should present no difficulties, but in reverse you might want to pass your pack to a partner (10,102'; 37.32573°N, 118.85213°W).

For the final 1.2 miles to the JMT you are ostensibly back on a "real" trail, but it is infrequently maintained. Beyond the scramble you cut across the top of a polished slab shelf high above the river and enjoy your final unbroken views of Seven Gables' northern face. Continuing down broken slabs, the trail leads into the first continuous lodgepole pine forest since the base of the Hilgard Branch. Occasionally near the creek and otherwise to its north, the trail reaches a junction where you reunite with the JMT. The junction is located on slabs-and-sand near some lovely campsites.

At the junction, turn right (north) and stroll through lush stands of lodgepole pine quite far east of the river corridor; there are no trailside campsites through here. Eventually, you reach two channels of the Hilgard Branch, both of which are a sandy-bottomed wade at moderate to high water levels. A little beyond these crossings you reach the junction with the trail ascending the Hilgard Branch to Lake Italy, where you close the loop part of this trip, continuing north (straight ahead) on the JMT/PCT. Now back on familiar trail, you retrace the 2.0 miles to the Bear Creek Trail junction, where you find campsites (8,912'; 37.36829°N, 118.88992°W).

DAY 5 (Bear Creek to Bear Dam Junction, 9.1 miles): Retrace your steps.

Walking through the Bear Lakes Basin near Little Bear Lake   Photo by Elizabeth Wenk

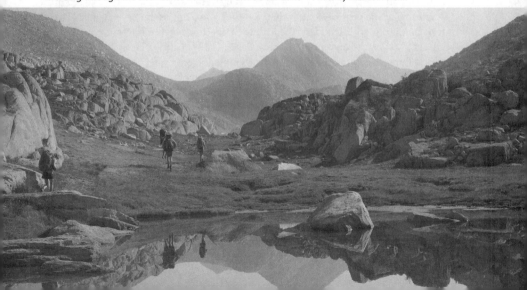

see
maps on
p. 46–47

trip 6 **Medley Lake**

Trip Data: 37.30666°N, 118.85469°W; 32.8 miles,
part cross-country; 4/1 days

Topos: *Mount Givens, Florence Lake, Mount Hilgard*

HIGHLIGHTS: This moderate hike follows the Bear Creek corridor upstream, forking off along the South Fork Bear Creek to the beautiful and serene basin holding Sandpiper and Medley Lakes. While the hike joins the busy John Muir Trail (JMT)/Pacific Crest Trail (PCT) for a short section, opportunities abound to find solitude and quiet campsites just off the trail. The alpine campsites found around Medley Lake can serve as idyllic base camps for side trips that explore the rugged terrain surrounding this water-filled granite basin.

HEADS UP! *The first mile of the four-wheel-drive road to Bear Diversion Dam was burned in the 2020 Creek Fire, but the landscape upstream was spared.*

DAY 1 (Bear Dam Junction to Twin Falls, 5.9 miles): Follow Trip 5, Day 1 to Twin Falls (8,119'; 37.36253°N, 118.93179°W).

DAY 2 (Twin Falls to Medley Lake, 9.8 miles): Upstream, the river is no less showy, but the trail now diverges north around a granite dome and away from its course and you'll sadly miss a trio of spectacular pothole pools and the river's continually chuting, cascading, bubbling flow. But the streamside terrain becomes rougher and the trail follows an easier route high above the creek, only dropping back to the banks of Bear Creek after 2.5 miles.

Climbing south alongside a seasonal tributary, you soon bend east along a creeklet beside which the landscape is marshy in early summer and brightly colored with water-loving flowers through most of August. The ensuing miles are hard, hot walking on a sunny afternoon. The trail continues up nominally forested passageways between bluffs and slabs, but the soils are thin and the sparse tree cover provides little shade. The tree cover further lessens until suddenly, around 8,900 feet, you emerge into a fabulous landscape of bare slabs decorated by weathered junipers. You climb to the shoulder of a ridge and then turn to the northeast to follow a trough between two rounded ribs. (*Note:* For the previous 0.75 mile, the trail trends well north of the route plotted on the USGS 7.5' topo maps.) Beyond, the trail descends an unwelcome 200 feet into a verdant lodgepole-pine-and-aspen forest, crosses a robust tributary, and soon reaches the banks of Bear Creek.

As soon as you approach the riverbank, campsites appear on benches and in lodgepole pine flats overlooking the vivacious river. Unlike the campsites 0.6 mile ahead at the JMT junction, these usually offer solitude. Beyond the campsites, continue through an often-boggy stretch of trail, past wet meadows, and soon reach large campsites, Old Kit Camp, under lodgepole pine cover, the final campsites for about 2 miles. The junction with the JMT is now just around the corner.

Turn right from the Bear Creek Trail onto the JMT (and PCT), paralleling the banks of Bear Creek southbound. The gradient of rollicking Bear Creek is lower here and the trail much less rocky—the coming miles are delightfully easy walking, mostly beneath lodgepole pine cover. Note that, until the Hilgard Branch junction in 2.0 miles, camping is currently prohibited between the trail and the river. Bear Creek, in stretches lined by granite slabs, contains enticing swimming holes when the water is low and striking cascades when the water is high. Eventually, the lodgepole forest gives way to broken slabs with dry sedge patches and you round a small knob to reach a sign for LAKE ITALY, marking the start of a rarely maintained trail left (east) up the Hilgard Branch (Trip 5).

This trip continues ahead (south) along the JMT/PCT, soon crossing a pair of channels (the Hilgard Branch), both of which are sandy-bottomed wades at moderate to high water levels. The track continues to be nearly level, and the walls of Bear Creek's canyon open wide. You are strolling through lush stands of lodgepole pine quite far east of the river corridor. As you emerge onto slabs, you pass a few campsites and reach the signed junction with the trail that ascends the East Fork Bear Creek to the Seven Gables Lakes and on toward the Bear Lakes Basin (left; southeast; Trip 5). The JMT continues right (southwest) and immediately drops to ford Bear Creek. This is a notoriously difficult early-season ford, transitioning to a long rock hop in mid to late summer. If the crossing is too dangerous, hikers continue 0.5 mile up the East Fork Trail, then head cross-country to cross the east and south forks of Bear Creek separately; you would reunite with the described route at Lou Beverly Lake.

Once across Bear Creek, the trail climbs through open lodgepole pine forest, switchbacking between slabs and a few short bluffs. This generally rocky ascent ends with a decomposing-log crossing of the West Fork Bear Creek at the north end of Rosemarie Meadow. Passing a few campsites, you reach a junction about 400 feet past the creek, where the JMT continues right (south; your return route), while you branch left (east) on a narrow trail, signposted for Lou Beverly and Sandpiper Lakes.

The little-used but perfectly serviceable trail sets off through lush lodgepole pine forest carpeted with dwarf bilberry and red mountain heather and sporting a few hemlocks. Soon it climbs onto broken slabs, looping east and then south toward Lou Beverly Lake. Dropping just slightly off the low ridge, the trail reaches the western shore of marshy, grassy Lou Beverly Lake, where you may find a flock of Brewer's blackbirds.

The trail loops around Lou Beverly Lake's southern shore, steps across its inlet (sometimes a wade), and begins a steady climb, with Seven Gables towering straight ahead. This strenuous climb is brief and temporarily eases as the route jogs toward the south. After passing a tumbling waterfall, the trail veers sharply north and makes a final, steep ascent to gain the lip of the glacial bench above. Upon reaching the top, you have no doubt you're nearing the alpine—whitebark pine have replaced the lodgepoles and expansive meadows and slabs stretch away from you. The trail follows the contour of the hillside south and presently arrives at the outlet of Sandpiper Lake. A few sandy patches make plausible campsites, but most of the ground is grassy, and better options lie ahead. Campsites along the lake's northwest shore are most easily reached by fording the creek here, while those to the southwest are more efficiently reached by looping around the lake's eastern and then southern shores, the route described here.

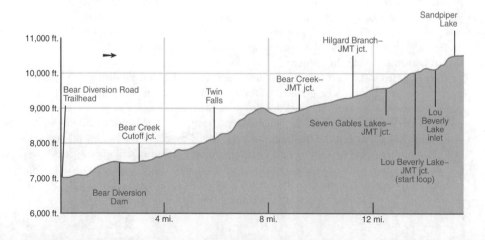

At Sandpiper Lake's southeastern corner, the trail vanishes and the final distance to camp is cross-country. Along the southern shore, you must navigate past some minor granite lumps, bypassed in part at lake level and elsewhere by climbing up and down the slab knobs. You then cut back toward the inlet creek, best jumped across near the outlet of the next tarn south. Climbing briefly, you reach the top of a bedrock knob with many sandy flats that make good campsites with stunning views in every direction (10,533'; 37.30666°N, 118.85469°W; no campfires). To the south is an abstract mingling of water and slab, speckled with sandy flats that make fine campsites—as long as you are 100 feet from water. I recommend picking a splendid perch near the given waypoint and then continuing your explorations without your pack to ensure your camp activities stay well clear of the ubiquitous water. While the smaller lakes do not contain fish, some of the deeper, bigger ones were once stocked with golden trout. The vistas from the ridge to the west at sunset are well worth the climb.

MEDLEY LAKE OR LAKES?

While only a single lake is given the moniker "Medley Lake" on the USGS 7.5' topo maps, it seems fitting to consider the collection of water bodies in this surreal basin to be a musical medley. Even a persistent explorer may become frustrated trying to follow the sinuous shoreline of the lakes, but ultimately one passes locations where one lake ends and the next starts—for there will be a *very* short stream segment that flows a few inches downhill and you'll indeed notice a change in water level. In fact, Medley Lake, as labeled on the topos, is actually several lakes. The granite underlying this astounding basin must be quite impermeable, for every minor depression is filled with water, many with neither an inlet nor outlet and therefore only recharged by snow or thunderstorms. Staring at an aerial photo you'll notice one slightly longer cleft—the main creek channel that must be fracture delineated. Otherwise you'll just see the most convoluted lake shapes linked together by low-angle polished granite slabs. Absolutely leave time to explore the Medley basin, and hopefully also to climb to big, deep, stark Three Island Lake another step up.

DAY 3 (Medley Lake to Bear Creek via Marie Lake, 8.0 miles, part cross-country): While it is possible to retrace your steps, an easy 1.9-mile cross-country segment across to Marie Lake lets you experience some new terrain on the return. From your campsite, continue southeast toward the prominent ridge to the west. Your goal is to cross the ridge at 10,800 feet, right where the top flattens (37.30447°N, 118.86230°W). You wind your way west across the slab landscape, following sandy passageways that present themselves and quite likely having to

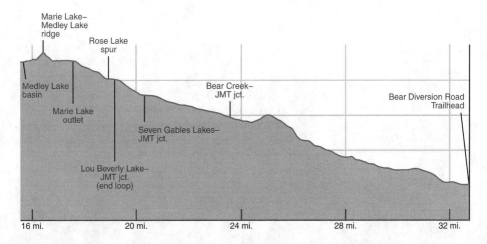

backtrack a few steps when an unexpected tarn appears in front of you or there is a bluff to circumvent. Once at the base of the ridge, you turn south and zigzag upward on the steepening slabs, staying east of the nose of the ridge and always finding sandy shelves that lead upward. Suddenly the terrain flattens and you are on a broad slab shelf with outstanding views east, west, and north. To the west, massive Marie Lake sits perched on a shelf—had glacial erosion proceeded slightly differently, it would have drained down the South Fork Bear Creek, not the West Fork. To the east you get a near-aerial view of the Medley Lake area backdropped by Seven Gables. And to the north you see the length of Bear Creek past Seven Gables to Recess Peak and Mount Hilgard and beyond to the Silver Divide.

Continuing just south of due west, the terrain is not too steep as you work your way down more sandy benches toward Marie Lake. As the slope eases, you walk across slab and then meadow to the lake. Approaching the lakeshore, turn north (right) and encircle the lake counterclockwise. You'll pick up a use trail by the time you reach the north end of the lake, although it is superfluous in the sand-and-grass terrain you traverse. There are some small campsites beneath lodgepole and whitebark pines near the north end of the lake, but camping is prohibited near the JMT corridor. Looping back south, you reach the JMT near the Marie Lake outlet.

Turn north (right) to follow the JMT back down to Rosemarie Meadow. The trail first leads down broken slabs and then into hemlock forest. Most memorable is an incised bedrock corridor with a mosaic of rectangular feldspar crystals. Soon you reach the edge of Rosemarie Meadow, offering campsites in stands of trees along the eastern border. Passing a left-hand (west) trail to Rose Lake, you continue right (north) on the JMT. Toward the north end of the meadow you close the brief loop part of this hike and retrace your steps from here to the JMT–Bear Creek Trail junction, selecting one of the campsites a short distance down Bear Creek.

DAY 4 (Bear Creek to Bear Dam Junction, 9.1 miles): Retrace your steps from Day 1 and part of Day 2.

Granite slab campsite near Medley Lake   Photo by Elizabeth Wenk

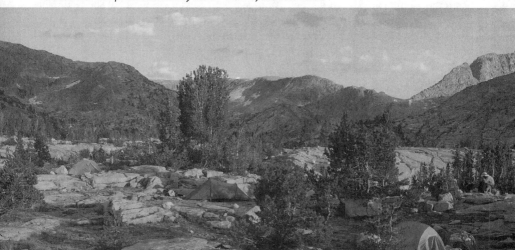

trip 7   Bear Creek to Florence Lake

Trip Data: 37.30666°N, 118.85469°W (Medley Lake);
35.0/31.0 miles; 4/1 days

Topos: *Mount Givens, Florence Lake, Mount Hilgard, Ward Mountain*

see maps on p. 46–47

HIGHLIGHTS: This popular shuttle trip traverses the length of Bear Creek's canyon, takes in pristine alpine scenery at Medley Lake and Marie Lake, descends past more subalpine lakes along Sallie Keyes Creek, and eventually reaches Blayney Hot Springs. The last miles of the trip tour wildflower-carpeted meadows before arriving at Florence Lake. It's an excellent longer trip for the intermediate hiker.

HEADS UP! *The exact routing described involves several miles of cross-country travel and is not recommended for beginners. However, you can easily bypass Medley Lake, continuing along the JMT from Rosemarie Meadow to Marie Lake, eliminating the cross-country leg and reducing the trip distance by 2.3 miles.*

HEADS UP! *The first mile of the four-wheel-drive road to Bear Diversion Dam was burned in the 2020 Creek Fire, but the landscape upstream was spared.*

SHUTTLE DIRECTIONS: From the Lake Edison/Florence Lake Y-junction, head right (southeast) on Florence Lake Road/FS 7S01 for 5.9 miles to the overnight parking lot. Vermilion Valley Resort often runs a once-a-day shuttle service between the Lake Edison area trailheads and Florence Lake. Call ahead to see if you can arrange a car shuttle at either the start or end of your trip.

DAY 1 (Bear Dam Junction to Twin Falls, 5.9 miles): Follow Trip 5, Day 1 to Twin Falls (8,119'; 37.36253°N, 118.93179°W).

DAY 2 (Twin Falls to Medley Lake, 9.8 miles): Follow Trip 6, Day 2 to Medley Lake (10,533'; 37.30666°N, 118.85469°W; no campfires).

DAY 3 (Medley Lake to Blayney Hot Springs, 10.2 miles, part cross-country): From your campsite, continue southeast toward the prominent ridge to the west. Your goal is to cross the ridge at 10,800 feet, right where the top flattens (37.30447°N, 118.86230°W). You wind your way west across the slab landscape, following sandy passageways that present themselves and quite likely having to backtrack a few steps when an unexpected tarn appears in front of you or there is a bluff to circumvent. Once at the base of the ridge, you turn south and zigzag upward on the steepening slabs, staying east of the nose of the ridge and always finding sandy shelves that lead upward. Suddenly the terrain flattens and you are on a broad slab shelf, with outstanding views east, west, and north. To the west, massive Marie Lake sits perched on a shelf—had glacial erosion proceeded slightly differently, it would have drained down the South Fork Bear Creek, not the West Fork. To the east you get a near-aerial view of the Medley Lake area backdropped by Seven Gables. And to the north you see the length of Bear Creek past Seven Gables to Recess Peak and Mount Hilgard and beyond to the Silver Divide.

Continuing just south of due west, the terrain is not too steep as you work your way down more sandy benches toward Marie Lake. As the slope eases, you walk across slab and then meadow to the lake. Approaching the lakeshore, you have the choice to encircle the lake in either direction. Looping south is ostensibly about 0.25 mile shorter, but only if you stay inland of the tortuous shoreline and climb over a series of shallow slab ribs. Northbound, you get to walk near the lakeshore, enjoying the stupendous lake throughout. So, I suggest you turn north (right) and encircle the lake counterclockwise. You'll pick up a use trail by the time you reach the north end of the lake, although it is superfluous in the sand-and-grass terrain you traverse. There are some small campsites beneath lodgepole and whitebark pines near the north end of the lake, but camping is prohibited near the JMT. Looping back south, you reach the JMT near the Marie Lake outlet. You turn left (south), while right (north) leads back down Bear Creek toward Rosemarie Meadow (Trip 6).

After skirting the west side of Marie Lake, you begin the final sandy climb to Selden Pass, an almost quaint slot between boulders and bluffs (10,926'). From the pass, you continue down a sheltered trough, prickly granite gilia coloring the cliff bases. Switchbacks lead to a straightaway beside a creeklet, bound for Heart Lake with tiny, exposed tent sites. Continuing south, beside Heart Lake's outlet, the trail crosses it twice en route to the Sallie Keyes Lakes. The meadow corridors are alight with alpine wildflowers—little elephant's head, alpine shooting star, tundra aster, and alpine gentian each appear in season.

Crossing the narrow isthmus separating the two upper Sallie Keyes Lakes, you continue along the second lake's western shore, sauntering alongside elegant spiral-trunked lodgepole pine. The flat-topped lump to the west, a shallow moraine, offers abundant campsites, including some trailside options as you approach the second lake's outlet. This shallow lake has pleasant swimming temperatures if you need a break. The trail crosses the outlet and continues due south, bypassing the third Sallie Keyes Lake before swinging east, crossing seasonally marshy terrain, and then climbing over a sand-and-gravel lump, a moraine. Here, a few feet south of the trail, is a worthwhile overlook of the valley, offering a stunning view of the South Fork San Joaquin River's U-shaped, glacially carved valley. Dropping to an elongate moraine-dammed meadow with a seasonal tributary, the trail skirts across a shallower moraine tongue before switchbacking down its chinquapin-and-boulder covered south side into lodgepole pine forest that leads to Senger Creek. Nearby you'll find some small campsites, but respect posted RESTORATION signs.

You now begin a long, dry drop into the South Fork San Joaquin canyon far below. The grade is continuous, with no benches for camping. The open slope is mostly covered by greenleaf manzanita bushes and whitethorn. As you descend, look for a small lake lying at the base of the opposite canyon wall. Blayney Hot Springs is just north of this lake. Zigzagging to and fro, the trail finally enters stands of trees—an eclectic assemblage, including aspen, red fir, lodgepole pine, junipers, and/or Jeffrey pine, that fluctuates continually with exposure. Crossing onto red metamorphic soils, you reach a junction where the JMT continues left (southeast), while straight ahead (right; south) is the trail toward Florence Lake, also coined the "MTR cutoff" by JMT/PCT hikers, who are taking this track to resupply on food at nearby Muir Trail Ranch.

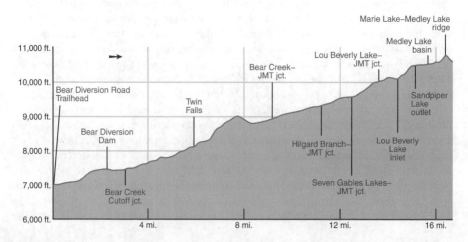

A steep, dusty descent mostly beneath forest cover leads to a four-way junction where right (west) leads to Florence Lake, straight ahead (south) to Muir Trail Ranch and Blayney Hot Springs, and left (east) back to the JMT and on to the Kings Canyon National Park boundary (Trips 8, 9). Continue straight ahead, then keep left where a lateral right drops to private Muir Trail Ranch. Winding through aspen glades just beyond the eastern boundary of the ranch you'll approach campsites near the South Fork San Joaquin. Be sure to pick a legal site—signs indicate which locations are acceptable (for example, 7,658'; 37.23501°N, 118.88021°W; no campfires). Many of the best sites—and the hot springs—are on the south side of the river, only accessible at low to moderate flows. There are additional campsites 0.3 mile upstream on the river's north side. This is not a river that can be crossed in early summer! Blayney Hot Springs is a delightful location, but I hesitated making it a night's destination in this edition—this location is currently hugely impacted by JMT and PCT hikers resupplying on food at Muir Trail Ranch and then spending the night in the vicinity. They camp here—and you probably will as well—because there aren't any other big campsites for many miles in any direction. Please be ultraconscious of Leave No Trace principles here and rangers' restoration efforts.

Beyond the campsites on the far side of the river is the trail crossing Shooting Star Meadow to the public pool at Blayney Hot Springs. Since the muddy pool is very susceptible to erosion, please enter and exit the pool carefully. Just beyond the willows is a magical little lake where you can go swimming. "Warm Lake" is the result of moraines and springs that come together to form this body of water, far below the usual elevation of Sierra lakes. The entire meadow and hot springs area is fragile; minimize your impact.

MUIR TRAIL RANCH

Muir Trail Ranch (MTR) is a family-owned guest ranch. The ranch provides a food-resupply service that is very popular with long-distance JMT and PCT hikers. See muirtrailranch.com for more details. They have a tiny store and water faucet, but their toilets and café are only available to overnight guests.

DAY 4 (Blayney Hot Springs to Florence Lake, 9.1 miles, or 5.1 miles with a ferry ride): Return 0.35 mile north to the signed trail toward Florence Lake and turn left (west). This trail stays well above the valley on a sunstruck traverse across talus slopes. You cross first Senger Creek and then Sallie Keys Creek, each on logs. You look down upon the verdant, tree-sheltered valley where Muir Trail Ranch sits, grateful when your trail drops to the valley

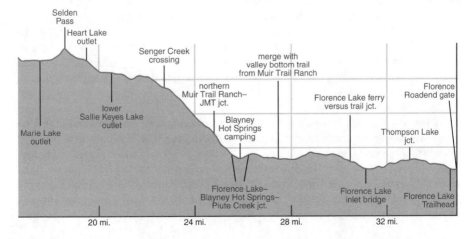

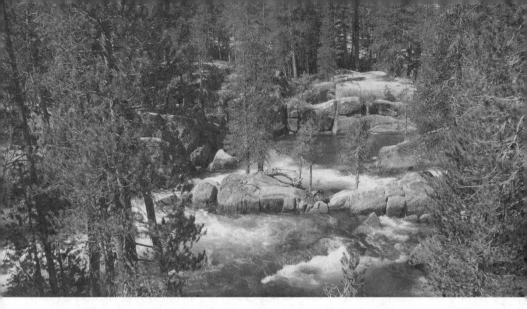

Bear Creek   Photo by Elizabeth Wenk

floor after 1.25 miles. Merging with a trail that comes from Muir Trail Ranch, you continue west. (You can also drop to MTR from the spur near the campsites and take the valley bottom route for the first miles through their property.) Here, and several times later on, you cross paths with a broader dirt track that Muir Trail Ranch uses to bring in supplies.

The trail follows the northern edge of massive, marshy Blayney Meadows, although the curtain of lodgepole pine and aspen between the trail and the meadow generally block your view across it. Now beyond the Muir Trail Ranch property, you could camp in the forest at the meadow's edge. Onward, you cross Alder Creek as you gradually ascend through lush aspen and lodgepole pine forest to Double Meadow, diving in and out of several of its lobes. Toward the end of Double Meadow, the trail climbs onto slabs beginning a mile-long lumpy meander through joint-defined corridors, alongside pocket meadows where moisture is trapped, and over bedrock.

It leads to a junction signposted for the FLORENCE FERRY LANDING (versus Florence Lake Trailhead), where you have a choice. If the timing works, I'd recommend the ferry, which leaves the east (trail) end of the lake on the hour, every odd hour, and sometimes more frequently. See florence-lake.com for more details. The right-trending spur trail leads 0.5 mile to the ferry landing—the distance increasing in drought years when the water level in Florence Lake, a reservoir, is lower and the ferry can't reach its normal wharf.

If hiking to the trailhead, continue ahead (left; west and then south) to a bridge across the South Fork San Joaquin River. Standing on the bridge watching the river surge into the lake is impressive. This is often your last water source before the trailhead, so fill a water bottle. Onward, the trail passes campsites alongside the river that are very popular with hikers and anglers who've taken advantage of the ferry and have carried their gear less than a mile to camp in this lovely setting. You then cross Boulder Creek, sidle across granite outcrops, and gradually climb 200 feet above the lake. The setting is delightful—a giant body of water, slabs everywhere, and occasional shade from tall Jeffrey pines, unusually straggly junipers, and the occasional lodgepole pine and white fir. Less delightful is the relentless, hot sun as you look enviously at boaters on the lake. You pass a junction for the near-abandoned trail to Thompson Lake and continue along benches to the northwestern end of the lake. Here you reach the trailhead, landing on a paved Southern California Edison Company road that you follow the final 0.3 mile uphill to a locked gate (7,343'; 37.27665°N, 118.97636°W). Now you continue a short distance farther to the parking lot or leave your pack and fetch the car!

Florence Lake Trailhead 7,343'; 37.27665°N, 118.97636°W

Destination/ GPS Coordinates	Trip Type	Best Season	Pace & Hiking/ Layover Days	Total Mileage	Permit Required
8 Martha Lake 37.09862°N 118.74304°W	Out-and-back	Mid to late	Leisurely 6/1	39.4/ 47.4	Florence Lake
9 Red Mountain Basin 37.14063°N 118.81912°W (Disappointment Lake)	Out-and-back	Mid to late	Leisurely 6/1	44.4/ 52.4	Florence Lake
7 Bear Creek to Florence Lake (in reverse of description; see page 59)	Shuttle	Mid to late	Moderate 4/1	35.0/ 31.0	Florence Lake (Bear Diversion as described)

INFORMATION AND PERMITS: This trailhead is in Sierra National Forest. Permits are required for overnight stays and quotas apply. Details on how to reserve permits are available at fs.usda.gov/detail/sierra/passes-permits. For advance reservations (60% of quota), there is $5-per-person reservation fee, while walk-up permits (40% of quota) are free. Permits can be picked up at 29688 Auberry Road, Prather, CA 93651; if you call 559-855-5355 in advance, they will leave your permit in a dropbox. Permits can also be picked up in person at the Eastwood Forest Service Office at the corner of Kaiser Pass Road and CA 168, at Huntington Lake or at the High Sierra Visitor Information Station, 15.7 miles along Kaiser Pass Road (shortly before the Lake Edison–Florence Lake split). If you plan to use a stove or have a campfire, you must also have a California campfire permit, available from a forest service office or online at preventwildfireca.org/campfire-permit. Along the South Fork San Joaquin River, campfires are prohibited below 7,800 feet, which includes locations near Blayney Meadows, and above 10,000 feet. In Kings Canyon National Park, campfires are prohibited above 10,000 feet. In Red Mountain Basin, campfires are prohibited within 0.25 mile of Disappointment Lake, Rae Lake, and Fleming Lake. Bear canisters are not required but are strongly encouraged.

DRIVING DIRECTIONS: From the intersection of CA 168 and CA 180, just east of Fresno, take CA 168 northeast through Clovis and up into the foothills, to the community of Shaver Lake. Here, continue straight along CA 168 to Huntington Lake (versus right along Dinkey Lakes Road to Courtright Reservoir), and reach a T-junction near the community of Lakeshore, 67.5 miles from CA 180. Here CA 168 ends, and Huntington Lake Road leads left around the lake's north shore, while Kaiser Pass Road/FS 80 branches right. Turn right onto Kaiser Pass Road and drive 16.7 miles over Kaiser Pass to a fork, where left leads to Lake Edison and Mono Hot Springs and right to Florence Lake. Turn right onto Florence Lake Road/FS 7S01 and drive 5.9 miles to the trailhead parking lot. Beyond, you can drop down and right toward a picnic area and gate, behind which the trailhead departs, or down and left to the store and ferry.

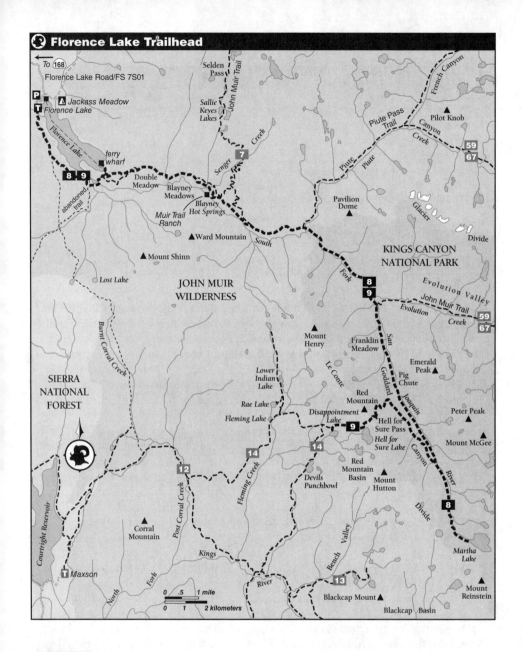

trip 8   **Martha Lake**

> **Trip Data:** 37.09862°N, 118.74304°W; 39.4/47.4 miles; 6/1 days
>
> **Topos:** *Florence Lake, Ward Mountain, Blackcap Mountain, Mount Henry, Mount Goddard*

HIGHLIGHTS: Beyond Muir Trail Ranch, this trip visits remote backcountry in the northwestern corner of Kings Canyon National Park. The scenery along South Fork San Joaquin River is stunning, with a parade of thrilling cataracts, cascades, and waterfalls visible from the trail. The long journey up the river culminates in a splendid crescendo at Martha Lake, a large alpine lake cradled in a rocky cirque basin nearly surrounded by craggy peaks and ridges. Along the way, sore backpackers can soak their weary bones in the soothing waters of Blayney Hot Springs.

HEADS UP! *You can save a total of 8.0 miles of uninspiring hiking along the shore of Florence Lake with arrangements for a ferry ride across the lake. The different distances shown above and in the Day headers below reflect this (with ferry/without). Note that the distance in the elevation profile below is without the ferry.*

FERRY
Rather than backpack the first 4 miles, you could purchase a ticket ($15 one-way, $28 round-trip in 2019) at the store and take advantage of the ferry ride across Florence Lake (see florence-lake .com for more information). From 8:30 a.m. to 5 p.m., the ferry makes a minimum of five scheduled trips (more on weekends) across the lake and back. From the ferry dock at the far end of the lake, climb uphill over barren granite slopes for a half mile to the junction with the trail around Florence Lake. For your return, there's a radiophone near the dock, from which you can call the store for your ride back.

DAY 1 (Florence Lake Trailhead to near Pacific Crest Trail (PCT)/John Muir Trail (JMT) junction, 5.7/9.7 miles): If you've elected not to take the ferry, follow the paved road through the picnic area, down to the lake, and along the west shore to the beginning of singletrack trail (7,357'; 37.27341°N, 118.97433°W), where a set of stairs leads into the John Muir Wilderness. Proceed generally south across gently rolling terrain beneath mixed forest. The trees part enough on occasion to allow for views across Florence Lake of the dam and the granite walls above the far shore, as well as more distant Mount Shinn and Ward Mountain to the southeast. Reach a junction with the Burnt Corral Meadow Trail signed for THOMPSON LAKE, 2.0 miles from the locked gate.

Continue ahead (southeast) at the junction, traveling above the southwest arm of the lake and then downhill to a junction marked only by a cairn with a lateral to the Burnt Corral Meadow Trail, 1.6 miles from the previous junction. Go ahead (east) here to cross over a tributary stream, followed by a short stroll to a more substantial bridge spanning the South Fork San Joaquin River at 3.5 miles from the trailhead. Lodgepole-shaded campsites are spread along both banks of the river. From the bridge, head upstream and briefly follow the trail along the river until a moderate, half-mile climb over granite slabs leads to the ferry dock lateral, 4.0 miles from the trailhead.

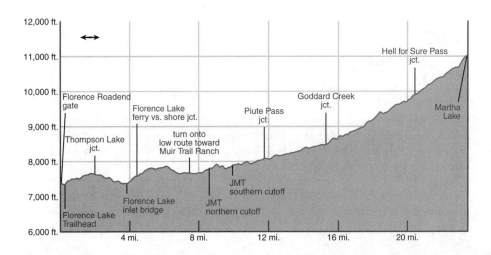

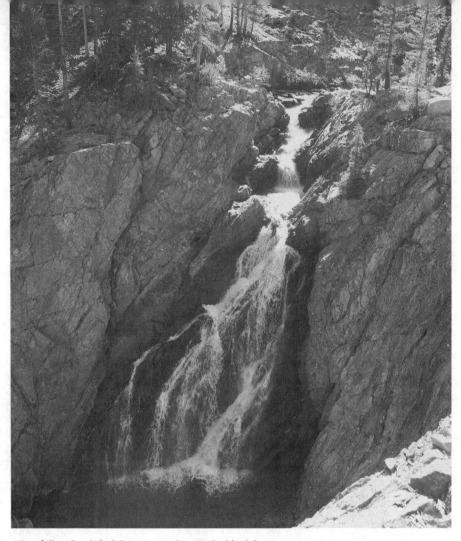

Waterfall on South Fork San Joaquin River in Goddard Canyon   Photo by Mike White

JEEP ROAD

Keen eyes will spy a primitive jeep road beyond the southeast end of the lake. Muir Trail Ranch, 2.5 miles upstream, uses an old army personnel carrier to transport guests along this road, which parallels and occasionally coincides with the route of the hiking trail. Such activity would seem incompatible with the idea of wilderness, but the family-owned operation has been in business for more than 50 years and was grandfathered into the 1964 Wilderness Act.

From the ferry junction, turn right (east) and climb over granite slabs and up dry gullies for a mile to the edge of pastoral Double Meadow. After skirting the meadow, the trail crosses a seasonal stream lined with grasses and wildflowers and then makes a gradual descent to a crossing of Alder Creek, where sheltered campsites are found on the far bank. A short distance past the creek is a lateral to better campsites near the river at Lower Blayney Campground. Past this junction, the broad expanse of Blayney Meadows momentarily springs into view, but the path quickly veers away in favor of a forested route that bypasses the meadows.

About 2.5 miles from the ferry dock, you pass through a gate at the fenced boundary of privately owned Muir Trail Ranch. The route across the ranch property may be difficult to distinguish amid a maze of dusty stock trails and the churned-up jeep road. Farther down the road, pay close attention to makeshift signs that direct you away from the road and onto singletrack trail to the left. Proceed southeastward through open terrain and light forest on gently graded trail to crossings of Sallie Keyes and Senger Creeks. A moderate climb of a hillside, followed by a lightly forested traverse, leads to a chain gate.

MUIR TRAIL RANCH

Although the presence of a resort seems inconsistent with a designated wilderness area, Muir Trail Ranch is hiker friendly. For a fee, packages can be held at the ranch for JMT and PCT thru-hikers. On the rare occasion when the ranch is not completely booked, usually only in early June, backpackers can purchase an overnight stay complete with three meals. Unfortunately, single meals are not available to nonguests. For more information, check out the ranch's website at muirtrailranch.com.

Beyond the gate, you continue across an open hillside in cadence to the rhythmic sound of a Pelton wheel that generates electricity for the ranch below. Reach an open knoll and then drop to a signed junction of a lateral accessing the ranch and Blayney Hot Springs.

BLAYNEY HOT SPRINGS

To visit the hot springs, turn right (south) and proceed a mere 75 feet, where the trail divides again—follow the path on the left marked HOT SPRINGS and pass overused campsites to the north bank of South Fork San Joaquin River. Ford the broad stretch of the river (difficult in early season) and reach more overused campsites on the far bank. Beyond the campsites, a use trail crosses Shooting Star Meadow to access the public pool at Blayney Hot Springs. Please enter and exit carefully, as the muddy pool is very susceptible to erosion.

Just beyond a patch of willows is "Warm Lake," a magical little gem of a swimming hole that is the result of an unlikely combination of moraines and springs having come together far below the usual elevations common for Sierra lakes. This area is very fragile, so please minimize your impact by being a good steward of this healing place.

Return to the junction and head southeast on gradually rising trail through light forest to a well-signed four-way junction with a steep lateral to the JMT/PCT climbing northbound (straight ahead) toward Selden Pass. Go right (southeast), as the main trail continues to parallel the now-unseen river upstream through a scattered forest of aspens, lodgepole pines, and Jeffrey pines. Pass a stagnant pond and reach an extensive camping area that occupies a forested bench above the river (7,790'; 37.22761°N, 118.86616°W; no campfires), 5.7 miles from the ferry dock, a third of a mile prior to a junction with the JMT (7,893'; 37.22577°N, 118.86123°W).

DAY 2 (JMT/PCT Junction to Goddard Canyon Trail Junction, 5.7 miles): Now on the southeast-trending JMT, follow the course of the river through a mixture of metamorphic slabs and conifers, with fine views of the South Fork San Joaquin over the next couple of miles or so. Just prior to the confluence of Piute Creek with the river is a junction with the Piute Pass Trail, 7.8 miles from the ferry dock. Go ahead (briefly east) and immediately find a steel bridge that spans the tumultuous creek and crosses the border into Kings Canyon National Park. A number of good campsites can be found on a flat near the junction, bordered by chaparral and partially shaded by widely scattered Jeffrey pines.

Hike upstream on a gradual, exposed climb around John Muir Rock and then draw nearer the river flowing through a narrow channel of dark rock. About 1.5 miles from the Piute Pass Trail junction, enter the cool forested glade of aspens and pines misnamed Aspen Meadow. While there is no semblance of a meadow here, there are a few sheltered campsites.

Leave Aspen Meadow behind and continue to follow the river upstream on a gradual, mile-long climb of a narrow and exposed section of the canyon. Cross a steel bridge over the river to a small, forested flat, where a use trail leads shortly downstream to shady campsites. Now on the south side of the river, pass through a gate near more campsites, walk through wildflower gardens, and ford a vigorous stream draining several tarns below Le Conte Divide. Reach campsites shaded by a mixed forest of aspens, lodgepole pines, and junipers near the signed junction with the Goddard Canyon Trail (8,487'; 37.19281°N, 118.79504°W).

From the junction, head either right (south) a short distance up the Goddard Canyon Trail, or left (briefly east, then north) across the river on the JMT's wooden bridge to fine campsites where you can hear the soothing South Fork San Joaquin.

DAY 3 (Goddard Canyon Trail Junction to Martha Lake, 8.3 miles): If necessary, return to the junction and take the Goddard Canyon Trail southward. Climb moderately through a light forest of lodgepole pines a half mile to Franklin Meadow, where tall aspens dot a picturesque, wildflower-laden grassland bisected by gurgling rivulets. A couple of primitive campsites are near the south end of the meadow just above the river.

Follow the trail away from the meadow and the river for a while on a gradual-to-moderate climb through the trees. Soon, the narrowing walls of the canyon force the path up the hillside and along an ascending traverse above the river. Pass more campsites on a narrow bench overlooking the river on the way to a lush hillside well watered by a series of rivulets and carpeted with willows, aspens, and wildflowers, including paintbrush, clover, coneflower, columbine, and heather. Visible across this verdant meadowland is Pig Chute, where a seasonal stream pours down a narrow, rocky cleft beside a dark, knife-edged protrusion of rock. Farther up the trail, a spectacular waterfall spills into an emerald pool.

For a while, the trail heads upstream with fantastic views across Goddard Canyon of the cascading river plunging down a narrow, deep, rocky cleft. Along the way, pass two more waterfalls as scenic as any to be found in the High Sierra and cross several flower-lined streams spilling across the trail.

Near the confluence with North Goddard Creek, the canyon widens, allowing the river to slow down and broaden. Stroll through meadowlands for a fine view of both river canyons separated by a low rock dome. A short, moderate climb leads to an obscure junction with the Hell for Sure Pass Trail, 5.1 miles from the JMT junction. A few primitive campsites shaded by a grove of trees can be found a short distance beyond the junction, near a creek crossing. Continue ahead (south-southeast) on the Goddard Canyon Trail.

Now the upper part of Goddard Canyon spreads out in subalpine splendor on an ascent of lush meadowlands, unbroken except for an occasional stunted pine or small clump of willows. Pockets of lupine and heather accent the green meadow as you gaze south and southeastward toward the mighty hulks of Mount Goddard and Mount Reinstein. Eventually, the path grows indistinct, but the route upstream along the South Fork is obvious on the way to its birthplace beneath the Le Conte and Goddard Divides. Flowers cover the slopes, including daisy, shooting star, and paintbrush.

After crossing the outlet stream from Lake Confusion, which is high above, begin a moderately steep, straightforward cross-country ascent over grassy benches and granite slabs to the lip of the basin holding Martha Lake. From there, a short, easy stroll leads to the west shore of the austere, rockbound lake (11,032'; 37.09862°N, 118.74304°W; no campfires).

AT MARTHA LAKE

A smattering of small pocket meadows almost softens the predominantly barren, rocky shoreline of the lake. Situated above timberline near the convergence of three divides—Goddard, Le Conte, and White—the lake is located in a truly alpine environment. The dark, rugged flanks of Mount Goddard (13,368') tower 2,500 feet over the northeast shore, while Mount Reinstein (12,604') provides a fine backdrop to the south. Although developed campsites are virtually nonexistent, resourceful backpackers will be able to find sandy spots suitable for pitching a tent in various locations around the shoreline. Anglers can ply the waters in search of rainbow and golden trout. For cross-country enthusiasts, Martha Lake is also the western gateway into some of the most coveted off-trail terrain in the High Sierra: directly east lies the mysterious realm of Ionian Basin, a trip through which is considered a Sierra classic. Mountaineers may want to tackle the Class 2–3 route up the southeast ridge of Mount Goddard.

DAYS 4–6 (Martha Lake to Florence Lake Trailhead, 19.7/23.7 miles): Retrace your steps.

trip 9 Red Mountain Basin

see map on p. 64

Trip Data: 37.14063°N, 118.81912°W; 43.5/51.5 miles; 6/1 days
Topos: *Florence Lake, Ward Mountain, Blackcap Mountain, Mount Henry, Mount Goddard*

HIGHLIGHTS: Red Mountain Basin offers backpackers the type of scenery for which the High Sierra is famous: alpine peaks, glacier-scoured terrain, and sparkling lakes highlight this rugged area on the west side of the Le Conte Divide. A bounty of picturesque lakes—some near the trail and others a short, easy cross-country jaunt away—make excellent base camps for the exploration of the extensive basin. Travelers can expect to find solitude on this multilayer journey along the lightly used trails necessary to reach Red Mountain Basin.

HEADS UP! *You can save 4.0 miles of uninspiring hiking along the shore of Florence Lake by arranging for a ferry ride across the lake (see details on page 65). Note that the distance in the elevation profile on page 70 is without the ferry.*

DAY 1 (Florence Lake Trailhead to near JMT/PCT Junction, 5.7 miles): Follow Trip 8, Day 1 to near the JMT/PCT junction (7,790'; 37.22761°N, 118.86616°W; no campfires).

DAY 2 (JMT/PCT Junction to Goddard Canyon Trail Junction, 5.7 miles): Follow Trip 8, Day 2 to campsites near the Goddard Canyon Trail junction (8,487'; 37.19281°N, 118.79504°W).

DAY 3 (Goddard Canyon Trail Junction to Disappointment Lake, 10.8 miles): Return to the junction and take the Goddard Canyon Trail southward. Climb moderately through a light forest of lodgepole pines 0.5 mile to Franklin Meadow, where tall aspens dot a picturesque, wildflower-laden grassland bisected by gurgling rivulets. A couple of primitive campsites are near the south end of the meadow just above the river.

Follow the trail away from the meadow and the river for a while on a gradual-to-moderate climb through the trees. Soon, the narrowing walls of the canyon force the path up the hillside and along an ascending traverse above the river. Pass more campsites on a narrow bench overlooking the river on the way to a lush hillside well watered by a series of rivulets and carpeted with willows, aspens, and wildflowers, including paintbrush, clover, coneflower, columbine, and heather. Visible across this verdant meadowland is Pig Chute, where a seasonal stream pours down a narrow, rocky cleft beside a dark, knife-edged protrusion of rock. Farther up the trail, a spectacular waterfall spills into an emerald pool.

For a while, the trail heads upstream with fantastic views across Goddard Canyon of the cascading river plunging down a narrow, deep, rocky cleft. Along the way, pass two more waterfalls as scenic as any to be found in the High Sierra and cross several flower-lined streams spilling across the trail.

Near the confluence with North Goddard Creek, the canyon widens, allowing the river to slow down and broaden. Stroll through meadowlands for a fine view of both river canyons separated by a low rock dome. A short, moderate climb leads to an obscure junction with the Hell for Sure Pass Trail, 5.1 miles from the JMT junction. A few primitive campsites shaded by a grove of trees can be found a short distance beyond the junction, near a creek crossing.

Turn right (west) at the junction and begin a 4.0-mile, stiff jaunt toward Hell for Sure Pass. After a half-mile, switchbacking climb, the trail follows a gentle 2.0-mile traverse heading northwest across the west wall of Goddard Canyon. This trail is only lightly maintained, designated by the park as a "minimally-developed" trail, and in sections can be difficult to discern. Near the end of the traverse, you hop across a creek draining the slopes below the pass. A short distance beyond this initial crossing, begin an 1,150-foot climb generally following the north side of creek's drainage on the way to austere Hell for Sure Pass (11,321'; 37.14590°N, 118.79807°W).

The views of Goddard Canyon have been stunning since you left the Goddard Canyon Trail, but they reach a climax at the pass, opening up to the west over sprawling Red Mountain Basin. While the route from Goddard Canyon to Hell for Sure Pass has consumed 4.0 miles of hiking, the trail down into Red Mountain Basin plunges rapidly to Hell for Sure Lake, tightly winding 500 feet down a steep gully to the north shore of the 10,782-foot lake. Tucked into a stunning cirque immediately below Le Conte Divide, the lake is surrounded by polished granite slabs that sparkle in the sunlight of a typically clear Sierra sky. Tiny pockets of meadow make feeble attempts to break up the otherwise rocky slopes of the basin. A few campsites are scattered around the north shore, and fishing is reported to be good for medium-size brook trout.

From Hell for Sure Lake, descend a hillside of granite slabs, pass by some small tarns, and step over a sparkling stream on the way to an unmarked lateral heading south and leading

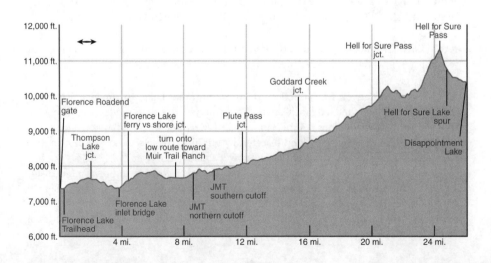

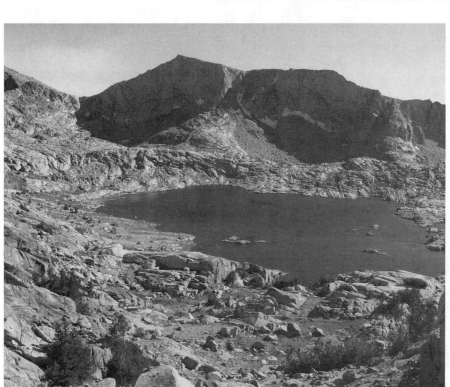

Descending to Hell for Sure Lake in Red Mountain Basin   Photo by Mike White

shortly to Disappointment Lake (10,368'; 37.14063°N, 118.81912°W; no campfires). Backdropped by Mount Hutton and the craggy Le Conte Divide, the lake is as attractive as any in the High Sierra, with alternating sections of meadow and sandy beach ringing the north shore and rolling granite slabs along the south shore. Fine campsites with grand views of the surrounding terrain will reward tired backpackers. A healthy population of brook trout should satisfy anglers.

EXPLORING RED MOUNTAIN BASIN

Red Mountain Basin offers many alternatives for spending extra days exploring the region. Several lakes are easily accessible by connecting trails, and many other lakes can be visited via easy cross-country routes. Due to the lengthy approaches necessary to reach the basin, you're unlikely to encounter too many other backpackers. For peak baggers, Red Mountain is a straightforward Class 1 climb from Hell for Sure Pass.

DAYS 4–6 (Disappointment Lake to Florence Lake Trailhead, 22.2/26.2 miles): Retrace your steps. A radiophone is available near the ferry landing for arranging your return via the ferry across Florence Lake.

CA 168 WEST SIDE TO DINKEY CREEK ROAD TRIPS

Dinkey Lakes Road accesses trails radiating from a pair of giant reservoirs in the North Fork Kings watershed, Courtright Reservoir to the north and Wishon Reservoir to the south. The small North Fork Kings drainage is an often-forgotten corner of the Sierra, but it has on display a splendid granite landscape, including rugged peaks, cirque lakes, rounded domes, and expansive meadows. The elevation gain is generally moderate, adding to the region's appeal. The trailheads described here are Cliff Lake, Maxson, and Woodchuck. Cliff Lake Trail leads from the west shore of Courtright Reservoir into Dinkey Lakes Wilderness, offering endless lakeshores for camping. Maxson Trail leads from the east shore of Courtright Reservoir into John Muir Wilderness and a collection of high-elevation, remarkably verdant lake basins. Woodchuck Trail departs from just beyond Wishon Reservoir's dam, climbing east to its own set of splendid lakes and offering access to Blackcap Basin, the headwaters of the North Fork Kings. Rancheria Trailhead out of Wishon Reservoir has been omitted, for many of the trails that branch off the main Rancheria Trail are in disrepair or lead to particularly remote, challenging areas (for example, Blue Canyon and Tehipite Valley); these are all worth a visit, but are better suited to hikers piecing together their own long, challenging loops, rather than following a set itinerary.

Trailheads: Cliff Lake

Maxson

Woodchuck

Looking down onto Courtright Reservoir from the summit of Dogtooth Peak   Photo by Elizabeth Wenk

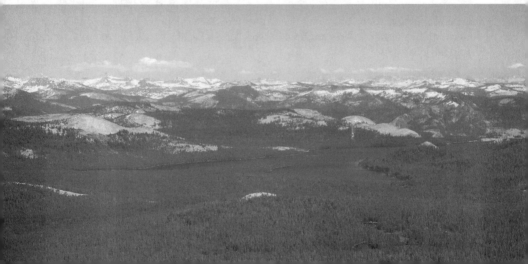

Cliff Lake Trailhead (Courtright Reservoir, Dinkey Lakes)

8,453'; 37.10612°N, 118.98764°W

Destination/ GPS Coordinates	Trip Type	Best Season	Pace & Hiking/ Layover Days	Total Mileage	Permit Required
10 Cliff Lake 37.14208°N 119.04240°W	Out-and-back	Mid to late	Leisurely 2/1	10.6	Cliff Lake
11 Dinkey Lakes 37.15931°N 119.06673°W (Island Lake)	Semiloop	Mid to late	Leisurely 3/1	21.1	Cliff Lake

INFORMATION AND PERMITS: This trailhead is in Sierra National Forest. Permits are required for overnight stays and quotas apply. Details on how to reserve permits are available at fs.usda.gov/detail/sierra/passes-permits. For advance reservations (60% of quota; reservable starting in January each year), there is a $5-per-person reservation fee, while walk-up permits (40% of quota) are free. Permits can be picked up at 29688 Auberry Road, Prather, CA 93651; if you call 559-855-5355 in advance, they will leave your permit in a dropbox. Permits can also be picked up in person at the Dinkey Lakes Forest Service Office, located a short distance north of Dinkey Lakes Road, 11.8 miles past Shaver Lake. If you plan to use a stove or have a campfire, you must also have a California campfire permit, available from a forest service office or online at preventwildfireca.org/campfire-permit. Campfires are prohibited above 10,000 feet. Bear canisters are not required but are strongly encouraged.

DRIVING DIRECTIONS: From the intersection of CA 168 and CA 180, just east of Fresno, take CA 168 northeast through Clovis and up into the foothills, to the community of Shaver Lake, a distance of 46.8 miles. Then turn right onto Dinkey Creek Road and follow it for 25.8 miles to a Y-junction where left leads to Courtright Reservoir and right to Wishon Reservoir; note it has changed names several times along the way and is now called McKinley Grove Road. Head left onto Courtright Way/FS 10S16 and continue 7.4 miles to a three-forked junction where you take the far left-hand choice. Still on Courtright Way/FS 10S16, continue an additional 2.5 miles to the Cliff Lake Trailhead, the parking area located to the left of the road. There are four bear boxes, but no water or toilets at the trailhead.

| trip 10 | ## Cliff Lake |

see map on p. 74

Trip Data: 37.14208°N, 119.04240°W; 10.6 miles; 2/1 days

Topos: *Courtright Reservoir, Dogtooth Peak, Ward Mountain.*

HIGHLIGHTS: Splendid subalpine scenery keeps hikers company as they enjoy this easy trip to a lake nestled under sheer granite cliffs and ledges. An optional (and, in part, exposed) climb of Dogtooth Peak adds adventure and provides a stunning panorama.

HEADS UP! *A stretch of trail south of Cliff Lake was burned in the 2020 Bullfrog Fire, but the Cliff Lake campsites are untouched.*

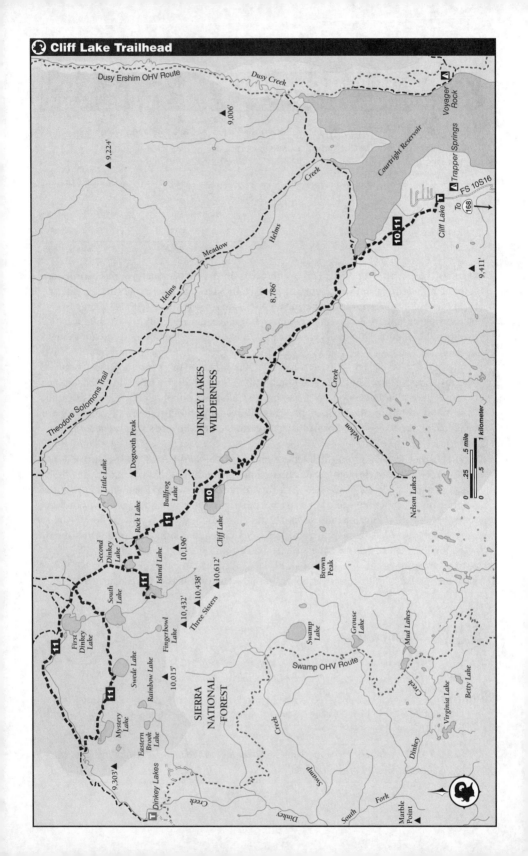

DAY 1 (Cliff Lake Trailhead to Cliff Lake, 5.3 miles): Leaving the trailhead, the path descends gradually northwest toward Courtright Reservoir, traversing down a slope under the shade of red fir and lodgepole pine. Ignore an old road that bisects the trail at 0.2 mile and continue northwest, briefly crossing open slab, but mostly ensconced in deep conifer shade and crossing two marshy areas on a pair of wooden boardwalks. At 0.9 mile you approach Courtright Reservoir's shore, turn more westerly to follow its northwest finger, cross a minor tributary, enter Dinkey Lakes Wilderness, and soon thereafter reach the banks of Nelson Creek, 1.4 miles from the trailhead.

THE ORIGIN OF *DINKEY*

One might assume that the name *Dinkey* refers to the dozens of small, unnamed, and unrecognized lakes within the wilderness area. But locals will tell you the 1863 legend of a tiny dog named Dinkey. On an outing with his owner, an aggressive grizzly bear charged. Dinkey, reportedly "no bigger than a rabbit," attacked, biting the hind leg of the massive grizzly. The bear swiped, and, in a flash, Dinkey was lifeless. Yet Dinkey's bravery was not in vain. By distracting the grizzly, Dinkey allowed his owner enough time to grab his gun and kill the bear. Local legend and Dinkey Lakes Wilderness honor small-but-mighty Dinkey to this day.

In early season, Nelson Creek has a formidable flow and must be crossed about 0.1 mile upstream, where its flow is shallower and less turbulent and the base less bouldery. Once across the creek, you promptly reach a junction, where you turn left (west) to ascend Nelson Creek, while right (east) is signposted for Helms Meadow. After nearly a mile through almost flat forest, some places dry and sandy and elsewhere lush with more understory vegetation, the trail climbs a steeper 200 feet, then resumes a gentle upward trajectory, reaching its next junction at the 3.1-mile mark. Here, you continue straight (northwest), toward Cliff Lake. Left (southwest) leads 1.9 miles to Nelson Lakes (good camping) and right (northeast) leads 1.5 miles to the Helms Meadow Trail. Continuing up along Cliff Lake's unnamed outflow, you walk at the base of an open, dry, bouldery slope of moraine deposits populated by western white pine, red fir, and lodgepole pine. The trail's grade steepens as it turns southwest and ascends a sunnier south-facing slope cloaked with red-barked mat manzanita and elegant western white pine. North-trending again, the trail switchbacks up glacial deposits with chinquapin emerging beneath just about every boulder. Enjoy views toward Courtright Reservoir and the granite domes bordering its shores, while farther east, the desolate, sawtooth, granite peaks of the Le Conte Divide are visible above Blackcap Basin; Mount Goddard is the notable dark, pyramidal-shaped peak. Meanwhile, Brown Peak (10,350'), Nelson Mountain (10,220'), and Eagle Peak (10,318') rise above the Nelson Lakes cirque on the southern skyline.

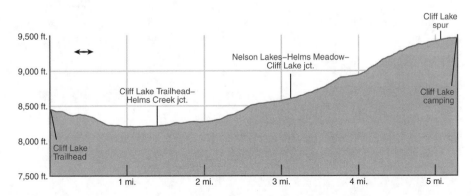

Ahead, you reach a flat, sandy expanse and soon an unsigned junction due east of Cliff Lake's outlet (9,442'; 37.13993°N, 119.03939°W). You head left (northwest) to drop to Cliff Lake's shore, while the right (more northerly) branch continues to a saddle, from which you can access Dogtooth Peak, and then descends to Rock Lake (Trip 11). *Note:* The trail's current location is east of that shown on USGS 7.5' topo maps; the main trail has been rerouted to stay on the sandy flat high above the lakeshore. But you drop down and find many pleasant campsites on sandy soil between lodgepole pine and western white pine (for example, 9,456'; 37.14208°N, 119.04240°W). There are additional sites in the flat near the inlet. A 400-foot sheer granite escarpment—the eponymous "cliff"—encircles half the lake and defines this gorgeous lake's ambiance.

DAY 2 (Cliff Lake to Cliff Lake Trailhead, 5.3 miles): Retrace your steps.

SUMMITING DOGTOOTH PEAK

As you'll read below, the final 40-foot ascent to Dogtooth Peak's summit is exposed and a little tricky. But even if you have no intention of "bagging" the actual summit, this is a worthwhile side trip—just plan to stop at either Point 10,179 (the subpeak you pass over) or on the broad ledge before the final scramble. These destinations offer excellent (and different) views, and the corridors and notches beneath Dogtooth Peak's summit are worth a visit themselves.

To begin this trip, return to the previous junction (9,442'; 37.13993°N, 119.03939°W) and take the main trail north across sandy flats high above Cliff Lake. After 0.4 mile, the trail passes the right-branching (east-trending) trail to Bullfrog Lake. Continue left (northwest), climbing up a sandy, bouldery slope to the prominent saddle where various sandy use trails trend right (northeast), leading upslope toward Dogtooth Peak (saddle: 9,903'; 37.15003°N, 119.04884°W).

You climb northeast up a dry slope with scattered whitebark pine, then turn east and continue just north of Point 10,179. Already now, you're offered brilliant views north across the lower San Joaquin River drainage to Kaiser Peak and beyond to the Ritter Range and the peaks in southern Yosemite.

Dropping 150 feet to the saddle between Point 10,179 and Dogtooth Peak, you climb again, now bound for Dogtooth Peak's collection of smooth, pinkish spires. Your summit is the northernmost point. You bypass the stand-alone southern spire and the broad saddle to its north and continue east, staying just south (right) of a very unappealing pile of giant talus blocks until you reach the base of steep outcrops. By now—if not before—you'll hopefully have stumbled upon a use trail that winds east and north up sandy strips between whitebark pine and boulders at the base of the cliff. This leads seamlessly east up a hidden corridor between two of Dogtooth's highest teeth to a broad ledge east of the true summit.

You follow the ledge as far as you can, stopping when there are 700-foot cliffs ahead (and below you); above is the final 40-foot Class 3 scramble. As with all climbing, down is harder than up, so only continue if you know you can reverse the climb. It is a series of steep blocks, broken by ledges and cracks. From the summit you are rewarded with splendid views in all directions.

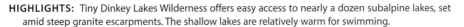

trip 11   ## Dinkey Lakes

see map on p. 74

Trip Data: 37.15931°N, 119.06673°W (Island Lake);
21.1 miles; 3/1 days
Topos: *Courtright Reservoir, Dogtooth Peak*

HIGHLIGHTS: Tiny Dinkey Lakes Wilderness offers easy access to nearly a dozen subalpine lakes, set amid steep granite escarpments. The shallow lakes are relatively warm for swimming.

HEADS UP! *A stretch of trail south of Cliff Lake was burned in the 2020 Bullfrog Fire, but the rest of Dinkey Lakes Wilderness was untouched.*

DAY 1 (Cliff Lake Trailhead to Island Lake, 7.6 miles): Leaving the trailhead, the path descends gradually northwest toward Courtright Reservoir, traversing down a slope under the shade of red fir and lodgepole pine. Ignore an old road that bisects the trail at 0.2 mile and continue northwest, briefly crossing open slab, but mostly ensconced in deep conifer shade and crossing two marshy areas on a pair of wooden boardwalks. At 0.9 mile you approach Courtright Reservoir's shore, turn more westerly to follow its northwest finger, cross a minor tributary, enter Dinkey Lakes Wilderness, and soon thereafter reach the banks of Nelson Creek, 1.4 miles from the trailhead.

In early season, Nelson Creek has a formidable flow and must be crossed about 0.1 mile upstream where its flow is shallower and less turbulent and the base less bouldery. Once across the creek, you promptly reach a junction, where you turn left (west) to ascend Nelson Creek, while right (east) is signposted for Helms Meadow. After nearly a mile through almost flat forest, some places dry and sandy and elsewhere lush with more understory vegetation, the trail climbs a steeper 200 feet, then resumes its gentle upward trajectory, reaching its next junction at the 3.1-mile mark. Here, you continue straight (northwest), toward Cliff Lake. Left (southwest) leads 1.9 miles to Nelson Lakes (good camping) and right (northeast) leads 1.5 miles to Helms Meadow. Continuing up along Cliff Lake's unnamed outflow, you walk at the base of an open, dry, bouldery slope of moraine deposits of western white pine, red fir, and lodgepole pine. The trail's grade steepens as it turns southwest and ascends a sunnier south-facing slope cloaked with red-barked mat manzanita and elegant

First Dinkey Lake   Photo by Elizabeth Wenk

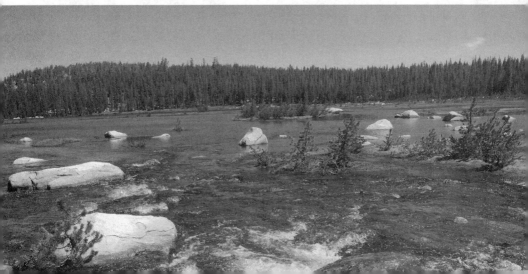

western white pine. North-trending again, the trail switchbacks up glacial deposits with chinquapin emerging beneath just about every boulder. Enjoy views toward Courtright Reservoir and the granite domes bordering its shores, while farther east, the desolate, sawtooth, granite peaks of the Le Conte Divide are visible above Blackcap Basin; Mount Goddard is the notable dark pyramidal-shaped peak. Meanwhile, Brown Peak (10,350'), Nelson Mountain (10,220'), and Eagle Peak (10,318') rise above the Nelson Lakes cirque on the southern skyline.

Ahead, you reach a flat, sandy expanse and an unsigned junction due east of Cliff Lake's outlet (9,442'; 37.13993°N, 119.03939°W). Staying right (north), you cross sandy flats high above Cliff Lake and after 0.4 mile pass the right-branching (east-trending) trail to Bullfrog Lake. Continue left (northwest), climbing up a sandy, bouldery slope to a prominent saddle. In early to midsummer, note the small pink-flowered plants with cylindrical succulent leaves. This species, quill-leaf lewisia, grows only in the Dinkey Lakes Wilderness, around nearby Crown Pass and Chuck Pass, and in the Siskiyou Mountains of far northwestern California—a rather peculiar distribution. Soon you attain the saddle (9,903') between the Three Sisters and Dogtooth Peak; see page 76 for details on how to summit Dogtooth Peak.

As you drop onto the steep north-facing slope above Rock Lake, the tree composition abruptly shifts; you switchback down under dense hemlock cover, reaching the lake after 0.4 mile. Rock Lake is set beneath steep exfoliating slabs but offers many flat campsites along its northern shore (and fishing for brook trout), with additional options near the southeast corner. The path skirts Rock Lake's eastern bank, crosses the outflow, and soon reaches a marked junction with a right-branching (northeast-trending) side trail to Little Lake.

LITTLE LAKE

A 0.9-mile side trail leads from Rock Lake to Little Lake. Turning right (northeast) at the Rock Lake junction, the trail descends a broad draw, densely forested with hemlock and lodgepole pine. Reaching the valley floor, the trail turns more easterly, coming closer to the creek connecting Rock Creek to Little Lake. The narrow, sinuous trail leads right to brilliant campsites scattered along Little Lake's northern shore. Little Lake is backdropped by the towering, serrated ridgeline of Dogtooth Peak and until midseason waterfalls splash into the lake, while shallow bays entice you for a near-shore swim. Come dusk and dawn, small rainbow and brook trout aggressively feed on the myriad of insects.

Onward toward Island Lake, you take the left (west) branch, climbing just slightly to cross a saddle out of Rock Lake's narrow basin and into the much bigger Dinkey Lakes

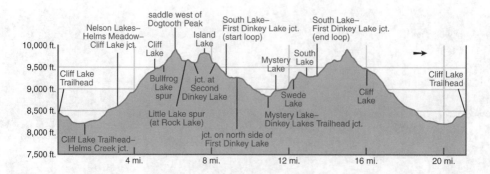

basin. You quickly drop to Second Dinkey Lake and loop around its eastern shore to abundant north-shore campsites under tall lodgepole pine. At the lake's northwestern corner is a junction, where you turn left (south) toward Island Lake, while right (north) leads downstream to First Dinkey Lake, tomorrow's route.

The final 0.55 mile to Island Lake's north-shore campsites are along a narrower trail. You begin by skirting Second Dinkey Lake's west shore and then ascending a steep, eroded trail up a sheltered draw. The ascent moderates at the base of granite bluffs, the trail skirting the base of the rocky outcrops until you cross a minor saddle into Island Lake's basin.

Perched in a broad granite basin with open westward views, Island Lake is often considered the crown jewel of Dinkey Lakes Wilderness. The trail skirts the lake's northeastern and then northwestern shores. There are campsites at the northern tip (9,827'; 37.15288°N, 119.06239°W; mileage to here) and also in broad flats west of the lake. All offer stunning views of Dinkey Wilderness's highest peaks, the three towering granite monoliths of the Three Sisters: 10,432 feet, 10,438 feet, and 10,612 feet. True to the lake's name, there are many tiny one-rock islands, a few with bonsai lodgepole pine. The islands are a popular destination for swimmers braving the frigid water. Fishing is fair for golden trout.

BEYOND ISLAND LAKE

The terrain surrounding Island Lake, bare granite slabs and broad open forests, is excellent for cross-country exploring. Fingerbowl Lake (9,680'), nestled west of Island Lake, can be reached easily by crossing the broad granite rib west of Island Lake. Less than a quarter mile away, Fingerbowl Lake is a small, deep, round lake fringed on one side by a marshy outlet and on the other by scree spilling off the Three Sisters' escarpment. From Island Lake, the Three Sisters escarpment looks impassable at first glance, but the ridge's high point can be reached by following Island Lake's mapped inlet southeast to a saddle and then turning southwest to climb a ridge to the summit.

DAY 2 (Island Lake to South Lake, 5.3 miles): From Island Lake, return to the junction near Second Dinkey Lake's outlet. Turn left (north), closely following the western banks of Dinkey Creek as it quietly cascades from Second Dinkey Lake to First Dinkey Lake. After a moderate, 0.6-mile descent, the track reaches a junction (9,305'; 37.16349°N, 119.06093°W), at which this trip's loop section begins. While the loop can be taken in either direction, this trip takes hikers counterclockwise, in order to finish the day at one of the higher-elevation lakes. It must also be noted that in reverse, tonight's destination is only 0.6 mile distant, while in the described direction you walk 4.1 miles with more than 400 feet of elevation gain and loss. So you might sensibly decide to walk to South Lake, establish a camp, and then complete the 4.7-mile loop part of this trip with only a water bottle and snacks. You'll have to walk the 0.6-mile segment between South Lake and this junction two extra times but have far less distance with a pack.

As described, counterclockwise, continue straight ahead (northwest) toward the broad, marshy, east end of First Dinkey Lake (9,239'), bound by bogs and meadows that host a vigorous population of mosquitoes well into summer. As you approach the eastern inlet creek, you walk across sandy soils with an astonishing density of young lodgepole pine. The barren ridge of the Three Sisters is visible beyond the southern shore. Crossing the inlet, the trail arcs around the lake's grassy north shore, meeting a four-way junction among boulders near the northwestern corner. You stay left (west) signposted for Willow Meadow, while straight ahead (northwest) leads to Coyote Lake and right (east) leads to Rock Meadow.

The trail begins a gradual descent along Dinkey Creek, following its heath-bound banks downward. In places, the water glides down open slabs, but the 1.6 miles to the next junction are mostly a forested walk. At this junction, you turn left (south) toward Mystery Lake, while right (straight ahead; west) leads to the Dinkey Lake Trailhead near Willow Meadow. Indeed, you are just 1.4 miles from the trailhead here and most groups you meet will have entered Dinkey Lakes Wilderness from this trailhead.

Turning toward Mystery Lake, you must immediately ford Dinkey Creek, a wet crossing at high flows, but not a dangerous one. The trail then crosses Mystery Lake's outlet and proceeds to climb steeply, but briefly, zigzagging up 150 feet just east of the outlet (not to the west as shown on USGS 7.5' topo maps). Once at Mystery Lake's outlet, the main trail turns sharply left (east), while use trails diverge in all directions. The best campsites at this heavily used lake are along its north side; bypass the many illegal sites and choose one that is at least 100 feet from water. Mystery Lake's shoreline is splendid: lots of shallow polished slab ribs and peninsulas on which to sit and admire its open basin.

The north-shore trail continues through bouldery lodgepole pine forest and across marshy meadow tentacles, crossing the eastern inlet, skirting additional wet meadows, and finally climbing a steep 250 feet to Swede Lake via tight switchbacks beside the bubbling creek. Swede Lake offers many lodgepole pine–shaded campsites along its western and northern sides but lacks Mystery Lake's showy lakeside slabs. Proceeding across the outlet and around the lake's northern tip, the trail ascends again, climbing to the broad ridge separating Swede Lake and South Lake. A slight descent leads into South Lake's basin. South Lake also offers an abundance of lodgepole pine–shaded campsites (9,297'; 37.15931°N, 119.06673°W) and views to the steep escarpments that separate this subalpine lake from Island Lake and Fingerbowl Lake, sitting in the next basin above. Indeed, South Lake's deep, alluring, emerald waters are fed by a waterfall rushing down from Island Lake.

DAY 3 (South Lake to Cliff Lake Trailhead, 8.2 miles): The main trail crosses South Lake's outlet just north of the lake; take note, for use trails also follow its west shore back to First Dinkey Lake. The trail briefly descends alongside the outlet creek and then begins a northeasterly traverse across rocky, sandy slopes. USGS 7.5' topo maps show an old trail routing that crossed through boggy meadows just east of First Dinkey Lake, but the trail was long ago rerouted to stay above the fragile meadow communities; oddly the trail is indistinct in a few key places—you more or less want to traverse with minimal elevation loss and will quickly reach the trail connecting First Dinkey Lake and Second Dinkey Lake at the junction where you began the loop on Day 2. At this junction, close the loop and turn right (southeast). Retrace your steps, skipping the side trip to Island Lake.

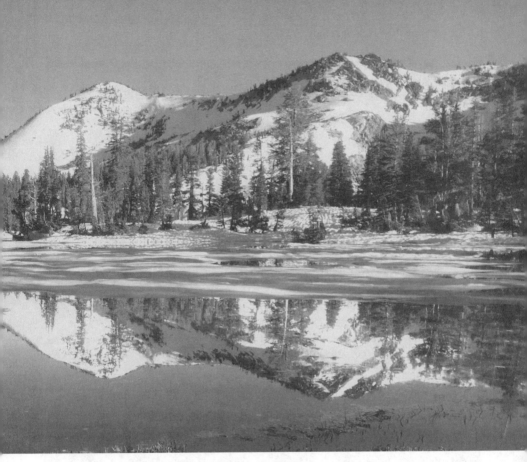

Island Lake in July of a high-snow year   Photo by Elizabeth Wenk

ALTERNATIVE ROUTE VIA HELMS MEADOW

Instead of returning the way you came, you could take the Helms Meadow Trail on the return. This route is 10.3 miles (from South Lake to the trailhead) versus 8.2 for the described route, but with less elevation gain. By late summer Helms Creek will be dry and Helms Meadow parched, but this is a beautiful early-summer walk. And the stunning views of Dogtooth Peak from Helms Meadow are alone worth taking this alternative.

From the junction 0.6 mile east of South Lake (9,305'; 37.16349°N, 119.06093°W), you take the north-trending trail toward Rock Meadow, and then turn northeast in 0.7 mile onto the Helms Meadow Trail (junction at 9,309'; 37.17218°N, 119.05902°W). This junction is poorly signed—make sure you take the trail toward Helms Meadow, not Rock Meadow. You head down Helms Creek to Helms Meadow on a serviceable but sparingly used trail (3.6 miles), taking the time to step into the meadow and stare up at Dogtooth Peak. Continuing across endless meadows, through sandy flats, and ultimately down a forested slope, you reach your next junction near where Helms Creek flows into Courtright Reservoir (2.7 miles) and turn right (west) to cross Helms Creek. A 1.4-mile leg across fantastic granite slab leads along Courtright's northern shore back to Nelson Creek, where you reunite with the described route for the final 1.4 miles to the car.

Maxson Trailhead (Courtright Reservoir)
8,106'; 37.08288°N, 118.96228°W

Destination/ GPS Coordinates	Trip Type	Best Season	Pace & Hiking/ Layover Days	Total Mileage	Permit Required
12 Post Corral Meadows 37.12066°N 118.89665°W	Out-and-back	Mid	Leisurely 2/0	14.2	Maxson (Courtright)
13 Bench Valley Lakes 37.07867°N 118.79976°W (Guest Lake)	Out-and-back	Mid	Moderate, part cross-country 6/1	33.0	Maxson (Courtright)
14 Red Mountain Basin 37.12877°N 118.82930°W (Devils Punchbowl)	Semiloop	Mid	Moderate 6/2	32.1	Maxson (Courtright)

INFORMATION AND PERMITS: This trailhead is in Sierra National Forest. Permits are required for overnight stays and quotas apply. Details on how to reserve permits are available at fs.usda.gov/detail/sierra/passes-permits. For advance reservations (60% of quota; reservable starting in January each year), there is a $5-per-person reservation fee, while walk-up permits (40% of quota) are free. Permits can be picked up at 29688 Auberry Road, Prather, CA 93651; if you call 559-855-5355 in advance, they will leave your permit in a dropbox. Permits can also be picked up in person at the Dinkey Lakes Forest Service Office, located a short distance north of Dinkey Lakes Road, 11.8 miles past Shaver Lake. If you plan to use a stove or have a campfire, you must also have a California campfire permit, available from a forest service office or online at preventwildfireca.org/campfire-permit. Campfires are prohibited above 10,000 feet and within 0.25 mile of most lakes in the Red Mountain Basin area. Bear canisters are not required but are strongly encouraged.

DRIVING DIRECTIONS: From the intersection of CA 168 and CA 180, just east of Fresno, take CA 168 northeast through Clovis and up into the foothills, to the community of Shaver Lake, a distance of 46.8 miles. Then turn right onto Dinkey Creek Road and follow it for 25.8 miles to a Y-junction where left leads to Courtright Reservoir and right to Wishon Reservoir; note it has changed names several times along the way and is now called McKinley Grove Road. Head left onto Courtright Way/FS 10S16 and continue 7.4 miles to a three-forked junction where you take FS 9S38 (the far right-hand choice). Continue 1.2 miles, crossing the dam at the spillway to reach the paved Maxson Trailhead parking lot.

trip 12 Post Corral Meadows

see map on p. 84

Trip Data: 37.12066°N, 118.89665°W; 14.2 miles; 2/0 days
Topos: *Courtright Reservoir, Ward Mountain*

HIGHLIGHTS: This trip is an excellent choice for a weekend excursion. The route winds past the granite domes surrounding Courtright Reservoir, traverses sunny subalpine meadows, and climbs through open forests of pine. With moderate elevation gain, easy terrain, and an abundance of campsites, this is a fine selection for beginners.

DAY 1 (Maxson Trailhead to Post Corral Creek crossing, 7.1 miles): Leaving the trailhead from the west side of the parking lot, head north, descending along the marked trail for 300 yards until merging with the Dusy Ershim OHV Route. This wide, dusty road descends briefly and then levels out over dirt and open granite slabs. After about 1 mile, you reach a signed junction near Maxson Meadow. While the OHV route heads left, your route bears right (northeast).

Leaving the road behind, follow singletrack tread across the meadow and back under forest cover. Gently ascending, the path follows and crosses a stream near the 2-mile mark, just before entering the signed John Muir Wilderness. Ascend a forested hillside to the crest of a rise to the signed Hobler Lake–Post Corral Meadows junction (8,882'; 37.12287°N, 118.94050°W). Take the right fork eastward.

The trail is briefly wide and flat and then begins to descend moderately through more pines on short switchbacks. Where the sandy trail leaves the forest, cross a seasonal creek and enter Long Meadow. The picturesque meadow is appropriately named and makes an excellent lunch and water stop. The small stream draining Long Meadow may be low during late season but may still provide water. If you got a late start, there are several campsites (8,571'; 37.12680°N, 118.92401°W) on the small, short rise to the north of the meadow that offer good wind protection.

After reaching the mouth of Long Meadow, the route traverses the length of the field and then gently descends back into the trees. Here, reach a signed junction with the nearly vanished Burnt Corral Creek Trail, which heads north. The sign is easily missed when heading east along this route. Continue ahead (east) and don't be concerned if you do not see the junction. Stroll next to the stream to a ford after about 0.75 mile.

The trail then drops back into more lodgepole pine, gradually descends, and turns toward the south. When the trail reaches a short wooden bridge and flattens, the ford of Post Corral Creek is another mile ahead. Although difficult to spot at first, there are several quiet campsites tucked into the pines along this section of trail. If the sites at Post Corral are full, you can backtrack to this area to find seclusion.

Just before the ford of Post Corral Creek, a granite boulder field opens on the right (west) side of the trail. There are several obvious campsites here (8,200'; 37.12066°N, 118.89665°W), at the edge of the encroaching forest. At the ford of Post Corral Creek, a wide granite slab eases gently into the water, making an idyllic dinner site.

DAY 2 (Post Corral Creek crossing to Maxson Trailhead, 7.1 miles): Retrace your steps.

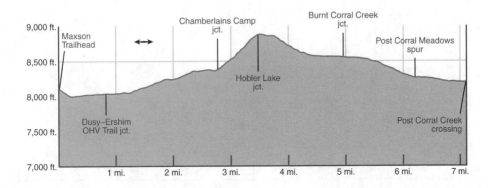

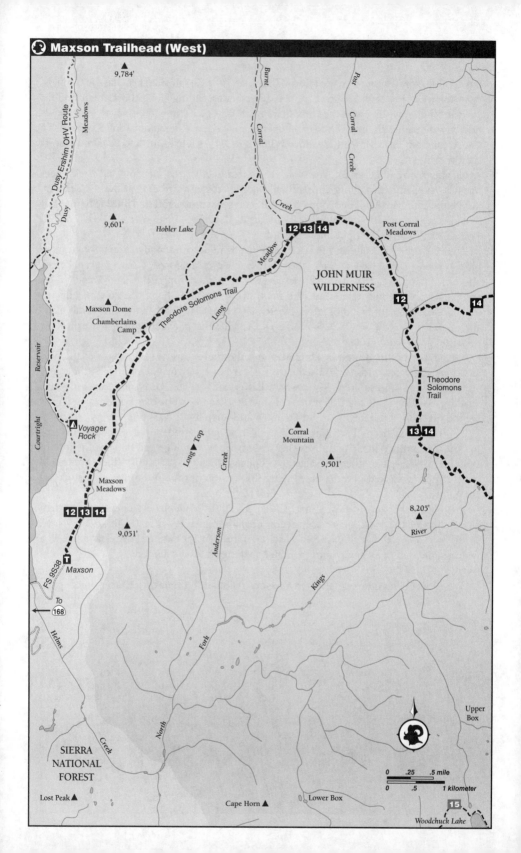

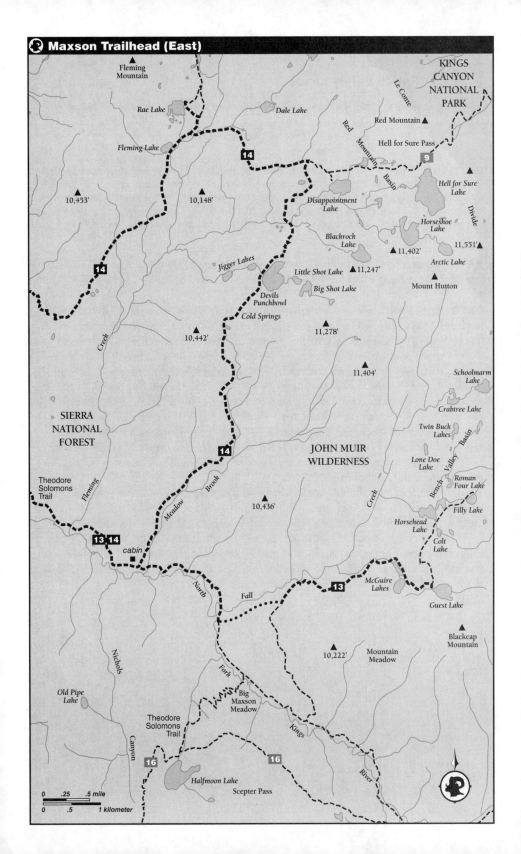

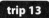 **trip 13**   **Bench Valley Lakes**

see
maps on
p. 84–85

Trip Data: 37.07867°N, 118.79976°W (at Guest Lake);
33.0 miles; 6/1 days

Topos: *Courtright Reservoir, Ward Mountain, Blackcap Mountain,
Mount Henry*

HIGHLIGHTS: This trip traverses the lush, forested meadows surrounding Corral Mountain and offers sweeping vistas of granite domes along North Fork Kings River. The path then ascends through serene meadows carpeted in wildflowers to the stark alpine beauty of the Bench Valley basin. The many small lakes and cliffs in this hanging valley offer fishing, rock climbing, and rich alpenglow at sunset. Since most of the trail follows marked, easy terrain, this trip makes a great choice for a longer yet moderate outing.

DAY 1 (Maxson Trailhead to Post Corral Creek crossing, 7.1 miles): Follow Trip 12, Day 1 to campsites near the Post Corral Creek crossing (8,200'; 37.12066°N, 118.89665°W).

DAY 2 (Post Corral Creek crossing to North Fork Kings River, 4.4 miles): Shortly after fording Post Corral Creek (wet in early season), the Hell for Sure Pass Trail heads left at a signed, three-way junction. Go right (south), following a sandy trail. After a half mile, the trail climbs out of the pines and passes larger granite boulders and sandy open flats. The route then makes a short descent and winds through more meadow and sandy forest for the next 2 miles.

After the trail gains a ridge and turns to the southeast, the vista opens dramatically, with sweeping views through the trees across the granitic North Fork Kings River canyon. The trail follows a sandy wash down short switchbacks and then meets low-angle granite slabs near the river. There are many relaxing lunch spots here, along with plenty of water and several refreshing swimming holes farther down the trail to the south. There are many campsites near this juncture if a short day is in order. Fishing along the river is good for brook, brown, and rainbow trout.

From here, the trail continues southeastward and reenters ubiquitous pine forest. On the left side of the path, yellow-green lichen coats house-size granite boulders nestled among the trees, while ferns and dense thickets of manzanita carpet the forest floor.

After a meandering half mile, the trail comes to a moderate clearing with a California Cooperative Snow Survey log cabin next to a waterfall and a large pool in the river. The trail exits the left side of this clearing to the southeast and continues on another 0.3 mile to the signed Devils Punchbowl/Big Maxson Meadow Trail junction (8,210'; 37.08158°N,

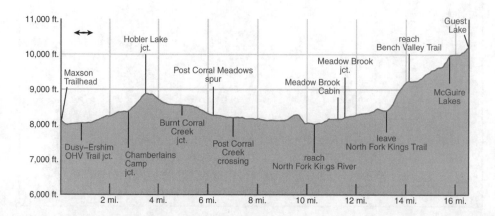

118.85809°W). There are several superb campsites just before the signed junction, across the granite slabs, next to the river on the west side of the trail (8,198'; 37.08147°N, 118.85862°W).

DAY 3 (North Fork Kings River to Guest Lake, 5.0 miles, part cross-country): The trail leaves the signed Devils Punchbowl/Maxson Meadow junction by the right fork (southeast), staying parallel with the North Fork Kings River. After crossing several small branches of Meadow Brook, the tread heads up a short set of stone stairs and crosses open granite slabs near a large pool. The normally rough granite has been worn down by the passage of the water, and several of the pools make for great swimming holes.

The path continues southeast and climbs gently up dirt and loose rock for about a mile until reaching the rocky ford of Fall Creek (wet in early season). Follow the trail 0.2 mile after the last ford of the creek to the point where a faint trail turns to the left (east) from the main trail; from here, the main trail goes far out of your way and is 2.4 miles longer. So take the angler's use trail. It's indistinct near the bottom, but many ducks become apparent as it climbs higher. If you lose the trail, head cross-country generally east-northeast up the hill parallel with the creek, keeping Fall Creek about 200 yards away on your left side. The trail is steep and occasionally loose, so exercise caution while ascending. At the top, find expansive views all the way back down the valley.

Once you reach the low-angle granite slabs at the top, the route levels off and once again enters dense lodgepole forest. Shortly thereafter, the route joins the main trail ascending from Big Maxson Meadow and begins a lazy traverse through 2 miles of beautiful foliage and dense ferns. In early summer, shooting star, penstemon, larkspur, monkshood, monkeyflower, columbine, wallflower, and paintbrush line the path. In late season, the ferns turn yellow, carpeting the forest floor with broad brushstrokes of color.

After traversing the forested meadow, the trail starts to climb again and culminates with a short but steep climb to the rim of the McGuire Lakes. The meadow-lined banks of the lake appear suddenly and make a welcome rest stop after the strenuous climb. From the vantage of the lake's shores, it becomes apparent that this point is the entrance to a hanging

Horsehead Lake is one of the many lakes to explore above Guest Lake.   Photo by Elizabeth Wenk

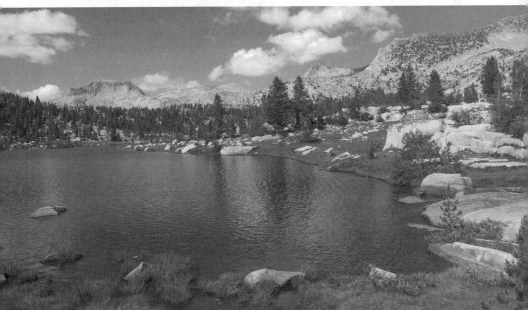

valley. Rising proudly to the southeast is Blackcap Mountain, its dark volcanic summit just barely visible above the granite blocks that sit outlined like a dark sentinel against the vibrant red alpenglow at sunset.

HANGING VALLEYS

Hanging valleys occur when a tributary glacier carves a valley more slowly than does the larger adjacent glacier. Over time, the larger glacier's valley floor will be well below the tributary glacier's valley. The tributary's valley is left "hanging" high on the wall of the main valley once the glaciers melt, and the tributary's stream drops, often from a lake, into the deeper main valley in the form of cascades and waterfalls. Yosemite's Bridalveil and Yosemite Falls are classic examples of this process. McGuire Lakes sit in one of a series of such hanging valleys that line the flanks of the Le Conte Divide.

The trail skirts the lake, curving north and then south along the lake through sparse pine and large granite boulders. After the footpath veers east and crosses a short ridge, Guest Lake is visible straight ahead. There are comfortable campsites on the south side of Guest Lake among the large boulders and more sites along the north bank in the trees (10,195'; 37.07867°N, 118.79976°W; no campfires). If these sites are crowded, consider continuing on the fisherman's trail another mile north to Horsehead Lake, where a few campsites dot the southeast shore. Guest Lake offers good fishing for brook trout.

EXPLORING BENCH VALLEY

If your itinerary allows time for a layover day, Guest Lake makes a fantastic base camp from which to explore the rest of the Bench Valley lakes. A wonderful day hike follows the angler's use trail northward to Horsehead Lake, and then explores Roman Four Lake, Twin Buck Lakes, and Schoolmarm Lake. Anglers will encounter brook and rainbow at Horsehead Lake, brook at Roman Four Lake, rainbow at West Twin Buck Lake (East Twin Buck Lake is barren), and small rainbow at Schoolmarm Lake. There is also wonderful bouldering on the granite outcroppings surrounding Guest Lake. Rock climbers will be tempted to explore the inviting cracks bisecting the towering granite walls overhead. The climbing here is of such quality that the walls would surely be crowded, were it not for the high price of admission.

DAYS 4–6 (Guest Lake to Maxson Trailhead, 16.5 miles): Retrace your steps.

Bedrock pools along the North Fork Kings River   Photo by Elizabeth Wenk

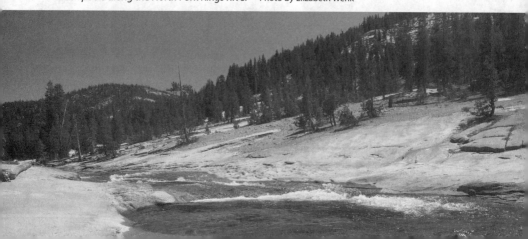

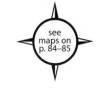

see maps on p. 84–85

trip 14   **Red Mountain Basin**

Trip Data: 37.12877°N, 118.82930°W (at Devils Punchbowl);
32.1 miles; 6/2 days

Topos: *Courtright Reservoir, Ward Mountain,*
Blackcap Mountain, Mount Henry

HIGHLIGHTS: This trip takes an old sheepherder's route, known as the Baird Trail, from the subalpine meadows at Post Corral Creek to the stunning alpine scenery surrounding Devils Punchbowl, a lake in remote Red Mountain Basin, which provides a good base camp for exploring the basin. The trek then descends via Meadow Brook, one of the Sierra's most picturesque subalpine meadows, offering spectacular views of the North Fork Kings River.

DAY 1 (Maxson Trailhead to Post Corral Creek crossing, 7.1 miles): Follow Trip 12, Day 1 to campsites near the Post Corral Creek crossing (8,200'; 37.12066°N, 118.89665°W).

DAY 2 (Post Corral Creek crossing to Rae Lake, 5.2 miles): Top off water supplies here; today's route gains 1,600 feet in about 5 miles with no reliable water source.

After leaving the campsites, head east to ford Post Corral Creek (wet in early season) and shortly arrive at a junction; to the right, the Blackcap Basin Trail leads to Red Mountain Basin, but you turn left (east) on Hell for Sure Pass Trail. The route then begins to climb the ridge separating the drainages of Post Corral Creek and Fleming Creek. The first mile moderately ascends under shady pine cover, but shortly thereafter the trail steepens over dynamited slabs.

Continue up the obvious path to the small, wooded flat before reaching switchbacks leading up the last few hundred feet to the ridgeline. The trail turns toward the northeast and begins a gentler ascent up the forested north flank of Fleming Creek's canyon.

After 1.5 miles, the track turns north and ascends steep, rocky switchbacks to gain the meadows surrounding small, photogenic Fleming Lake. Here, the landscape takes on a definite subalpine character with less tree cover and more exposed granite boulders and slabs.

The path crosses Fleming Lake's outlet and soon comes to a junction with a trail at the foot of a long meadow dotted with colorful wildflowers. Turn left (north) here and climb to a shaded hillside junction with the short spur trail leading to Rae Lake (9,909'; 37.15288°N, 118.84802°W; no campfires). Idyllic campsites lie beneath the trees on the north banks of the lake, where anglers will find good fishing for brook trout.

DAY 3 (Rae Lake to Devils Punchbowl, 3.6 miles): Return to the junction and turn left (east) to continue on Hell for Sure Pass Trail, shortly fording Fleming Creek. The path then begins a 500-foot ascent that starts on a tree-covered slope with patches of meadow and wildflowers. With the terrain growing dry and sandy, the trail gains a ridgetop and briefly turns south to cross open meadows and seasonal creeks before heading east again.

In another mile, find the signed junction with a trail to Devils Punchbowl next to a tall, gray stump. Turn right (south) and pass a small lake before dropping 300 feet to reach East Fork Fleming Creek. The trail crosses at a rocky ford (wet in early season) and then climbs 300 feet to the low ridge on the north side of Devils Punchbowl. Good campsites are located on the east side of the lake (10,122'; 37.12877°N, 118.82930°W; no campfires), which is quite popular with both hikers and anglers. The outlet plummets in dramatic fashion over the lip of the basin on the way down steep cliffs to Jigger Lakes below, highlighting an outstanding view of the terrain to the west. This fine location makes a great spot for a layover day, as the rugged terrain of Red Mountain Basin on all sides begs for exploration.

DAY 4 (Devils Punchbowl to North Fork Kings River, 4.7 miles): From the north side of the lake, the trail heads south along the granite walls that dam the lake. Midway along the ridge, you can spy the small Jigger Lakes below and to the west. At the southwest corner of Devils Punchbowl, the trail makes several short switchbacks to gain a saddle before turning to the south and beginning a 2,000-foot descent to the North Fork Kings River.

The descent begins with a 200-foot sandy slope leading to lush meadows at the head of Meadow Brook. In the next mile, the path skirts the west side of the meadows, threading past lavender shooting star, purple Sierra gentian, and monkeyflower. The views from this section of trail are breathtaking: with the meadow in the foreground, you can see all the way to the far side of the North Fork Kings River drainage. There are many idyllic lunch spots to enjoy this meadow's beautiful setting.

After this pleasurable mile, the grade steepens and turns southwest away from the creek, angling down a forested moraine. The next mile descends continuously, where stands of red fir, Jeffrey pine, and quaking aspen welcome you back to lower elevations. The path levels out on open granite slabs at the bottom of the grade and reaches a signed junction with the Blackcap Basin Trail (8,210'; 37.08158°N, 118.85809°W). Wonderful campsites lie on the banks of the North Fork Kings River past this junction, west of the trail (8,198'; 37.08147°N, 118.85862°W).

DAY 5 (North Fork Kings River to Post Corral Creek crossing, 4.4 miles): From the junction, turn right (west) along the North Fork Kings River, passing a California Cooperative Snow Survey log cabin next to a waterfall and a large pool in the river, soon curving northwest and shortly fording Fleming Creek. Cross a forested flat, descend a little to slabs near the river, and then climb an open hillside to a ridgetop with fine views over the North Fork Kings River.

Descend from the ridge and follow the sandy, undulating trail winding through forest and small meadows for 2.0 miles to a ford of an unnamed creek. Meet the Red Mountain Basin Trail at the junction near Post Corral Creek. Turn left (northwest) here and ford Post Corral Creek to find the good campsites of Day 1 (8,200'; 37.12066°N, 118.89665°W) at the end of the loop section.

DAY 6 (Post Corral Creek crossing to Maxson Trailhead, 7.1 miles): Retrace your steps from Day 1 of this trip.

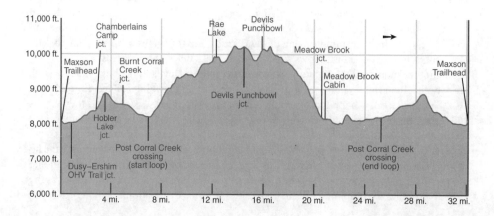

Woodchuck Trailhead (Wishon Reservoir)

6,680'; 36.99585°N, 118.96378°W

Destination/ GPS Coordinates	Trip Type	Best Season	Pace & Hiking/ Layover Days	Total Mileage	Permit Required
15 Woodchuck Lake 37.04349°N 118.88339°W	Out-and-back	Early to late	Moderate 2/1	19.6	Woodchuck
16 Blackcap Basin 37.04383°N 118.75756°W (Portal Lake)	Out-and-back	Mid to late	Moderate 5/2	42.8	Woodchuck
17 Crown Lake 37.03623°N 118.84912°W	Semiloop	Early to late	Leisurely 4/1	29.3	Woodchuck

INFORMATION AND PERMITS: This trailhead is in Sierra National Forest. Permits are required for overnight stays and quotas apply. Details on how to reserve permits are available at fs.usda.gov/detail/sierra/passes-permits. For advance reservations (60% of quota; reservable starting in January each year), there is a $5-per-person reservation fee, while walk-up permits (40% of quota) are free. Permits can be picked up at 29688 Auberry Road, Prather, CA 93651; if you call 559-855-5355 in advance, they will leave your permit in a dropbox. Permits can also be picked up in person at the Dinkey Lakes Forest Service Office, located a short distance north of Dinkey Lakes Road, 11.8 miles past Shaver Lake. If you plan to use a stove or have a campfire, you must also have a California campfire permit, available from a forest service office or online at preventwildfireca.org/campfire-permit. Campfires are prohibited above 10,000 feet and within 300 feet of Woodchuck Lake and within 600 feet of Crown Lake. Bear canisters are not required but are strongly encouraged.

DRIVING DIRECTIONS: From the intersection of CA 168 and CA 180, just east of Fresno, take CA 168 northeast through Clovis and up into the foothills, to the community of Shaver Lake, a distance of 46.8 miles. Then turn right onto Dinkey Creek Road and follow it 25.8 miles to a Y-junction where left leads to Courtright Reservoir and right to Wishon Reservoir; note it has changed names several times along the way and is now called McKinley Grove Road. Head right and continue 4.0 miles along the McKinley Grove Road to the Woodchuck Trailhead, located up a short spur on your left just 0.4 mile after you pass the Spillway day-use area beyond the Wishon Dam. This is 1.1 miles *before* the spur road that Google Maps has programmed as the Woodchuck Trailhead; that road is locked and is a private staging point for the local pack station.

see map on p. 92

trip 15   ## Woodchuck Lake

Trip Data: 37.04349°N, 118.88339°W; 19.6 miles; 2/1 days
Topos: *Rough Spur, Courtright Reservoir*

HIGHLIGHTS: Woodchuck Lake is a hidden gem—perfect for swimming, fishing, relaxing, or exploring. Its setting is gorgeous, even by the Sierra's lofty standards, with an escarpment to the east and just a minor ridge constraining its long western shore and a broad sandy beach on its northern side. The only downside is the predominately viewless walk to reach it.

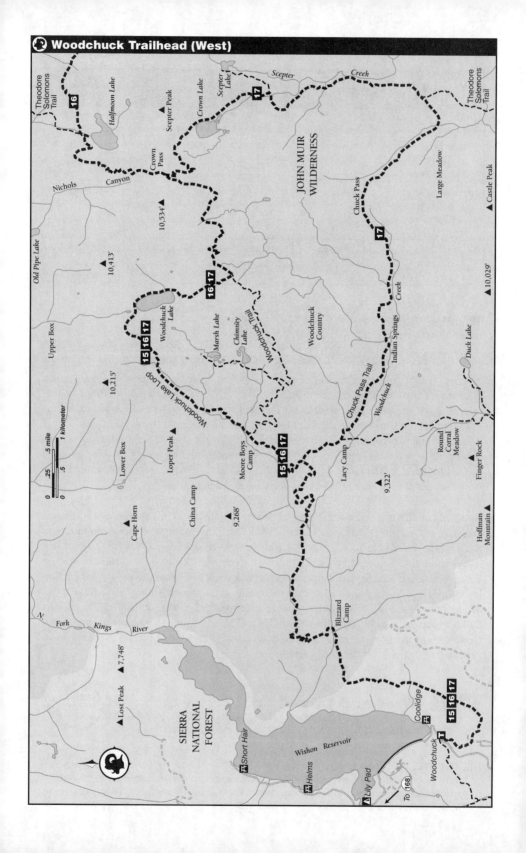

Woodchuck Trailhead (West)

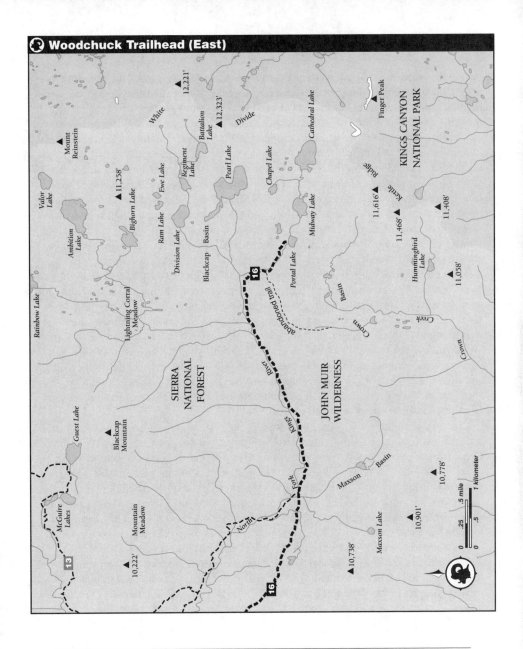

HEADS UP! *In many books the distance to Woodchuck Lake is significantly underestimated; 9.8 miles to its northern tip is an accurate measurement.*

DAY 1 (Woodchuck Trailhead to Woodchuck Lake, 9.8 miles): From the Woodchuck Trailhead, the trail launches into a steep, sinuous ascent up a dry, scrubby slope. After this 0.5-mile stint up a spur you reach a dirt road—leading to a pack station staging area—along which you jog 40 feet right (south), before a sign directs you left (east) onto the continuing trail. Now trending more easterly, the ascent continues, the shrubs soon yielding to a forest of incense cedar, white fir, and sugar pine (the latter easily identified by its large cones and its five needles per bundle). Rounding the head of a broad draw, the trail turns north, beginning a long ascending traverse across a remarkably lush slope. A succession of rivulets irrigates the slope, with the trail repeatedly weaving between redstem dogwood, Sierra currant, lupine, mugwort, and thickets of bracken fern. Although the slope remains steep, the trail's grade slowly flattens as it undulates across a slope high above Wishon Reservoir; only broken glimpses of the water are on offer. Once 2.5 miles from the car, the trail rounds a spur, the end of Woodchuck Creek's moraine, and turns due east; you briefly have views north toward Lost Peak (8,476') and other granitic domes, before diving back under forest cover. Just beyond, you enter John Muir Wilderness and continue along a minor shelf, slowly converging with Woodchuck Creek. Easterners mistook the Sierra's marmots for the East's woodchucks and gave the area its erroneous name, Woodchuck Country, which has stuck.

After crossing a series of seeps, the trail loops around a white fir–shaded shelf, Blizzard Camp (now so overgrown and strewn with downed logs that just a few tent sites exist), and drops to ford Woodchuck Creek, 3.2 miles from the trailhead. The crossing is in a safe location but requires caution in early season, especially with its rocky base. A well-graded ascend ensues, first across a sandy flat (campsites) and then up through open white fir and ponderosa pine forest, transitioning to a lodgepole pine, white fir, and Jeffrey pine forest with increasing elevation. Stretches are dry, with slabs near the surface, while elsewhere you walk alongside flower-edged seeps and trickles. You're offered sporadic views south across Woodchuck Creek toward Hoffman Mountain, but mostly follow forested corridors. After crossing a substantial tributary, you brush close to Woodchuck Creek (and campsites) and then climb more steeply alongside a second tributary to a junction, 3.3 miles beyond your ford of Woodchuck Creek. You continue left (north) toward Crown Pass, while right (southeast) leads to Lacy Camp and Chuck Pass (Trip 17).

Crossing a minor creek on a plank bridge, the trail climbs to a moraine crest and continues switchbacking up a ridge, leading into the drainage of the first Woodchuck Creek tributary you crossed. Here, the trail has been rerouted to the southeastern side of a seasonally boggy meadow, walking at the base of volcanic outcrops. You look across the expanse of meadow dotted with shooting stars, western bistort, and corn lilies, but remain well east of the locale marked as "Moore Boys Camp" (now just a little-used campsite with a large campfire ring) as you proceed to a junction that lies about 650 feet northeast of the location indicated on the USGS 7.5' maps. Here, 7.5 miles from the trailhead, you continue left (northeast) toward Woodchuck Lake, while right (east) leads to Crown Pass.

Your trail first traverses lush lodgepole pine forest carpeted with dwarf bilberry and knee-high western blueberries, the latter providing a delightful treat in late summer. Alpine prickly currant encircles many of the tree bases. Ambling along, you enjoy the abundant wildflower

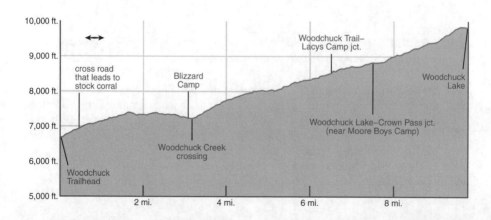

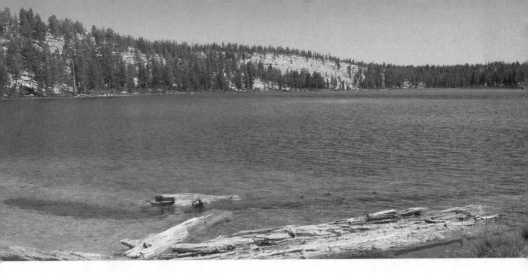

Woodchuck Lake   Photo by Elizabeth Wenk

color and early-summer birdsong (and mosquito buzz) on offer. Slowly the slope increases and this stretch of trail, unlike what you walked earlier today, has not been regraded or rerouted—and where the terrain is steep, so is the trail. Climbing diligently beneath Loper Peak, underfoot is alternately moist and dry, shifting in tandem with the depth of soil over-lying buried granite slabs. Then, quite suddenly, the ground is dry and sandy with small outcrops, boulders, stragglier lodgepole pine, and some big western white pine. You feel like you're rolling onto a shelf and see Woodchuck Lake ahead, a large, oval lake with gorgeous blue water, sandy beaches, and ample camping along both its western (for example, 9,825'; 37.04349°N, 118.88339°W; no campfires within 300 feet of the lake) and northern sides. Hopefully you have scheduled at least one layover day here. You'll notice on a topo map that Woodchuck Lake seems to sit on a shelf, not in a basin, and indeed along the western side just a minor ridge constrains the lake, giving it a wonderful open feel.

DAY 2 (Woodchuck Lake to Woodchuck Trailhead): Retrace your steps from Day 1.

AN ALTERNATIVE RETURN ROUTE

If you want to turn this trip into a semiloop, you can return via the main Woodchuck Trail, possibly spending a night at Chimney Lake to split the return journey. Without a detour to Chimney Lake, this route is 2.5 miles longer, adding 1 mile round-trip to visit Chimney Lake. For longer trips, such as to Honeymoon Lake, Crown Lake, or beyond, see Trips 16 and 17.

The trail continues around the east side of Woodchuck Lake, walking close to its meadow-fringed shore, then cuts across the delicate meadows along the lake's southern inlet and climbs gently through sandy terrain to reach the Woodchuck Trail after 1.3 miles. Here, you turn right (southwest) to reach Chimney Lake, while left (northeast) leads to Crown Pass. The descent to the Chimney Lake junction is 1.9 miles, much longer than the routing depicted on the USGS 7.5' maps, leading through open lodgepole pine and western white pine forest, past a volcanic spur, and down an open, sandy spur to the junction. Chimney Lake lies just under 0.5 mile to the north, a pleasant forest-ringed lake with a rugged escarpment to its east; there are ample campsites along its northwestern side. The trail segment between the Chimney Lake junction and the "near Moore Boys Camp junction" is 1.5 miles, also notably longer than shown on old topo maps. It is correspondingly pleasantly graded, as it passes a cinder cone and continues down through an open forest of lodgepole pine, white fir, red fir, and western white pine. Slowly you approach the junction near Moore Boys Camp where you rejoin the route described in Day 1.

trip 16 Blackcap Basin

see maps on p. 92–93

Trip Data: 37.04383°N, 118.75756°W (Portal Lake);
42.8 miles; 5/2 days

Topos: *Rough Spur, Courtright Reservoir, Blackcap Mountain*

HIGHLIGHTS: One of a dozen High Sierra lakes within Blackcap Basin, Portal Lake occupies a step in a glacial staircase. Although the official trails end at Portal Lake, this really is just the "portal" to begin exploring vast Blackcap Basin and beyond; every one of the broad, often shallow lakes occupying the higher steps in Blackcap Basin is worth visiting. This is a landscape of exquisite scenic beauty at the west edge of the Le Conte Divide and Kettle Ridge, deep in the heart of John Muir Wilderness.

DAY 1 (Woodchuck Trailhead to Woodchuck Lake, 9.8 miles): Follow Trip 15, Day 1 to Woodchuck Lake (9,825'; 37.04349°N, 118.88339°W; no campfires within 300 feet of the lake).

DAY 2 (Woodchuck Lake to Halfmoon Lake, 5.1 miles): The trail continues around the east side of Woodchuck Lake, walking close to its meadow-fringed shore, then cuts across the delicate meadows along its southern inlet. It soon crosses the inlet (contrary to the old route plotted on maps) and climbs gently through sandy terrain out of Woodchuck Lake's basin. After 1.3 miles you reach the signed junction with the Woodchuck Trail and turn left (northeast) toward Crown Pass, while right (southwest) leads back toward Wishon Reservoir.

You climb gently up a meadow corridor abloom with shaggy lupine in midsummer and step onto broken slab, staring south at another lupine-covered meadow and small tarn. Note as well the reddish rock, where overlying basalt deposits altered the granite. Your route continues across barren granite slopes, looping around the southern end of a ridge. In early to midsummer, note the small pink-flowered plants with cylindrical succulent leaves. This species, quill-leaf lewisia, grows only around Crown Pass, Chuck Pass, and in the Dinkey Lakes Wilderness—and in the Siskiyou Mountains of far northwestern California, a rather peculiar distribution. While the trail once took the direct route over a pair of ridges toward Crown Pass, it now loops around the head of a minor drainage and then continues south to cross the second ridge where it is shallower. Suddenly the gentle slabs and sandy corridor give way to a dramatic vista to the southeast. Peaks as distant as the Kaweah summits in Sequoia National Park are readily visible, as are the major summits of the Great Western Divide. Mount Harrington, a small but unmistakable peak along the Monarch Divide, sticks out like a thumb behind the turrets decorating the Gorge of Despair.

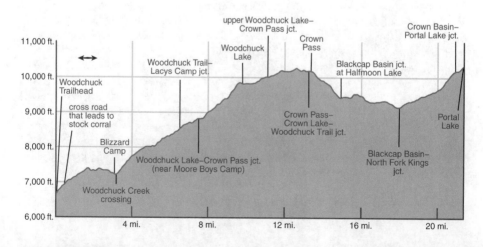

DETOURS FROM CROWN PASS

For exhilarating views you can head cross-country to one of three locations: Peak 10,534, the unnamed summit 0.4 mile west of the pass; Scepter Peak; or the knob just 0.1 mile east of the pass. While the knob offers the best views to Crown Lake, the two more distant points vie for the best "big" vista. Scepter Peak has the better view into Blackcap Basin, but otherwise they offer similar panoramas. You can see peaks from the Yosemite boundary south to the Kaweahs in Sequoia National Park.

From the vista point, the trail bends north, walking at the bluff-forest boundary. Slowly the slope's angle lessens and you approach a junction, where right (due south) leads to Crown Lake (Trip 17), while you stay left (straight ahead, north). You are now on the Theodore Solomons Trail (TST), a route designated as a midelevation alternative to the John Muir Trail, but rarely thru-hiked. In just 0.1 mile you reach Crown Pass (10,188'), a broad sandy saddle. If you have time on your return (or now), the 0.8-mile detour east to Scepter Peak or one of the other nearby knobs is well worth the effort; see the sidebar above. Continuing north, the trail tread is a little awkward for the first time, as you wind down a narrow, in-places-eroded gully. Although you sense open vistas to the east, trees mostly block your view; finally a break in the timber lets you gaze down upon Halfmoon Lake, a beautiful, intricately shaped, meadow-and-slab-ringed lake, and glimpse the dark pyramidal tip of Mount Goddard. Continuing, the rocky path descends toward Halfmoon Lake, moderately at first and then on steep switchbacks under western white and lodgepole pines. Halfmoon Lake is set in an amphitheater of granite walls and offers good swimming and fishing for brook and rainbow trout. There are scattered campsites all around the northwestern lobe of the lake, with the nicest selection near the outlet (for example, 9,439'; 37.05221°N, 118.84995°W), with views straight across the water to Scepter Peak's escarpment.

DAY 3 (Halfmoon Lake to Blackcap Basin, 6.5 miles): A short distance beyond Halfmoon Lake, the main trail, the TST, continues due north toward Big Maxson Meadow, while you turn right (east) onto a less-used spur toward Blackcap Basin. The route-finding is easy, but as of 2019 this trail hasn't been maintained in some years. Over the 3.0 miles to the North Fork Kings you will step across many a downed tree and most likely pause on occasion to make sure you've correctly distinguished between the trail and a drainage gully. Your route loops around the top of a spur extending north off Scepter Peak and then follows a shelf halfway between the Scepter Pass ridge and the valley floor, created by one of the successive glaciations; there are steep slabs above and below your shelf, but you are walking on pleasantly angled, sandy soils in an open forest, where the standard lodgepole pine are occasionally replaced by stately stands of red fir (in more sheltered draws) and western white pine (in deep soils). You never see the steep terrain downslope but repeatedly have a chance to admire the exfoliating slabs shedding above you. In a notch among them is Scepter Pass, a commonly used route in the late 1800s, allowing shepherds the quickest and easiest access from the North Fork Kings into the Crown Creek drainage and on to the Middle Fork Kings. Ultimately, your trail drops off the shelf to reach the banks of the North Fork Kings at a junction, where you turn right (east) to ascend the North Fork Kings into Blackcap Basin, while left (northwest) leads down the river toward Big Maxson Meadow and onto Maxson Trailhead at Courtwright Reservoir. It is the longer but probably more traveled route toward Blackcap Basin and is described up to the Red Mountain Basin junction, 1.95 miles downstream, as part of Trip 14.

If you're searching for a campsite, the best nearby choices are near this junction, either a short way up- or downstream. Thereafter, there are few options for many miles. You're following the south side of the river and a steep, rugged crest rises straight above you, while across the river the terrain is astonishingly bright white, perfectly polished granite slabs that extend on and on. The gentle but steady ascent is mostly under lodgepole pine shade, but it also traverses areas swept by avalanches, where vigorous willow thickets thrive. Your trail is easy to follow but awkward until late in the summer, for endless upslope seeps flow across—and along—the narrow tread. The track is always close to the river, the sound of flowing water increasing and diminishing with the gradient; the North Fork Kings, sometimes cascading down the granite slabs and elsewhere meandering through meadows, contains a healthy population of golden, brook, and brown trout. Brisk and incredibly refreshing swimming holes scoured smooth by the crystalline river will rejuvenate weary hikers.

About 2 miles beyond the last junction, the gradient increases markedly as you climb from the valley bottom toward Blackcap Basin proper. The trail then turns south, ascending the North Fork tributary that leads to Portal Lake and you soon emerge from the lodgepole pine shroud into a lovely subalpine meadow. Here is a nearly vanished junction: just a line of rocks marks the start of what was once a trail to Crown Basin (right; west); another old shepherd route, it is easy to follow, but a "trail" is only occasionally visible. Your route continues upstream (left; southeast), steps up briefly, and then reaches a second meadow, where you must ford the creek. This is best done where you first reach the meadow and the creek is pinched between bedrock. The trail may be faint through the meadow, but you'll

Looking down on Pearl and Division Lakes from high in Blackcap Basin   Photo by Elizabeth Wenk

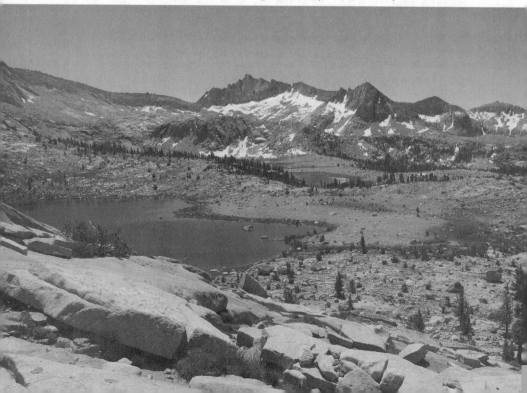

quickly pick it up again and continue winding upstream. Climbing up benches and over slabs, the trail leads to Portal Lake, where you'll find some small campsites to either side of the outlet (10,332'; 37.04383°N, 118.75756°W; no campfires). Portal Lake is a small lake with shallows at its north end and an escarpment to the south.

EXPLORING BLACKCAP AND CROWN BASINS

The described route ends at Portal Lake because this is the end of the trail, but calling this "Blackcap Basin" is rather disingenuous. Having walked for three days and more than 20 miles to get here, make sure you have spare time to explore upward, with or without your pack. Portal Lake is the lowest of about a dozen lakes in Blackcap Basin, a series of remarkably flat granite-slab-and-sand shelves with steeper steps between. The lakes sit on these shelves, many positioned like infinity pools, with barely a bedrock rib to block your downcanyon views. To most easily access the upper lakes, from Portal Lake proceed a short distance northeast to an unnamed amoeboid lake (excellent camping). Continue northeast toward a treed ramp that leads to Pearl Lake. From Pearl Lake, easy terrain leads north to Division Lake, northeast up another forested ramp to Regiment Lake (and onto Battalion Lake). Alternatively, from Pearl Lake you can head south along a convenient shelf to Chapel Lake and the phenomenally flat shelf with Midway Lake (excellent but exposed camping). To reach Crown Basin, follow the gentle, sloping ridge southwest above Portal Lake and continue along the open granite slabs south to several shallow unnamed lakes. From there, follow Crown Creek downstream. If you have a full day free, consider an ascent of Blackcap Mountain, a talus-free summit with wide-ranging views.

DAYS 4–5 (Blackcap Basin to Woodchuck Trailhead, 21.4 miles): Retrace your steps. With a lighter pack and better acclimation, many hikers will choose to spend just two days retracing their steps. You may understandably want to spend another night at Woodchuck Lake, but otherwise, at the junction due south of Woodchuck Lake, stay left (southwest) to take an alternate route via Chimney Lake, described in a sidebar on page 95. If you bypass Chimney Lake, this route is 0.2 mile shorter than the described route; if you visit Chimney Lake, it is 0.8 mile longer than the route via Woodchuck Lake.

trip 17 **Crown Lake**

see map on p. 92

    Trip Data: 37.03623°N, 118.84912°W; 29.3 miles; 4/1 days
    Topos: *Rough Spur, Courtright Reservoir, Blackcap Mountain.*

HIGHLIGHTS: This loop leads you through a piece of the Sierra known as Woodchuck Country, reasonably gentle forested terrain broken by a succession of meadows. Moisture is usually abundant until late summer and wildflowers color both the forest floor and meadow expanses. If you have spare time, the terrain around Crown Pass offers good opportunities for off-trail exploring.

DAY 1 (Woodchuck Trailhead to Woodchuck Lake, 9.8 miles): Follow Trip 15, Day 1 to Woodchuck Lake (9,825'; 37.04349°N, 118.88339°W; no campfires within 300 feet of the lake).

DAY 2 (Woodchuck Lake to Crown Lake, 4.6 miles): The trail continues around the east side of Woodchuck Lake, walking close to its meadow-fringed shore, then cuts across the delicate meadows along its southern inlet. It soon crosses the inlet (contrary to the old route plotted on maps) and climbs gently through sandy terrain out of Woodchuck Lake's basin. After 1.3 miles you reach the signed junction with the Woodchuck Trail and turn left (northeast) toward Crown Pass, while right (southwest) leads back toward Wishon Reservoir.

You climb gently up a meadow corridor abloom with shaggy lupine in midsummer and step onto broken slab, staring south at another lupine-covered meadow and small tarn. Note as well the reddish rock, where overlying basalt deposits altered the granite. Your route continues across barren granite slopes, looping around the southern end of a ridge. In early to midsummer, note the small pink-flowered plants with cylindrical succulent leaves. This species, quill-leaf lewisia, grows only around Crown Pass, Chuck Pass, and in the Dinkey Lakes Wilderness—and in the Siskiyou Mountains of far northwestern California, a rather peculiar distribution. While the trail once took the direct route over a pair of ridges toward Crown Pass, it now loops around the head of a minor drainage and then continues south to cross the second ridge where it is shallower.

Suddenly the gentle slabs and sandy corridor give way to a dramatic vista to the southeast. Peaks as distant as the Kaweah summits in Sequoia National Park are readily visible, as are the major summits of the Great Western Divide. Mount Harrington, a small but unmistakable peak along the Monarch Divide, sticks out like a thumb behind the turrets decorating the Gorge of Despair. From the vista point, the trail bends north, walking at the bluff-forest boundary. As the upslope slabs vanish, the slope's angle lessens and you approach a junction, where you turn right (due south) toward Crown Lake, while left (straight ahead, north) leads onto Crown Pass and Halfmoon Lake (Trip 16). Crown Pass is an easy 0.1 mile north of this junction and since this is a short day, you may want to head to the pass and climb one of the excellent vista points to either side; see the sidebar "Detours from Crown Pass" on page 97 for details.

You are now on the Theodore Solomons Trail (TST), a little-used route designated as a midelevation alternative to the John Muir Trail. From the junction, the trail descends a steep sandy, bouldery slope of western white pine. Soon you drop into a grassier lodgepole pine forest, the gradient easing as you turn to the northeast and begin a long gradual traverse to the valley floor. After crossing the northern edge of the massive, multilobed meadow, you reach a lodgepole pine stand just north of Crown Lake. Here, under forest cover, are Crown Lake's best campsites (9,762'; 37.03623°N, 118.84912°W; no campfires within 600 feet of the lake), although options also exist on the shallow rib west of Crown Lake. Looking at a map, you'll notice Crown Basin and Crown Creek are in a separate drainage to the east, while Crown Lake's outlet flows into Scepter Creek. All these "Crowns" were named after Crown Rock, a long way south; its summit rocks bear resemblance to a crown.

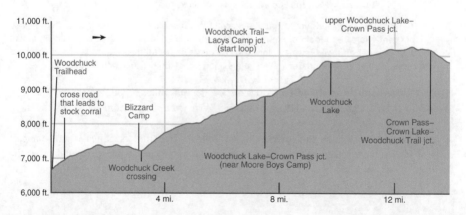

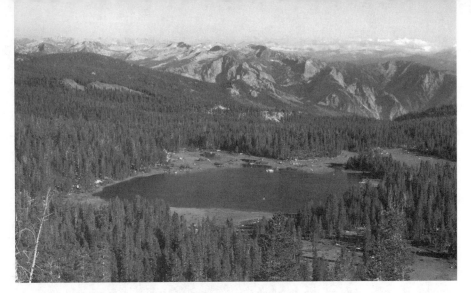

View of Crown Lake from the ridge east of Crown Pass   Photo by Elizabeth Wenk

DAY 3 (Crown Lake to Indian Springs, 6.4 miles): Continuing around Crown Lake's eastern shore, you walk beneath steep slabs that rise up to Scepter Peak. The trail becomes somewhat indistinct as it crosses the southern marshlands below Crown Lake, but it is easy to relocate the trail along the east side of the unnamed outlet creek. Descend easily in moderate forest, at first lodgepole but later mixed with western white pine. Intermittent marshy patches inter-rupt the trail's loose duff surface as the path descends gently south beside this creek.

At the unmarked junction with the Scepter Lake Trail (9,527'; 37.02351°N, 118.84142°W), you turn right (west) to cross the creek, while left (east) leads to Scepter Lake on a faint trail (nice campsites; easy to explore off-trail toward Scepter Pass). The coordinates are given, for this junction is about 0.1 mile (and 100 feet elevation) above the location depicted on USGS 7.5' topo maps; the trail has been rerouted to loop west around the meadow below. So you continue west, traversing high above the valley bottom, slowly bending south, then southeast to reunite with the old trail. Now along Scepter Creek, the trail is sometimes right at the marshy meadow's edge and elsewhere swings west of the creek into the fring-ing lodgepole pine forest. After crossing a pair of side tributaries (notable for their boggy pocket meadows), the trail climbs gently and you note volcanic outcrops upslope. As you pass these, and just before you drop to a grassy tarn, grab your camera and head left (east), upslope, to the ridge for a splendid view toward the Cirque Crest and Monarch Divide.

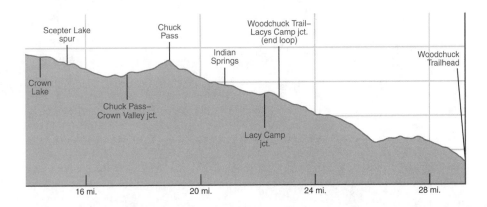

Kettle Dome is the nearby dome that stands high above the landscape, while Tehipite Dome is low down and barely visible. Climbing back into forest, you imperceptibly cut onto a moraine crest and reach a junction with the Chuck Pass Trail back toward Wishon Reservoir; you turn right (southwest) onto this trail, while left (south) is the TST's continuing route toward Crown Valley.

The Chuck Pass Trail climbs to a shallow ridge, again with remnant basalt outcrops, and then loops northwest alongside a small creek. Under lodgepole pine cover, the trail climbs moderately up the southwest side of the creek and its fringing meadow finger. As you near the ridge, the landscape is slightly more bouldery and western white pine becomes more common, but you never break above the trees—even Chuck Pass (9,640') offers no view.

Onward, the rocky trail leads down through parklike, spacious stands of lodgepole pine, western white pine and red fir on a set of steep, dusty switchbacks to the headwaters of Woodchuck Creek. Soon, the trail passes above a rocky, snag-strewn meadow, remaining on sandier soils to the north, then ducking into lusher forest. Along this enjoyable, mostly gentle walk, both the forest and meadows boast a tapestry of wildflower colors and aromas. As you approach Indian Springs, the terrain steepens and the trail has been rerouted; it loops considerably north of the old route to avoid damaging the meadow grasses. Through lush, spring-fed forest, you slowly drop toward Indian Springs, approaching the meadow's northern edge. The best campsites are near the northwestern corner of the meadow on a shallow sandy lump between the meadow and Woodchuck Creek with young lodgepole pine (8,901'; 37.00479°N, 118.88692°W). There are additional trailside sites once past the meadow boundary, near where a campsite symbol is marked on USGS 7.5' topo maps (8,915'; 37.00524°N, 118.88734°W).

DAY 4 (Indian Springs to Woodchuck Trailhead, 8.5 miles): The trail continues west, quickly crossing a tributary scoured bare by a debris flow in the 1990s and still strewn with tree trunks. One more downward step leads to the broad, flat valley that extends to Lacy Camp. In places you walk through bouldery, grassy lodgepole pine forest and elsewhere the ground is strewn with smaller boulders from past flood events. There are abundant wildflowers throughout, especially prettyfaces, wandering fleabane, and mariposa lilies. Shortly you reach a junction near the locale marked as "Lacy Camp," where you turn right (north) to return to Wishon Reservoir via the Woodchuck Trail, while left (south) leads to Round Corral Meadow and onto the Rancheria Trail (signposted for Finger Rock).

Climbing briefly, you reach the ruins of an old cabin and cut across a sandy flat and down a minor drainage, back to the Woodchuck Trail. Here, you reunite with your route from Day 1 and retrace the final 6.5 miles to the trailhead.

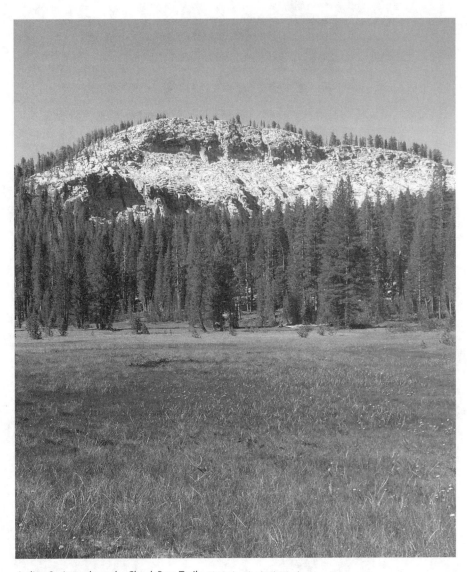

Indian Springs along the Chuck Pass Trail   Photo by Elizabeth Wenk

CA 180 TRIPS

CA 180 ends at Roads End, near Cedar Grove, in the South Fork Kings River Valley. A long, broad, vertical-walled glacial canyon rivaling Yosemite Valley in grandeur, it is the main west-side starting point for backpacking trips into Kings Canyon National Park. Just as the landscape parallels Yosemite Valley, so do elevation profiles for trips starting in the Cedar Grove environs—they all start with a steep, sustained, switchbacking climb to surmount the valley walls. Included here are the Lewis Creek, Copper Creek, and Roads End Trailheads. The very challenging Lewis Creek and Copper Creek Trails lead up steep, narrow creek drainages to the crest of the Monarch Divide and a selection of stunning lakes cradled in cirques to either side of the ridge. The trail from Roads End quickly forks, with one branch leading up the South Fork Kings to Paradise Valley and Woods Creek and the other up Bubbs Creek. A south-trending side valley off Bubbs Creek, East Creek, leads to East Lake and Lake Reflection. The Copper Creek, Woods Creek, and Bubbs Creek Trails all lead to the John Muir Trail (JMT), providing lots of scope for loop trips. The famous Rae Lakes Loop links the Woods Creek and Bubbs Creek valleys together, while Trip 20 provides a challenging loop linking the Middle Fork and South Fork Kings Rivers.

Trailheads: Lewis Creek

Copper Creek

Roads End

From the base of the Copper Creek Trail, you'll enjoy beautiful views of the South Fork Kings River and the Sphinx.   Photo by Elizabeth Wenk

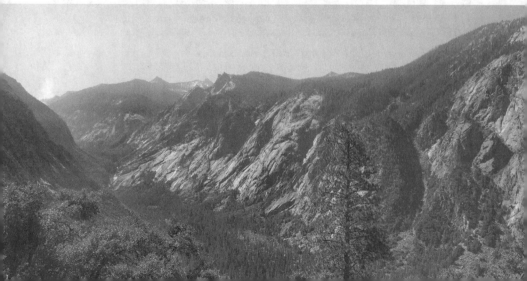

Lewis Creek Trailhead				4,553'; 36.80043°N, 118.69132°W		
Destination/ GPS Coordinates	**Trip Type**	**Best Season**	**Pace & Hiking/ Layover Days**	**Total Mileage**	**Permit Required**	
18 Volcanic Lakes 36.89644°N 118.63492°W (Volcanic Lake 9,702)	Shuttle	Mid to late	Strenuous 5/1	30.0	Lewis Creek *(Copper Creek in reverse)*	

INFORMATION AND PERMITS: The Lewis Creek Trailhead is in Kings Canyon National Park. Permits are required for overnight stays and quotas apply. Permits can be reserved up to six months in advance at recreation.gov/permits/445857, with additional details at nps .gov/seki/planyourvisit/wilderness_permits.htm. For both advance reservations (67% of quota) and walk-up permits (33% of quota), there is a $15-per-permit processing fee and a $5-per-person reservation fee. Both reserved and walk-up permits for this trailhead must be picked up in person at the Roads End Permit Station, open 7 a.m.–3:30 p.m. daily. This is located at the far eastern end of Kings Canyon, so-called Roads End, 6.8 miles east of the Lewis Creek Trailhead. Campfires are prohibited above 10,000 feet and in Granite Basin. Bear canisters are not required but are strongly encouraged.

DRIVING DIRECTIONS: From the CA 99–CA 180 interchange in Fresno, take CA 180 east into Kings Canyon National Park. After 54.3 miles you pass the Kings Canyon National Park entrance station and then at 56.0 miles reach a T-junction where you turn left, still on CA 180. Continue another 28.9 miles to the Lewis Creek Trailhead; the trailhead is on the left (north) side of the road, and the parking area, with vault toilets and bear boxes, is to the south. However, you must continue an additional 6.8 miles east along CA 180 to pick up your wilderness permit at the Roads End Permit Station before returning to the trailhead.

see maps on p. 106– 107

trip 18   ## Volcanic Lakes

> **Trip Data:** 36.89644°N, 118.63492°W (Volcanic Lake 9,702); 30.0 miles; 5/1 days
> **Topos:** *Cedar Grove, Slide Bluffs, Marion Peak, the Sphinx*

HIGHLIGHTS: This adventurous, rigorous trip climbs steeply to the stark alpine beauty of the Monarch Divide, separating the gigantic chasms formed by the South and Middle Fork Kings Rivers. Upon climbing to the ridge, you are rewarded with wide views of summits far to the north and south, with those toward the Black Divide and Palisades particularly striking. The Volcanic Lakes are a gem nestled beneath the northern Monarch Divide escarpment—barren, yet remarkably accessible. You need decent off-trail navigation skills to complete this hike but will be rewarded with surprisingly easy cross-country walking. The long climb from the Lewis Creek Trailhead is the most arduous part.

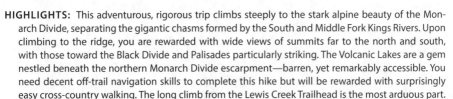

HEADS UP! *This is a very demanding route, with more than 6,000 feet of elevation gain and a fair amount of cross-country travel. This trip should be attempted by strong, experienced hikers only. The first day is a long, hot climb—pick up your permit the afternoon before or be in line by 6:45 a.m.*

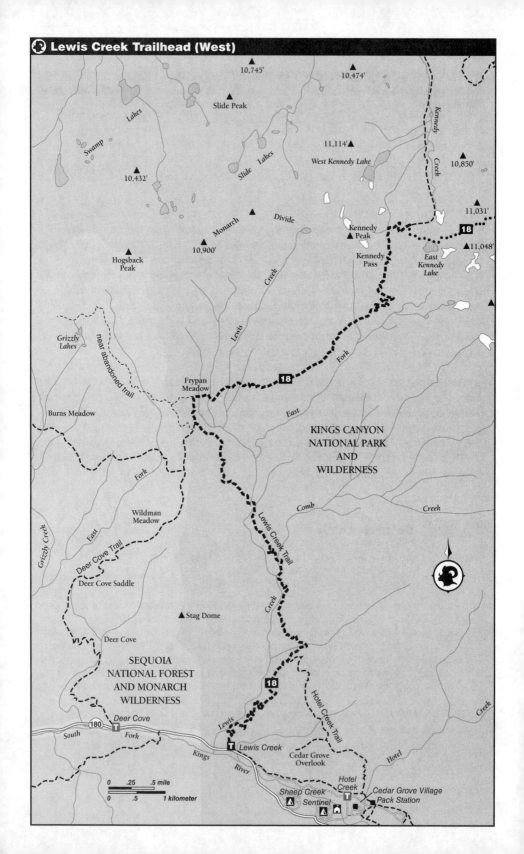

10,745'

10,474'

▲ Slide Peak

Lakes

Swamp

11,114'▲

West Kennedy Lake

Kennedy Creek

10,850'▲

▲ 10,432'

Slide Lakes

11,031'▲

18

▲ Monarch *Divide*

Kennedy Peak

▲11,048'

10,900'

Kennedy Pass

East Kennedy Lake

▲ Hogsback Peak

▲

Grizzly Lakes

near abandoned trail

Lewis

Fork

Frypan Meadow

18

Burns Meadow

East

KINGS CANYON NATIONAL PARK AND WILDERNESS

Fork

Wildman Meadow

Comb

Creek

Grizzly Creek

East

Deer Cove Trail

Lewis Creek Trail

Deer Cove Saddle

Creek

▲ Stag Dome

Deer Cove

SEQUOIA NATIONAL FOREST AND MONARCH WILDERNESS

18

Hotel Creek Trail

Deer Cove

180 T

South *Fork*

Lewis

Cedar Grove Overlook

Hotel

Creek

T Lewis Creek

Kings *River*

Hotel Creek

Cedar Grove Village Pack Station

0   .25   .5 mile

0   .5   1 kilometer

Sheep Creek Sentinel T

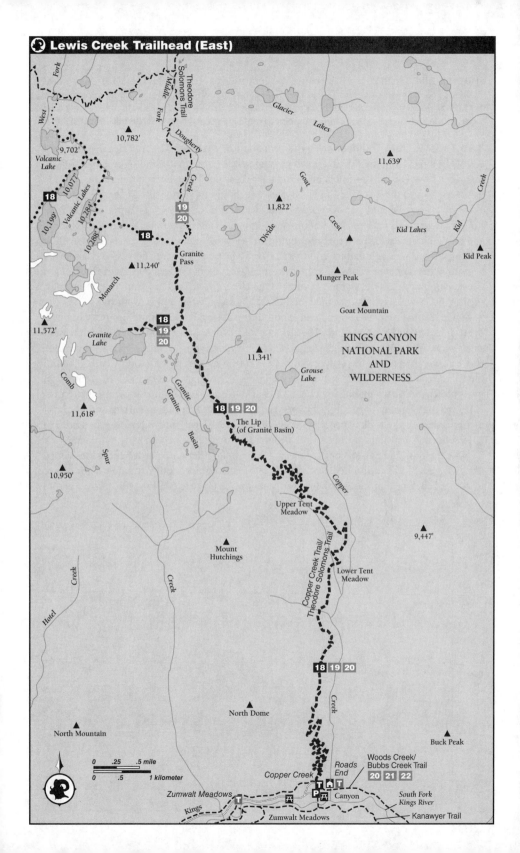

West Fork

Middle Fork

Theodore Solomons Trail

Dougherty Creek

Glacier Lakes

▲10,782'

▲9,702'

Volcanic Lake

▲11,639'

18

10,077'

Volcanic Lakes

10,284'

19
20

▲11,822'

Goat Crest

Kid Lakes

Kid Creek

10,199'

10,288'

18

Granite Pass

Divide

Munger Peak

Kid Peak ▲

▲11,240'

Monarch

Goat Mountain

▲11,572'

Granite Lake

18
19
20

▲11,341'

Grouse Lake

KINGS CANYON
NATIONAL PARK
AND
WILDERNESS

Comb

Granite

Granite Basin

18 **19** **20**

The Lip
(of Granite Basin)

▲11,618'

Copper

Spur

▲10,950'

Upper Tent
Meadow

▲9,447'

Mount
Hutchings

Copper Creek Trail/
Theodore Solomons Trail

Lower Tent
Meadow

Hotel Creek

Creek

Creek

18 **19** **20**

North Dome ▲

Buck Peak ▲

North Mountain ▲

0   .25   .5 mile

0   .5   1 kilometer

Copper Creek

Roads
End

Woods Creek/
Bubbs Creek Trail

20 **21** **22**

Zumwalt Meadows

1

Canyon

South Fork
Kings River

Kings

Zumwalt Meadows

Kanawyer Trail

SHUTTLE DIRECTIONS: The end point is the Copper Creek Trailhead, located along CA 180 near Road's End, 6.8 miles east of the Lewis Creek Trailhead. Although there is no shuttle service to link the two trailheads, there is sufficient hiker traffic to make hitching a ride realistic. An alternative would be to bring a bicycle to stage at the endpoint to retrieve the car—it an easy, slightly downhill ride.

DAY 1 (Lewis Creek Trailhead to Frypan Meadow, 6.1 miles): The trail heads north, just across the street from the parking lot, bypassing a little-used right-trending trail that follows the valley floor eastward. Almost all of today's hike is up slopes burned at least once in the past decades and there is little shade—this ascent should be started as early as possible. Just a few incense cedar and ponderosa pine survived the most recent conflagration, the 2015 Rough Fire, and you are mostly walking among regrowing manzanita, Fremont's silktassel, and mountain misery, shrubs that resprout from below-ground storage organs following fire. Fortunately, just enough mature conifers survive to be a seed source and young conifers are beginning to regenerate. The trail traverses and zigzags across steep slopes high above Lewis Creek, climbing 1,250 feet in the 1.9 miles to the Hotel Creek Trail junction. Right leads past the Cedar Grove Overlook into the Hotel Creek drainage, while you stay left (north).

While the first miles were steep and exposed, you at least made upward progress, but now the trail frustratingly drops nearly 100 feet to cross a Lewis Creek tributary beneath pleasant sugar pine, white fir, and incense cedar shade. Onward, you sidle back to the steep slope above Lewis Creek, gaining only modest elevation to a crossing of Comb Creek. Though there are scattered trees still surviving, including occasional dense stands of conifers, in most places mountain mahogany carpets the ground. This sticky, low-growing shrub provides welcome ground cover, but the aroma can be overwhelming in early summer and if it encroaches on the trail, expect sticky legs. The Comb Creek ford was elegantly rebuilt in 2018 following a spring washout, but you should anticipate wet feet in early summer.

Now the trail makes a steeper climb up a spur, before flattening as it approaches a ford of Lewis Creek, a beautiful bedrock stream with enticing pools downstream—a good spot to cool off before continuing to Frypan Meadow. Rock blocks allow you to hop across

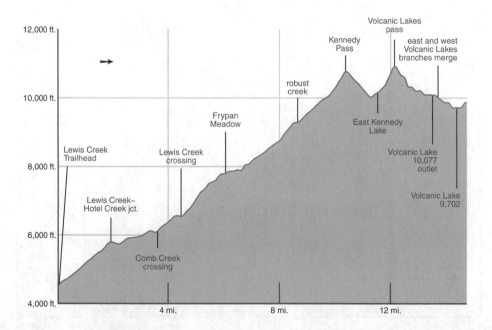

on all but the highest flows. Beyond, the trail again diverges from the steep-walled creek corridor and you resume your steady climb through an endless sea of mountain misery. As before, many trees are dead, but everywhere a few seed trees have survived—you may not have shade, but do be thankful the ecosystem is able to regenerate. The track climbs another 1,250 feet in the final 1.6 miles to Frypan Meadow—the most sustained climb yet, with a few particularly steep, rockier stretches. At 7,500 feet the mountain misery cover suddenly subsides—you are approaching its maximum elevation—only to be replaced by the pricklier mountain whitethorn and taller greenleaf manzanita. Here, your view south toward Roaring River, Glacier Ridge, the Great Western Divide, and Cloud Canyon begins to open, a teaser for tomorrow's vistas. And suddenly the trail is flatter with sugar pine, white fir, red fir, and Jeffrey pine as you follow a Lewis Creek tributary. Passing an unmarked, barely noticed track west to Wildman Meadow (the best route to the Grizzly Lakes), you drop a little and wade through waist-high vegetation at the base of welcome Frypan Meadow. A large campsite with a bear box is nestled beneath conifer cover on the meadows western side—a lovely location beside the verdant, flower-filled meadow (7,808'; 36.85348°N, 118.69864°W).

DAY 2 (Frypan Meadow to East Kennedy Lake, 5.4 miles): Don't be misled by today's modest mileage—this is probably a harder day than Day 1, even though there is nominally less elevation gain. The trail ascends 3,000 feet in the 4.3 miles to Kennedy Pass and the trail's condition is rougher. It is also imperative that you fill your water bottles, for the last 1,500 feet are waterless.

From the main Frypan Meadow camping area, the trail continues briefly north and passes an old sign pointing to the Grizzly Lakes; the first 0.3 mile of this spur trail does not exist, but as soon as you cross into Sierra National Forest you pick up the Deer Cove Trail, which is still maintained. After the Grizzly Lakes sign, the trail to Kennedy Pass bends right (east), crosses the creeklet that flowed by camp, and begins a leisurely climb eastward under tall pines, the

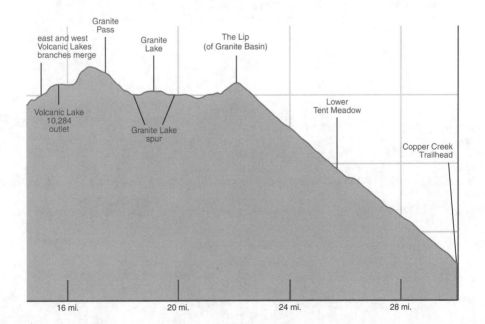

landscape only slightly burned here. Crossing a flattish rib, there are more places you could camp, your last for several miles. The trail then quickly drops to cross a second small creek, then larger Lewis Creek at the top of small falls; take care here at high flows. The path next makes several switchbacks, rounding the southwestern spur off Kennedy Mountain.

At about 8,300 feet, 0.65 mile past Lewis Creek, all semblance of tree cover vanishes and the ascending traverse carries you across a slope filled with greenleaf manzanita and whitethorn. The views south to the southern Great Western Divide, Kaweah Peaks, and Silliman Crest are outstanding. At 8,500 feet you enter a slope of scrubby aspen, seasonal trickles, and a wildflower display that is a highlight of this trip; nowhere is the expression "riot of color" more appropriate, with the astounding flower display persisting into August. For nearly a mile you climb up flower-choked slopes, the giant red paintbrush, Canada goldenrod, large-flowered collomia, and California coneflower all waist high and abundant, joined by close to 50 other species. Birds of prey circle overhead, attracted to numerous rodents living in the thick vegetation.

At 8,900 feet the trail is suddenly indistinct due to fallen logs and the abundant vegetation; moreover, the foot traffic disperses, exacerbating the problem. If you lose the trail, head straight up to a cluster of lodgepole pine and Jeffrey pine, where you sense there is also diminishing vegetation (9,282'; 36.86295°N, 118.67143°W). Here you pick up the trail and continue traversing northeast up the gradually drying slope past some near-dependable springs and a usually flowing tributary of East Fork Lewis Creek to a shelf with lodgepole and western white pines; this is the first flat place to camp since Frypan Meadow and offers some lovely sites. Onward, the trail steepens again and the forest cover thins. For the first mile there are ever-scrawnier lodgepole pine with a sprinkling of western white pine, but then the trees transition to multistemmed whitebark pine.

The trail continues diligently switchbacking up through a band of trees, to broad, flat-topped Kennedy Pass (10,781'). You are rewarded with a view over the Middle Fork Kings River's canyon into northern Kings Canyon National Park. Adventurers with spare energy

The eastern Volcanic Lakes basin is broad and open.   Photo by Elizabeth Wenk

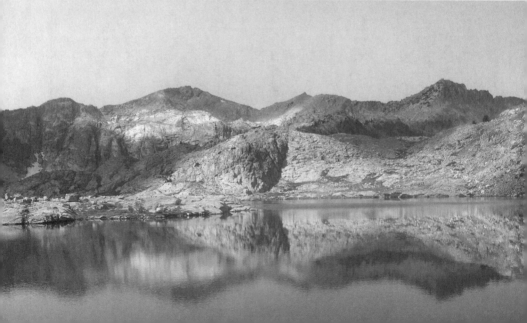

could continue another 1,000 feet west along the ridge to the summit of Kennedy Peak for even more exceptional views; the terrain is very easy.

Tight, eroded switchbacks carry you down the north side of Kennedy Pass, although they are often covered by a late-lasting snowbank; then take care on this short but difficult slope. After just a 150-foot descent you reach a small tarn, not plotted on the USGS 7.5' topo maps, and spy another tarn farther downslope. Above this first tarn lies a regal campsite perched like a throne, from which you can view Kennedy Pass above and the tarns below. An alternative campsite is the sandy flats beside a cluster of whitebark pine north of the second tarn with outstanding views across the Middle Fork Kings. However, do note the tarns and the stream plotted on the topo maps can dry out in late summer.

As you approach the second tarn, the trail turns sharply eastward and disappears over the edge of Kennedy Canyon. Near the top, the trail is well built, with sturdy steps, now so little used that even slow-growing alpine plants are creeping onto the tread. The trail winds its way down a sandy passageway between steep polished slabs, then suddenly all but vanishes at 10,050 feet, just before you reach the first trees (36.88042°N, 118.65617°W). This is a cue to cut due south across slabs to an elongate tarn. There are several pleasant tent sites among slabs along the north side of the tarn—better sites than are found at more enclosed East Kennedy Lake. Follow the north bank of this lakelet eastward, climbing slabs to deep, clear East Kennedy Lake. Although a stunning location, there are only a few, quite small single-tent campsites at East Kennedy Lake itself, either on the knob northwest of the outlet (10,189'; 36.87856°N, 118.65350°W; no campfires) or on the rib rising northeast of the lake.

DAY 3 (East Kennedy Lake to Volcanic Lake 9,702, 2.9 miles, all cross-country): East Kennedy Lake sits on a bench, with cliffs rising above and below the lake. The terrain is inhospitable except due east, where a pleasant, sandy, not-too-steep ramp leads to the Volcanic Lakes. You wind your way upward, zigzagging up either the sandier slope where red mountain heather and sedges hold the soil in place or along the slab, as you prefer. Scattered lodgepole and whitebark pines cling to the rocks. An 800-foot climb over 0.6 mile leads to a broad sandy pass and you stare down to the western Volcanic Lakes (10,923'; 36.87975°N, 118.64516°W). Just left of the shallow saddle is an excellent viewpoint, where you can see Mount Gardiner, Arrow Peak, the Palisades, and the Sierra Crest beyond.

This is a good place from which to consider your alternatives for your next night's campsite. The two big western lakes are gorgeous but offer few camping alternatives. The two main eastern lakes, currently hidden from view, have some flatter, sandier areas that are better for camping. You can reach them by going either south past the uppermost lakes or north, walking down the western fork and then up the eastern one, the route described here. There are virtually no trees in the upper basin, so if you are seeking a less stark campsite, descend to Volcanic Lake 9,702. The description includes the route there because a tour of the Volcanic Lakes must include a detour to this beautiful destination whether or not you camp at it.

The key to descending to Volcanic Lake 10,199 (the lake directly below you) is to trend northeast, reaching its shores most of the way to its outlet. The terrain is much steeper descending due east. Initially you descend through sand with a few scattered trees, but then you drop alternately to small grassy benches and across slabs, mostly avoiding any talus as you ramp down to reach the lakeshore about 600 feet before the outlet. The terrain is now easy as you walk beside vegetation on broken slab and gravel next to the lake. Onward, you follow the western bank of the outlet creek to Volcanic Lake 10,077 and follow its western shore as well. The water is superbly clear—you can admire big slabs of rock on the lake's bottom far from shore. At the outlet of the second lake are some small campsites beneath the first lodgepole pine.

Continuing another 0.2 mile down the western side of the outlet stream, you'll notice the eastern fork merging from the right. Not long after they merge, cross to the eastern bank and you'll likely find some traces of a use trail. Nearby are some good campsites, more sheltered than those at the upper lakes, and a good choice if you don't want to carry your pack down an unnecessary 300 feet to Volcanic Lake 9,702. You continue down, not far from the creek bank, through thickening lodgepole pine forest, looping around the north side of a tarn and then jutting south across open slab back toward the creek corridor where sandy passageways wind between the steeper bluffs; the landscape is steeper if you stay farther north. You drop to the shores of pleasant Volcanic Lake 9,702 and follow them north, with heath species, including dwarf bilberry and Labrador tea, underfoot. At the northern end of the lake is a broad flat—in places sand and slab and elsewhere are lodgepole pine groves—with ample campsites (9,717'; 36.89644°N, 118.63492°W). This is a gorgeous staging spot for fishing or exploring.

TAKING A TRAIL TO GRANITE PASS

If you don't want to continue the cross-country route, you could follow the West Fork Dougherty Creek 0.4 mile downstream (north) to pick up the trail linking Kennedy Canyon to Dougherty Creek. Staying on the east (right) side of the creek, you walk through forest and down easy broken slabs, reaching the trail on the east side of a small tarn. Turning right (east) you follow the Kennedy Canyon Trail 2.2 miles to the Granite Pass Trail, then turn right (south) and continue 2.9 miles to rejoin the described route atop Granite Pass. I'd strongly recommend the off-trail route—the eastern Volcanic Lakes are a treat and the cross-country walking is easier than what you completed yesterday.

DAY 4 (Volcanic Lake 9,702 to Granite Lake, 4.7 miles, part cross-country): For the cross-country route, retrace your steps 0.7 mile uphill to where the eastern and western branches of the Volcanic Lakes split. Now stay left to ascend the eastern fork, crossing to the southwestern side of the seasonal creek in a flat at 10,100 feet. Climbing through meadows colored by alpine shooting stars and tundra aster, you reach a pair of tarns with small tent sites. Beyond the tarns, recross the creek and climb slabs just beside the drainage, the terrain rapidly flattening again beside an unmapped amoeboid tarn. Pleasant but circuitous slab-and-grass walking winds along the eastern shoreline of Volcanic Lake 10,284 as you round a series of sharp, steep knobs. You'll pass additional sandy flats where you could camp. As you walk, be sure not to miss the black-and-white banded rock, flow patterns of light and dark minerals that seem like a misplaced superhighway. This, like all the rock in the basin, is diorite that solidified deep underground early in the formation of the Sierra's granite—none of the rock is of volcanic origin. Hopefully you'll have several hours to explore the basin before continuing to Granite Pass. The east side of Volcanic Lake 10,288 boasts a sandy beach and two points of rock jutting into the clear water, calling out for a swimming stop.

The ramp to Granite Pass departs from near the northeastern corner of Volcanic Lake 10,288 (around 36.88079°N, 118.62630°W), climbing 400 feet to a shelf. This is the broadest, more vegetated ramp rising above the lake; although steep, it is straightforward walking. Once in a perched, shallow trough, turn right (south), quickly reach a small tarn, and then turn east again, climbing another gully for 100 feet to reach a broad, rolling landscape that leads the final 0.6 mile to Granite Pass. Once on this plateau, you trend just south of due east, descending a most gradual 200 feet. In early season, tarns here making camping plausible, but they will generally be dry by mid-July. And soon you are back on the Monarch Divide at Granite Pass (10,655'; 36.87808°N, 118.61093°W).

After a lengthy break to enjoy the views north one last time, you head south on the Copper Creek Trail down a narrow coarse-grained sandy gully, completing nearly 20 tight switchbacks to reach the meadowed lands below. Here you are greeted by streamside blue-bell, Sierra saxifrage, and violets, before ducking into a moist lodgepole pine glade. A short downcanyon jaunt leads to a junction with a spur trail leading right (west) to Granite Lake. Granite Lake is an unnecessary 0.75-mile detour, but it is such a stunning spot, you should carry your pack toward the lake to spend the night—for after all, isn't spending time at gorgeous out-of-the-way lakes the reason you've taken this trip? The narrow, sinuous trail stays on the north side of Granite Creek, climbing up broken slabs and past some spectac-ularly thick-trunked lodgepole pine. While there are few established sites at Granite Lake, sandy nests exist on benches north (10,118'; 36.86554°N, 118.61962°W; no campfires) and east of the lake, with brilliant views of the deep, island-dotted lake ringed on three sides by marvelous granite walls.

DAY 5 (Granite Lake to Copper Creek Trailhead, 10.9 miles): Your final day is the longest, but it is predominately downhill. Moreover, the only campsites are in the first 2.0 miles and at Lower Tent Meadow, 4.3 miles from the end. Most parties will reach Lower Tent Meadow and just keep rolling down the hill, although this is a good campsite if your knees need to split the descent over two days.

Retrace your steps to the Copper Creek Trail and turn right to continue south through Granite Basin. You initially skirt a giant meadow, around whose perimeter there are addi-tional campsites if you didn't want to detour to Granite Lake with a full pack. Over the 2.2 miles to The Lip of Granite Basin, you climb just 350 feet, mostly in the final half mile, but these miles are neither quick nor flat. Instead the narrow, incised trail winds through lodgepole pine flats and across broken slabs, slowly diverging from Granite Creek. The creek bottom has enticing meadows and lakelets if you have more free time for exploring. Ultimately, your trail resolves into switchbacks, climbing 200 feet up a sandy slope of bright white granite to the spur that divides Granite Creek from Copper Creek. From here, you see two prominent peaks to the east, Mount Clarence King, on the left, and Mount Gardiner.

Over the final 8.0 miles to the trailhead, you drop more than 5,000 feet. Fortunately the trail is mostly sandy or on forest duff, with little cobble fill to navigate. You begin with 1,300 feet of switchbacks first through lodgepole and western white pine forest, and later into red fir stands, that drop you to Upper Tent Meadow, which offers neither tent sites nor a meadow—it is a steep, vegetated creek corridor that provides a chance to fill your water bottles. Trees cannot establish along the creek due to repeat avalanches, while the sea of mountain whitethorn and greenleaf manzanita below is the aftermath of a 1980 fire. You'll notice some Jeffrey pine beginning to shade out the whitethorn; it will be more than two decades before the slopes you ascended on the Lewis Creek Trail reach this stage of eco-logical succession. Continued descent, in part along a moraine crest, brings you to Lower Tent Meadow, the final campsites before the trailhead. There is a bear box here (7,842'; 36.82983°N, 118.58054°W).

In Lower Tent Meadow you cross the Upper Tent Meadow tributary and begin a long descending traverse across the eastern base of Mount Hutchings, now in white fir forest. More distant peaks have now vanished from view, but to the southeast you still see Cross Mountain, Mount Farquhar, the Sphinx, and the Avalanche Pass area. You step across multiple seasonal trickles, each with colorful flowers—geranium, Coulter's fleabane, coneflower, and crimson columbine and now and again cross open shrubby slopes that bespeak past fires. Switchbacks commence once you are 2.1 miles from the end of the trail, zigzagging down a hot south-facing slope where scattered live oak, black oak, and occasional ponderosa and pinyon pines provide insufficient shade; the rest of the slope is shrub covered. The walls grow around you until you are finally at the valley floor trailhead (5,049'; 36.79636°N, 118.58379°W).

Copper Creek Trailhead (at Roads End)

5,049'; 36.79636°N, 118.58379°W

Destination/ GPS Coordinates	Trip Type	Best Season	Pace & Hiking/ Layover Days	Total Mileage	Permit Required
19 Granite Lake 36.86554°N 118.61962°W	Out-and-back	Early to late	Strenuous 3/1	21.8	Copper Creek
20 Middle Fork–South Fork Kings River Loop 37.01697°N 118.58339°W (Devils Washbowl)	Loop	Mid to late	Strenuous 9/1	78.7	Copper Creek (Woods Creek in reverse)
18 Volcanic Lakes (in reverse of description; see page 105)	Shuttle	Mid to late	Strenuous 5/1	30.0	Copper Creek (Lewis Creek as described)

INFORMATION AND PERMITS: The Copper Creek Trailhead is in Kings Canyon National Park. Permits are required for overnight stays and quotas apply. Permits can be reserved up to six months in advance at recreation.gov/permits/445857, with additional details at nps .gov/seki/planyourvisit/wilderness_permits.htm. For both advance reservations (67% of quota) and walk-up permits (33% of quota), there is a $15-per-permit processing fee and a $5-per-person reservation fee. Both reserved and walk-up permits for this trailhead must be picked up in person at the Roads End Permit Station, open 7 a.m.–3:30 p.m. daily. This is located at the far eastern end of Kings Canyon, so-called Roads End, just 500 feet before you reach the Copper Creek Trailhead parking area—park your car and walk back for your permit. Campfires are prohibited above 10,000 feet and in Granite Basin. Bear canisters are required along the Woods Creek drainage and strongly encouraged in all locations.

DRIVING DIRECTIONS: From the CA 99–CA 180 interchange in Fresno, take CA 180 east into Kings Canyon National Park. After 54.3 miles you pass the Kings Canyon National Park entrance station and then at 56.0 miles reach a T-junction where you turn left, still on CA 180. Continue another 35.7 miles to Roads End. Here there are two parking areas: one to the south servicing the Roads End Trailhead (Woods Creek and Bubbs Creek) and also the day-use trail to Zumwalt Meadows and one to the north, adjacent to the Copper Creek Trailhead. There are a toilet and garbage receptacles between the two, a water tap at the permit station, and bear boxes at both parking lots.

trip 19 Granite Lake

see map on p. 117

Trip Data: 36.86554°N, 118.61962°W; 21.8 miles; 3/1 days
Topos: *The Sphinx, Marion Peak*

HIGHLIGHTS: The South Fork Kings River's valley is comparable to Yosemite Valley in many ways, but without the crowds. Granite Basin is perched high above the north rim of this valley, with a setting definitely worthy of a king—or a queen. The climb out of the valley is arduous, but once you experience the matchless scenery and excellent fishing at Granite Lake, the memory of the difficult ascent will soon fade away.

HEADS UP! *Because the canyon walls are so steep, the Copper Creek Trail climbs out of the canyon very quickly—5,000 feet in a mere 6.0 miles. This ferocious ascent, often exposed to blazing sunshine, is suitable only for the backpacker in top shape. With a starting elevation just barely over 5,000 feet, plan on a very early start to try and beat the heat.*

DAY 1 (Copper Creek Trailhead to Lower Tent Meadow, 4.3 miles): The Copper Creek Trail begins on the north side of the parking loop (5,036') under tall pines but all too soon leaves the shady pines behind on a hot climb up the north wall of Kings Canyon. Canyon live oaks provide insufficient shade for the first 1.25 miles of ascent to the first stream. The granite walls reflect much sunlight and, on a typically hot summer's day, hiking up this trail produces the sensation of being baked in a glaring furnace. Despite the intense heat, this route has been well used for centuries.

The first set of switchbacks gains 1,400 feet and then the trail swings into Copper Creek's canyon, where the path is partially shaded under a mixed forest of Jeffrey pines, incense cedars, and white fir (although sugar pines are present here, too, they are mostly dead).

The trail crosses several previously burned slopes with a healthy covering of manzanita. So intense is the heat radiating from the sandy tread across these slopes that imagining the forest floor is still smoldering is quite easy. Soon, the trail reaches a large aspen- and brush-covered clearing. Hop over a couple of rivulets in this well-watered clearing and then reenter forest cover on the way to the next creek crossing. Just after the crossing, the path arrives at Lower Tent Meadow Camp (7,842'; 36.82983°N, 118.58054°W), with five designated campsites and a bear box. *Note:* Be forewarned that Lower Tent Meadow is the only decent place to camp from here to Granite Basin.

DAY 2 (Lower Tent Meadow to Granite Lake, 6.6 miles): Continuing a northward, now moderate climb, the trail passes through a brush-choked slope, the aftermath of a 1980 fire. After two long switchbacks, the path nears the creek in a wide avalanche swath where only low-lying shrubs and a profusion of wildflowers are allowed to grow. The trail switchbacks again and nears the creek for the last time (9,100'); fill your water bottles here.

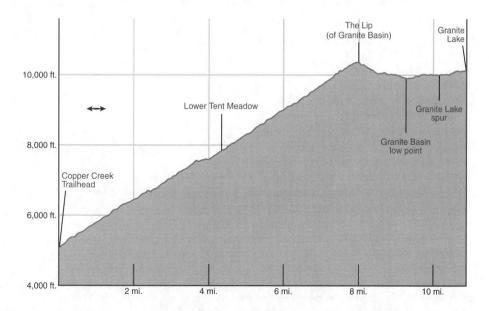

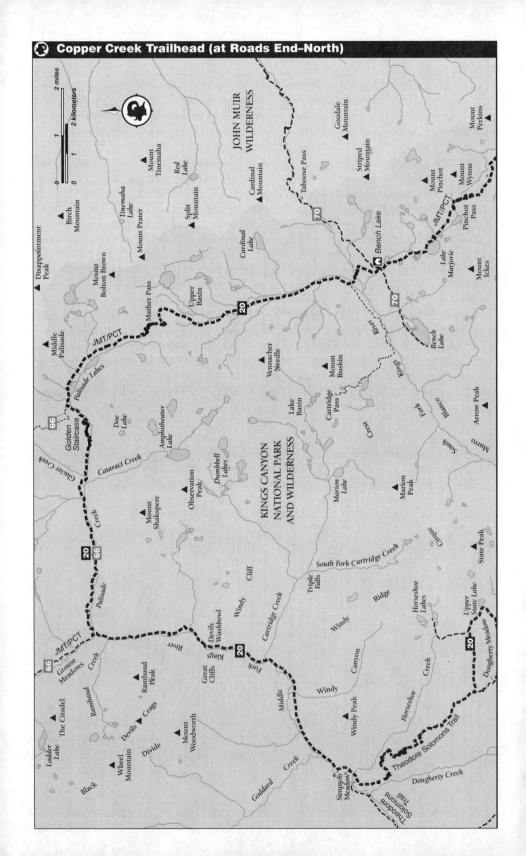

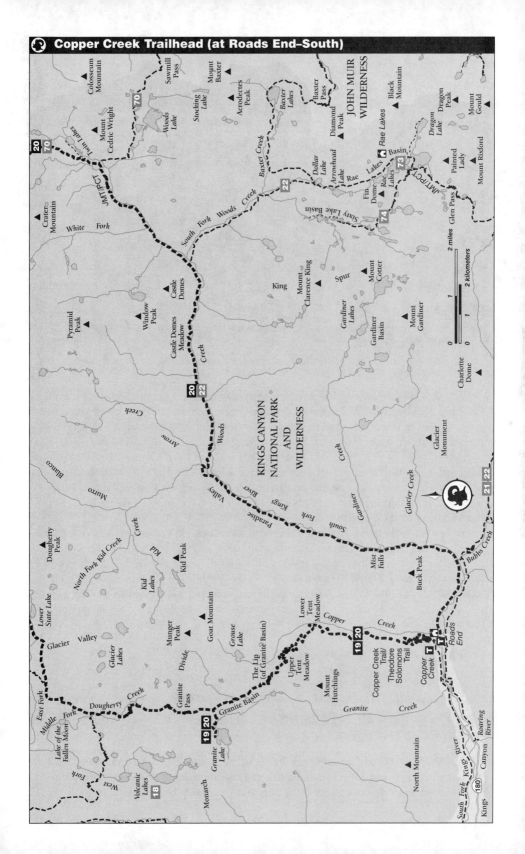

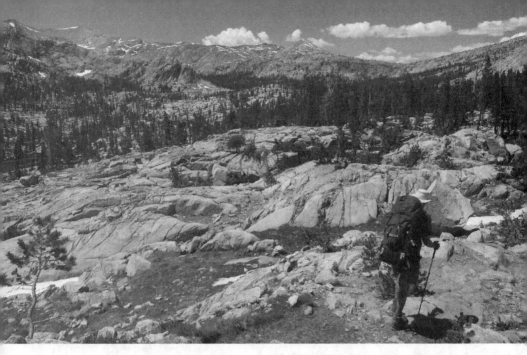

Reaching Granite Basin after the hard climb up the Copper Creek Trail   Photo by Elizabeth Wenk

Enter shady red fir forest and begin a long series of switchbacks that angle northwest as the trail climbs 1,300 feet up a bedrock ridge dividing Copper and Granite Creeks. En route, cross a belt of western white pines and then lodgepole pines along the ridgetop. From here, you see two prominent peaks to the east, Mount Clarence King, on the left, and Mount Gardiner.

A short, winding descent leads through a drift fence and down toward Granite Basin, filled with delightful tarns and irregular-shaped meadows. The trail avoids the floor of the basin in favor of an undulating traverse across a lodgepole-shaded hillside above. Parties interested in camping at locations within the basin other than Granite Lake must leave the trail and head cross-country.

Just beyond the large meadow at the north end of the basin, in a pocket of willows, reach a signed junction with a lateral to the lake. Turn left (west) and follow this lateral over a stream and past a couple of seldom-used campsites on a gradual ascent toward the lake. Hop over the seasonal inlet and arrive at campsites along the north shore of Granite Lake (10,118'; 36.86554°N, 118.61962°W; no campfires). The island-dotted lake nestles in a rocky basin below the cliffs of the Monarch Divide. Sparse pines offer little shelter for the smattering of campsites scattered around the lakeshore. Anglers can test their skill on fair-size brook trout.

DAY HIKING FROM GRANITE LAKE

A layover day at Granite Lake offers so many choices for farther wanderings that you might want to stay a week or more. Leaving your backpack behind, a day is long enough to explore several Volcanic Lakes (Trip 18) or State Lakes (Trip 20), or the unnamed lakes in lower Granite Basin. Also within easy reach are the Glacier Lakes and the two unnamed lakes just northeast of Granite Pass.

DAY 3 (Granite Lake to Copper Creek Trailhead, 10.9 miles): Retrace your steps. Backpackers wishing to avoid the 10.9-mile, one-day hike out should plan on two days and a stay at Lower Tent Meadow, which is the only viable campsite between Granite Basin and the trailhead.

trip 20   Middle Fork–South Fork Kings River Loop

Trip Data: 37.01697°N, 118.58339°W (Devils Washbowl);
78.7 miles; 9/1 days

Topos: *The Sphinx, Marion Peak, Slide Bluffs, North Palisade,
Split Mountain, Mount Pinchot, Mount Clarence King*

see maps on p. 116–117

HIGHLIGHTS: This spectacular trek introduces you to the wondrous, truly regal terrain along two forks of the mighty Kings River. Indeed, just about every step of the walk is fit for a king, passing many splendid lake basins and walking beneath towering walls and rugged summits, including the world-renowned Palisades. Only a single layover day is suggested not because of a lack of exquisite locations to while away your time, but because 10 days of food is as much as most people can fit in a bear canister!

HEADS UP! *Backpackers must be in top shape for this trip. It includes a difficult, 5,000-foot ascent in 6.0 miles along the Copper Creek Trail and then another long climb up Palisade Creek to Mather Pass. If you don't want to carry 9 (or more) days of food, suggested options include combining Days 1 and 2, combining Days 2 and 3, or completing the final three days over two, breaking for the night near the Woods Creek suspension bridge.*

HEADS UP! *The Palisade Creek crossing just before you reach the John Muir Trail (JMT) (on Day 5), cannot be crossed during peak snowmelt, generally through mid-July in an "average" year or later in a year with a late-melting snowpack. There is a somewhat safer crossing a mile above the official trail junction, necessitating a cumbersome cross-country section along the south bank of Palisade Creek.*

DAY 1 (Copper Creek Trailhead to Lower Tent Meadow, 4.3 miles): The trail departs from the back of the trailhead parking lot, immediately launching into a 1,400-foot climb up insufficiently shaded switchbacks. Copper Creek, the trail's namesake, remains tantalizingly out of reach on the entire ascent, here flowing down a steep, incised course east of the trail. Scattered live oak, black oak, and even more occasional ponderosa and pinyon pines provide just dots of shade, with greenleaf manzanita, whiteleaf manzanita, and silktassel occupying the rest of the slope. The granite walls reflect much sunlight, and on a typically hot summer's day, hiking up this trail produces the sensation of being baked in a glaring furnace—be in the permit line at 6:45 a.m., so that you can be hiking by 7:30, or ascend the distance to Lower Tent Meadow in the late afternoon. Slowly you feel higher relative to the valley walls and can measure your progress by the changing shape of the Sphinx rising to the south.

After 2.1 miles, the trail transitions to a long ascending traverse across the eastern base of Mount Hutchings. Here the ponderosa pine and incense cedar provide more shade, soon joined by the first white fir and some still-living sugar pine. Taking regular breathers, turn around to enjoy the expanding view southeast to Cross Mountain, Mount Farquhar, the Sphinx, and the Avalanche Pass area. You step across a sequence of seasonal creeklets, brightly colored by water-loving wildflowers, including geranium, Coulter's fleabane, coneflower, and crimson columbine. Beyond, cross a more substantial creek at 7,500 feet and cut through a thicket of redstem dogwood, aspen, and willows. Exiting the dense vegetation, you land in a blue-green sea of prickly mountain whitethorn, marking the location of a past fire, and then transition back to white fir forest. You welcome the next creek crossing, for just beyond is Lower Tent Meadow, with adequate camping and a bear box (7,842'; 36.82983°N, 118.58054°W). While not the most inspiring of campsites, it is the only decent place to camp until Granite Basin, a farther 5.5 miles up the trail with an additional 2,500 feet of elevation gain to add to the 2,800 feet you've already climbed; if it is early in the day and you're keen to continue, maybe take a long break and continue up in the late afternoon.

DAY 2 (Lower Tent Meadow to Granite Lake, 6.6 miles): Above Lower Tent Meadow, you quickly climb out of forest cover into an expanse of mountain whitethorn and greenleaf manzanita, the aftermath of a 1980 fire. Climbing along the slope of a moraine, you'll notice some Jeffrey pine beginning to shade out the whitethorn, but it will be many decades before these saplings are big enough to shade the trail. Long switchbacks lead back and forth, twice taking you close to the perennial creek flowing through so-called Upper Tent Meadow, a steep, vegetated creek corridor (and avalanche chute) that provides a chance to fill your water bottles but offers no tent sites and is not a meadow. Above the second brush with the creek, the trail leads into standing red fir forest, the understory bare, and up another flight of switchbacks. Elegant western white pines grace the ridges and lodgepole pines replace the red fir as you complete your long climb and cross the ridge connecting Mount Hutchings to the Cirque Crest, a saddle referred to as The Lip (of Granite Basin).

Steep sandy switchbacks wind tightly down the northwest side of the saddle toward Granite Basin, dropping about 400 feet. The downhill may be welcome, but this is slow walking along a narrow, often incised trail with embedded rocks. The trail works its way across a landscape of broken slabs with splendid views down on Granite Basin, a valley of delightful tarns and irregularly shaped meadows. If you wish to camp along the Granite Creek corridor, you must leave the trail and go cross-country, for the trail avoids the valley floor in favor of an undulating traverse across the lodgepole-shaded hillside above.

After a little over a mile, the trail sidles up to a side creek, your low point within Granite Basin, and begins a gentle climb alongside its drainage, soon crossing it. Continuing across a shallow saddle, the trail emerges beside a broad, seasonally marshy meadow, with hidden Granite Lake nestled on a shelf farther west. There are campsites under lodgepole pine

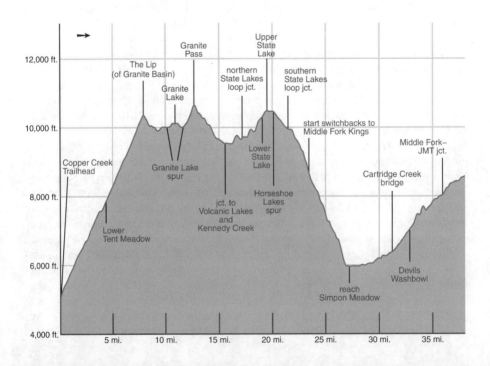

cover at the meadow's edge. Just past the end of the meadow is a junction with the spur trail left (west) to Granite Lake. The narrow, sinuous trail stays on the north side of Granite Creek, climbing up broken slabs and past some spectacularly thick-trunked lodgepole pine. While there are few established sites at Granite Lake, sandy nests do exist on benches north (10,118'; 36.86554°N, 118.61962°W; no campfires) and east of the lake, with brilliant views of the deep, island-dotted lake ringed on three sides by marvelous granite walls.

DAY 3 (Granite Lake to Lower State Lake, 8.2 miles): Retrace your steps to the junction with the Copper Creek Trail and turn left (north), crossing the meadow-rimmed creek corridor and then leaving the forest behind for a steep, rocky, 0.6-mile climb up a narrow gully toward Granite Pass (10,655') on the Monarch Divide. Granite Pass is remarkably flat and offers possible campsites if seasonal tarns still hold water. The views north are superlative, with massive Mount Goddard far to the left and the sharp-toothed ridges of Mount Woodworth and the Black Divide in the center. North Palisade, rising above 14,000 feet, marks the right-hand edge. Looking south you see the serrated profile of distant summits, including the Great Western Divide and the Kaweah Peaks Ridge.

The trail then begins a zigzagging descent past a series of meadow-covered benches rimmed by granite walls, approaching Middle Fork Dougherty Creek several times along the way. The river pauses its descent three times to meander through marshy meadows, beautiful to gaze down upon from the trail, but only the third, spanned by a pair of drift fences, offers campsites. Just beyond, the trail turns west and drops down steeper slabs, the creek tumbling to its north. As the terrain moderates, you continue north through mostly open lodgepole pine forest, hopping over the creek three times and passing numerous places where you could camp. At 2.9 miles from Granite Pass, you reach a junction with the minor trail that leads past the lower Volcanic Lakes and onward over Dead Pine Ridge and up Kennedy Creek to Kennedy Pass.

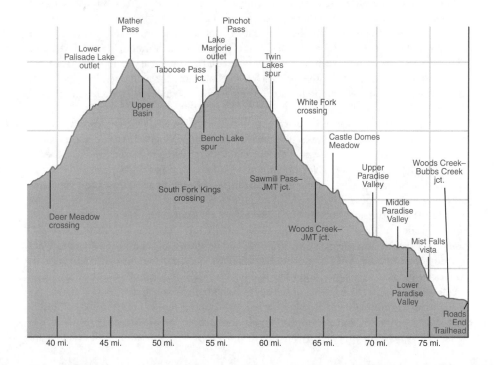

Continue north, stepping across a creek flowing toward Lake of the Fallen Moon. After a minor ascent up a ridge cloaked in moraine debris—and chinquapin, which commonly grows on these bouldery deposits—you drop to a lush pocket meadow nestled beside a second moraine crest and find a trail junction. Right (east), the recommended route, leads to the lovely State Lakes, but if you're in a hurry to reach Simpson Meadow, staying straight (north) is 2.8 miles shorter—just realize that it is another 7.4 miles to Simpson Meadow and your last water and camping until then is at the East Fork Dougherty Creek crossing in 0.7 mile.

Turn right (east) at the junction, onto a lateral trail that loops past the State Lakes. Briefly following the wet corridor, you climb up and over the minor moraine and drop to another moist passageway trapped behind a third moraine crest. Here you pass a good-size meadow filled with wildflowers, including shooting star, Kelley's lily, and arrowleaf ragwort, then climb to the crest of this moraine. Continue along it, until you approach the mouth of lovely Glacier Valley (and the moraine is truncated) and drop to the banks of its creek, crossing it on rocks. Then traverse to East Fork Dougherty Creek, the vigorous stream plummeting downslope from Lower State Lake, crossed on a log.

A moderately steep climb north of the stream leads up a hillside to gently rising, flower-dotted terrain below the lower lake. Soon, you reach the northwest shore of Lower State Lake (10,250'; 36.92481°N, 118.57345°W; no campfires). Backdropped by the impressive cliffs of the Cirque Crest, the lower lake offers a few lodgepole pine–shaded campsites along the north shore and others to its west. Fishing is usually excellent for good-size golden and rainbow trout, probably because the lake sees so few anglers.

DAY 4 (Lower State Lake to Cartridge Creek, 12.2 miles): Continuing your loop, you follow the trail up to the upper State Lake, where there are many additional campsites under lodgepole pine cover. This is another good-looking lake, edged by dwarf bilberry mats and with a more open feel. Beyond the route is less traveled—pay attention to the i-blazes carved in trees to ensure you are on the route as you first continue across lodgepole pine flats and then amble up sandy slopes to the top of a prominent moraine crest. Here you'll pass a junction with the lateral to the Horseshoe Lakes (also a worthwhile detour, but you're probably out of time), and turn left (west) to return to the main trail to Simpson Meadow. This next trail segment is even more seldom traveled and it is easy to lose the tread; the trail stays just a little north of the moraine crest, continuing through open lodgepole pine forest. If you were to lose the trail, just continue west and you'll know when you intersect the Simpson Meadow–bound trail.

Continuing to the main trail, turn right (north) to begin a 4,000-foot descent over 5.3 miles. (Going left here would take you down to East Fork Dougherty Creek, a year-round stream, in 0.3 mile; this is the segment of the main trail that you bypassed by taking the lateral through the State Lakes.) Northbound, the gradient is, at first, gentle, passing through open, gravelly, exceedingly dry lodgepole pine forest. The gradient increases and you begin dropping more purposefully, but still through gravel and sand—as pleasant a descent for your knees as is possible. At 9,420 feet, just before the trail completes its first switchback among eroded outcrops, take the time to stop and enjoy the view—this is the best vista point on the descent, staring down into the Middle Fork Kings and across to the Black Divide, now so much closer than from Granite Pass. This trail is a historic route, used by American Indians, shepherds, and early white Sierra explorers before you, the only "easy" way to cross the Monarch Divide until the JMT was built across Mather Pass.

The trail continues down the ridgecrest under scattered conifer cover until 8,660 feet. It then departs onto the west side of the spur, initiating broader switchbacks down a brushy slope: an expanse of mountain whitethorn and greenleaf manzanita—and resident fox

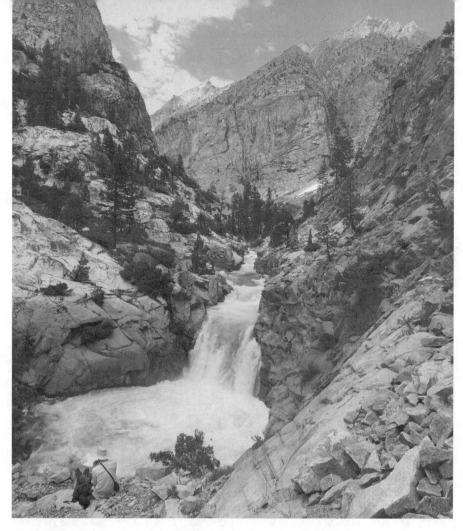

Devils Washbowl   Photo by Elizabeth Wenk

sparrows—with few mature trees. This slope and indeed most of the terrain between here and the east end of Simpson Meadow was charred to varying degrees by a lightning-caused fire that burned slowly for weeks in 1985. Then, as now, park service policy recognized fire as a normal part of forest ecology. It allows natural fires to run their course in the backcountry, clearing away the understory and providing the light required for seedlings to establish. Periodic fire is important to release nutrients from dead plant matter back into the soil, provided that when a fire ignites it isn't too intense and enough mature trees survive to provide a seed source. As of this update, both Jeffrey pine and western white pine are reestablishing, with some trees growing through the shrub cover.

The tread is still pleasant and sandy as the trail drops into a stand of mature white fir and Jeffrey pine at 7,800 feet. The trail cuts east across the steep slope on a long, gradual traverse. The occasional rockier stretches are narrow bands of moraine deposits left as the massive glacier down the Middle Fork Kings melted away. Overall, the trail is in quite decent condition—well maintained and as of this writing reasonably well used, as it is part of two named routes that currently are attracting many hikers: the Theodore Solomons Trail, that travels from Yosemite to southern Sequoia National Park, staying generally far west of the crest, and the Big SEKI Loop that links a selection of Kings Canyon and Sequoia National Parks' showiest trails (and is coincident with your route for more than 60 miles).

Around 7,200 feet, turning west, you'll have a brief view to the Obelisk and Tehipite Dome, two impressive domes guarding the north side of Tehipite Valley, far to the west. Meanwhile, Windy Peak now appears high above to the northeast. By 7,000 feet you'll notice a change in tree composition, with black oak, ponderosa pine, and incense cedars replacing the firs and Jeffrey pine. This community should also include sugar pine, but most have died following the 2012–16 drought. The final 600 feet to the valley floor are uncomfortable on the knees—here there are steep, rocky switchbacks that are incised by runoff. And so, with a sigh of relief you exit a thicket of incense cedar and black oak and arrive in a sagebrush flat that marks the far western extent of Simpson Meadow (5,960'). Here you will discover a sign that reads GRANITE PASS 12, with no indication of where other directions lead.

THE TRAIL TO TEHIPITE VALLEY
A bridge once spanned the Middle Fork Kings River a third of a mile downstream from where the trail reaches Simpson Meadow. It was washed out in 1982 and the park service has yet to contemplate rebuilding this structure. Those who wish to visit magnificent Tehipite Valley, 12 miles to the west, have to make a wet ford of the Middle Fork. This often-dangerous crossing should only be envisaged in mid- to late season after runoff drops and is best done upstream where the river is broader and slower. The trail down the Middle Fork Kings to Tehipite Valley is used more by bears than humans, and the climb from Tehipite Valley to Crown Valley is notoriously overgrown—but the rewards of overcoming these hurdles (and braving the numerous rattlesnakes) are well worth the effort.

Curving upstream (right; eastward), the trail stays some distance south of the creek, mostly in the forest fringing the meadow. It passes as old packer's camp, crosses Horseshoe Creek, and continues to a junction where a use trail darts across the meadow (5,965'; 36.97095°N, 118.63157°W). This is one of many trails that lead to the riverbank and is a decent place to ford the flow. And for you whose route remains on the south bank of the Middle Fork, it is a place to immerse yourself in Simpson Meadow, see the Middle Fork, and easily imagine why shepherds flocked to this valley. Also, fishing for rainbow trout in the Middle Fork is good. At high flows, the river's water will be far above your head and span the entire river channel, while by mid-September it may be just knee deep, meandering down the center of expansive cobble bars. There are many different places you could camp at the edge of Simpson Meadow, but a 78-mile trip without food resupply probably necessitates a few more miles today. Wait here, in the shade of the black cottonwood, until the midday heat has abated and then continue the final 3.6 miles to campsites near Cartridge Creek.

ALLUVIAL PROCESSES IN GODDARD CREEK'S CANYON
Where Goddard Creek pours into the Middle Fork, the Middle Fork's channel has been pushed right to the foot of Windy Peak by the sediments deposited by Goddard Creek's debouching from its canyon. This process is widespread within the canyon of the Middle Fork Kings River: farther upstream, the river flows on the far north side of the canyon floor opposite the alluvial fan at the base of Windy Canyon.

After passing another spur that leads to the river, the trail jogs briefly north where Simpson Meadow pinches closed, passes yet another northbound spur, and then continues upcanyon, gaining little elevation as it begins to contour around the base of Windy Peak, opposite the cleft of Goddard Creek's canyon. Nearby, on stream terraces, you'll spy more good campsites. You continue upstream, walking across volcanic talus that spills down the face of Windy Peak, comprised of a dark-colored rock called dacite that is similar in chemical composition to granite.

Crossing small alluvial fans dissecting the face, you continue to the massive alluvial fan that spills out of Windy Creek. The trail gradually cuts across this shadeless slope of boulders, cobble, and gravel. Near its center grow some bands of black oak that thrive in coarse, well-drained soils; here they probably have well-aerated soils but are able to tap into the groundwater at depth. Continuing past scattered black oak and through thickets of mountain whitethorn, the trail crosses many seasonally dry channels and then the main Windy Canyon creek in a thicket of vegetation.

Ahead the trail turns northeast for the final leg to Cartridge Creek and here the canyon is steeper and narrower. You traipse across a near-continuous sequence of alluvial fans spilling down the face of Windy Ridge, all densely vegetated with shrubs and some with thickets of black oak. Shifting to an exposed bedrock slope directly above the water, you reach Cartridge Creek, crossed high up on a stout bridge. A few more steps lead to a big, lovely campsite beneath stately incense cedar, white fir, and ponderosa pine. This is your last decent multitent campsite until you intersect the John Muir Trail (JMT) in 4.7 miles (6,426'; 36.99823°N, 118.58901°W).

DAY 5 (Cartridge Creek to Palisade Creek near Deer Meadow, 8.6 miles): From Cartridge Creek to Palisade Creek, the rocky Middle Fork canyon is impressively steep and narrow, guarded over by the Great Cliffs to the north and Windy Cliffs to the south. The trail generally follows a rocky ledge high above the incised, channeled river, oscillating from concave drainage to convex slope time and again. Along the first miles, the rock to either side is part of the metavolcanic Goddard pendant and erodes into angular ribs along bedding planes, forming the imposing walls that hem you in.

Passing a narrow cleft in the wall to the north, you are then suddenly back in granite with a new sight to behold, Devils Washbowl (7,017'; 37.01697°N, 118.58339°W). Here the Middle Fork is channeled over a lip, dropping into a circular basin. In late summer it invites a swim—for some—but during early-summer runoff you can imagine this whirling, seething washbowl cleaning the dirtiest of clothes. Above and below are more spectacular falls and cataracts set in the granite gorge.

Leaving this tumult of water behind, the trail continues its ascent over rock and across a talus field to ford the unnamed creek draining the cirques beneath Mount Shakspere and Observation Peak. A rock platform has been built across the flow, allowing the water to spread thinly, and it is easily crossed. After fording the main channel, continue across the broad alluvial fan that is bisected by a giant, generally dry debris flow channel and gaze upward at the seasonally memorable falls spilling down cliffs to the south. The flora around these tributary fords deserves attention for its lushness—wildflowers along these streams include Leichtlin's mariposa lily, cinquefoil, Kelley's lily, lupine, crimson columbine, and elderberry.

Turning due north, you cross onto talus and climb far above the river's banks. The canyon is steep, with many cliffs, and the trail builders have picked the best route through this difficult terrain. For nearly a mile the undulating trail is far above the river, but then cuts a route across bedrock and the ubiquitous brushy alluvial fans closer to the water's edge. The underfooting is rocky until the approach to Palisade Creek, where the grade levels and then curves through a packer camp on the way to the flower-lined stream. The ford is preceded by a return to timber cover, a forest of Jeffrey, lodgepole, and western white pine and white fir.

The bridge across Palisade Creek has been gone since the 1980s and will not be replaced anytime soon. Wade the swift, rolling, ice-cold waters about 50 feet upstream from its confluence with Middle Fork Kings River. The ford is difficult at any time during the summer and may be dangerous in early season; this is a crossing to ask about when you pick up your permit because you might otherwise find yourself having to walk off-trail just over a mile up the southern bank of the river before you reach a safe crossing site (at about 8,400 feet where the creek meanders through a small meadow)—or retrace your steps. After successfully fording the creek, head east across the lodgepole-shaded flat on a use trail to meet the JMT near some campsites.

Turn right (east) onto the JMT (and coincident PCT) and begin paralleling Palisade Creek upstream on an 11-mile, 4,000-foot climb to Mather Pass, which you will split over two days. Although less confined than the stretch of the Middle Fork Kings you just walked, you're still in a steep-walled canyon with granite walls towering overhead. Avalanches regularly pour down every gully on the north wall and the trail skirts around one alluvial fan after another, the ones here mostly covered in scrubby aspen; at least now the canyon is broad enough that the trail can loop around rather than over these fans. Much of the first 3 miles up Palisade Creek was burned in the 2002 lightning-started Palisade Fire; fallen logs crisscross the landscape, and young trees are establishing. Vegetation has grown rapidly and in places with sufficient water there are lush grass and colorful flower displays. Campsites are limited—look beneath surviving stands of lodgepole pine for the best options. Crossing through some particularly colorful meadows, the trail enters more continuous lodgepole pine forest and crosses the creek draining the Palisade Basin on large rocks. Just beyond are spacious campsites under lodgepole pine cover, Deer Meadow. The trail then loops slightly north to bypass a marshy expanse and crosses well-irrigated wildflower gardens before reentering forest cover, then fording many-channeled Glacier Creek. Beyond are more large campsites beneath red fir and lodgepole pine cover, a good staging point for tomorrow's stiff climb (8,890'; 37.05456°N, 118.51910°W).

Castle Domes along the Woods Creek Trail   Photo by Elizabeth Wenk

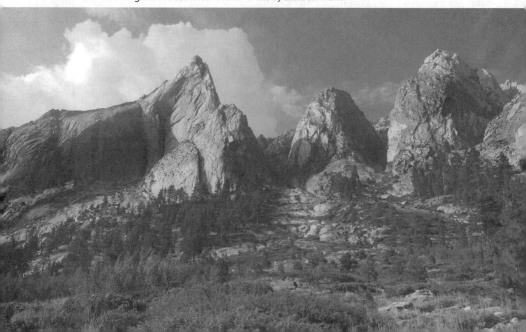

DAY 6 (Palisade Creek near Deer Meadow to South Fork Kings, 12.2 miles): Just a short distance past the campsites, you exit forest cover and begin an exposed 1,500-foot climb up switchbacks known as the Golden Staircase. Impressively built walls form the foundation for the switchbacks that make for a steep climb up a much steeper headwall. Completed in 1938, this was the last section of the JMT to be constructed. For stretches, the trail is dry and rocky, while elsewhere, small seeps provide water and nourish colorful flowers. During required breathers turn west to look downcanyon to the Black Divide, the serrated Devils Crags marking its southern end. The route-finding required to build this trail is phenomenal; notice how tight switchbacks take you up one joint-defined gully, only to have it dead-end in cliffs. The trail then traverses seamlessly to the next passable gully, letting you work your way up the face. The grade finally eases as the trail loops closer to Palisade Creek and crosses a polished bedrock knob. Passing small meadows and winding between rounded bluffs, the trail climbs to the outlet of the lower Palisade Lake. Here you'll find a large selection of currently overused campsites with brilliant views of the 14,000-foot Palisade Peaks.

Onward, the trail follows the lake's shore for a length and then zigzags upward, following benches across steeper bluffs. As you approach the upper Palisade Lake, you step across a succession of streamlets and reach some broader shelves well above lake level. Here you'll find a selection of small, exposed campsites beneath whitebark pine krummholz. Beyond, the trail continues its journey south across sandy-rocky slopes with scattered trees, then walks among meadowed creek corridors before tackling the headwall to Mather Pass. By 11,200 feet the trail is unpleasantly rocky, switchbacking up a seemingly endless, amazingly barren talus slope of bouldery moraines left by the last of the Pleistocene glaciers, the trail mostly filled with angular riprap. Hopefully, the occasional patches of Sierra primroses will be in bloom, distracting you with bursts of intense magenta.

Finally you reach the pleasantly broad top of Mather Pass, named for Stephen Mather, the first head of the National Park Service. Looking at the awe-inspiring view to the north, you see the full length of the North and Middle Palisade Peaks, with six points that extend above the 14,000-foot mark. To the southeast is Split Mountain, the southernmost of the Palisade fourteeners and the easiest of the peaks to ascend. You also look south across Upper Basin, the headwaters of the South Fork Kings and a delightfully flat slab basin cradling endless tarns. Two elongate strips of sand, moraine remnants, offer possible campsites, with others tucked wherever there is unvegetated sand.

In comparison to the long climb up the north side of Mather Pass, on the south side you have just nine switchbacks down the headwall, a long traverse across a sandier slope, a few final sandy switchbacks, and after just over a mile reach the first tarns. (The upper switchbacks can hold late snow—take care along this notoriously steep, icy stretch.) Sauntering onward, the trail follows the first of the morainal sand lumps and then traverses to the second, crisscrossing rivulets that will soon coalesce into the South Fork Kings. At 10,840 feet you cross to the western bank of the nascent river and enter lodgepole pine forest, continuing a pleasantly graded walk with nary a switchback. The slope is generally too angled to offer camping until you are below 10,400 feet, but then many options emerge, including large streamside campsites where an old trail once climbed to Taboose Pass (10,180'; 36.97435°N, 118.44280°W; no campfires).

DAY 7 (South Fork Kings to Twin Lakes, 8.0 miles): Today's suggested mileage is more modest and the walking easier. With an ever-lighter pack and better fitness you could easily continue farther down Woods Creek. However, unless you are trying to squeeze the next three days into two, there is no reason to rush downward. You begin with a short downward jaunt through lodgepole pine forest, passing an unmarked spur, an old trail that continues down the South Fork Kings and up over Cartridge Pass.

CARTRIDGE PASS AND SOUTH FORK KINGS

Your route follows the only possible trail loop to link the Middle and South Fork Kings Rivers. The old Cartridge Pass Trail used to provide another alternative, crossing the Monarch Divide at Cartridge Pass, traversing Lake Basin to Marion Lake and descending Cartridge Creek to where you camped on Day 4. While the trail from your current location along the South Fork Kings to the summit of Cartridge Pass can still be followed, the trail down Cartridge Creek has mostly vanished and is now a challenging off-trail route. The trail was popular for several decades in the early 1900s, as increasing numbers of Sierra Club groups sought to follow the crest-parallel "John Muir Trail", but the lack of a trail up the Golden Staircase forced them to detour west. Meanwhile, following the South Fork Kings itself to Paradise Valley has always remained a challenging cross-country route, eschewed even by seasoned Sierra explorers, for it includes several miles of willow-covered boulder hopping where the canyon walls pinch together.

Staying on the JMT, you quickly reach a notorious South Fork Kings crossing. Take care and walk upstream a stretch if the current is too swift. (If northbound hikers have mentioned this is a difficult crossing, you can much more easily cross at the last night's campsite and then follow the eastern riverbank south to here.) Ahead, a stiff switchbacking climb leads to an eastbound (left) junction with the current trail to Taboose Pass (Trip 70); the JMT stays right (south). Stepping across the creek draining Lake Marjorie, you reach a second junction where right (west) leads to Bench Lake (Trip 70) while the JMT continues left (again, south). Walking up shallow, open slopes above the creek and a lake, you may spy a large white tent to the east; this is the sometimes-staffed Bench Lake Ranger Station.

Continuing up the base of a sandy-gravelly moraine, you soon cut to its crest, where there are campsites near a tarn, and then drop back onto slabs near a creek crossing. A short traverse across slabs leads to a second creek, the outflow from Lake Majorie. Heading west (right) here leads to campsites alongside the two lakelets downstream of Lake Marjorie. Onward, the trail continues across sandy strips and over low-angle slabs, passing just the occasional whitebark pine to reach Lake Marjorie itself, a wonderful big, deep, round, vibrant lake. Talus spills into its western shores, while you are walking across delightful alpine turf and passing a final few Spartan campsites.

Zigzagging upward, you look down upon two more talus-bound lakes and soon a third. Your upward climb leads across rills and past endless well-irrigated alpine wildflower gardens. Nearly devoid of talus or cobble, the JMT carries you south to Pinchot Pass, ultimately squiggling up tight switchbacks to surmount the final blocky headwall (12,132').

From the summit, you have a brilliant view north to steep granite peaks, with the dark tip of distant Mount Goddard just visible. Farther northeast are the rugged Palisades. To the south is giant Colosseum Peak and cliffier Mount Cedric Wright, behind which the Woods Lake basin sits. While the pass is on granodiorite, the summit of Mount Wynne rising just to your east, as well as Mount Pinchot to the northeast and Crater Mountain to the southwest, are composed of ancient metamorphic rocks. The small patches of white in the otherwise red rock are bits of marble, the remains of ancient sea creatures.

You navigate down the south side of the craggy headwall and then cross flower-strewn alpine meadows, stepping across streamlets. Once you are past the uppermost meadows, the JMT curves east to traverse above an enchanting series of ponds and lakes. The trail once followed the meadow corridor downstream but has been rerouted to protect the fragile alpine turf. You continue winding south beneath Mount Perkins, reaching your first trailside campsite beside a small tarn on a morainal ridge with lodgepole pine. Below you sit the Twin Lakes and behind them Mount Cedric Wright. Descending more steeply, you approach the Twin Lakes outlet and good campsites (10,528'; 36.90687°N, 118.39867°W; no campfires). (There are campsites ahead both at the Sawmill Pass junction and along the JMT farther downstream, if you seek more shelter or want to complete some extra miles.)

DAY 8 (Twin Lakes to Upper Paradise Valley, 9.6 miles): Continuing along the JMT, after 0.5 mile, you pass the signed junction to the Sawmill Pass Trail (left, south); a few exposed campsites lie on the bench just east of this junction, across the multistranded creek. Descending more steeply now, the JMT drops into the sunstruck, southwest-trending canyon of Woods Creek, approaching the creek near a campsite at 9,800 feet, then following the creek's northern bank. The trail tread is generally rocky, mimicking the landscape, especially as it cuts across the base of a bedrock rib, composed of deformed granitoid rocks that are crisscrossed by darker-colored dikes. Weathered foxtail pine and juniper grow atop the bluffs and the stream cascades down its gorge.

Where the terrain flattens you cross an expansive alluvial fan, bisected by the White Fork. This creek is usually a trivial crossing, but it is, at times, notoriously swift and dangerous due to its bouldery bed. Continuing down the rugged canyon, you cross back onto lighter-colored granite as you reach the cascading outflow from the Window Peak drainage, while to your left, Woods Creek is now splashing vigorously down chutes. A length through greenleaf manzanita with scattered junipers and Jeffrey pine leads to a prominent junction. Here the JMT turns left (south) to cross Woods Creek on an impressive suspension bridge (Trip 22), while you stay right (west).

You continue downstream along Woods Creek, the Castle Domes looming to the north and the King Spur to the south. Sandy patches among the dark slabs offer view-rich campsites from which to admire the Castle Domes, bulbous domes and steep-fronted fins of rock divided by chasms. At Castle Domes Meadow the valley broadens, but the terrain is alternatively too vegetated or rocky to camp. Looping around a meadow lobe, the trail climbs to avoid steep riverside slabs, only dropping back to riparian red fir forest around 7,800 feet; nearby are some small campsites. The valley's character remains the same: lots of dry-site shrubs on slopes, occasional stands of conifers, and steep commanding granite walls. With continued descent, lodgepole pine and red fir are replaced by black oak, white fir, and ultimately incense cedar.

Soon you curve onto a west-facing slope that leads back into the South Fork Kings River drainage, landing in a dense, moist, valley-bottom forest, scattered with giant boulders from past floods. A final 0.15 mile up along the South Fork Kings takes you to a major bridge—or currently a pair of bridge pilings, for the bridge was washed out in 2017 and its replacement is still in progress as of 2020. Crossing the river, hopefully on a bridge again, you reach an expansive camping area with a bear box (6,940'; 36.86993°N, 118.51652°W). Arrow Creek falls is just visible on the eastern canyon wall.

DAY 9 (Upper Paradise Valley to Roads End, 9.0 miles): Your final day follows the South Fork Kings back to Cedar Grove. From here to the trailhead you may only camp in the designated camping areas in Upper Paradise Valley, Middle Paradise Valley (2.25 miles southwest), and Lower Paradise Valley (an additional 1.0 mile southwest). You drop just 300 feet over the miles to Lower Paradise Valley, walking mostly beneath a pleasant white fir canopy, although occasionally crossing a scrubbier, burned slope. The river is notably bigger, now the combined flow of the upper South Fork Kings and Woods Creek, but by late summer there are plenty of play spots, especially near the Middle Paradise Valley campsites.

At the west end of Lower Paradise Valley you pass a gigantic log jam, and suddenly the trail plunges down the steeper, narrowly V-shaped canyon. The route ahead was initially impassable for stock and a trail climbed west from Lower Paradise Valley across the rugged spur to join the Copper Creek Trail near Lower Tent Meadow. Today's trail hugs the base of the precipitous walls, almost always walking past talus deposits—sometimes rocks deposited by alluvial fans and elsewhere from rockfall overhead. The trail is well built to negotiate these obstacles; in one location there is even a causeway to work through house-size boulders. But the descent is still tough on your feet and knees. Sometimes you are beneath a canopy of black oak, live oak, white fir, and incense cedar and elsewhere in the open, while the tumbling river course is mostly well below you. The river's roar loudens as you approach Mist Falls and follow a few switchbacks to its base, where a spur trail leads to the river's banks. At high flow, the mist is so voluminous that you barely see the waterfall itself. Of this stretch of trail, Bolton Brown, an early Sierra mountaineer, commented in 1896, "It is as difficult as useless to specify the finest parts. It is all splendid." Hopefully you agree.

After one more downward pitch you are back in a flat valley-bottom forest and walk an easy mile to the junction with the Bubbs Creek Trail. Here you stay right (west) and complete the final leg to the trailhead. Initially you are under a lush canopy wandering past giant boulders, vestiges of past rockfall, but all too soon you emerge onto an objectionably wide, hot, dusty trail that leads to the car (5,020'; 36.79461°N, 118.58290°W).

A beautiful ponderosa pine along the South Fork Kings　　Photo by Elizabeth Wenk

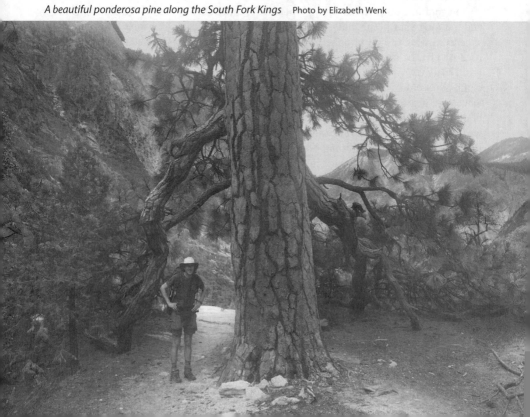

Cedar Grove Roadend Trailhead

5,020'; 36.79461°N, 118.58290°W

Destination/ GPS Coordinates	Trip Type	Best Season	Pace & Hiking/ Layover Days	Total Mileage	Permit Required
21 Lake Reflection 36.70521°N 118.44313°W	Out-and-back	Mid to late	Moderate 4/1	29.6	Bubbs Creek
22 Rae Lakes Loop 36.80638°N 118.39796°W (Middle Rae Lake)	Semiloop	Mid to late	Moderate 6/1	40.7	Woods Creek (Bubbs Creek in reverse of description)
20 Middle Fork–South Fork Kings River Loop (in reverse of description; see page 119)	Loop	Mid to late	Strenuous 9/1	78.7	Woods Creek (Copper Creek as described)

INFORMATION AND PERMITS: The trailhead is in Kings Canyon National Park. Permits are required for overnight stays and quotas apply. Permits can be reserved up to six months in advance at recreation.gov/permits/445857, with additional details at nps.gov/seki/plan yourvisit/wilderness_permits.htm. For both advance reservations (67% of quota) and walk-up permits (33% of quota), there is a $15-per-permit processing fee and a $5-per-person reservation fee. Both reserved and walk-up permits for this trailhead must be picked up in person at the Roads End Permit Station, open 7 a.m.–3:30 p.m. daily. This is located at the far eastern end of Kings Canyon, so-called Roads End, conveniently located at your trailhead—park your car and pick up your permit. Campfires are prohibited above 10,000 feet. Bear canisters are required.

DRIVING DIRECTIONS: From the CA 99–CA 180 interchange in Fresno, take CA 180 east into Kings Canyon National Park. After 54.3 miles you pass the Kings Canyon National Park entrance station and then at 56.0 miles reach a T-junction where you turn left, still on CA 180. Continue another 35.7 miles to Roads End. Here there are two parking areas: one to the south servicing the Roads End Trailhead (Woods Creek and Bubbs Creek) and also the day use trail to Zumwalt Meadows and one to the north, adjacent to the Copper Creek Trailhead. There are a toilet and garbage receptacles between the two, a water tap at the permit station, and bear boxes at both parking lots.

see map on p. 132

trip 21   Lake Reflection

Trip Data: 36.70521°N, 118.44313°W; 29.6 miles; 4/1 days
Topos: *The Sphinx, Mount Clarence King, Mount Brewer*

HIGHLIGHTS: Those who appreciate the serenity of high, alpine lake basins will find this trip to the upper reaches of East Creek a rewarding choice. Excellent fishing amid spellbinding surroundings makes this a fine trip for anglers. Nonanglers can while away the time simply soaking up the country.

HEADS UP! *Bears are a serious problem in this area and bear canisters are required for trips on any portion of the popular Rae Lakes Loop out of Cedar Grove. The area around Lake Reflection can be quite windy.*

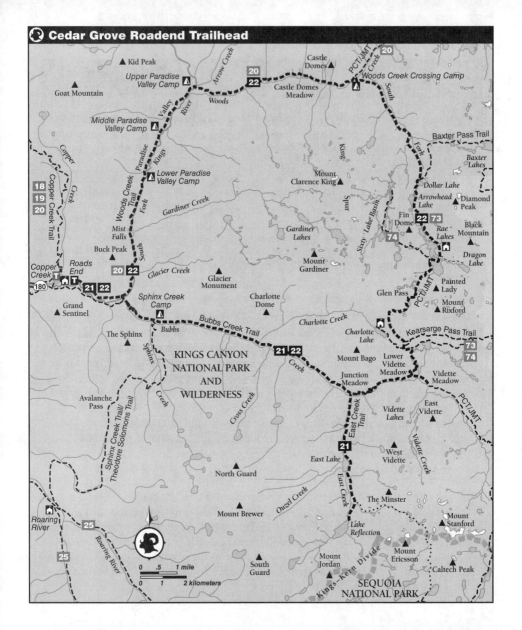

DAY 1 (Cedar Grove Roadend Trailhead to Charlotte Creek, 7.2 miles): Since the climb is hot and dry, an early start is highly recommended. From the paved road-end loop (5,036'), the wide, sandy trail heads generally east through a mixed forest of ponderosa pines, incense cedars, black oaks, sugar pines, and white fir. Soon, the shade is left behind amid a sparse cover of ponderosa pines.

EARLY HISTORY
The balmy climate characteristic of the gently sloping canyon floor made Kings Canyon a favorite of Native Americans, who camped here from spring to fall. Foraging parties of Yokuts established spur camps along Bubbs Creek at many of the same spots currently used by modern-day backpackers.

Soon, the trail enters a shady, dense forest of alders, white firs, ponderosa pines, and sugar pines on the way to a junction with the Woods Creek Trail, branching north. Head right (southeast) at the junction and cross a steel bridge over South Fork Kings River just below its confluence with Bubbs Creek. Past the bridge is another junction, where the Kanawyer Loop and Bubbs Creek Trails meet. Continue ahead (southeast) up the Bubbs Creek Trail and follow a series of short, wood bridges across braided Bubbs Creek.

> **PINYON PINES**
>
> Along the climb up Bubbs Creek, you may notice a rarity for this side of the Sierra: pinyon pines. This single-needle pine, quite common to the lower elevations on the east side of the Sierra, has a distinctive spherical cone, the fruit of which is the tasty pine nut. Most noticeable about the cone is the very thick, blunt, four-sided scale.

A moderate climb leads to the first of many switchbacks climbing away from the floor of the canyon and up the Bubbs Creek drainage.

The stiff ascent offers fine views for the panting backpacker down into the dramatic, U-shaped South Fork Kings River canyon. On the south wall of Bubbs Creek canyon, the dominating landmark is the pronounced granite point named the Sphinx. To the east, Sphinx Creek cuts a sharp-lipped defile on the peak's east shoulder.

Above the switchbacks, the moderately ascending trail heads into tall, shady conifers on the way to a junction with the southbound Sphinx Creek Trail. Continue ahead (east) here to Sphinx Creek Camp (6,280'). Excellent campsites with bear boxes are here on either side of Bubbs Creek; to access the southbank sites, turn right (south) toward Avalanche Pass, cross the creek on a wooden bridge, and almost immediately turn left to reach them.

From Sphinx Creek Camp, continue ahead, eastbound on the Bubbs Creek Trail, traveling in and out of mixed forest for the next few miles. Well past the crossings of a trio of tiny brooks, ford Charlotte Creek and reach a path that leads to pleasant, tree-shaded campsites (bear box; 7,360'; 36.77103°N, 118.48478°W) near the bank of Bubbs Creek. Fishing may be good for brown, brook, rainbow, and golden-rainbow hybrid.

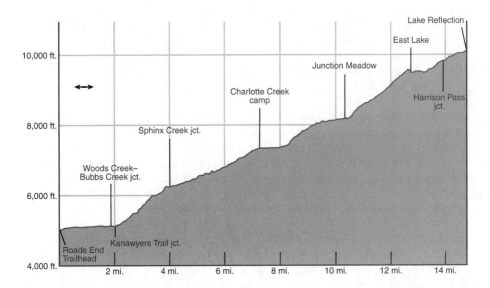

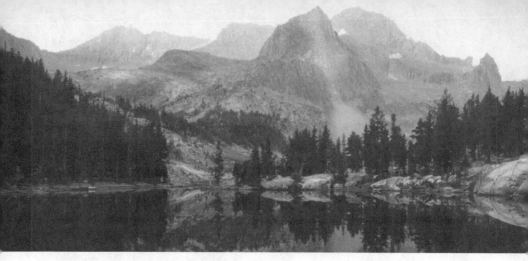

Lake Reflection   Photo by Elizabeth Wenk

DAY 2 (Charlotte Creek to Lake Reflection, 7.6 miles): Alternating stretches of lush foliage and dry slopes greet you for the next few miles on a steady ascent away from Charlotte Creek. Across periodic clearings, Mount Bago looms above the north side of Bubbs Creek's steep-walled canyon. Reach some campsites, stroll through a gap in a drift fence, and pass a horse camp on the way to lengthy Junction Meadow (8,190'), carpeted with lush grasses, wildflowers, and ferns. Near the far end of the meadow is a signed junction with the East Creek Trail.

Turn right (south) and follow the East Creek Trail across the dense foliage of the meadow to a wet ford of Bubbs Creek (difficult in early season). Past the creek, the trail ascends East Creek's canyon via rocky switchbacks zigzagging through a sparse-to-moderate cover of lodgepoles, western white pines, firs, and aspens. The red metamorphic rocks of Mount Bago dominate the vista to the north, with Mount Gardiner coming into view just behind. As you reach the top of the first rise, look for the peaks of the Kings–Kern Divide. Anglers may find small rainbow and brook trout in East Creek; the fish in East Lake may be a bit larger.

Following a brief stretch of moderate climbing, the trail crosses a bridge over East Creek and then climbs steadily along the east bank. The grade gets steeper where the trail enters a forest of pines and firs. After the ford of an unnamed, fern-lined stream, the grade eases near the outlet of East Lake. Fortunate hikers may spot one of the many mule deer that frequent East Lake's picturesque, grass-fringed waters. The trail rounds the east shore to good campsites in dense forest near the head of the lake. The barren, unjointed granite walls rising on either side—especially Mount Brewer on the west—provide an impressive backdrop.

At the head of East Lake, you pass a large campsite with a bear box. Beyond, the trail climbs steadily south past a drift fence and through rock-broken stands of lodgepole and foxtail pine. Just before crossing a 50-yard rockpile, bypass an unsigned junction with the cross-country route toward Harrison Pass. Beyond this talus slope, the easy grade traverses many wet areas along the east side of East Creek to good campsites beside the little lake below and at the northeast end of Lake Reflection (10,072'; 36.70521°N, 118.44313°W; no campfires). Anglers should find good fishing for golden, rainbow, and hybrids. When breezes fail to stir the lake's surface, the tableau of peaks reflected in the mirrored waters is a memorable scene of a scope seldom matched in the Sierra. At the head of the cirque basin, all side excursions are straight up, but your effort is repaid by great views and a sense of achievement shared by many mountaineers.

DAYS 3–4 (Lake Reflection to Cedar Grove Roadend Trailhead, 14.8 miles): Retrace your steps to the trailhead.

see map on p. 132

trip 22 **Rae Lakes Loop**

Trip Data: 36.80638°N, 118.39796°W; 40.7 miles, 6/1 days
Topos: *The Sphinx, Mount Clarence King*

HIGHLIGHTS: This fine and very popular trip circles King Spur. The scenery en route is dramatic enough to challenge the most accomplished photographer or artist as the trail ascends the glacially carved canyon of South Fork Kings River, visits the exceptionally beautiful Rae Lakes, makes a breath-taking ascent of Glen Pass, circles beneath the towering ramparts of the Videttes and Kearsarge Pinnacles, and then returns down the canyon of dashing Bubbs Creek.

HEADS UP! *See nps.gov/seki/planyourvisit/rae-lakes-loop.htm for the latest informa-tion on and regulations affecting this heavily visited area. Due to heavy use, camping at Arrowhead Lake, Dollar Lake, and each of the Rae Lakes is restricted to a single night. There is a two-night limit at Charlotte Lake. In Paradise Valley, camping is limited to designated sites at three camps (two-night limit). Crafty bears have made the use of approved bear canisters mandatory on this route. Along the Rae Lakes, the permanent metal food-storage boxes are reserved for use by thru-hikers on the Pacific Crest Trail (PCT) and John Muir Trail (JMT) only. Campfires are not permitted above 10,000 feet.*

DAY 1 (Cedar Grove Roadend Trailhead to Middle Paradise Valley Camp, 6.7 miles): From the paved road-end loop (5,036'), the wide, sandy trail heads east through a mixed forest of ponderosa pines, incense cedars, black oaks, sugar pines, and white firs. Soon, the shade is left behind as a result of a previous fire. The trail enters a shady, dense forest of alders, white firs, ponderosa pines, and sugar pines on the way to a junction with the Bubbs Creek Trail on the right, where, in a few days, you'll close the loop.

For now, turn left (north) on the Woods Creek Trail along the river, which, in this stretch, is broad and peaceful, and ascend moderately under a cover of conifers, alders, black oaks, and live oaks. In sunny spots, slopes are covered with chaparral, including silk-tasseled mountain mahogany and manzanita. Soon, the river swirls, leaps, and pools through a nar-row channel, and the canyon walls soar on both sides. Open granite slabs offer opportunities for rest stops with excellent views downcanyon to the Sphinx and Avalanche Peak. Soon reach Mist Falls, a spectacle of tumbling whitewater in early season that becomes sedate and subdued by late season. Most day hikers will be left behind above the falls.

The trail continues climbing to the lower end of Paradise Valley, while the river dashes straight down the canyon. The grade eases to gentle once the trail curves into Paradise Valley (6,640'), beneath a mixed forest cover of lodgepole pine, red fir, Jeffrey pine, and a smattering of aspen and juniper. Soon arrive at Lower Paradise Valley Camp, with desig-nated campsites, a pit toilet, and bear boxes. Proceed on a gentle stroll alongside the sedate river to Middle Paradise Valley Camp (6,641'; 36.84777°N, 118.53577°W), with more des-ignated campsites and bear boxes.

DAY 2 (Middle Paradise Valley Camp to Woods Creek Crossing Camp, 7.9 miles): Con-tinue upstream (north) on easy trail through alternating stands of mixed conifers and clearings with awesome views of the steep-walled canyon. A moderate stretch of climbing followed by another gentle stroll near a flower-filled meadow leads to Upper Paradise Val-ley Camp (6,190'), with more designated sites and bear boxes. *Note:* Immediately beyond the camp, the bridge that provided a straightforward crossing to the east side of South Fork Kings River, upstream from its confluence with Woods Creek, was washed out during the winter of 2016–17. The bridge is scheduled to be replaced in the 2021 summer season. Without the bridge, the ford of the river can be extremely hazardous, especially in early season—check with the park service regarding current conditions.

Now on the north side of Woods Creek, the trail curves east, rising steeply at first and then following an undulating ascent eastward on a moderate grade up the canyon, crossing two unnamed tributaries along the way. Wind through Castle Domes Meadow, named for the obvious landmarks to the north. Stands of water-loving quaking aspen dot the banks of Woods Creek.

Away from the meadow, the underfooting is alternately sandy and rocky as the trail climbs. The forest cover includes more and more lodgepole pines, corresponding to the increase in altitude. Where the path meets the PCT/JMT, turn right (south) and soon cross roaring Woods Creek on a swaying suspension bridge, built in 1988 and dubbed the "Golden Gate of the Sierra." (Obviously, this crossing would be extremely difficult without the bridge). On the creek's south side, find overused but welcome, fair-to-good campsites beneath Jeffrey and lodgepole pines with bear boxes nearby (8,520'; 36.87340°N, 118.43762°W). Although campfires are legal, most of the available firewood is usually gone by midsummer at this popular stop along the PCT/JMT.

DAY 3 (Woods Creek Crossing Camp to Rae Lakes, 6.3 miles): Follow the JMT/PCT southeast to begin the long climb up South Fork Woods Creek. Juniper and red fir provide forest cover on the way past several adequate campsites along the creek to the left.

Presently, the trail rounds the base of King Spur, leaves forest cover, and begins a hot, exposed climb up South Fork Woods Creek, staying well above the stream. Legal campsites are almost nonexistent along this stretch of the JMT/PCT up to the junction with the trail to Baxter Pass. Resist the temptation to pitch a tent on the inviting patches of alpine grass along the way: These pockets of grass can live for decades—some clumps are known to be more than 50 years old—but can't survive repeated use by campers.

Jump over the rivulet that hurries down from Lake 10,296 and enter an open, rocky area. Beyond, a wooden span provides an easy crossing of a boggy meadow. Pass through a drift fence, ascend a rocky ridge, and then pass by a pair of fair campsites near the crossing of a willow-and-flower-lined stream that drains Sixty Lake Basin. Across the canyon, Baxter Creek stitches a ribbon of water down a rock-ribbed slope.

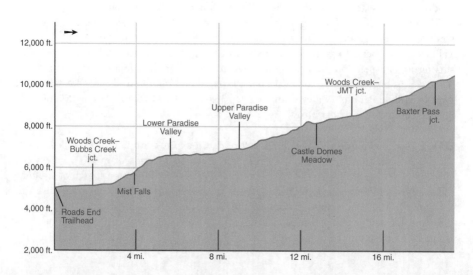

A mile-long ascent through diminishing forest cover affords fine views ahead of the peaked monolith of Fin Dome, heralding the approach to the beautiful Rae Lakes. To the right (southwest) are the impressive steel-gray ramparts of King Spur. In contrast, the massive, sloping Sierra Crest in the east is made up of much darker granitic rocks. Finally, ascend a low, rounded spur and reach a junction with the Baxter Pass Trail, just north of Dollar Lake, where the sign indicates the trail is not maintained; indeed it is difficult to follow in places. The setting of jewellike Dollar Lake is magnificent; lodgepoles crowd the shore amid granite outcroppings, and Fin Dome, along with some blackish spires beyond, provides a jagged backdrop for the mirrored surface of the lake.

Go ahead (south) at the junction, pass west of Dollar Lake and some small ponds, and then ford South Fork Woods Creek below Arrowhead Lake. Continue up the canyon on the east side of the lake chain. The long black striations seen along the face of Diamond Peak and the ridge that extends to the north are metamorphosed lava—one of the few remaining bits of volcanic evidence to be found in this area.

With the familiar landmark of distinctive Fin Dome in sight, pass a lateral to campsites with a bear box on the north side of Arrowhead Lake and continue above the east side of the lake. Climb high above the creek through widely scattered lodgepole pines past a small, unnamed lake on the way to the Rae Lakes. Campsites and bear boxes are found near the lower two lakes (Middle Rae Lake: 10,610'; 36.80638°N, 118.39796°W; no campfires), and a summer ranger station tucked into the trees above the second lake (10,620'; 36.81093°N, 118.40005°W) sometimes provides emergency services. The highest lake's shores are rocky-marshy and offer no good camping, but higher Dragon Lake does offer suitable campsites (see Day 4).

RAE LAKES

A camp at one of the Rae Lakes should be among the best and longest remembered of the trip, simply because of the extraordinary views: the rugged granite Fin Dome reflected in the still waters of the lake; the jagged King Spur beyond; and, if you are camped at one of the higher lakes, multicolored Painted Lady to the south. Glistening slabs of granite and pockets of verdant, flower-sprinkled meadow surround the island-dotted lakes. Despite the area's popularity, fishing may be good for brook and rainbow trout.

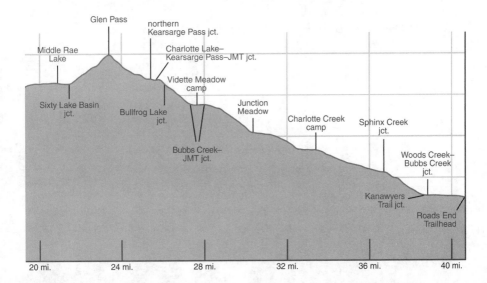

DAY 4 (Rae Lakes to Vidette Meadow Camp, 6.8 miles): The gently ascending trail goes south from the middle lake and, after just 0.1 mile, passes an old trail that heads east to more secluded camping around Dragon Lake. Stay on the PCT/JMT here. The path then bends west around the north shoreline of the highest of the Rae Lakes (10,541'), fords the creek at the narrow "isthmus" separating the near-rockbound highest lake from the rest of the chain (on logs), and comes to a junction with a well-trod trail into Sixty Lake Basin, an extremely worthy destination for a layover day (also see Trip 74).

From the Sixty Lake Basin junction, turn left (south) on the JMT/PCT and begin the climb toward Glen Pass, following switchbacks through diminishing pockets of vegetation to a tarn-filled bench covered with talus. A winding ascent leads to the crest of a ridge and then a short traverse to 11,978-foot Glen Pass. The view from the pass is somewhat disappointing when compared to other High Sierra passes, but there is a fine, farewell glimpse of the Rae Lakes.

A winding, rocky descent switchbacks past a pair of green, rockbound tarns on the way to a crossing of a seasonal stream with a pair of poor campsites nearby. The trail continues the descent through an extensive boulder field until more hospitable terrain appears where the trail veers southeast. The grade eases on a descending traverse across a whitebark and foxtail pine–covered hillside above Charlotte Lake. Gaps in the pines allow brief views of the lake and granite Charlotte Dome farther down Charlotte Creek. At 2.3 miles from the pass, reach a junction with a connecting trail to Kearsarge Pass. Go right (south), staying on the JMT/PCT, and soon breaking out of the forest to fine views of Mount Bago. Stroll across a sandy flat to a four-way junction. From here, the Kearsarge Pass Trail heads northeast and the Charlotte Lake Trail heads northwest 0.8 mile to the lake, with excellent campsites (two-night limit) and a seasonal ranger station.

Go straight ahead on the JMT/PCT and head southeast, away from the sandy flat and over a low rise. Follow tight switchbacks downhill through open forest to a junction with the Bullfrog Lake Trail, which climbs northeast to the extremely picturesque lake (no camping). Continue ahead (south-southwest, then southeast) on the descent, crossing Bull-frog Lake's outlet twice on the way to Lower Vidette Meadow and a junction with Bubbs Creek Trail. At the junction, turn left (east), remaining on the JMT/PCT, ford the outlet of Bullfrog Lake again, and after 0.4 mile arrive at the good and possibly crowded campsites at Vidette Meadow Camp (9,542'; 36.75925°N, 118.40699°W) along Bubbs Creek and near

View south to Center Basin, East Vidette, and toward Forester Pass   Photo by Mike White

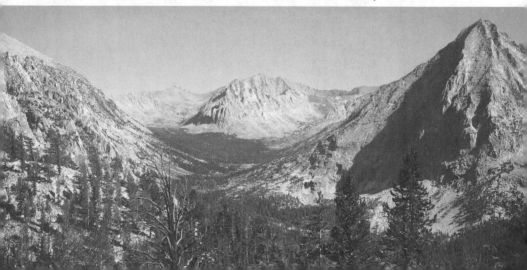

beautiful Vidette Meadow; the bear box that was previously available here is currently locked. Fishing for brook and rainbow trout is reported to be fair.

DAY 5 (Vidette Meadow Camp to Charlotte Creek, 5.8 miles): Retrace your steps 0.4 mile to the junction of the JMT/PCT and the Bubbs Creek Trail. Turn left (west), make a short descent, and pass to the north of Lower Vidette Meadow. Excellent campsites with a bear box are nestled beneath lodgepole pines along the fringe of the meadow. Leaving the gentle grade near the meadows, the trail begins a more pronounced descent along the now tumbling creek plunging down the gorge. Break out into the open momentarily near a large granite hump that provides an excellent vantage point for surveying the surrounding terrain.

Head back into the trees and continue down the canyon, generally west, stepping over numerous meadow-lined rivulets along the way. Periodic switchbacks mark the descent, along with occasional views of the topography above East Creek, including such notable landmarks as Mount Brewer, North Guard, and Mount Farquhar. The stiff, protracted descent eventually eases near the grassy, fern-filled, and wildflower-covered clearing of Junction Meadow (8,190'). Reach the signed junction with the East Creek Trail heading south to East Lake and Lake Reflection (Trip 21). Overnighters can find passable campsites a short way down the trail on either side of the ford of Bubbs Creek; additional campsites are farther down Bubbs Creek, past the large horse camp at the west edge of Junction Meadow.

Go right (ahead, northwest) at this junction. Away from the meadow, the moderate descent resumes as you stroll alongside turbulent Bubbs Creek through a moderate forest, composed primarily of firs. After nearly 2 miles of steady descent, Bubbs Creek mellows, and gently graded trail leads through a grove of aspens on the way to the ford of Charlotte Creek. Just before the ford, a path leads to pleasant, tree-shaded campsites (bear box; about 7,360'; 36.77103°N, 118.48478°W) near the bank of Bubbs Creek. Fishing may be good for brown, brook, rainbow, and golden-rainbow hybrid trout to 10 inches.

DAY 6 (Charlotte Creek to Cedar Grove Roadend Trailhead, 7.2 miles): The trail continues descending gradually for a while past Charlotte Creek, as you hop across a trio of streams and stroll through shoulder-high ferns, before Bubbs Creek returns to its tumultuous course down the gorge. A steady, moderate descent follows the tumbling stream over the next several miles before arriving at Sphinx Creek Camp and a junction with the Sphinx Creek Trail.

From here, continue ahead (west, downstream) on the Bubbs Creek Trail to a lengthy series of switchbacks that drop to the floor of Kings Canyon. At the bottom of the canyon, follow a series of short, wood bridges over multibranched Bubbs Creek, go ahead (northwest) at the next junction, cross a steel bridge over South Fork Kings River, and soon reach a signed junction with the Woods Creek Trail. The loop closes here.

From the junction, go left (west) to retrace your steps 1.9 miles to the trailhead.

PINYON PINES

Along the climb up Bubbs Creek, you may notice a rarity for this side of the Sierra: pinyon pines. This single-needle pine, quite common to the lower elevations on the east side of the Sierra, has a distinctive spherical cone, the fruit of which is the tasty pine nut. Most noticeable about the cone is the very thick, blunt, four-sided scale.

CA 198 (GENERALS HIGHWAY) TRIPS

Generals Highway winds through parts of Sequoia National Forest and along the western edge of Sequoia National Park, passing the Sierra's most famous sequoia grove, the Giant Forest. From the Generals Highway, a number of spur roads travel a short distance east to roadend trailheads. The trailheads described in this book are all distinguished by midelevation starts, making for more moderate ascents than the Cedar Grove (CA 180) Trips. They offer both nearby lake destinations and quite easy access to the rugged peaks along the Great Western Divide, a crest that divides southern Kings Canyon National Park and all of Sequoia National Park in half.

Four trailheads are included in this book: Big Meadows, Twin Lakes (Lodgepole Campground), Wolverton Corral, and Crescent Meadow. Big Meadows Trailhead lies in Sequoia National Forest and leads into little Jennie Lakes Wilderness, split between the South Fork Kings River and North Fork Kaweah watersheds. Departing from the Lodgepole Campground, the Twin Lakes Trail similarly leads through conifer forest to lake basins on the Silliman Crest, the Kings River–Kaweah River divide. It is also the departure point for the longest hike in this book, Trip 25, which takes advantage of the easy terrain in this corner of Kings Canyon National Park to access two remote glacial canyons, Cloud Canyon and Deadman Canyon, and the rugged landscapes beyond. Two trails depart from the Wolverton Corral, the Lakes Trail and a popular connector to the Alta Trail. The Alta Trail, described here, traverses high above the Middle Fork Kaweah to reach perched Alta Meadow and nearby Alta Peak, while the Lakes Trail (not included) accesses overused (but gorgeous) Pear Lake. It is not included primarily because permits cannot be reserved, making it difficult to plan this as your destination. Finally, the High Sierra Trail leaves from Crescent Meadow in the Giant Forest, cutting a magnificent path dominated by canyons and gorges through the southern High Sierra, then leading to the summit of Mount Whitney.

Trailheads: Big Meadows

Twin Lakes (Lodgepole Campground)

Wolverton Corral

Crescent Meadow

Big Meadows Trailhead   7,612'; 36.71749°N, 118.83378°W

Destination/ GPS Coordinates	Trip Type	Best Season	Pace & Hiking/ Layover Days	Total Mileage	Permit Required
23 Jennie Lakes 36.68169°N 118.76322°W (Jennie Lake)	Semiloop	Early to mid	Leisurely 3/0	18.6	self-registration at trailhead

INFORMATION AND PERMITS: This trailhead is in Sequoia National Forest: Hume Lake Ranger District, 35860 East Kings Canyon Road, Dunlap, CA 93621; 559-338-2251, fs.usda .gov/sequoia. You can self-register for entry into Jennie Lakes Wilderness at the trailhead. You must also have a California campfire permit (available at ranger stations or online at preventwildfireca.org/campfire-permit) in order to have a campfire or use a stove. If you plan on entering Sequoia and Kings Canyon National Parks from Jennie Lakes Wilderness for an overnight stay, you must have a valid permit from the parks (picked up at Kings Canyon Visitor Center in Grant Grove). Bear canisters are not required but are strongly encouraged.

DRIVING DIRECTIONS: From the CA 99–CA 180 interchange in Fresno, take CA 180 east into Kings Canyon National Park. After 54.3 miles you pass the Kings Canyon National Park entrance station, and then at 56.0 miles reach a T-junction where you turn right onto Generals Highway/CA 198. Drive south along Generals Highway 6.4 miles to Big Meadows Road/FS 14S11. Turn left (northeast) and drive 3.5 miles to the Big Meadows Trailhead parking lot, equipped with vault toilets.

trip 23   Jennie Lakes

see map on p. 142

> **Trip Data:** 36.68169°N, 118.76322°W (Jennie Lake); 18.6 miles; 3/0 days
>
> **Topos:** *Muir Grove, Mount Silliman*

HIGHLIGHTS: A peaceful alternative to the popular backcountry in adjacent Kings Canyon National Park, this stroll through Jennie Lakes Wilderness leads backpackers along rushing streams, through shady forests, and across flower-filled meadows to a pair of pleasant lakes with craggy backdrops.

DAY 1 (Big Meadows Trailhead to Weaver Lake, 3.4 miles): A sign near the restroom points the way to the start of the trail heading southeast up a wooded hillside and across the paved access road. A short descent leads to a wooden bridge across a sluggish stretch of Big Meadows Creek to a trail register. From there, gradually traverse the base of a granite hump, and then curve along a delightful, spring-fed tributary of Big Meadows Creek. Through a mixed forest of red firs, lodgepole pines, and Jeffrey pines, briefly follow this stream south to a ford.

Away from the crossing, the trail makes a moderate climb around an exposed ridge with a momentary view over lupine and manzanita of Monarch Divide and Shell Mountain. Continuing the arc around the ridge, you pass verdant Fox Meadow and then climb to a streamside junction, 2 miles from the trailhead, where the loop part of this trip begins.

Head left (northeast) across the stream from the junction into signed Jennie Lakes Wilderness and follow the path eastward through alternating sections of scattered to light forest and shrub-covered clearings. After 1.1 miles, reach a junction with the lateral to Weaver Lake.

Turn right (east and then south) onto the lateral and wind uphill through mixed forest sprinkled with boulders 0.3 mile to Weaver Lake (8,709'; 36.70489°N, 118.79776°W). The whitish granite of Shell Mountain creates a fine backdrop, mirrored in the lake's usually

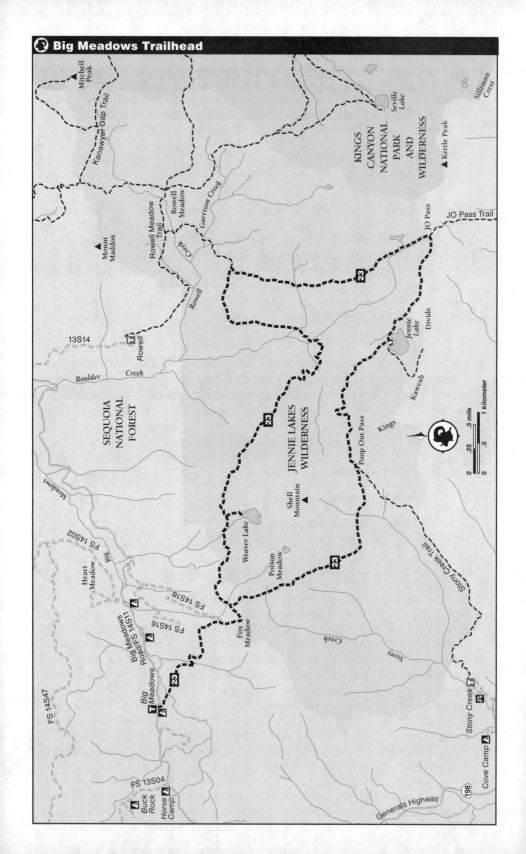

placid surface. Campsites pepper the shoreline, the least crowded of which seem to be above the south shore amid a grove of conifers. Anglers will be tempted by the resident brook trout, but the easily reached lake appears to be heavily fished.

DAY 2 (Weaver Lake to Jennie Lake, 8.8 miles): Retrace your steps 0.3 mile from Weaver Lake to the junction, and turn right (northeast) to follow less-used tread on a moderate climb toward Rowell Meadow. Proceed through a mixed forest of firs, lodgepole pines, and western white pines across a pair of saddles and then down to the head of Boulder Creek's canyon. After multiple crossings of the creek's tributaries, climb northward up the west-facing wall of the canyon. Shade from a scattered-to-light forest greets you where the path bends east over the crest of a ridge and then descends to a Y-junction with the trail to Rowell Meadow.

Turn sharply right at the junction to head south on a gradual climb to the crest of a rise. From the rise, descend gently, then moderately, enjoying occasional glimpses of Shell Mountain through the trees and crossing back over a lushly lined tributary of Boulder Creek. A lengthy climb follows, past slabs and boulders and across a small stream draining a hidden pond 0.1 mile east of the trail. Eventually, the ascent leads to JO Pass (9,444') and a junction, 2.5 miles from the Rowell Meadows junction.

Turn right (west) and follow the crest of an undulating ridge until switchbacks lead northwest down the hillside, from which you have momentary views of Jennie Lake through the trees. At 1.4 miles from JO Pass, find a junction with the short lateral to the lake and turn left (south). Like Weaver Lake, Jennie Lake (9,057'; 36.68169°N, 118.76322°W) is backdropped by impressive granite cliffs and rimmed by a light forest of red firs and lodgepole pines. Jennie Lake is larger than Weaver Lake. Overnighters can locate decent campsites on either side of the driftwood-choked outlet. Anglers may have better luck here than at Weaver, since Jennie is twice as far from the nearest trailhead and fishing pressure should be quite a bit less.

DAY 3 (Jennie Lake to Big Meadows Trailhead, 6.4 miles): Retrace your steps along the lateral to the main trail, turn left (northwest), and follow a gentle decline before making an ascending westward traverse with fine views of the Monarch Divide along the way. Following the traverse, a steep, winding climb concludes at Poop Out Pass (9,140'). A short descent from the pass brings you to a junction with the Stony Creek Trail.

Turn right (west) at the junction and make a moderate descent across the southern slopes of Shell Mountain to a crossing of a nascent, twin-channeled tributary of Stony Creek. From the creek, a gradual ascent around the nose of a ridge leads to a traverse across the west slope of Shell Mountain. Mostly open terrain allows excellent views of Big Baldy, Chimney Rock, and, if the ubiquitous haze miraculously abates, the San Joaquin Valley.

Return to forest cover as the track curves north-northwest, crosses a brook, and follows a moderate descent across a second rivulet to Poison Meadow. Past the meadow, cross a third little stream, exit the signed Jennie Lakes Wilderness, and soon arrive at the junction where you close the loop. Turn left (south) and retrace your steps 2 miles to the trailhead.

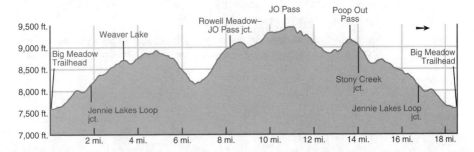

Twin Lakes Trailhead
(Lodgepole Campground)
6,778'; 36.60580°N, 118.72289°W

Destination/ GPS Coordinates	Trip Type	Best Season	Pace & Hiking/ Layover Days	Total Mileage	Permit Required
24 Ranger Lake 36.66749°N 118.69607°W	Out-and-back	Mid to late	Moderate 2/1	20.0	Twin Lakes
25 Deadman and Cloud Canyons 36.61860°N 118.50105°W (Colby Pass)	Semiloop	Mid to late	Strenuous 11/2	113.4	Twin Lakes

INFORMATION AND PERMITS: This trailhead is in Sequoia National Park. Permits are required for overnight stays and quotas apply. Permits can be reserved up to six months in advance at recreation.gov/permits/445857, with additional details at nps.gov/seki/planyour visit/wilderness_permits.htm. For both advance reservations (67% of quota) and walk-up permits (33% of quota), there is a $15-per-permit processing fee and a $5-per-person reservation fee. Both reserved and walk-up permits for this trailhead must be picked up in person at the Lodgepole Visitor Center, open 7 a.m.–3:30 p.m. daily. This is located toward the western side of the complex at Lodgepole. Campfires are prohibited above 10,000 feet in Kings Canyon National Park, above 9,000 feet in Sequoia National Park when west of the Great Western Divide, and above 10,000 feet in Sequoia National Park when east of the Great Western Divide. Bear canisters are not required but are strongly encouraged.

DRIVING DIRECTIONS: From the CA 99–CA 180 interchange in Fresno, take CA 180 east into Kings Canyon National Park. After 54.3 miles you pass the Kings Canyon National Park entrance station and then at 56.0 miles reach a T-junction where you turn right onto Generals Highway/CA 198. Drive south along Generals Highway 24.6 miles, then turn left toward the Lodgepole Visitor Center and Lodgepole Campground. After just 0.2 mile turn left into the visitor center parking lot to obtain your permit. All facilities you need are available within the store-and-visitor-center complex. Afterward, drive your car an additional 0.4 mile along the Lodgepole Road, past the campground entrance station to a large overnight parking area with bear boxes. The trailhead itself is another 0.2 mile to the east: continue along the campground road, cross the Marble Fork Kaweah, pass the Tokopah Trailhead, and then find the Twin Lakes Trailhead on your right.

trip 24   Ranger Lake

see map on p. 146

Trip Data: 36.66749°N, 118.69607°W; 20.0 miles; 2/1 days
Topos: Lodgepole, Mount Silliman

HIGHLIGHTS: Crossing the Silliman Crest on the boundary between Sequoia and Kings Canyon National Parks, this trip terminates at picturesque Ranger Lake. En route, the trail passes through fir forests, skirts flowery meadows, traces rambling brooks, and passes between a pair of shallow lakes whose inviting waters tempt dusty hikers. If 10.0 miles and 3,850 feet of elevation gain is too stiff a day, you can easily break the trip over two days, staying at either the campsites near the JO Pass junction or at Twin Lakes, crossing Silliman Pass on Day 2.

DAY 1 (Twin Lakes Trailhead [Lodgepole Campground] to Ranger Lake, 10.0 miles): The trailhead is toward the back of the Lodgepole Campground, marked with a large placard: you cross the Marble Fork Kaweah on a bridge (toward sites 151–214), pass the trailhead to Tokopah Falls, and then just before the campground road forks find the signed Twin Lakes Trailhead. The trail loops behind campsites and slowly bends from north to west, beginning a long climb up the moraine confining the valley from the north. It is a wide trail, constructed at a pleasant grade, mostly under a cover of ponderosa pine, incense cedar, and white fir, with an occasional sugar pine. Only the continued traffic noise below is a deterrent. Rounding the corner north into the Silliman Creek drainage, the trail continues to a junction, where left (west) leads to Wuksachi Lodge and you continue straight ahead (north). *Note:* This trail is not mapped on USGS 7.5' topos.

The trail continues a gentle ascent, winding through a mixed-conifer forest to reach Silliman Creek. This creek cuts down the center of a big, bouldery steep channel—a rock hop by midsummer, but a very dangerous crossing at high flow. Continuing, the trail zigzags out of the Silliman Creek drainage, cuts across a steep slope, and curves into the tributary exiting Cahoon Meadow. Passing a small campsite at the meadow's edge, the first legal site on the trail, the trail ascends a ridge through dry white fir forest. The trail then cuts more to the north, angling in and out of a series of minor, seasonal streamlets as it continues up pleasant forest duff and across sand toward Cahoon Gap. Excepting the flower-dotted banks of brooks, the west-facing slope is dry and open, with lower montane white fir transitioning to upper montane red fir by the time Cahoon Gap is attained (8,662').

Crossing the broad forested saddle, the trail leads down through a handsome forest of mature red fir and lodgepole pine to a dependable, unnamed tributary of East Fork Clover Creek (with campsites). Stepping across the creek and sidling around the tip of another moraine, a quarter mile farther you reach a junction, where a trail to JO Pass leads left (north), while you stay right (northeast). Just a short distance down the JO Pass Trail is a campsite with a bear box.

Your route continues through a flat with abundant downed trees (and live ones) to a generally easy ford of East Fork Clover Creek and soon begins a long climb up-valley to the Twin Lakes. It is a broad canyon, bordered, again, by a pair of moraines. The trail swings from side to side, occasionally positioned near the creek, where you watch water gush down bedrock, but mostly continuing up through mixed-conifer forest farther to the north. Stretches have been burned, with some mature trees surviving and lots of young lodgepole pine and red fir growing in. The last half mile to the timbered flats around Twin Lakes is a steeper, hotter switchbacking ascent—tough at the end of an already long climb.

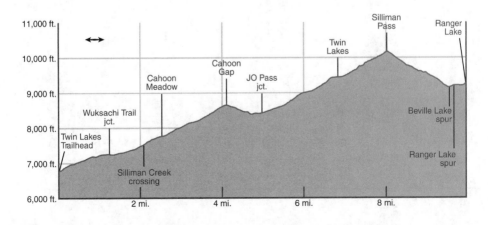

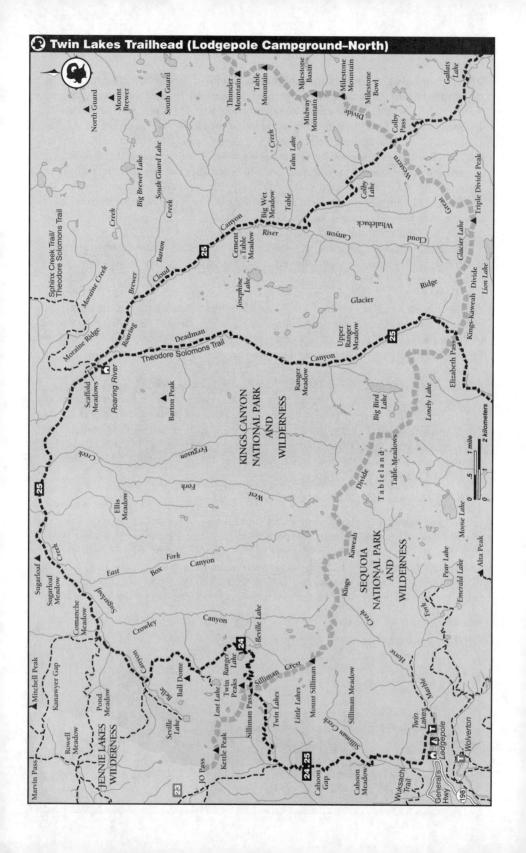

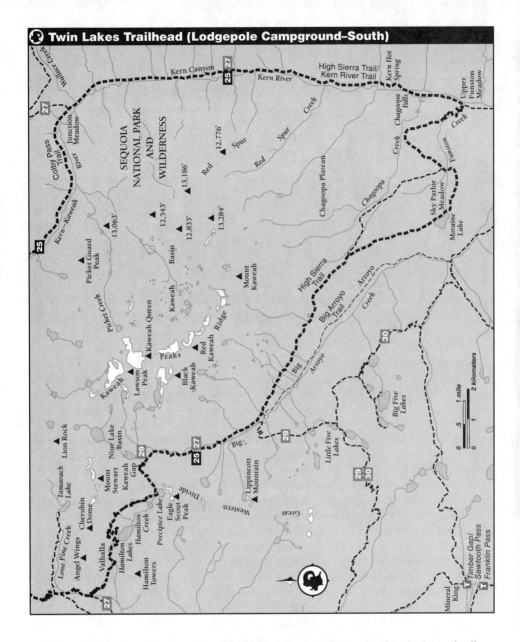

At least the open stretches here are a high tide of floral colors. And suddenly the trail rolls over into the flat basin holding the Twin Lakes. Reaching the first campsites, you pass a spur left (north) to a pit toilet and then continue along the isthmus between the two lakes, quickly reaching many more campsites and a bear box (9,447'; 36.65852°N, 118.71521°W; no campfires). The southern lake is much larger and deeper and from its shores you are staring at steep, bright white granite cliffs exfoliating slabs at a prodigious rate. These are beautiful campsites but can be very crowded.

A forested swath to the northeast is the only plausible route toward the crest, and the trail ascends it, completing 24 switchbacks to climb the requisite 750 feet to Silliman Pass. At the base you are in red fir forest, rapidly transitioning to lodgepole pine and then western white pine on the summit. Flowers are showy throughout, including patches of Sierra bleeding

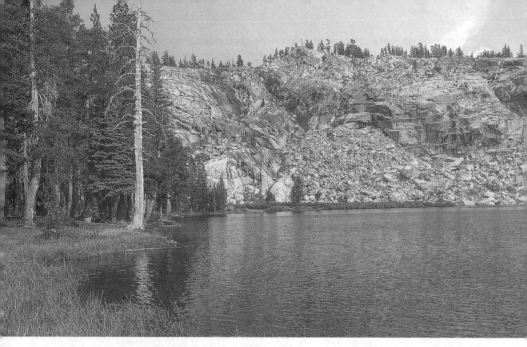

Twin Lakes   Photo by Elizabeth Wenk

heart, twinberry, green leaved raillardella, and pink alumroot, all appreciating the moisture from a spring flowing down the slope. The view of two large "pillars" of exfoliating granite to the north (the base of Twin Peaks) dominates the horizon throughout. Despite these distractions you'll be pleased to reach the broad sandy pass (10,172'). From Silliman Pass, there's a decent view of flat-topped Mount Silliman to the south, the heavily wooded Sugarloaf Creek drainage to the northeast, the Great Western Divide to the east, and the barren flats of the Tableland to the southeast. For a grander version of this vista, consider climbing an additional 200 feet north to the easy summit of Twin Peaks, where you'll stand above the trees.

Dropping down the west side of Silliman Pass, you are now in Kings Canyon National Park, having crossed the divide between the Kaweah River and the Kings River watersheds. Switchbacks lead down a steep slope of magnificent western white pine, around the base of an old rock glacier, and down forested slopes. The trail then crosses onto granite slabs that extend north and east to the edge of a precipitous drop—from this superb vista you are staring straight down on Ranger Lake and have a sublime view north to the Monarch Divide, Black Divide, and all the way to the Palisade Peaks on the Sierra Crest and east to distinctly pyramidal Mount Brewer. The trail then trends south until it can finish its descent down broken slabs, soon reaching a junction where right (southeast) leads to lovely but marshy Beville Lake (no campsites); you continue left (north).

In just a few minutes you reach a second junction, where right (east) leads onward to Comanche Meadow, while you stay left and make a short jaunt north to Ranger Lake. There are excellent campsites on the northwest, north, and east sides of the lake, the first two with bear boxes (9,262'; 36.66749°N, 118.69607°W at the north end). Those to the northwest are nestled within a big, dense red fir stand, while those to the north and east are in open sandy sites. Ranger Lake's setting is splendid, with the steep Silliman Crest to the south. A quick walk to the top of the rib to the north provides excellent views. And angling is good in the area. If you have a layover day, consider Lost Lake as a destination.

DAY 2 (Ranger Lake to Lodgepole Campground Trailhead, 10.0 miles): Retrace your steps.

trip 25   Deadman and Cloud Canyons

Trip Data: 36.61860°N, 118.50105°W (Colby Pass);
113.4 miles; 11/2 days

Topos: *Lodgepole, Mount Silliman, Sphinx Lakes,*
Triple Divide Peak, Mount Kaweah, Chagoopa Falls

HIGHLIGHTS: This is a long and unforgettable trip of stunning beauty and immense rewards—and one less traveled because of its length and the remoteness of its principal destinations: Deadman, Cloud, and Kern Canyons, and the canyon of the Kern–Kaweah River. It will be the trip of a lifetime for many, so schedule as many layover days as your food-carrying ability allows. Because of its length, we don't recommend this trip for beginners.

HEADS UP! *Fitting sufficient food in a bear canister is one of this trip's greatest challenges. The campsites suggested for Days 1 and 2 both have a bear box where you could place excess food. This reduces to 11 the number of days of food you have to fit in your canister—or 9 without layover days. There are no bear boxes along Deadman Canyon, so you'd have to then complete a very difficult 17.3 miles to the next bear box, at Upper Hamilton Lake. Instead, make sure your bear canister holds your remaining food. See wild-ideas.net for large canister rental (or purchase) options.*

HEADS UP! *The 2020 Rattlesnake Fire burned several miles in the Kern River Canyon near Kern Hot Spring. As this book goes to press, it is unknown if this fire killed many mature conifers or mostly cleared brush.*

HEADS UP! *The days on this trip vary significantly in length, from 6.8 to 15.8 miles. This trip has some long stretches without good campsite options for a large party, which made it impractical to divide this hike into all 8- to 10-mile days, as would be ideal. And so, if you follow the suggested itinerary, you will have a mix of longer and shorter days. A small group will have no difficulty finding campsites every few miles along the route.*

ALTERNATIVE TRIP 25 ROUTES
An alternative for those with less time is to make this a shuttle trip: From Roaring River Ranger Station, head to Deadman Canyon and over Elizabeth Pass to the Lone Pine Creek junction as described. Then take the Over the Hill Trail to Bearpaw Meadow when you meet the High Sierra Trail. Take the High Sierra Trail west to its trailhead at Crescent Meadow, which is a few miles south of Lodgepole and serviced by a free shuttle bus that runs throughout the day. This will probably be a six-day trip. An alternate start would be to hike to Roaring River from Road's End in Cedar Grove, ascending the Bubbs Creek Trail to Sphinx Creek and then continuing up Sphinx Creek over Avalanche Pass. Although only 15.7 miles to Roaring River (versus 23.0 on the described route), Sphinx Creek is a very tough climb.

DAY 1 (Twin Lakes Trailhead [Lodgepole Campground] to Ranger Lake, 10.0 miles): Follow Trip 24, Day 1 to Ranger Lake (9,262'; 36.66749°N, 118.69607°W).

DAY 2 (Ranger Lake to Roaring River Ranger Station, 13.0 miles): Return to the junction with the main trail and turn left (east) onto it, dropping 350 feet, first across slabs and then through predominately lodgepole pine forest. Ball Dome rises prominently on a ridge to the north. After climbing over a minor ridge, the trail drops to a wet creek corridor where it meets a lateral left (west) to Lost Lake. Keep Lost Lake in mind as a camping destination for your return trip; it lies just 0.5 mile off the main route and has campsites that rival those at Ranger Lake (and a bear box). Crossing the trickle, colorfully vegetated with the likes of Kelley's lily and marsh marigold, you proceed down parallel to the drainage, thereafter cutting down and across a low moraine where prickly chinquapin grows among the bouldery glacial deposits. The trail slowly encircles Ball Dome, beginning a generally flat walk north, alternating between dry, sandy, rocky stretches (minor moraine crests) and lush meadow and forest (where the moraines raise the water table). Ultimately you drop down steeper slopes (yet again a moraine) to Belle Canyon and cross Sugarloaf Creek, a broad, shallow wade at high flows but sometimes dry. Just beyond the main creek channel you reach a junction, where you turn right (northeast) to follow Sugarloaf Creek to Comanche Meadow, while left (west) leads to Rowell Meadow and the 1.2-mile spur to Seville Lake (more camping).

Turning northeast, you pass some small campsites (if there is still water in the creek), cross a smaller secondary river channel, and proceed just out of sight of the river. After a brief section in live lodgepole pine forest, you emerge into a landscape of mostly dead trees. The Williams Fire burned here in 2003, killing the majority of trees. Lodgepole pines have thin bark and are easily killed; you walk past extensive flats of dead trees where even the small branches are still intact, but the trees are dead. The moist ground is strewn with trunks, saplings, and a plethora of flowers, fireweed, arrowleaf ragwort, common yellow monkeyflower, and mountain strawberry among the most common. Similar landscape continues to the next junction, at the edge of Comanche Meadow, where left (west) is again signposted for Rowell Meadow and you turn right (east) toward Roaring River, 7.6 miles away, not 9 miles as the sign proclaims.

Walking east at the southern boundary of verdant, flower-filled Comanche Meadow, a veritable marsh in spring, you pass a large campsite with a bear box and soon jog north to step across the Williams Canyon tributary. Among white fir, chinquapin, mountain whitethorn, and broken slabs, the trail now drops nearly 500 feet to the far western end of Sugarloaf Valley, passing a drift fence near the bottom of the grade. To the south Sugarloaf Creek and its more robust south fork merge into a substantial river. Sugarloaf Valley follows the course of an old glacier and its base is comprised of sandy-gravelly glacial sediments, a slog to walk through when they are dry. For about a mile, you diverge from the creek and walk across dry flats with scattered Jeffrey pine and shrubs. The landscape here mostly avoided the 2003 blaze but was burned in 1975 and is still recovering. You soon pass a spur left (north) to a large campsite (and bear box) at the edge of Sugarloaf Meadow, popular with stock users, and amble around the front of 800-foot-tall Sugarloaf Dome. This steep, smooth, round dome is more resistant than the surrounding rock and withstood the onslaught of ice, leaving an aesthetic granite island protruding above the rolling landscape.

The trail continues to parallel the creek, now close to your side again so you can savor the riparian corridor's tall black cottonwood, abundant bird life, and expansive cobble bars that are submerged only by spring flows. Presently, the trail drops to cross the creek, a wide, shallow ford, with more campsites just beyond. You continue west, crossing a pair of minor ridges, undoubtedly very eroded moraine remnants, and alternating between conifer cover—mostly lodgepole pine with some white fir and occasional Jeffrey pine—and scrubbier patches of mountain whitethorn and greenleaf manzanita. After 1.5 miles you ford Ferguson Creek (more campsites) and then round a more prominent moraine and drop down a hot, dry, previously burned slope into the Roaring River drainage. Where you reach the river's bank you pass a stock drift fence and some sandy campsites. The final 1.0 mile to the Roaring River Ranger Station is an exposed walk beside the river, across sandy flats and past outcrops, ascending beside the sometimes-roaring river at a gentle grade. As you walk, looking across the river, you see a knob where the stock camp and bear box are located (hikers may also camp here) and Scaffold Meadows, some parts reserved for NPS grazing, and other sections a designated public pasture. Looping around a small meadow lobe, you arrive at a junction, with the sometimes-staffed Roaring River Ranger Station just a few steps to the right (south). Left (northeast) leads quickly to the main hiker camping area (7,397'; 36.71279°N, 118.58626°W) with bear box and pit toilet—the latter a fantastic hollowed-out tree trunk. Fishing for rainbow and some golden trout is fair to good. At the aforementioned junction, right is also the direction up Deadman Canyon to Elizabeth Pass (tomorrow's route), while left leads across a bridge to a second junction and the trails southeast up Cloud Canyon and over Colby Pass (your return route) and north over Avalanche Pass to Cedar Grove.

DAY 3 (Roaring River to Upper Ranger Meadow, 6.8 miles): Today you begin the loop part of the trip, walking past the Roaring River Ranger Station toward Deadman Canyon. The trail quickly veers away from the river, following a shelf east, then turning south where the Deadman Canyon creek and Roaring River divide. You continue south along the western bank of the unnamed creek, walking through quite dense mixed-conifer forest; even the forest floor is brightly colored with seasonal wildflowers, including wild strawberries, crimson columbine, and wandering fleabane. You pass a drift fence, and, once you're 1.8 miles beyond the ranger station, ford the creek for the first of four times, a shallow wade or rock hop. You continue past meadows, across short stretches of slab, and through forest, now mostly lodgepole pine with a few magnificent red firs in the mix. Only rarely are there appealingly flat, unvegetated places for a tent. And all the while, the valley walls are growing taller—such steep, unfractured bedrock that barely a tree has established on the slopes. Passing a decent campsite, you reach a dry sagebrush flat in which there is a wooden grave marker (8,400'; 36.67276°N, 118.57308°W); the canyon's namesake lies here. You continue beneath aspen and lodgepole pine, past wildflower gardens at the meadow's edge that are thigh-high rainbows of color, and 0.25 mile later cross the creek again, most of the time a broad wade.

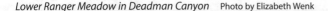

Lower Ranger Meadow in Deadman Canyon   Photo by Elizabeth Wenk

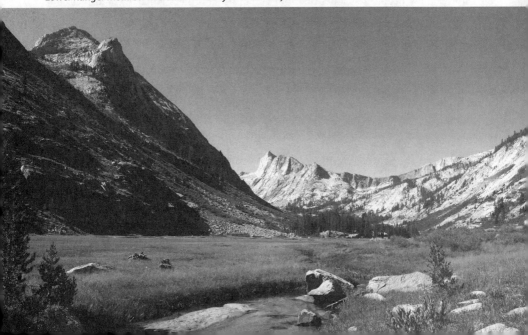

THE GRAVE IN DEADMAN CANYON

The citation on the grave reads: HERE REPOSES ALFRED MONIERE, SHEEPHERDER, MOUNTAIN MAN, 18– to 1887. But it's a mystery now. Nobody knows who Alfred Moniere was or why he died. At least two major versions of the story exist: The occupant was murdered nearby, or he died of illness before his partner could complete the two-week round-trip to and from Fresno to bring back a doctor. Still, as Wilderness Press author Jeff Schaffer put it, no pharaoh in all his power and glory ever enjoyed a more magnificent setting for his tomb than does this unknown soul.

Just beyond the grave you find tree cover thinning and then vanishing rather unexpectedly, since you are only at 8,500 feet and the southern Sierra treeline is above 11,000 feet. Excepting a few locations, trees simply don't grow in Deadman Canyon. The walls are astoundingly unjointed bedrock, barely disintegrating into talus, much less soil. Even the valley bottom is essentially a thin veneer of soil atop impervious bedrock, which stops water from draining downward and the soils are too wet for conifers to establish. You'll also notice that side creeks are mostly absent, but there are tiny seeps everywhere irrigating near-continuous wildflower gardens. In Deadman Canyon, the precipitous, glacier-smoothed canyon walls most certainly dominate the experience. At 0.6 mile above the second ford, the trail climbs alongside a dramatic, green-water, granite-slab chute. Not long after you are staring at a giant meadow, Ranger Meadow (or "Lower Ranger"), a five-star location (even by the Sierra's high standards) with endless flowers—especially tall corn lilies, Bigelow's sneeze-weed, orange sneezeweed, and giant red paintbrush—as foreground for your mountain photographs. The creek follows hairpin-meanders down the center of the grassy expanse, while oxbow lakes to the edge mark a long-ago course. Looking upcanyon, the cirque holding Big Bird Lake is clear on the west wall. A mile after you first reach the meadow, you pass possible campsites, sandy patches atop a small knob between the trail and river.

Beyond this campsite, the trail resumes its ascent over duff and sand, through stands of lodgepole and clumps of aspen. Below a forested bench, the creek again streams down broad granite slabs and soon thereafter you ford the creek for a third time, now a simpler rock hop. Now begins a steadier 300-foot climb; the trail here is narrow and incised as you climb up through willows and flower thickets to a lodgepole pine–forested flat, the

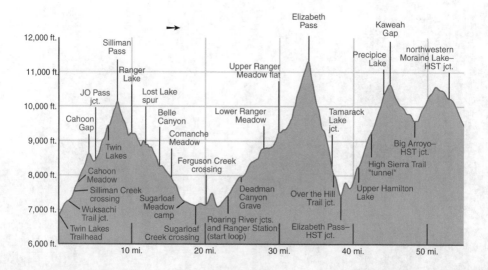

Upper Ranger Meadow flat. Here are some splendid campsites at the edge of slabs (9,238′; 36.63216°N, 118.58376°W; no campfires), with sublime views both up- and downcanyon, including awesome glimpses of the headwall of the Deadman Canyon cirque. Fishing for rainbow, brook, and hybrids is good. A cross-county route to Big Bird Lake takes off west across the creek here, becoming a well-worn tread as it ascends the slope south of the lake's outlet, a worthwhile afternoon jaunt.

Today's distance was short and its elevation gain modest, but only be tempted to continue upward if it is not yet lunchtime, for there are very few campsites along the next 7.4-mile stretch and none for big groups. Moreover, the following day's hike is a tough one: the 2,200-foot ascent to Elizabeth Pass is followed by a 3,200-foot descent to Lone Pine Creek. It is mostly very steep terrain and the trail is, in places, faint and "unbuilt," especially on the south side of Elizabeth Pass.

DAY 4 (Upper Ranger Meadow to Lone Pine Creek, 7.4 miles): Leaving the campsites, the trail ascends gently through boulders, with Upper Ranger Meadow to the west. Low-growing willows line the stream, and clumps of wildflowers dot the green expanse. The trail skirts the meadow turf, walking across gravel that has been carried down from slopes to the east. It is striking how there are still no talus fans in this canyon—the integrity of the rock here is extraordinary. Walking past coyote mint, woolly sunflower, and mountain pride penstemon, the trail begins a switchbacking ascent once 1.6 miles above the campsites. Pleasant zigzags and a continued traverse suddenly morph into a wet, incised track that dives into a jungle of flowers and climbs steeply through a cliff band. Nowhere else at the head of the valley is there enough soil covering the cliffs to even allow upward passage! Nearly lost beneath the fireweed, Kelley's lilies, and streamside bluebell, the trail cuts to the top of a dramatic series of cascades and falls. You are now in the broader upper basin—although the walls are no less breathtaking.

The trail cuts across the top on the falls and then follows a line of rocks across polished slab, before beginning a zigzagging route upward, alternatively on slab and across alpine heath. You may notice vestiges of an old trail to the side, but the current route is always well delineated and obvious. Everywhere there is water irrigating the arctic willows, red mountain heather, and dwarf bilberry that carpet the ground—for like in the lower canyon,

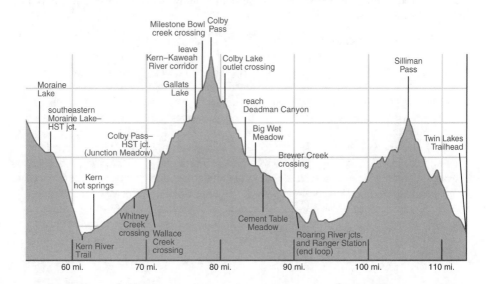

the rock is so massive that water flows across the surface, rarely vanishing down fractures. Ahead the trail switchbacks up a single talus strip that covers the underlying slab, the tread filled with riprap, angular cobble fill. The hiker may look longingly at the smooth granite slabs to the side, but for stock this trail construction makes good sense. Twenty-one switchbacks later you reach the top of the talus field and dart west onto red and gray metamorphic rock to complete the final length to the pass. Here there is a Spartan campsite or two, as long as snowmelt trickles provide water. A final four short zigzags lead to Elizabeth Pass for a well-earned break (11,391'). Looking east, you see where the arc of metamorphic rock you are standing on next intersects the crest near an old copper mine site. Now in the Middle Fork Kaweah drainage, brilliant granite slabs again greet you to the south, while to the west a thin sliver of Moose Lake is visible at the edge of the Tableland.

From the pass, the initially sandy trail drops straight down the strip of metamorphic rock, a steeply sinuous trail that winds more than zigzags. To either side rise the most amazing fins of bright white granite. About half a mile beyond the pass, among endless trickles of water, the trail briefly fades, and you must pay attention to cairns to avoid dropping too low. Ultimately, you drop 1,100 feet in the first 0.8 mile and then begin a slightly more moderate traverse west, transitioning onto granite slabs. Dropping again, first down a sandy rib and then back west, the trail crosses the bedrock-chiseled outlet of Lonely Lake above a series of cascades. The path continues southwest, resolving into switchbacks once positioned on a broad slope of gravelly soil, cobble, and shrubs that lets you bypass the cliff bands. Zigzagging down between juniper-covered ribs, the descent provides amazing views to Lion Rock and Mount Stewart. Finally, your weary knees reach the valley floor and a junction where left (east) leads up Lone Pine Creek to Tamarack Lake and right (south) leads downstream toward the High Sierra Trail. The only campsites until Upper Hamilton Lake, 3.6 miles distant, are 0.25 miles up the trail toward Tamarack Lake; turn left and proceed across the bouldery floodplain, densely colored with Sierra bleeding heart. Across the creek you'll find big sandy flats beneath scattered red fir, perfect for campsites (8,129'; 36.58492°N, 118.59360°W). (*Note:* The distance from the junction is not included in the mileage.)

DAY 5 (Lone Pine Creek to Nine Lake Basin, 8.3 miles): Return to the Elizabeth Pass Trail junction, turn left (south), and descend another 0.2 mile to a junction, where the described route continues left (south), while right (southwest) is the Over the Hill Trail to Bearpaw Meadow.

SHUTTLE OPTION: TO CRESCENT MEADOW

For hikers who wish to cut this trip short by taking the High Sierra Trail to Crescent Meadow, take the right fork southwest at the Over the Hill Trail junction; this 2.1 mile segment meets the High Sierra Trail at Bearpaw Meadow. Follow this trail up exposed granite slopes and into conifer cover, traversing above a steep cliff band ("over the hill") and then down into forest near Bearpaw Meadow. Around this trail's high point, there are outstanding eastward views up Lone Pine Creek to Triple Divide Peak and, farther on, up toward Kaweah Gap. Upon reaching the High Sierra Trail, left (east) leads 0.1 mile to the Bearpaw Ranger Station and right (west) 0.1 mile to a second junction. From here, you can descend south 0.2 mile to the well-used Bearpaw Meadow Campground (with water taps, toilets, and bear boxes) or turn right (northwest) to continue 11.2 miles on the High Sierra Trail to the Crescent Meadow Trailhead. There are campsites with bear boxes at Buck Creek (in 1.1 miles), Ninemile Creek (in 2.4 miles), and Mehrten Creek (in 5.3 miles). The last legal campsites are near the westernmost tributary of Panther Creek, 2.9 miles from the trailhead. See also Days 1 and 2 of Trip 27 for details. From Crescent Meadow, a free shuttle bus leads back to Lodgepole.

Your route south along Lone Pine Creek continues down the steep, enclosed canyon, the walls radiating heat on a summer's day. Where the trail skirts east, some small falls hide themselves in an alcove, only noticed if you turn around once back along the creek. Walking through dense, tall vegetation beside Lone Pine Creek, you reach a junction with the High Sierra Trail, where you turn left (east) to ascend toward Hamilton Lake and Kaweah Gap, while right (southwest) leads to Bearpaw Meadow.

As in Deadman Canyon, the granite is stupendous—polished, unfractured walls shaped into exquisite spires and arêtes guarding Hamilton Creek. The trail climbs brushy switchbacks and then begins traversing across steep rock slabs; you are thankful for the well-constructed trail. The final climb to a ford of Hamilton Creek is overshadowed on all sides by Valhalla's mighty rock: Angel Wings, the sheer granite fins to the north; Cherubim Dome, the more massive dome to the northeast; the Hamilton Towers, the sharply pointed granite sentinels atop the south wall; and, of course, the wall's avalanche-chuted sides. The creek is crossed at the lip of a waterfall, requiring care at moderate to high flows, and then ascends switchbacks up a brushy slope. A traverse leads above the vegetation-choked basin holding Lower Hamilton Lake—don't expect to find camping here—and then upstream to Upper Hamilton Lake, where slabs spill straight into the lake's depths. Just set back from the lake are justifiably popular campsites (and a bear box and pit toilet)—a worthy goal for Night 4 if you have the energy to continue the additional miles. Views from the campsites, including the silver waterfall ribbon at the east end, are superlative, and fishing for brook, rainbow, and golden is fair to good.

Angel Wings is one of the most impressive features in Valhalla.   Photo by Elizabeth Wenk

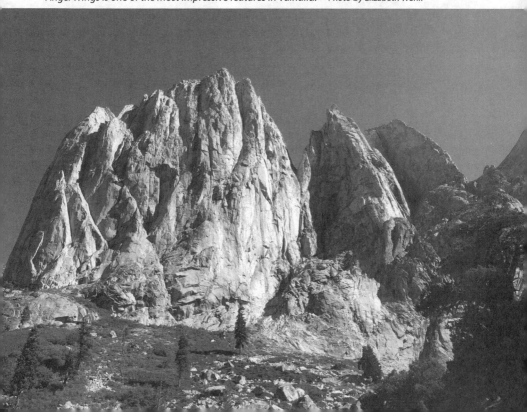

Staring at the walls rising above Upper Hamilton Lake you again thank the trail construction crew; the ascent is an engineering marvel—albeit distinctly not "leave no trace"— with the trail literally blasted across vertical cliff sections. You ford Hamilton Lake's outlet creek (on logs), leave the lakeside cluster of red fir, and begin a steep 2,500-foot climb to Kaweah Gap. For the first 800 feet, the trail ascends a slope that is predominantly mountain whitethorn and greenleaf manzanita, with seasonal wildflowers providing vivid touches of color. Notice the succulent liveforever growing from rock cracks. The occasional juniper, clinging to life in small soil pockets, provides momentary shade. The trail then begins an eastward traverse, particularly impressive as it cuts in and out of sheer-walled chasms in the canyon walls. The first two notches are arresting, the third unbelievable, as the trail dives into a tunnel and disappears deep into a notch; the excellent trail tread is essential here. The traverse, of course, offers unceasing views of Upper Hamilton Lake and the dramatic walls of Valhalla; this truly is a hall guarded over by the gods.

Thereafter, the trail doubles back, turning slowly to the south as it ascends across just slightly less sheer walls below Mount Stewart. Endless rills—none plotted on maps—irrigate the slopes all season. It is no exaggeration to call it a rainbow of color, with early-season marsh marigolds, Lewis monkeyflower, marsh checkerbloom, and Sierra bleeding heart replaced by orange sneezeweed, fireweed, and lupine as summer advances. Marmots abound, splayed across boulders and seemingly enjoying the surroundings as much as you do. You pass a tarn with adequate campsites and your final otherworldly Valhalla views, and climb a final 400 feet to Precipice Lake (10,300'). Offering only small bivvy sites among talus, this lake is better suited to a long afternoon break. Situated at the foot of the near-vertical north face of Eagle Scout Peak, a serrated ridge marks the skyline. Halfway down the face is a shelf harboring late snow and reflective trickles of water dribble down the lower rock faces all summer, creating black water marks. The lake has little sediment, and boulders are visible in its depths.

Onward, after a short climb up talus, the trail traverses a meadow-and-tarn-filled alpine valley that segues remarkably gently to the summit of Kaweah Gap (10,711'), an unbelievably gentle gap in the monumental Great Western Divide. The Kaweah Peaks Ridge dominates the skyline to the east, while below and to the north is Nine Lake Basin and south you're staring straight down the U-shaped, glacially wrought Big Arroyo. Hikers with a penchant for exploring barren high country, or those interested in the good brook trout fishing, can detour across granite-slab-and-ledge routes north to Nine Lake Basin and its good but exposed campsites (Trip 29)—indeed, from this perch you could already select a sandy nook between the trail and the lowest lake.

Easy switchbacks lead down the eastern side of Kaweah Gap. If you plan to camp north of the trail, it is best to leave between 10,400 and 10,500 feet and strike north in search of campsites. Soon afterward, just as you reach the banks of the Big Arroyo, is a big campsite west (right) of the trail, atop an eroded moraine (10,369'; 36.55463°N, 118.54717°W; no campfires).

DAY 6 (Nine Lake Basin to Moraine Lake, 10.0 miles): Beyond, the trail begins its steady-to-moderate southward descent along the west side of the headwaters of the Big Arroyo. For the first mile, you walk along the sandy moraine, continually impressed by the views of the Black Kaweah to the east and Eagle Scout Peak to the west. Slowly there are more lodgepole pines, then bigger lodgepole pines, and the surrounding peaks rise higher. To the west, you pass a succession to impressively steep granite ribs dividing one cirque lake basin from the next. At 1.75 miles beyond the campsite you cross to the creek's east side and soon thereafter cross from unjointed granite onto the red, black, and white hues of metamorphic rock comprising the Kaweah Peaks. Numerous runoff streams cross the track,

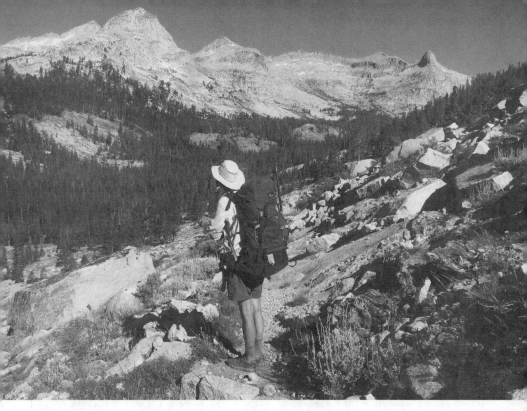

High Sierra Trail above the Big Arroyo   Photo by Elizabeth Wenk

even in late season, and the trail skirts many a small meadow. Under timber cover, you pass one good campsite with a fire ring at 9,635 feet and 0.25 mile later reach a junction, where the High Sierra Trail continues left (southeast), while right (south) leads past an old cabin to the main Big Arroyo campsite and bear box (9,518′; 36.51950°N, 118.53391°W), the trails to Little Five Lakes/Black Rock Pass (Trips 29 and 30), and down the Big Arroyo.

Your route, the High Sierra Trail, now embarks on a long, ascending traverse across the eastern wall of the Big Arroyo, angling onto the Chagoopa Plateau. West-facing, hot, and undulating, the trail feels like it gains more than the 1,000 feet it does in the coming miles. You begin in lodgepole pine forest, crossing a series of flower-bounded rivulets, then cross an expanse of dry slabs, before sidling across rib upon rocky rib, sagebrush, green-leaf manzanita, and chinquapin all more abundant than the sparse trees. In early summer, spreading phlox, wavyleaf paintbrush, and wooly sunflower all color the dry soils. Slowly gnarled foxtail pines appear on the rockiest slopes. At 10,300 feet, just before you cross a small stream, is your next possible campsite, and soon thereafter the grade starts to lessen as the trail reaches a shelf beneath Mount Kaweah, the massive mountain mirrored on the surface of a small seasonal tarn; nearby are more campsites when there is water.

Beyond, you suddenly "feel" like you are on the Kern Plateau—the gradient is gentle, the dominant trees are foxtails, and it is soft, sandy walking. Continuing around and then past the flank of Mount Kaweah, tree-interrupted views of the jagged skyline of the Great Western Divide accompany the descent to a broad meadow holding a Chagoopa Creek tributary. By the time you reach a trail junction at its southern edge, you have memorable views north to Mount Kaweah, Black Kaweah, and Red Kaweah. This stream should be permanent and there are campsites at the meadow's edge.

At this junction, the official High Sierra Trail continues left (southeast) toward Chagoopa Creek, while you turn right (south) toward Moraine Lake; the two routes reunite at the eastern edge of the Chagoopa Plateau. Your route is nearly a mile longer, but Moraine Lake is worth the extra distance. The descent over coarse granite sand slowly grows steeper amid dense stands of lodgepole and foxtail pines. At 9,970 feet, 0.9 mile past the junction, head toward the canyon lip for choice views down into the Big Arroyo and across to the drainages of Soda and Lost Canyon Creeks. Beyond, the descending trail again skirts away from the rim for 0.4 mile. Take care around 36.47691°N, 118.46049°W (9,790') where a plethora of stray footprints indicate that many hikers temporarily lose the track as it jogs back southwest and soon drops into a shallow draw. (*Note:* The trail here only loosely follows the line drawn on the USGS 7.5' topos.)

Continuing down through thickening lodgepole pine stands, in places with abundant deadfall, the gradient eases and quite suddenly Moraine Lake emerges through the trees. This splendid lake sits nestled between tongues of moraine debris, but, unlike many a moraine-dammed lake, it is large, deep, and stunning, albeit, like all moraine-dammed lakes, a little leaky. The main campsites (and bear box) are along the lake's northeastern shore (9,302'; 36.46229°N, 118.45459°W), although there are also small sites to the south that have the advantage of Kaweah Peaks Ridge views reflected in the lake's waters.

DAY 7 (Moraine Lake to Kern Hot Spring, 7.4 miles): After traversing a moraine just east of Moraine Lake and crossing the often-dry outlet, the trail descends moderately, then gently, passing an old stockman's cabin before reaching superb Sky Parlor Meadow, its boundaries delineated by moraine lobes. Here you have excellent views across this flower-filled grassland to the Great Western Divide and Kaweah Peaks. Expanses of dead lodgepole pine indicate a decades-ago fire, with abundant young trees growing in. Shortly after fording Funston Creek (sometimes dry) at the east end of the meadow, this trip's route rejoins the official High Sierra Trail route (merging from the left; northwest) and turning right (northeast) begins the moderate, then steep, descent to the bottom of Kern Canyon.

The trail first heads northeast, offering broken views east to the Rock Creek drainage and Mount Anna Mills and northwest toward the Red Spur. Continuing through burned, regenerating forest, the trail leads to the banks of Chagoopa Creek and a lovely little campsite garnering the sun's morning rays. Continuing down through Jeffrey pine, juniper, and greenleaf manzanita, the trail reaches a long, lush trough nestled between two granite ribs. The trail follows this convenient corridor south, then drops into the Funston Creek corridor. Quite suddenly, you're dropping steeply toward the Kern River—and enjoying the view south down the length of the unmistakably U-shaped Kern Canyon, the typical profile of glacially modified valleys. Kern Canyon's position is determined by the location of a fault and predates the Pleistocene glaciations by tens of millions of years, but the glaciers reshaped and deepened it. The final descent to the valley floor is accomplished via a series of steep, rocky switchbacks generally paralleling the plunge of Funston Creek. This slope was burned in 2013, and each eastward switchback leads onto the burned slope and the western ones back to surviving red fir stands in the riparian corridor.

Now on the floor of Kern Canyon, you reach a junction, where your route turns left (north), upstream, on the Kern River Trail, while right (south) leads downcanyon to the Kern River Ranger Station. The main Upper Funston Meadow campsites are a little to the south of this junction. The trail skirts the base of the canyon walls, first beneath a pleasant cover of white fir and incense cedar beside a sea of ferns and then across a talus slope to avoid willow thickets and stagnant water. Back beneath forest cover, you soon begin crossing many channels of Chagoopa Creek and emerge from forest cover onto extensive boulder-and-cobble bars, deposited by the Kern River during a long-ago flood. Turning around, you see Chagoopa Falls, a fury of plunging whitewater when the stream is full. Traversing the hot, exposed floodplain, the trail reaches a fine bridge across the Kern River. Once on the east side of the Kern, you again cross cobble deposits, this time a giant alluvial fan emanating from the mouth of Rock Creek some 0.5 mile ahead. You step across a side creek, one of Rock Creek's several channels, pass a campsite, and quickly reach a spur to Kern Hot Spring, 1.8 miles from the Kern River–High Sierra Trail junction (6,866'; 36.47815°N, 118.40623°W).

The hot spring consists of a single tub nestled in a small meadow—there is space for at most two people. It is a therapeutic treat for the tired and dusty hiker, as long as you arrive here ahead of anyone else! Just a dozen feet away from the 115°F pool, the great Kern River rushes past. Just to the north of the hot spring is a large designated campground spanning both sides of the trail, where you'll find bear boxes and a pit toilet (6,929'; 36.47936°N, 118.40586°W). While this is a fine campground, many people will choose to continue upstream, to shorten the following day. It is a relatively easy 7.5 miles to the large camping area at Junction Meadow.

DAY 8 (Kern Hot Spring to Gallats Lake, 12.5 miles): Continuing north, the route fords the northernmost—and largest—fork of Rock Creek on large rocks or logs (or a tricky wade) and traverses the gravelly canyon floor below the immense granite cliffs of the canyon's east wall. The next many miles of walking are defined by the 2,000-foot-tall cliffs confining the river; today's first miles are where the canyon is at its steepest and narrowest. You sense the presence of the precipitous granite whether in dense conifer forest or traversing the intermittent sandy flats. Stretches are flat and elsewhere the gradient is moderate, but never steep. In places the trail tracks the river's meanders, but more often it stays east and takes a straighter course, approaching the river's banks only occasionally. There are no large established camping areas, but at least once a mile you'll find a flat terrace with grandiose views that holds a few tents. About 3 miles past the hot spring you reach the base of Red Spur and the western cliff faces become craggier and even more phenomenal, especially in early summer as water pours down the gullies. At 7,860 feet (nearly 5.5 miles upstream of the hot spring) you cross Whitney Creek, draining the west side of Mount Whitney, often a long, bouldery wade.

A little farther and you sense the valley is opening, marking the final approach to Junction Meadow, the junction of the three upper forks of the Kern River, the Kern–Kaweah (once the West Fork Kern), the Kern itself (once the Middle Fork Kern), and Wallace Creek (once the East Fork Kern). You reach the Wallace Creek ford, currently crossed on a conveniently fallen giant lodgepole pine trunk that will hopefully provide safe passage for many years; otherwise, it can be a challenging wade. Just beyond, you reach the large Junction Meadow camping area (and bear box) spread across both sides of the trail (8,071'; 36.57729°N, 118.41374°W). Just past a little knob are more campsites and then, entering a sublime parklike grove of Jeffrey pine, you reach a junction. Here the High Sierra Trail (Trip 27) continues right (east) up Wallace Creek, while you turn left (west) to ascend to Colby Pass.

KERN TRENCH

The U-shaped trough of the Kern River, known as the Kern Trench, is remarkably straight for about 25 miles along the course of the Kern Canyon fault. The fault, a zone of structural weakness in the Sierra batholith, is more susceptible to erosion than the surrounding rock, and this deep canyon has been carved by both glacial and stream action. Many times, glaciers advanced down the canyon, shearing off spurs created by stream erosion and leaving some tributary valleys hanging above the main valley. At the base of steep walls, the glaciers also scooped and plucked at the bedrock, creating cirque basins in the granite, the depressions filling with water to become lakes when the glaciers melted and retreated.

The High Sierra Trail is designated as a "fully developed" trail by the National Park Service, while the trail over Colby Pass, like that over Elizabeth Pass, is maintained to a "moderately developed" standard. The trail is correspondingly narrower and less perfectly graded. Heading northwest through lodgepole pine and fir forest, the trail soon cuts across a cobble and gravel field toward the now-tiny Kern River; indeed, the Kern–Kaweah descending the Colby Pass corridor has the greater flow. Nonetheless, the Kern River is nearly always a wade, and a difficult one in early season.

Once across the river, you ascend a brushy slope, while the Kern–Kaweah flows down a blocky corridor of fractured rock. The trail is directed north, ultimately passing through a notch between an elongate dome and steep walls that has been called Kern–Kaweah Pass. Losing a little of your hard-earned elevation, you drop down a narrow slot to a bench and soon reach the river's edge at Rockslide Lake, a pair of crystal-clear, emerald-green watered pools partially dammed by rock fall. Continuing through aspens-and-lodgepole pine glades with lush vegetation and expanses of ferns, you soon start climbing again. Avalanches repeatedly tear down the slopes, and you pass both uprooted trees and ones sheared off many feet above the ground. Two waterfalls tumble down the wall to the south, exiting utterly remote Picket Creek basin and Kaweah Basin. Onward you climb up this delightful valley, sometimes on dry slab-and-sand slopes, repeatedly through seasonally boggy aspen scrub and elsewhere through lodgepole pine flats. The deep canyon lies between steep walls, Picket Guard Peak to the south and Kern Point to the north, but your gradient is only modest and there are sporadic flats with tent sites throughout.

As you approach 9,800 feet the persistent aspen scrub and avalanche debris suddenly yields to ever-more-pleasant walking across open slabs; just pay attention to the cairns to stay on route. Not long after, as you climb above the 10,000-foot mark the views open further and the trail turns more to the west—you've arrived at Gallats Lake, a giant marshy meadow with a persistent pool of water (i.e., the lake) in its southern corner. The bright white, supremely polished slabs at the far eastern edge offer extensive campsites (10,050'; 36.59485°N, 118.47120°W; no campfires) with sublime views upcanyon to Triple Divide Peak at the head of the Kern–Kaweah River and south to Picket Guard Peak. In the foreground are flat slabs and small domes, all polished to perfection. Fishing is good for golden trout. Sadly, the mosquitoes like the view of the meandering creek as well and until late July you may prefer to camp before or after this location! In 1897, the first explorers up this valley, William Dudley and companions, circumnavigated the Kaweah group, just as you have done (although not quite by your route), in order to ascertain that the Kaweah River, contrary to its name and the popular belief of the time, did not drain any part of the Kaweah Peaks Ridge. They determined that the Kaweah Peaks are a completely separate spur from the Great Western Divide. Indeed, Triple Divide Peak, at the head of the Kern–Kaweah River, marks the divide between the Kern, Kaweah, and Kings Rivers!

DAY 9 (Gallats Lake to Big Wet Meadow, 9.3 miles): Skirting the meadow's northern edge, and passing smaller, less showy campsites, the trail reenters lodgepole pine forest and climbs briefly to reach another flat. Here the trail parts ways with the Kern–Kaweah, as the river trends southwest up the main valley, while the trail climbs steeply toward Colby Pass. There are ample forested campsites nearby, including some across the creek.

Climbing a very stiff 500 feet beneath lodgepole pine shade, the gradient next eases in an alpine meadow with across-the-valley views back to the northern end of the Kaweah Peaks Ridge near Mount Lawson. There are a few tiny campsites here and bigger ones to the east—climb 200 feet up to an unseen moraine-top flat with an oval-shaped tarn. Continuing north through the meadow, you cross the creek just below where it forks, the right branch leading off-trail to Milestone Bowl (a worthwhile location to explore if you've budgeted spare days).

You now begin the final 1.1-mile climb to the summit of Colby Pass, a sinuous ascent, first past a final stand of foxtail and lodgepole pines and then up remarkably lushly vegetated slopes, along which you step across a rivulet three times. Low-growing willows, dwarf bilberry, and phyllodoce form a mat, with brightly colored Sierra ragwort, shooting stars, and alpine gentians emerging between. Soon you discover the source of moisture—a perched tarn with brilliantly clear blue water—and climb the final sandier slopes to Colby Pass (12,010'; 36.61860°N, 118.50105°W), named for one of the Sierra Club's early luminaries. Here there are excellent views back (south) toward Kaweah Peaks Ridge and north over Cloud Canyon to Palmer Mountain, framed by the canyon's walls.

The descent of the northwest side of Colby Pass is trying on the knees—you descend 700 feet in 0.5 mile, effectively down an active rockslide. The sandy slopes on the southeast side are but a pleasant memory as you work your way down cobble and around jutting boulders as you navigate the rocky slope. Near the top of the pass you might wistfully wish for a better trail, but looking back up from the first meadow you'll be impressed that a trail even exists up such a steep talus fan and realize how much better this route is than others nearby. A brief reprieve in a flat meadow and it's down again, although now following a vegetated slope of grass, sedge, willows, and a few whitebark pines to the banks of one of Colby Lake's inlet creeks. A descending traverse slowly leads to Colby Lake (10,584'), a scenic gem in a cirque high above Cloud Canyon's floor. Where the lake pinches closed, you'll pass small campsites beneath lodgepole pine stands and on slab. For those who love alpine conditions, the temptation to stop here is almost irresistible, especially because fishing for rainbow and brook is good.

At 1.9 miles below the pass, the trail crosses the lake's outlet and climbs steeply west of the drainage onto a bedrock rib that leads out of Colby Lake's hanging valley and onto a west-facing slope high above the next cirque. Descending steeply down broken slab, your attention will be continually drawn to striking Whaleback, a massive fin of granite with a skirt of talus at its base. Some gigantic foxtail pines cling to life on the slabs, most missing at least one spiral of bark from partially eroded roots. The descent leads to the flat valley bottom that you follow north, sometimes across polished slabs and elsewhere on a narrow, eroded trail beside endless flowers.

Soon after the trail fords the creek for a third time, it traverses around the northern tip of Whaleback—as with the Colby Lake hanging valley, the creek suddenly drops steeply and the trail needs to exit the canyon more gently. As you wind down between broken slabs and then loop westward to avoid steep bluffs, you're enjoying views north to Big Wet Meadow. A final southward leg, suddenly in red fir forest, leads to the floor of Cloud Canyon and you step across Roaring River on rocks. You have covered just 4.7 miles since Colby Pass, but dropping 3,000 feet on a narrow, rocky trail is not fast. These miles may have taken you longer than expected and, indeed, the 7.0 miles from here to Roaring River Ranger Station may take less time—the trail is constructed to a higher standard and you lose only another 1,600 feet of elevation.

Walking through a pleasant lodgepole pine and red fir forest, after just 0.2 mile you pass trapper Shorty Lovelace's cabin, a historic landmark and one of only two of his dozens of cabins remaining sufficiently intact that the park service has partially restored it. (It is located about 0.25 mile upstream of the site plotted on the USGS 7.5' topos.) Beyond, you pass your first sheltered campsite in many hours, a stock fence and then an unmissable round swimming hole with cascades above and below. A few more steps lead to a small boggy, flower-filled meadow, where you must cross Roaring River again, a broad, reasonably deep wade. (*Note:* Through here, the trail is not as plotted on USGS topo maps.) Soon you reach forested campsites that herald Big Wet Meadow's imminent arrival and come to the meadow's eastern edge. Now you marvel at the views up and down this wonderful glacier-carved valley, its floor eclipsed by nearly 3,000-foot walls. Whaleback dominates the upcanyon view. There are more good campsites nearby (for example, 8,757'; 36.66067°N, 118.53075°W).

DAY 10 (Big Wet Meadow to Comanche Meadow, 12.9 miles): From Big Wet Meadow, descend through lush lodgepole pine forest and meadows to ford Cunningham Creek, pass a lovely stand of mature aspens, and reach Cement Table Meadow, where you'll find an established campsite and many other choices within lodgepole pine forest. The amazingly dense, vegetated forest continues, the trees generally blocking the canyon views. The gradient slowly increases again once 2.1 miles past Big Wet Meadow and the terrain is a little drier. Continuing, you step across Barton Creek, unnoticed by midsummer, and then Brewer Creek, its approach marked by an impressive cobble fan the trail wiggles across. Ahead, the trail and river turn west, bordered to the north by a massive moraine, once deposited by Roaring River's glacier. As you slowly exit Cloud Canyon, the terrain is drier and a broad Jeffrey pine–dotted bench separates Roaring River from the trail; there are plenty of campsites if you trend toward the river in the lower-gradient areas. About 1.5 miles past Brewer Creek, Roaring River and the Deadman Canyon creek merge and the walls narrow again. A brief trot brings you to a junction where right (north) leads to Avalanche Pass (and Bubbs Creek), straight ahead (northwest) is a use trail to the Barton-Lackey Cabin (worth a look), and left (southwest) leads across Roaring River, on a bridge, back to the camping area and ranger station. At the ranger station you complete the loop part of the hike and turn right to retrace your steps 23.0 miles to the trailhead. If you have only one more night on the trail, it is recommended you walk as far as Comanche Meadow today (7,769'; 36.71081°N, 118.68400°W). If you have two nights, stop at either the Sugarloaf Creek crossing or Sugarloaf Meadow and then spend a second night at Lost Lake (0.5 mile up a spur trail; 9,158'; 36.67583°N, 118.70487°W), Ranger Lake, or Twin Lakes.

DAY 11 (Comanche Meadow to Twin Lakes Trailhead [Lodgepole Campground], 15.8 miles): Retrace your steps of part of Day 2 and Day 1 to the trailhead.

Lying not far off the trail, Lost Lake is a hidden gem.   Photo by Elizabeth Wenk

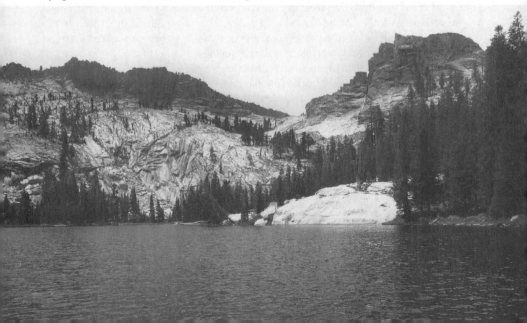

Wolverton Corral Trailhead				7,279'; 36.59663°N, 118.73427°W	
Destination/ GPS Coordinates	**Trip Type**	**Best Season**	**Pace & Hiking/ Layover Days**	**Total Mileage**	**Permit Required**
26 Alta Meadow 36.57919°N 118.66547°W	Out-and-back	Mid to late	Leisurely 2/1	11.8	Alta Trail

INFORMATION AND PERMITS: This trailhead is in Sequoia National Park. Permits are required for overnight stays and quotas apply. Permits can be reserved up to six months in advance at recreation.gov/permits/445857, with additional details at nps.gov/seki/planyour visit/wilderness_permits.htm. For both advance reservations (67% of quota) and walk-up permits (33% of quota), there is a $15-per-permit processing fee and a $5-per-person reservation fee. Both reserved and walk-up permits for this trailhead must be picked up in person at the Lodgepole Visitor Center, open 7 a.m.–3:30 p.m. daily. This is located toward the western side of the complex at Lodgepole. Campfires are prohibited above 9,000 feet in Sequoia National Park when west of the Great Western Divide and above 10,000 feet in Sequoia National Park when east of the Great Western Divide. Bear canisters are not required but are strongly encouraged.

DRIVING DIRECTIONS: From Visalia, drive east on CA 198 for 40 miles through Woodlake village, around Lake Kaweah, and through Lemon Cove, Three Rivers, and Hammond villages. Continue 17 more miles to Giant Forest and then about another 2.25 miles to the turnoff right (east) to the General Sherman Tree and to Wolverton. Turn toward Wolverton, avoid the General Sherman Tree turnoff, and follow this road to the parking loop at the end, 1.5 miles from the Generals Highway. The trailhead is on the upper side of the loop, easily distinguished by a large sign and a set of concrete stairs. There are bear boxes where you must store any bear-attracting items you're not taking with you.

trip 26 ## Alta Meadow

see map on p. 164

> **Trip Data:** 36.57919°N, 118.66547°W; 11.8 miles; 2/1 days
> **Topos:** *Lodgepole*

HIGHLIGHTS: Natural gardens and wonderful panoramas make the hike to Alta Meadow a treat, while the huge meadow itself—seasonally carpeted in wildflowers—is a delight to visit. Taking the trail up to Alta Peak is a popular day hike to an incredible view.

HEADS UP! *The exposure on the Alta Trail may trouble acrophobes. Also, a trail that once went across Alta Meadow to Moose Lake no longer exists—barely a use trail even across the meadow—and trying to follow the route is a frustrating exercise in bashing through deadfall and over animal trails. A better route to Moose Lake may be to go cross-country at or above treeline—a rough route for hardier hikers, especially for those who wish to loop over to Pear Lake.*

DAY 1 (Wolverton Corral Trailhead to Alta Meadow, 5.9 miles): Begin your hike on the Lakes Trail (7,279'; 36.59663°N, 118.73427°W) with a moderate-to-steep climb northward, first up the stairs and then up the duff trail under a dense fir forest, shortly passing a spur

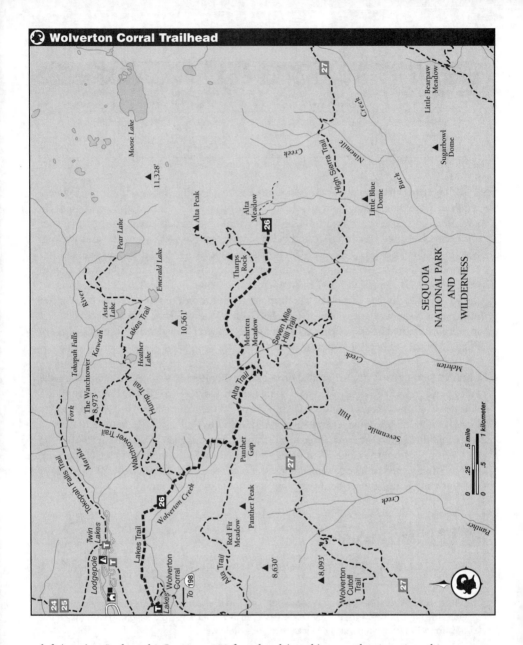

left (west) to Lodgepole. Continue 150 feet ahead (north) to another junction, this one on the right (south-southeast) signed for Long Meadow. Stay on the Lakes Trail (now eastward) as it travels this forested ridge. After about 0.75 mile, the path traverses above musical Wolverton Creek before descending into the meadow along the creek for a welcome and flowery break from the dense forest.

At 1.2 miles, the trail hooks right (southeast), where openings in the forest provide displays of abundant wildflowers. The grade steepens around 1.5 miles, and the path soon fords a stream. Around 1.8 miles, you reach a major junction (8,069'; 36.59294°N, 118.71010°W): the Lakes Trail turns left (north) toward Heather, Aster, Emerald, and Pear Lakes, while this trip continues ahead (east-southeast) toward Panther Gap. On the way to Panther Gap, the trail crosses numerous small streams. Beyond the last stream crossing at 2.3 miles, the trail climbs a steep switchback to Panther Gap (8,513'; 36.58439°N,

118.70553°W). Before continuing, take in the sublime views from the south edge of Panther Gap over unseen Middle Fork Kaweah River to Castle Rocks and the jagged peaks of the Great Western Divide. The gap also offers a couple of dry bivy sites. At the Panther Gap junction, the little-used continuation of the Alta Trail to Giant Forest heads west.

From the junction, turn left (east) on the Alta Trail toward Alta Meadow. After wandering to one side of the gap and then to the other, the trail settles into a gradual, ascending, eastward traverse of the south side of the ridge separating the Kaweah River's Middle and Marble Forks. The Alta Trail is a narrow, sandy, mostly exposed track perched as much as 5,000 feet above the Middle Fork, almost paralleling the famed High Sierra Trail (about 1,500 feet below on the same slopes; Trip 27).

Beyond a spring-fed garden, the path switchbacks up and then resumes the traverse, soon crossing a tiny meadow. At a signed but faint junction (8,997'; 36.58158°N, 118.69110°W) with the Seven Mile Hill Trail, a connector right (southeast) down to the High Sierra Trail, the Alta Trail bears left (east, then northeast), curves up, and soon reaches Mehrten Meadow, with a welcome creek, shade, and a few campsites. Ignore a use trail that darts right and steeply down to a creek crossing and eventually a tent spot; continue ahead (north and then east) to ford two forks of the creek, where you could perhaps take a well-earned rest.

From Mehrten Meadow onward, the Alta Trail is better shaded, the downhill slopes seem less precipitous, and the views are less frequent. The trail soon passes above a vigorous spring and then a hillside meadow. Nearing Tharps Rock, the track crosses a trio of seasonal streams and soon meets the trail to Alta Peak (9,304'; 36.58487°N, 118.67772°W) on the left in an open area with good views upslope to the peak. There are bivy sites near this junction.

Continue ahead (southeast) to Alta Meadow, now about a mile away. A hundred yards farther east, on the edge of the open area, the trail fords a stream and shortly passes a campsite just downhill. Beyond the previous junction, the path seems to deteriorate somewhat and crosses a runoff channel. Views here are splendid across open slopes down to Little Blue Dome and east toward the Great Western Divide.

Next the trail traverses above a great downslope sweep of granite (more superb views!) and then fords a year-round stream nourishing a very steep meadow. Just beyond, the maintained trail peters out at a sandy spot on a south-trending ridge on huge Alta Meadow's west side (9,356'; 36.57919°N, 118.66547°W; no campfires). This ridge has moderate forest cover and offers the best campsites at Alta Meadow. The best water source is the stream you just forded; water on this side of the meadow consists of inadequate seeps and scummy pools.

Note: Beyond here, the topo is badly out of date. The route across the meadow barely qualifies as a use trail and ends altogether a few yards into the trees on the meadow's east side. Campsites on that side have been virtually wiped out by deadfall, runoff, and overgrowth.

DAY 2 (Alta Meadow to Wolverton Corral Trailhead, 5.9 miles): Retrace your steps.

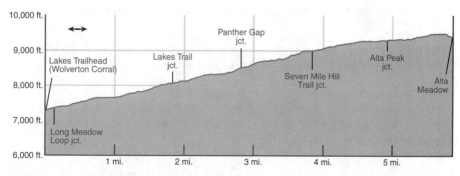

Crescent Meadow Trailhead   6,700'; 36.55458°N, 118.74888°W

Destination/ GPS Coordinates	Trip Type	Best Season	Pace & Hiking/ Layover Days	Total Mileage	Permit Required
27 High Sierra Trail 36.57856°N 118.29218°W (Mount Whitney)	Shuttle	Mid to late	Moderate (trans-Sierra) 9/3	68.0	High Sierra Trail

INFORMATION AND PERMITS: This trailhead is in Sequoia National Park. Permits are required for overnight stays and quotas apply. Permits can be reserved up to six months in advance at recreation.gov/permits/445857, with additional details at nps.gov/seki/planyour visit/wilderness_permits.htm. For both advance reservations (67% of quota) and walk-up permits (33% of quota), there is a $15-per-permit processing fee and a $5-per-person reservation fee. Both reserved and walk-up permits for this trailhead must be picked up in person at the Lodgepole Visitor Center, open 7 a.m.–3:30 p.m. daily. This is located toward the western side of the complex at Lodgepole. Campfires are prohibited above 9,000 feet in Sequoia National Park when west of the Great Western Divide and above 10,000 feet in Sequoia National Park when east of the Great Western Divide. Bear canisters are not required but are strongly encouraged.

DRIVING DIRECTIONS: From Fresno, take CA 180 east approximately 50 miles into Kings Canyon National Park and a junction with the Generals Highway. Turn south toward Giant Forest. Near the Giant Forest Museum, turn west toward Crescent Meadow onto narrow Crescent Meadow Road, a circuitous ribbon of old asphalt that then wanders south and east. Go past the Moro Rock junction to the parking lot and toilet at the end of the road, 2.5 miles from Generals Highway. If parking is hard to come by at Crescent Meadow, you can park your vehicle in the Giant Forest Museum lot and ride the free shuttle bus (Gray Route 2) to the trailhead.

trip 27   ## High Sierra Trail

see maps on p. 168– 169

Trip Data: 36.57856°N, 118.29218°W (Mount Whitney); 68.0 miles; 9/3 days

Topos: *Lodgepole, Triple Divide Peak, Mount Kaweah, Chagoopa Falls, Mount Whitney, Mount Langley*

HIGHLIGHTS: This dramatic trans-Sierra route follows the renowned High Sierra Trail from Crescent Meadow to Whitney Portal, visiting many classic Sierra points and crossing the Great Western Divide at Kaweah Gap and the Sierra Crest at Trail Crest, the Sierra's highest on-trail pass. From a junction near there, bagging Mount Whitney's summit is an integral part of this trip. The High Sierra Trail is the quintessential Sierra crossing—and there's plenty of fine fishing along the way.

HEADS UP! *Bear canisters are required on the Mount Whitney Trail. The U.S. Forest Service also asks hikers on Mount Whitney to pack out solid waste. You will be given a waste disposal bag when you pick up your permit at the Lodgepole Ranger Station.*

HEADS UP! *The 2020 Rattlesnake Fire burned several miles in the Kern River Canyon near Kern Hot Spring. As this book goes to press, it is unknown if this fire killed many mature conifers or mostly cleared brush.*

SHUTTLE DIRECTIONS: From CA 395 in Lone Pine, at the only stoplight, head west on Whitney Portal Road 13 miles to the large overnight parking lot near the end of the road (toilet, water, store, nearby campground). Note that the trailhead is a 6-hour drive from here.

DAY 1 (Crescent Meadow Trailhead to Mehrten Creek Camp, 6.0 miles): From the parking loop, circumvent the meadow on an asphalt path and begin climbing steadily and generally eastward through a forest of giant sequoias, sugar pines, and white firs. Soon after passing through junctions with the Crescent Meadow and Bobcat Point Trails, continue ahead (generally eastward) on the High Sierra Trail and break out of the trees onto open, chaparral-covered slopes high above the Middle Fork Kaweah River on the way to Eagle View overlook, where the view is indeed stunning: Moro Rock pops up nearby to the west, far below is the churning river, and to the east are the heavily glaciated peaks of the Great Western Divide.

The course of the trail does not follow a "natural" route, but instead makes a high traverse across the north wall of the Middle Fork Kaweah River's canyon. However, the traverse is not level: the trail undulates, usually just a 50-foot descent and ascent, but drops 300 feet as it descends to cross Panther Creek.

The trail, for now shady and nearly level, continues generally northeastward in a forest of ponderosa and sugar pine, black oak, incense cedar, and white fir, mixed with manzanita, whitethorn scrub, and much fragrant mountain misery (called kit-kit-dizze by the Miwok). Across the canyon, those impressive sentinels of the valley, Castle Rocks, fall slowly behind as the path marches up the canyon. After negotiating three switchbacks, resume the stroll and soon pass a junction with the Wolverton Cutoff, used mainly by pack stock.

Go ahead (north) from the junction. Legal camping begins just past this spot, at the point where a tributary of Panther Creek splashes steeply down granite—not that any campsites are yet apparent. Where another tributary of Panther Creek descends a loose slot to cross the trail at about 7,080 feet, look for campsites some 150 yards farther east in a shallow, forested draw below the trail. Spring-fed streams cross the trail in this vicinity late into the season. Yellow-throated gilia and mustang clover are abundant along the trail until late in the season. Climb over Sevenmile Hill and continue to the crossing of Mehrten Creek (7,653'; 36.57250°N, 118.68400°W), 6.0 miles from the trailhead. On the west side of the creek, a use trail leads steeply up the hillside to campsites with a bear box.

DAY 2 (Mehrten Creek Camp to Upper Hamilton Lake, 9.6 miles): Beyond Mehrten Creek, pass a junction with the Seven Mile Hill Trail, which provides a 2.2-mile connection to the Alta Trail, 1,300 feet above. Continue ahead, generally eastward.

From that junction, descend to a ford of an unnamed tributary and then climb steeply. Views to the south and southeast include the spectacular granite-dome formations of Sugarbowl Dome and Castle Rocks above the timbered valley floor. At each ford of the unnamed tributaries draining the slopes of Alta Peak, the trail passes precariously perched campsites. The next developed campsite with a bear box is 8.5 miles from Crescent Meadow, near Nine Mile Creek, the first branch of the twin-channeled tributary before Buck Creek. Beyond the streams, the trail bends around the mostly open slopes of Buck Canyon and then descends to a bridge over Buck Creek, where there is another campsite with a bear box.

A switchbacking climb leads up the forested east wall of Buck Canyon to the top of a low ridge and the signed 200-yard lateral south to Bearpaw Meadow Campground (7,650'; 36.56485°N, 118.62349°W; no campfires). There, viewless, very overused campsites sheltered by dense timber have bear boxes, pit toilets, and piped water.

In 0.1 mile, the trail reaches a junction with the northeast-bound Over the Hill Trail; stay on the High Sierra Trail curving south for a bit. Emergency services are usually available from the nearby A-frame ranger station. Not far away is Bearpaw High Sierra Camp.

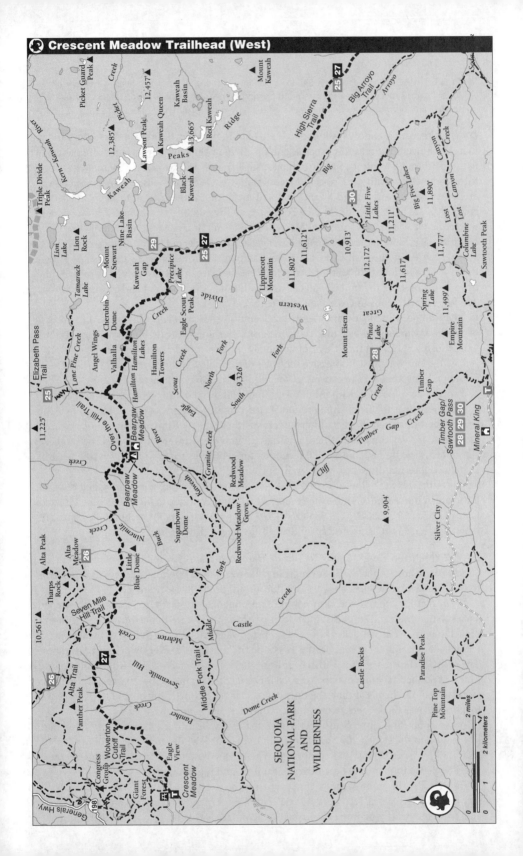

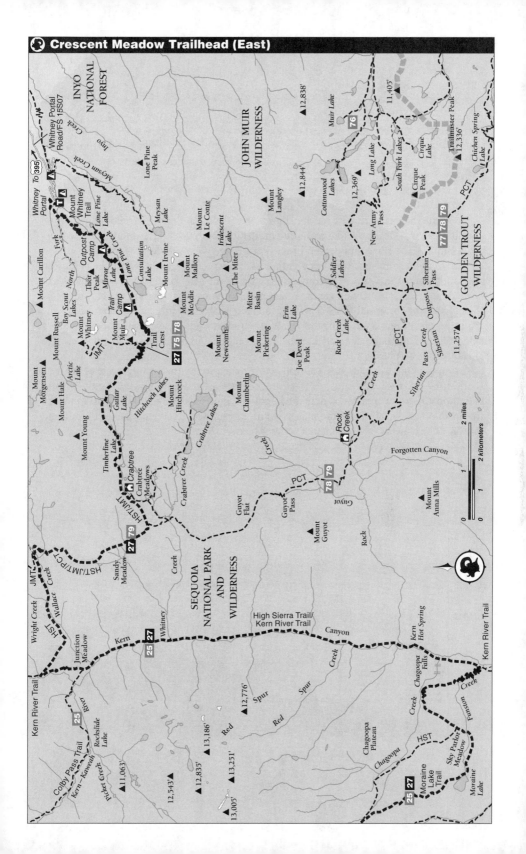

INYO NATIONAL FOREST

Whitney Portal Road/FS 15S07

To 395 Whitney

Whitney Portal

Mount Carillon ▲

North Fork

Lone Pine Creek

Lone Pine Peak ▲

JOHN MUIR WILDERNESS

Mount Russell ▲

Boy Scout Lakes

Arctic Lake

Mount Whitney ▲

Thor Peak ▲

Mirror Lake

Outpost Camp

Lone Pine Creek

Consultation Lake

Mount Irvine ▲

Mount Mallory ▲

Mount Le Conte ▲

Iridescent Lake

Meysan Lake

Mount Langley ▲

12,838'

11,405'

Muir Lake

76

Long Lake

Cirque Lake

South Fork Lakes

Trailmaster Peak ▲ 12,336'

Chicken Spring Lake

PCT

12,369'

Cirque Peak ▲

Cottonwood Lakes

12,844

New Army Pass

GOLDEN TROUT WILDERNESS

77 78 79

Mount Morgensen ▲

Mount Hale ▲

Mount Young ▲

Mount Whitney ▲

Mount Muir ▲

Trail Camp

JMT

Trail Crest

27 75 78

Mount McAdie ▲

The Miter ▲

Miter Basin

Mount Newcomb ▲

Mount Pickering ▲

Joe Devel Peak ▲

Erin Lake

Rock Creek Lake

Soldier Lakes

Outpost

Siberian Pass

Siberian Pass Creek

Siberian

11,257' ▲

PCT

Timberline Lake

Guitar Lake

Hitchcock Lakes

Mount Hitchcock ▲

Crabtree Lakes

Mount Chamberlin ▲

Creek

Rock Creek

Crabtree

JMT/HST

Crabtree Meadows

Crabtree Creek

Guyot Flat

Guyot Pass

Mount Guyot ▲

Rock Creek

78 79

PCT

Rock

Guyot

11,405'

Mount Anna Mills ▲

Forgotten Canyon

2 miles

2 kilometers

Wright Creek

JMT

Wallace Creek

HST

27 79

HST/JMT/PCT

Sandy Meadow

Whitney Creek

SEQUOIA NATIONAL PARK AND WILDERNESS

High Sierra Trail/ Kern River Trail

Kern Canyon

Kern Hot Spring

Chagoopa Falls

Kern River Trail

Junction Meadow

Kern River

Rockslide Lake

25

Kern River Trail

Colby Pass Trail

Kern—Kaweah

Picket Creek

11,063' ▲

Kern

25 27

12,776' ▲

Red Spur

Red Spur

Creek

Chagoopa Plateau

Chagoopa Creek

Chagoopa Creek

HST

Funston Creek

Sky Parlor Meadow

Moraine Lake Trail

Moraine Lake

25 27

13,186' ▲

12,835' ▲

13,251' ▲

13,005' ▲

12,543 ▲

BEARPAW HIGH SIERRA CAMP

At this backcountry lodge, like the famed High Sierra Camps of Yosemite, guests sleep in tent cabins and enjoy hot meals for breakfast and dinner (by reservation only). Unlike the claustrophobic backpackers' camp, Bearpaw's location on the edge of Middle Fork Kaweah River's canyon offers expansive views of the glacier-scoured surroundings, including such notable landmarks as Eagle Scout Peak and Mount Stewart on the Great Western Divide, the Yosemite-esque cleft of Hamilton Creek, and Black Kaweah above Kaweah Gap. A tiny "store" may offer snacks, batteries, and other needed supplies.

Continue the eastward trek on the High Sierra Trail, leaving the backcountry hubbub around Bearpaw Meadow and descending moderately through sparse stands of mixed forest. Rounding the slope and descending toward River Valley, the trail traverses a section blasted from an immense exfoliating granite slab. Views of clear-cut avalanche chutes on the south wall of the canyon accompany the descent to the bridge over wild, turbulent Lone Pine Creek. This stream cascades and plunges down a narrow, granite chasm below the culvert; the torrential force down the slender, V-shaped slot is clear evidence of the sculpting power of water. From the creek, the trail ascends an exposed slope, passing a side trail to Tamarack Lake and Elizabeth Pass (good campsites near the junction). Go ahead (southeast) here.

Continuing the steady ascent, you will be overwhelmed by the gigantic scale of the rock sculpted by ice, rock, and snow to the east and southeast. The final climb to the ford of Hamilton Creek is overshadowed by the mighty rock on all sides: the sheer granite wall to the north called Angel Wings, the sharply pointed granite sentinels atop the south wall, and its avalanche chutes—all are constant sources of awe.

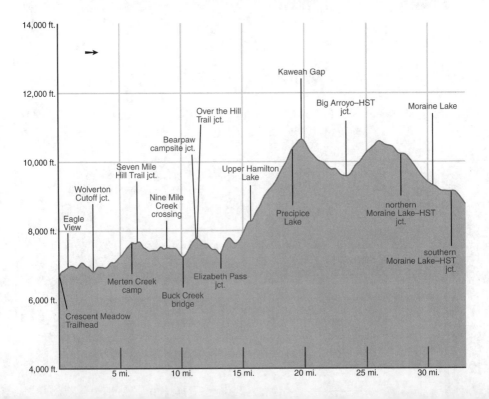

Under these heights, ford the creek a few hundred yards below the lowest Hamilton Lake and then climb steeply over shattered rock to good campsites at the northwest end of Upper Hamilton Lake (8,248'; 36.56416°N, 118.57866°W; no campfires; two-night limit at this overused lake). Views from the campsites, including the silver waterfall ribbon at the east end, are superlative, and fishing for brook, rainbow, and golden is fair to good.

DAY 3 (Upper Hamilton Lake to near Big Arroyo Trail Junction, 7.3 miles): Regain the High Sierra Trail and go generally east toward Kaweah Gap on a 2,500-foot climb that is something of an engineering marvel, with sections literally blasted out of a vertical cliff. Beginning at the northwest end of Upper Hamilton Lake, the trail ascends steadily up a juniper-and-red-fir-dotted slope with constant views of the lake and its dramatic cirque wall. Despite the rocky terrain, many wildflowers line this ascent, and among the manzanita and chinquapin, you may see lupine, yellow columbine, penstemon, Indian paintbrush, white cinquefoil, false Solomon's seal, and Douglas phlox.

After some doubling back, the trail turns south on a steep ascent to a point just above the north shore of Precipice Lake (10,300') at the foot of the near-vertical north face of Eagle Scout Peak. The jagged summits of the Great Western Divide dominate the skyline to the east during the final, tarn-dotted ascent to U-shaped Kaweah Gap, but on the approach, the equally spectacular ridges of the Kaweah Peaks come into view beyond. This colorful ridge dominates the view from Kaweah Gap (10,711'), which also includes the Nine Lake Basin watershed to the north.

From the gap, hikers ready to stop for the day can turn left (north), find a very easy cross-country route into Nine Lake Basin, and soon arrive at the roughly horseshoe-shaped first lake (10,462'; 36.55790°N, 118.54735°W; no campfires), with numerous fair-to-good

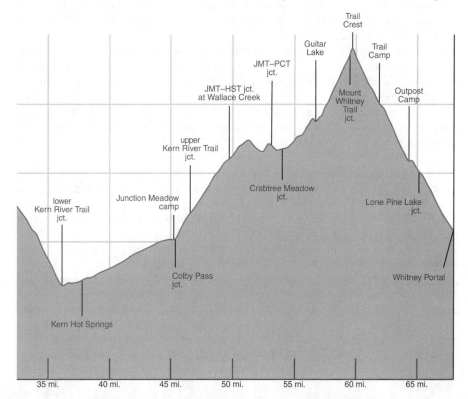

campsites and good fishing for brook trout. A base camp here makes a fine springboard for excursions to the increasingly secluded and dramatic lakes to the north and east. Climbers will find a wealth of steep faces west and east of this fine base camp.

For this trip, the trail continues a steady, moderate southward descent along the west side of Big Arroyo, fording to the east side of the creek midway down. Descend over unjointed granite broken by substantial pockets of grass and numerous runoff streams that continue to flow even late into the season. Open stretches afford fine views of U-shaped, glacially wrought Big Arroyo below, and the white, red, and black rocks of Black Kaweah and Red Kaweah Peaks to the east.

The route then reenters timber cover and arrives at some good campsites (9,637'; 36.52465°N, 118.53633°W) along the stream, about a quarter mile above the Little Five Lakes/Black Rock Pass junction (Trips 29 and 30). Fishing in the creek for brook trout should be fair to good, but anglers with extra time should take the 2-mile side trip to Little Five Lakes to enjoy fine angling for golden trout.

DAY 4 (Big Arroyo Trail Junction to Moraine Lake, 7.5 miles): Continue ahead (southeast) past the Little Five Lakes junction. The High Sierra Trail begins a long, moderate ascent along the north canyon wall of Big Arroyo. This route parallels the course of a trunk glacier that once filled Big Arroyo, overflowed the benches on either side, and contributed to the main glacier of Kern Canyon. The track climbs the wall of this trough amid sparse timber and a bounty of wildflowers tucked between sagebrush, manzanita, and chinquapin; the most colorful flowers include columbine, bright Indian paintbrush, and purple lupine.

The grade eases near the mirrored surface of a tarn, and then, swinging away from the lip of Big Arroyo, the trail begins a gradual descent through alternating stretches of timber and meadow. Tree-interrupted views of the jagged skyline of the Great Western Divide accompany the descent on the way to a trail junction in a meadow on the south side of a tributary of Chagoopa Creek.

Leave the official High Sierra Trail route at this junction and turn right (south) through meadows filled with clumps of shooting stars. This descent grows steeper over coarse granite sand amid dense stands of lodgepole and foxtail pine, with superlative views down into Big Arroyo to the drainages of Soda and Lost Canyon Creeks. This steadily down-winding trail leads to the wooded shores of Moraine Lake (9,302'; 36.46229°N, 118.45459°W). Good campsites on the south side of the lake provide views across the water of the Kaweah Peaks, along with nearby gardens of wild azalea.

DAY 5 (Moraine Lake to Kern Hot Spring, 7.4 miles): After traversing a moraine just east of Moraine Lake, the trail descends moderately, then gently, passing an old stockman's cabin before reaching superb Sky Parlor Meadow, with excellent views back across this flower-filled grassland to the Great Western Divide and Kaweah Peaks. Shortly beyond the ford of Funston Creek, at the east end of the meadow, this trip's route rejoins the official High Sierra Trail route, turns right, and begins the moderate, then steep, descent to the bottom of Kern Canyon.

Along the initial descent, lodgepole pine is replaced by lower-altitude white fir and Jeffrey pine; farther down, the trail descends steeply through manzanita and snowbush beneath an occasional juniper or oak. The unmistakably U-shaped Kern Canyon is typical of glacially modified valleys. The final descent to the valley floor is accomplished via a series of steep, rocky switchbacks generally paralleling the plunge of Funston Creek.

Now on the floor of Kern Canyon, the route turns north, upstream, on the Kern River Trail, drops into a marshy area, and then crosses a talus slope. Then the trail leads gently upward through a forest of Jeffrey pine and incense cedar. High on the western rim of the canyon, look for Chagoopa Falls, a fury of plunging whitewater when the stream is full.

Past a manzanita-carpeted opening, the trail crosses the Kern River on a fine bridge and arrives at the south fork of Rock Creek. Then, around a point, the path leads to Kern Hot Spring (6,866'; 36.47815°N, 118.40623°W)—a therapeutic treat for the tired and dusty hiker. Although the cement tub screened by wood planks would appear crude by suburban backyard standards, here in the midst of the backcountry, Kern Hot Spring is a regal, heated paradise. Just a dozen yards away from the 115°F pool, the great Kern River rushes past. Just north of the hot spring, there is a large camping area, including a pair of bear boxes and a pit toilet (6,929'; 36.47936°N, 118.40586°W). Fishing in the Kern is good for rainbow and golden-rainbow hybrids.

DAY 6 (Kern Hot Spring to Junction Meadow, 7.5 miles): Continuing north, the route fords the upper fork of Rock Creek and traverses the gravelly canyon floor below the immense granite cliffs of the canyon's east wall. Past the confluence of Red Spur Creek, this route ascends gradually, sometimes a bit steeply, beside the Kern River, heading almost due north.

Big Arroyo   Photo by Elizabeth Wenk

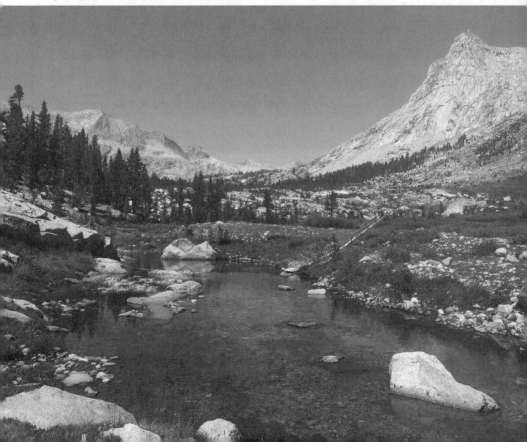

> **KERN TRENCH**
> The U-shaped trough of the Kern River, known as the Kern Trench, is remarkably straight for about 25 miles along the course of the Kern Canyon fault. The fault, a zone of structural weakness in the Sierra batholith, is more susceptible to erosion than the surrounding rock, and this deep canyon has been carved by both glacial and stream action. Many times, glaciers advanced down the canyon, shearing off spurs created by stream erosion and leaving some tributary valleys hanging above the main valley. The glaciers also scooped and plucked at the bedrock, creating basins in the granite, which later became lakes when the glaciers melted and retreated.

The walls of this deep canyon, from 2,000 to 5,000 feet high, are spectacular, with a number of streams cascading and falling down granite faces. (The fords of the stream draining Guyot Flat and Whitney Creek can be difficult in early season.) Beyond a log crossing of Wallace Creek, the trail enters a parklike grove of stalwart Jeffrey pines, providing a noble setting for the overused campsites at Junction Meadow (8,071'; 36.57729°N, 118.41374°W) on the Kern River, where fishing should be good for rainbow and some brook trout.

Day 7 (Junction Meadow to Crabtree Ranger Station, 8.7 miles): The trail leaves the parklike Jeffrey pines of Junction Meadow and heads north to ascend steeply on rocky underfooting over a slope covered by manzanita and currant. Over-the-shoulder views down Kern Canyon improve continuously, as the occasional Jeffrey, lodgepole, and aspen offer frames for the photographer composing a shot of the great cleft.

After 1.2 miles, reach a junction with the Kern River Trail, where your route turns right (southeast), back toward Wallace Creek's canyon. At 10,400 feet is another junction, this one with the John Muir Trail (JMT)/Pacific Crest Trail (PCT). Turn right (south) onto the JMT/PCT, which, in this area, is also the route of the High Sierra Trail. Immediately ford Wallace Creek (difficult in early season), pass some campsites, and then continue southward on generally gentle gradients through sporadic stands of lodgepole and foxtail pine.

At approximately 10,800 feet, reach a junction between the PCT, which continues south, and the JMT and High Sierra Trail, which both turn east here. Take the left fork east and follow the JMT/High Sierra Trail on a climb over a bench through lodgepole and foxtail pines, staying well above the north bank of Whitney Creek. About a mile from the PCT junction, come to a junction (campsites) with a lateral that drops to a ford of Whitney Creek and continues south through upper and lower Crabtree Meadows, eventually joining the PCT south of here.

Along this lateral, just across Whitney Creek, are a bear box and a junction with a lateral to Crabtree Ranger Station and the fair campsites nearby (10,640'; 36.56391°N, 118.34937°W; no campfires). Emergency services are sometimes available at the ranger station. Fishing in Whitney Creek is fair for golden trout.

DAY 8 (Crabtree Ranger Station to Trail Camp, 7.9 miles): From the vicinity of the ranger station, return to the JMT/High Sierra Trail and climb east along the north side of Whitney Creek to Timberline Lake, a small, irregular-shaped body of water most noted for reflecting the west face of Mount Whitney—a favorite subject of both amateur and professional photographers. The lake is closed to camping.

Skirt the north side of the lake and continue a gentle ascent past timberline into an alpine meadow on the way around Guitar Lake. Backpackers in search of overnight accommodations may find decent campsites near the "guitar's neck" and near the crossing of Arctic Lake's outlet.

Away from Guitar Lake, the trail climbs to a bench with some tiny ponds and poor camp-sites. Traverse an alpine meadow, and then start climbing on long, rocky switchbacks across the west face of Mount Whitney to a junction of the JMT/High Sierra Trail, which heads to the summit of Mount Whitney, and the Mount Whitney Trail from Whitney Portal.

SIDE TRIP TO MOUNT WHITNEY

To come all this way and not take the 2-mile trail to the summit of the highest peak in the lower 48 would be unforgivable. It's an integral part of the High Sierra Trail.

First, stash your heavy backpack into clefts of rock near the junction and don a day pack with the usual essentials. Then follow a steady climb along the west side of Whitney's south ridge, where the trail periodically enters notches with acrophobic vistas straight down the east face. As you ascend the rocky trail, sharp eyes will soon spy the summit hut, built for research purposes by the Smithsonian Institute in 1909. Nearing the final slope, the grade increases.

Cresting the broad summit plateau of jumbled slabs and boulders, the roof of the hut comes into view, and soon you find yourself at 14,505 feet (14,505'; 36.57856°N, 118.29218°W). Any adjective used to describe the incredible summit vista is grossly inadequate. Suffice it to say, the view from the highest point in the lower 48 is a complete, 360-degree panorama, with each bearing of the compass holding something extraordinary to discover—a just reward for the toil necessary to reach such a lofty goal. Be sure to record your name in the summit register near the hut before backtracking the 2 miles to the trail junction. Officially, the JMT ends (or begins) at the summit, but the High Sierra Trail continues. Alas, there is no solitude here: any halfway decent day sees dozens of hikers milling around the summit plateau.

If you took the side trip up Mount Whitney, retrace your steps to the junction with the main trail. From the junction, make a short climb up to Trail Crest (13,620') along the spine of the Sierra and on the boundary between Sequoia National Park to the west and John Muir Wilderness to the east. From Trail Crest, the Mount Whitney Trail angles east around the top of a steep chute before embarking on a seemingly interminable descent down about 100 tight switchbacks. Midway down is a shaded stretch of trail that routinely ices up, providing tenuous footing; a steel cable is usually in place to aid in negotiating this sometimes-tricky section. The demanding, 1,600-foot descent finally eases on the approach to Trail Camp, the highest legal camping area along the Mount Whitney Trail.

Hordes of expectant peak baggers may be camped in sandy sites between boulders at Trail Camp (12,025'; 36.56298°N, 118.27915°W; no campfires), which lends a somewhat circus-like atmosphere to the surroundings on a typical summer day. Despite the crowd, the alpine setting below the east face of the Whitney massif is spectacular. To the north is Wotan's Throne, with Pinnacle Ridge behind, and, to the south, 13,680-foot Mount McAdie and 13,770-foot Mount Irvine form a striking amphitheater for the icy waters of Consulta-tion Lake. Water is readily available from nearby streams and tarns.

DAY 9 (Trail Camp to Whitney Portal, 6.1 miles): Beyond Trail Camp, head east-northeast to descend some poured concrete steps and continue steeply down a granite trail, wit-nessing ivesia, currant, creambush, and gooseberry growing in between the boulders. The outlet of Consultation Lake cascades down a ravine southeast of the trail. Ford Lone Pine Creek and pass tiny Trailside Meadow (no camping), carpeted with lush grasses and bright-ened by shooting stars, paintbrush, and columbine. Beyond the meadows, the trail refords Lone Pine Creek and then switchbacks down to sparse timber, finally leveling out near Mirror Lake (10,650'; no camping), cradled in a cirque beneath the south face of Thor Peak.

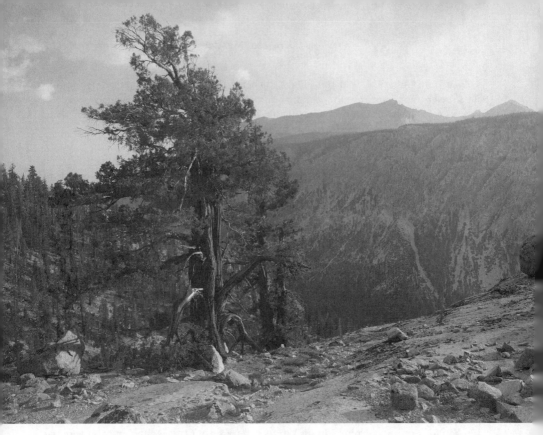

Gorgeous junipers on the climb along Wallace Creek   Photo by Elizabeth Wenk

After fording Mirror Lake's outlet, the descent continues down a slope blooming with senecio, fireweed, pennyroyal, currant, mountain pride penstemon, Sierra chinquapin, Indian paintbrush, and creambush. Upon leveling out, the trail crosses Lone Pine Creek and enters a large meadow on the way to Outpost Camp (10,367'), which has several campsites.

From Outpost Camp, the trail crosses Lone Pine Creek, skirts a willow-lined meadow dotted with wildflowers, and then switchbacks down to a junction with a lateral to Lone Pine Lake (campsites). Ford Lone Pine Creek again and begin a final set of long, dusty switchbacks that pass through open areas of sagebrush, chinquapin, mountain mahogany, and other members of the chaparral community common to the east side of the Sierra.

Views down the V-shaped canyon of the Alabama Hills provide a fine diversion along the drop toward the trailhead. Exit John Muir Wilderness and soon reach the paved road loop at shady Whitney Portal (8,330'; 36.58691°N, 118.24019°W), where a hamburger and milkshake from the café should be a rewarding temptation after more than a week dining on trail food. In addition to the café, Whitney Portal offers campgrounds, restrooms, water, and a small store.

CA 198 TO MINERAL KING ROAD TRIPS

The narrow, windy Mineral King Road leads to the southwestern corner of Sequoia National Park. Ten different trails depart along Mineral King Road, including a cluster that radiates in all directions from the road-end parking lot. The road-end trails predominately lead toward the rugged Great Western Divide, a tall crest that bisects southern Kings Canyon and all of Sequoia National Parks. The trails to the west access lands mostly covered by coniferous forests, including some remote groves of giant sequoias. Just three of the Mineral King Road trailheads are included in this book—the Timber Gap and Franklin Pass Trailheads at the road's end and the Tar Gap Trailhead, located at the back of Cold Spring Campground. Timber Gap Trail leads across a low, forested pass into the Cliff Creek drainage. Franklin Pass Trail climbs steeply past the Franklin Lakes to Franklin Pass, on the Great Western Divide. Both of these trails, and the Sawtooth Trail (not included in this book), offer access to a series of lake basins on the eastern flank of the Great Western Divide and the Big Arroyo, one of the major forks of the Kern River. The Tar Gap Trail (and Atwell Trail, farther downcanyon) leads to the gentle forest-and-meadow landscape of the Hockett Plateau. Lying a little off the beaten track at the end of a dead-end road, Mineral King–area trails tend to be only moderately busy, with the crowds continuing toward Lodgepole.

Trailheads: Mineral King Roadend (Timber Gap and Franklin Pass)

Tar Gap

Mineral King Roadend Trailheads
(Timber Gap and Franklin Pass)   7,841'; 36.45329°N, 118.59673°W

Destination/ GPS Coordinates	Trip Type	Best Season	Pace & Hiking/ Layover Days	Total Mileage	Permit Required
28 Pinto Lake 36.48508°N 118.58071°W	Out-and-back	Mid to late	Moderate 2/1	16.4	Timber Gap
29 Nine Lake Basin 36.55790°N 118.54735°W	Out-and-back	Mid to late	Moderate, part cross-country 6/3	39.0	Timber Gap
30 Big and Little Five Lakes 36.48347°N 118.50679°W (lower Big Five Lake)	Loop	Mid to late	Moderate 6/2	38.7	Franklin Pass (Timber Gap in reverse)

INFORMATION AND PERMITS: These trailheads are in Sequoia National Park. Permits are required for overnight stays, and quotas apply. Permits can be reserved up to six months in advance at recreation.gov/permits/445857, with additional details at nps.gov/seki/planyour visit/wilderness_permits.htm. For both advance reservations (67% of quota) and walk-up permits (33% of quota), there is a $15-per-permit processing fee and a $5-per-person reservation fee. Both reserved and walk-up permits for these trailheads must be picked up in person at the Mineral King Ranger Station, open 8 a.m.–3:45 p.m. daily. Campfires are prohibited above 9,000 feet in Sequoia National Park when west of the Great Western Divide and above 10,000 feet in Sequoia National Park when east of the Great Western Divide. Bear canisters are not required but are strongly encouraged.

DRIVING DIRECTIONS: From the CA 99–CA 198 interchange in Visalia, take CA 198 east past Lake Kaweah and the town of Three Rivers, turning right onto the tiny Mineral King Road after 38.6 miles; this is 1.5 miles after you leave Three Rivers. This minor road is easily missed—if you cross the Kaweah River you've gone 1.6 miles too far. Follow a very slow, windy Mineral King Road 23.4 miles east to the Mineral King Ranger Station. After picking up your permit, drive an additional 0.8 mile uphill to the large roadend parking lot.

HEADS UP! *Be forewarned that some very aggressive marmots live at this trailhead, and they are infamous for chewing into car radiator hoses. People routinely wrap their cars in a large tarp as a marmot-deterrent; see nps.gov/seki/planyourvisit/marmots.htm for the current advice. Alternatively, park across the street from the ranger station, where the marmots won't bother your vehicle.*

---

trip 28   ## Pinto Lake

see maps on p. 180– 181

Trip Data: 36.48508°N, 118.58071°W; 16.4 miles; 2/1 days
Topos: *Mineral King*

HIGHLIGHTS: The fine scenery of the Cliff Creek drainage, the good camping, and the relatively warm swimming in Pinto Lake make this trip worthwhile in spite of the tough hike.

DAY 1 (Timber Gap Trailhead to Pinto Lake, 8.2 miles): From the trailhead, the route climbs north-northwest on manzanita-and-sagebrush-flanked trail to a junction. Turn left (north) and begin a relentless 1,600-foot climb up a southwest-facing slope that can be quite hot in midsummer. Fortunately, a good part of the climb is under red fir forest. At the top of some switchbacks, the trail leaves the trees and makes a long, ascending traverse toward Timber Gap. Before heading back into the trees just below the gap, turn around and take in the fine view downslope toward Mineral King Valley, and then conclude the ascent at the forested saddle of Timber Gap (9,511').

From the gap, the trail drops steeply on switchbacks through red fir forest toward a crossing of Timber Gap Creek, where a long swath of flower-filled meadow supplants the forest. The delightful garden is one of the largest and most vibrant in the Sierra. Soon, cross back over the creek and then hop over a number of lush, spring-fed rivulets on the way down the drainage. Eventually, the trail leaves Timber Gap Creek, rounds the nose of a ridge, and then switchbacks down toward Cliff Creek through dense coniferous forest. Immediately after a ford of Cliff Creek (difficult in early season), find tiny Cliff Creek Camp (7,125'), complete with a bear box, and a signed junction with the Black Rock Pass Trail. *Note:* There are no campsites between Cliff Creek Camp and the Pinto Lake area.

Turn right (southeast) and climb up Cliff Creek's canyon on the Black Rock Pass Trail through wildflowers, pockets of shrubs, and scattered firs, and across several meadow-lined rivulets. In early summer, the fine wildflower displays include mariposa lily, rein orchid, wild strawberry, monkeyflower, wallflower, corn lily, delphinium, yellow-throated gilia, and buckwheat.

Farther up the canyon, the trail emerges from the forest onto an extensive boulder field, under which the creek temporarily runs at lower flows. Ahead, the creek spills down a rock wall on the canyon's south side. Switchbacks lead upcanyon along the creek's north fork through dense willow, sagebrush, whitethorn, and bitter cherry, to a ford of Pinto Lake's outlet. Shortly after, reach an unmarked junction with a lateral on the right to well-used campsites on a forested bench just south of Pinto Lake (bear box; 8,726'; 36.48508°N, 118.58071°W; no campfires). Pinto Lake hides in a dense thicket of willows nearby, offering surprisingly pleasant swimming.

DAY 2 (Pinto Lake to Timber Gap Trailhead, 8.2 miles): Retrace your steps.

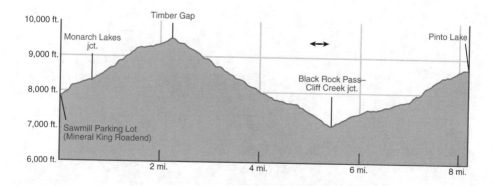

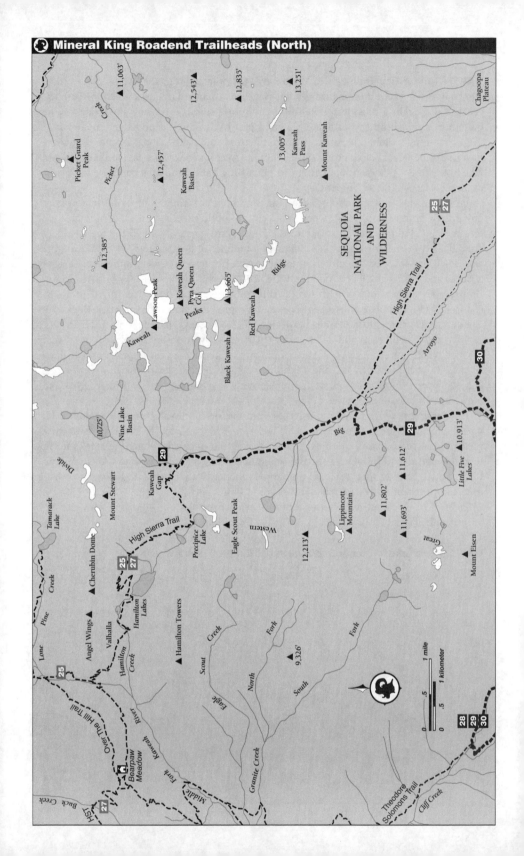

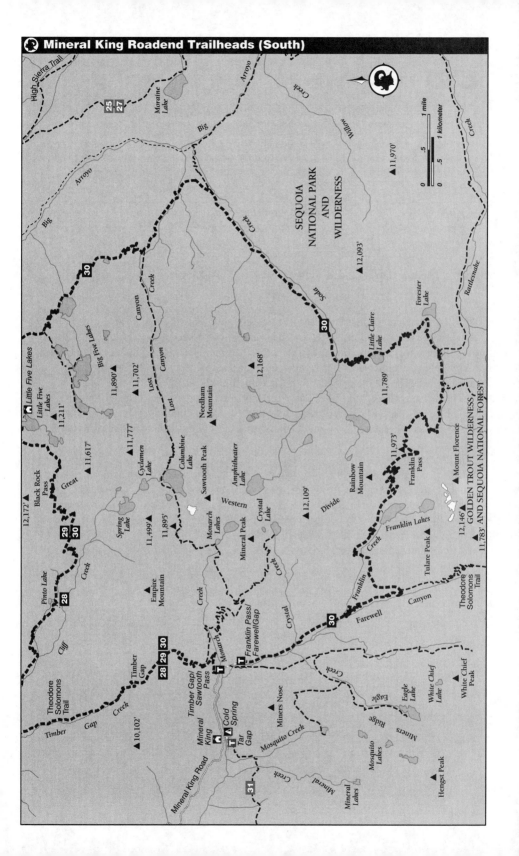

High Sierra Trail

Moraine Lake

25
27

Arroyo

Creek

Willow

SEQUOIA
NATIONAL PARK
AND
WILDERNESS

▲11,970'

1 mile

1 kilometer

.5

.5

0

0

Big

Arroyo

Big

30

Creek

Canyon

Creek

Canyon

Lost

Soda

30

▲12,093'

Forester
Lake

Little Claire
Lake

Rattlesnake
Creek

Little Five Lakes

Little Five
Lakes

11,211'▲

Big Five Lakes

11,890'▲

▲11,702'

Lost

Canyon

Needham
Mountain

12,168'

▲11,789'

12,172'▲

Black Rock
Pass

Great

▲11,617'

▲11,777'

Cyclamen
Lake

Columbine
Lake

Sawtooth Peak

Amphitheater
Lake

Rainbow
Mountain

▲11,973'

Franklin
Pass

29
30

Spring
Lake

11,499'▲

11,895'▲

Monarch
Lakes

Mineral Peak

Western

Crystal
Lake

Divide

12,109'

Mount Florence

12,146'▲
GOLDEN TROUT WILDERNESS,
AND SEQUOIA NATIONAL FOREST
11,783'▲

Pinto Lake

28

Cliff

Creek

Empire
Mountain

Creek

Crystal

Franklin

Creek

Franklin Lakes

Tulare Peak ▲

Theodore
Solomons
Trail

Theodore
Solomons
Trail

Timber
Gap

Creek

▲10,102'

28 29 30

Timber Gap/
Sawtooth
Pass

Franklin Pass/
FarewellGap

T

T

Monarch

Farewell

30

Canyon

Mineral
King

Cold
Spring

Tar
Gap

Miners Nose

Mosquito Creek

Creek

Eagle

Miners

Ridge

White Chief
Lake

White Chief
Peak

Mineral King Road

Timber
Gap

31

Mineral

Creek

Mosquito Creek

Mosquito
Lakes

Mineral
Lakes

Eagle
Lake

Hengst Peak ▲

see maps on p. 180– 181

trip 29   ## Nine Lake Basin

Trip Data: 36.55790°N, 118.54735°W; 39.0 miles; 6/3 days
Topos: *Mineral King, Triple Divide Peak*

HIGHLIGHTS: Nine Lake Basin offers seclusion that only cross-country destinations seem to possess. While hundreds tramp the High Sierra Trail, not more than a half mile away, and many throng to Little Five Lakes, through which this trip passes, few visit this wild basin, with its splendid lakes and majestic scenery.

HEADS UP! *The trail is relatively easy, and the route to the lowest lake in Nine Lake Basin is straightforward but trackless: just follow the outlet stream. Map-and-compass skills and some cross-country experience are prerequisites for exploring the basin's highest lakes.*

DAY 1 (Timber Gap Trailhead to Pinto Lake, 8.2 miles): Follow Trip 28, Day 1 to Pinto Lake (8,726'; 36.48508°N, 118.58071°W; no campfires).

DAY 2 (Pinto Lake to Little Five Lakes, 5.2 miles): From the camping area, regain the Black Rock Pass Trail. Start climbing across slopes covered with sagebrush, chinquapin, and willows. Early summer puts on quite a wildflower display, with forget-me-nots, paintbrush, lupine, phlox, wallflower, yampa, larkspur, senecio, and Bigelow sneezeweed. Soon, you encounter the first of many switchbacks leading to Black Rock Pass.

The interminable slog is made more tolerable by the incredible scenery along the way, including the cascades below Spring Lake and the classic chain of cirque lakes consisting of Spring Lake, Cyclamen Lake, and Columbine Lake, often still icebound in early summer.

> **PATERNOSTER LAKES**
>
> When books on Sierra geology discuss "paternoster lakes," a series of lakes in glacier-carved basins, strung like rosary beads one after the other on the stream connecting them, they often choose a photo of these very lakes (Spring, Cyclamen, and Columbine) to illustrate the concept.

Finally, the rocky path attains Black Rock Pass (11,630'), where the views are vast. To the east and southeast, the companion basins of Little Five Lakes and Big Five Lakes drop off

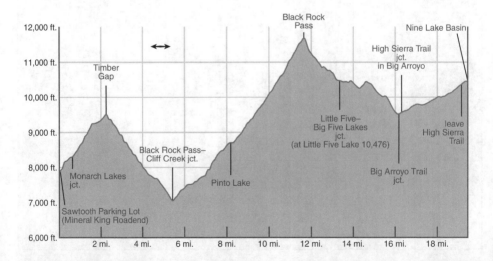

into Big Arroyo, and beyond this chasm rise the multicolored Kaweah Peaks. In the distant east is the 14,000-foot Whitney Crest, backbone of the Sierra.

From the pass, the zigzagging downgrade trends southeast and then angles northeast to pass above the highest of the Little Five Lakes, which actually comprise more than a dozen lakes. (When snow obscures the trail in early season, keep to the left so as not to end up off-route too far to the right and come out onto some cliffs.) A couple of Spartan campsites nestle in the rocks above the highest lake, which has a large tarn to the south. Just below the second of the Little Five Lakes, the trail fords the outlet and meets the trail to Big Five Lakes. Just south of this junction (10,482'; 36.49265°N, 118.53625°W; no campfires), overused campsites are huddled around a bear box, just east of a peninsula (no camping) and a bay. Stroll out onto the peninsula at sunset to catch the alpenglow on Kaweah Peaks Ridge. A summer ranger station across the bay may offer emergency services. The other lakes may offer more privacy.

DAY 3 (Little Five Lakes to Nine Lake Basin, 6.1 miles, part cross-country): Returning to the main trail, turn left (northeast) and continue down the Little Five Lakes chain to another ford of the stream that links them. Soon, the trail crosses the outlet of the northern cluster of Little Five Lakes.

After an easy rise out of the basin, the trail descends into Big Arroyo, a large canyon whose stream is a tributary of the Kern River. The route becomes increasingly steep as it turns northeast. Beyond a ford of Big Arroyo, reach a junction with an unsigned trail heading down Big Arroyo; there is a large campsite with a bear box at the junction. Head left (north), past an old cabin, and in just over 0.1 mile reach a second junction. Turn left (north) again, now on the High Sierra Trail, to ascend gently up this broad glacial valley past numerous potential campsites with great views of Lippincott Mountain and Eagle Scout Peak towering in the west, and metamorphic Black Kaweah and Red Kaweah piercing the eastern sky.

The trail fords Big Arroyo again and then climbs over grassy pockets and granite slabs toward Kaweah Gap, a distinctive low spot on the Great Western Divide to the northwest.

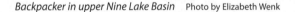

Backpacker in upper Nine Lake Basin   Photo by Elizabeth Wenk

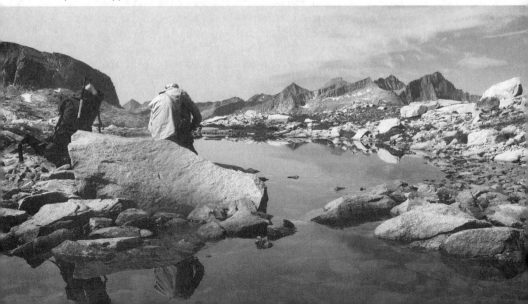

Where the High Sierra Trail swings west to Kaweah Gap, your cross-country route heads north into Nine Lake Basin and soon arrives at the roughly horseshoe-shaped first lake (10,462'; 36.55790°N, 118.54735°W; no campfires), with numerous fair-to-good campsites, good fishing for brook trout, and fine opportunities to explore this fascinating basin.

Days 4–6 (Nine Lake Basin to Timber Gap Trailhead, 19.5 miles): Retrace your steps.

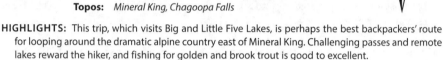

trip 30 ## Big and Little Five Lakes

see maps on p. 180– 181

> **Trip Data:** 36.48347°N, 118.50679°W; 38.7 miles; 6/2 days
> **Topos:** *Mineral King, Chagoopa Falls*

HIGHLIGHTS: This trip, which visits Big and Little Five Lakes, is perhaps the best backpackers' route for looping around the dramatic alpine country east of Mineral King. Challenging passes and remote lakes reward the hiker, and fishing for golden and brook trout is good to excellent.

HEADS UP! *You'll need to be in excellent shape in order to enjoy this challenging trip.*

DAY 1 (Franklin Pass Trailhead to Franklin Lakes, 6.1 miles): From the parking lot, return to Mineral King Road. Walk east and then south up the road to the pack-station access road, and then follow that road south-southeast up the canyon past the pack station and a sign indicating that you're now on the Franklin Lakes/Farewell Gap Trail. Continue past corrals and through the open terrain of the East Fork Kaweah River's valley. Gazing southeast, spot the prominent, V-shaped notch of Farewell Gap at the head of the canyon on the border of Sequoia National Park. Just right (west) of the road, the hurried waters of the river are hidden by a screen of willows. On the approach to Crystal Creek, scattered clumps of juniper and red fir contrast vividly with the ghost-white trunks of some cottonwoods.

Ford Crystal Creek and then branch left (south-southeast) onto a singletrack trail, as the road, closed to vehicles, veers right toward Soda Spring. Along the rocky trail, enjoy the fragrance of sagebrush, and between the sagebrush and gooseberry of these lower slopes, find spots of color provided by a variety of wildflowers, including paintbrush, fleabane, cow parsnip, and ipomopsis. A gradual-to-moderate climb leads to a ford of dashing Franklin Creek (difficult in early season) and the start of a steep, switchbacking, exposed climb, interrupted by an ascending traverse near the midpoint of the switchbacks. Above the switchbacks, reach a junction of the Franklin Lakes and Farewell Gap Trails.

Turn left (northeast) at the junction and follow the Franklin Lakes Trail on a long, ascending traverse across the northwest slopes of Tulare Peak. Here you will enjoy fine views down the Kaweah River's canyon to Mineral King and up to Farewell Gap. The contrast between the green hillside and the red of Vandever Mountain in the south is especially striking in the morning light. Enter a sparse forest of mature foxtail pines and cross red-hued, rocky slopes dotted with spring flowers and laced with tiny snowmelt rills, as the trail turns northeast into Franklin Creek's upper canyon. Drop briefly to a ford of willow-lined Franklin Creek and resume a switchbacking climb toward the lakes. Pass the first campsites along the creek just below the rock-and-concrete dam across the outlet of the lower lake.

Continue climbing on the trail as it rises well above the shore of Lower Franklin Lake to the first of a pair of paths that lead down to view-filled campsites (bear box; 10,377'; 36.42073°N, 118.55853°W; no campfires) notched into sandy ledges on the sloping hillside above the lake. The second path accesses campsites (bear box, pit toilet) near the east inlet about 400 feet above the lake. The popularity of the lakes, combined with the limited number of viable campsites, may lend more of a feeling of a trailer park than remote backcountry on busy summer weekends; don't expect solitude.

Backpackers who haven't expended all their energy on reaching the first campsites may escape some of the crowd by continuing another half mile to a bench between the lower and upper lakes. Campsites on the bench are treeless and exposed but see far fewer visitors. A short romp from the bench over boulders leads to Upper Franklin Lake (10,578'), directly below the cirque wall between Florence and Tulare Peaks.

VIEWS AND FISHING AT FRANKLIN LAKE

A bizarre conglomeration of colors appears in Upper Franklin Lake's dramatic cirque basin. To the northeast, the slopes of Rainbow Mountain are a study of gray-white marble whorls set in a sea of pink, red, and black metamorphic rocks. To the south, the slate ridge joining Tulare Peak and Florence Peak is a hue of chocolate red that sends photographers scrambling for viewpoints from which to foreground the contrasting blue of Lower Franklin Lake against this colorful headwall. Anglers should find the fishing for brook trout good at the lower lake and perhaps better at the upper lake.

DAY 2 (Franklin Lakes to Little Claire Lake, 7.5 miles): Away from Lower Franklin Lake, the trail rises steadily eastward and then climbs steep switchbacks. Views of the Franklin Lakes' cirque improve with elevation, with both lakes eventually coming into view. The ascent leaves forest cover behind as the trail crosses and recrosses a field of coarse granite granules dotted with bedrock outcropping. Despite the sievelike drainage of this slope, wildflowers abound. High up on the slope, two adjacent, year-round rivulets nourish gardens of yellow mimulus and lavender shooting stars. At windy Franklin Pass (11,760'), views are panoramic.

VIEWS AT FRANKLIN PASS

Landmarks to the northwest include Castle Rocks and Paradise Peak; to the east is the immediate unglaciated plateau above the headwaters of Rattlesnake Creek, as well as Forester Lake on the wooded bench just north of the creek. East of the Kern Trench and plateaus is Mount Whitney along the Sierra Crest.

The initial descent from the pass, unlike the westside ascent, zigzags down a slope mostly covered with disintegrated quartz sand and, oddly, sprinkled with small, wind-sculpted granite domes. Eventually, very widely scattered stunted pines begin to reappear prior to some switchbacks that lead down to a small meadow in the Rattlesnake Creek drainage (campsites in the vicinity; fine fishing). On the way, pass a signed junction with the faint Shotgun Pass Trail on the right. Skirt the meadow and continue downstream to a junction of the Soda Creek and Rattlesnake Creek Trails.

From the junction, go left (east-northeast) on the Soda Creek Trail. Walk through light, lodgepole pine forest on a gradual ascent to Forester Lake (10,190'), a little more than 3 miles from the pass. The lake is rimmed by grass and pine, with plenty of campsites spread around the shore. Fair-size brook trout should tempt the angler.

From the lake, head north for a moderate climb, interrupted briefly by a short stroll across a meadow-covered bench, leading to the top of a rise. From there, follow a moderate ascent to the sandy crown of a ridge dividing the Rattlesnake Creek and Soda Creek drainages. At this rounded summit, the crests of Sawtooth Ridge and Needham Mountain are easily visible to the north, and they remain in view as the trail descends moderately to the south end of Little Claire Lake. You may hear the effervescent burble of the Brewer blackbird and the raucous call of the Clark nutcracker as you skirt the east side of the lake to the good campsites on a sandy slope dotted with foxtail pines at the north end of Little Claire Lake (10,425'; 36.42417°N, 118.52117°W; no campfires). Fishing for brook trout may be excellent.

DAY 3 (Little Claire Lake to Big Five Lakes, 8.6 miles): The trail west of the outlet stream from Little Claire Lake follows well-graded switchbacks northward down a steep, forested slope for more than a mile. At the bottom of this 900-foot, precipitous, duff-and-rock slope, the route fords Soda Creek, descends gently over duff and sand through a moderate forest cover, and then becomes steeper. (Contrary to the 7.5' topo, the trail doesn't ford the creek again.) Marmots on the rocky slope south of the creek whistle excitedly as unexpected visitors pass by, but they usually fail to stir from their lookout posts unless travelers show more than passing interest.

During the next several miles of undulating descent through lodgepole forest and across dry slopes, usually well away from Soda Creek, the trail leads across occasional refreshing tributaries, one of which is spanned by a boardwalk, and passes a half-dozen campsites of uneven quality. Among the lodgepoles, notice an occasional whitebark pine and then red fir. Clumps of sagebrush fill gaps between the stands of timber, and nestled next to their aromatic branches are healthy patches of Douglas phlox and Indian paintbrush.

The appearance of Jeffrey pine heralds the approach to a signed junction with the route along the Sawtooth Pass Trail to the left (northwest) and a trail branching right down into Big Arroyo. Turn left on the Sawtooth Pass Trail. (Fortunately, the park service has rerouted what was once a steep, rocky, loose, hot, exposed ascent to the foot of Lost Canyon.)

Beyond a crossing of Lost Creek, the trail follows a zigzagging climb through light forest to a meadow with a nearby campsite. Past the meadow, a more moderate ascent continues up Lost Canyon to a junction with the trail to Big Five Lakes. From here, campsites with a bear box are a short distance farther up the Sawtooth Pass Trail near another crossing of Lost Creek.

However, today's route turns right (north) at the junction and follows switchbacks up a hillside covered with lodgepole pines and chinquapin. Reach a bench where a tepid tarn at

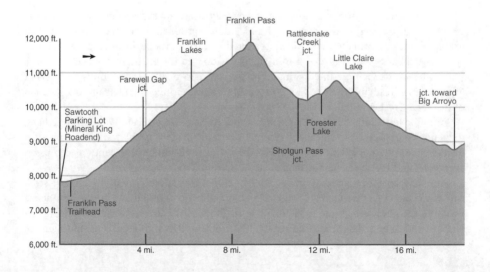

10,084 feet offers the possibility of a fine swim and secluded camping above the heather-lined shore. Beyond the bench, resume a moderate climb amid boulders and slabs to the apex of a ridge overlooking the Big Five Lakes' basin. A rocky, steep descent leads to the first of the lakes (9,834'; 36.48347°N, 118.50679°W), where backpackers can overnight at good campsites near the log-jammed outlet or along the north shore (9,853'; 36.48450°N, 118.50742°W).

DAY 4 (Big Five Lakes to Little Five Lakes, 3.1 miles): From the outlet of the lowest Big Five Lake, Lake 9,830, follow the trail around the north shore to an informal junction with a use trail to campsites and ahead to the next lake. Take the right-hand fork northwest and make a steep, zigzagging, mile-long climb to a T-junction with the trail to the upper Big Five Lakes (very beautiful, campsites) and the path to Little Five Lakes.

Turn right (north) and follow the Little Five Lakes Trail to the top of a ridge. The trail undulates for a dry mile, with periodic great views of Mount Kaweah, the Kaweah Peaks Ridge, and, at the ridge's west end, Red Kaweah and Black Kaweah.

The dry stretch ends when the trail dips to traverse a boardwalk over a small, intimate valley, where a stream flows at least until late summer. From this brook, climb for several hundred vertical feet through a moderate lodgepole forest, level off, and then gain sight of the main Little Five Lake, Lake 10,476, bordered by a large meadow. Soon, the trail reaches the north end of the lake (10,482'; 36.49265°N, 118.53625°W; no campfires), where overused campsites are huddled around a bear box. A summer ranger station may offer emergency services.

DAY 5 (Little Five Lakes to Pinto Lake, 5.2 miles): From the north end of Lake 10,476, follow the trail around the west shore and then climb moderately above the lake to the north before angling south to pass above the highest of the Little Five Lakes. Leaving the lakes behind, a zigzagging climb leads to 11,630-foot Black Rock Pass on the Great Western Divide.

Rocky switchbacks lead from the austere surroundings of the pass down into the more hospitable surroundings of some subalpine meadows near Cliff Creek. Find an unsigned junction with a use trail on the left that leads roughly south to shady campsites with a bear box (8,726'; 36.48508°N, 118.58071°W; no campfires). Nearby, Pinto Lake hides in a pocket of thick willows, offering surprisingly pleasant swimming.

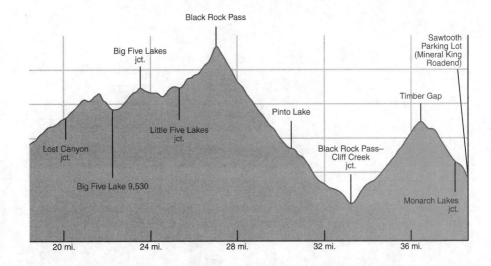

DAY 6 (Pinto Lake to Franklin Pass Trailhead, 8.2 miles): From the vicinity of Pinto Lake, the trail heads generally west-northwest down the canyon, crosses the lake's outlet, and then switchbacks down the north wall of the canyon, well above the course of Cliff Creek. At the bottom of this descent, reach a signed junction with the Timber Gap Trail near Cliff Creek Camp (campsites, bear box).

Turn left (southwest), immediately ford Cliff Creek (difficult in early season), and make a switchbacking climb up a hillside. Above the switchbacks, climb around the nose of a ridge into the drainage of Timber Gap Creek. Ascend the canyon; farther upstream, the trail crosses the main creek a couple of times in a splendid, flowery meadow. A final, switchbacking climb through red firs leads to aptly named Timber Gap (9,511').

Drop southeast away from Timber Gap, eventually breaking out of the trees to a tremendous view down into Mineral King's subalpine valley. After a while, a series of switchbacks descends through red firs before traversing open slopes to a junction with the Monarch Lakes–Sawtooth Pass Trail. Take the right fork southeast here. A steeper descent from there leads down to the roadend parking lot.

Little Five Lakes   Photo by Elizabeth Wenk

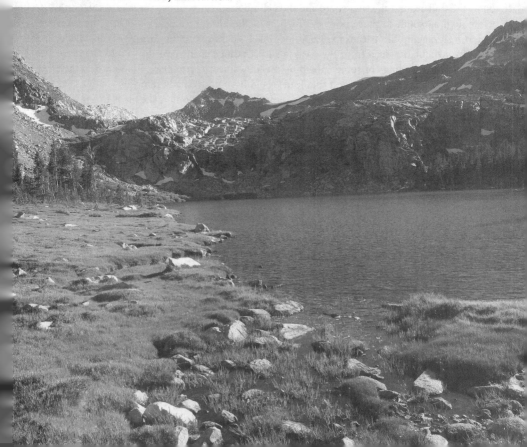

Tar Gap Trailhead (in Cold Spring Campground)
7,487'; 36.45082°N, 118.61402°

Destination/ GPS Coordinates	Trip Type	Best Season	Pace & Hiking/ Layover Days	Total Mileage	Permit Required
31 Hockett Lakes 36.35179°N 118.66756°W	Out-and-back	Early to late	Moderate 4/1	23.6	Tar Gap *(Atwell for alternative start)*

INFORMATION AND PERMITS: The trailhead is in Sequoia National Park. Permits are required for overnight stays, and quotas apply. Permits can be reserved up to six months in advance at recreation.gov/permits/445857, with additional details at nps.gov/seki/planyour visit/wilderness_permits.htm. For both advance reservations (67% of quota) and walk-up permits (33% of quota), there is a $15-per-permit processing fee and a $5-per-person reservation fee. Both reserved and walk-up permits for this trailhead must be picked up in person at the Mineral King Ranger Station, open 8 a.m.–3:45 p.m. daily. Campfires are prohibited above 9,000 feet in Sequoia National Park when west of the Great Western Divide. Bear canisters are not required but are strongly encouraged.

DRIVING DIRECTIONS: From the CA 99–CA 198 interchange in Visalia, take CA 198 east past Lake Kaweah and the town of Three Rivers, turning right onto the tiny Mineral King Road after 38.6 miles; this is 1.5 miles after you leave Three River. This minor road is easily missed—if you cross the Kaweah River you've gone 1.6 miles too far. Follow a very slow, windy Mineral King Road 23.4 miles east to the Mineral King Ranger Station. After picking up your permit, you can park across the street from the ranger station or retreat just 0.1 mile back downhill (west), parking your car across the street from the entrance to the Cold Springs Campground. Instead of bear boxes, there is a large wooden shed to store food and toiletries in, located in the parking area across from the ranger station. The actual Tar Gap Trailhead is located at the far western end of the campground, near some walk-in tent sites.

see map on p. 190

trip 31 ## Hockett Lakes

Trip Data: 36.35179°N, 118.66756°W; 23.6 miles; 4/1 days
Topos: *Mineral King, Silver City, Moses Mountain*

HIGHLIGHTS: This enjoyable hike takes travelers south to the striking Hockett Plateau. A pleasant walk leads past luxuriant subalpine meadows along the way to quiet and solitude at Hockett Lakes. This is a splendid late-spring (or early-summer) walk, before it is too hot and when the endless wildflowers are in full bloom. An alternate return route via the Atwell Trail leads past trailside sequoia trees growing interspersed with other conifer species and a view of dashing falls along the East Fork Kaweah River. This would be given as the main route, did it not have an extra 1,000 feet of elevation gain.

HEADS UP! *The 2020 Castle Fire burned just west of the Hockett Lakes basin. Call the Mineral King Ranger Station before your trip to determine if the fire's footprint extends to the lakes themselves; if it does, consider camping at Hockett Meadows and taking side trips to Evelyn Lake, Cahoon Rock, and the Hockett Lakes.*

DAY 1 (Tar Gap Trailhead to Horse Creek campsites, 7.9 miles): The route leaves the southwest end of Cold Spring Campground; follow the main access road through the campground

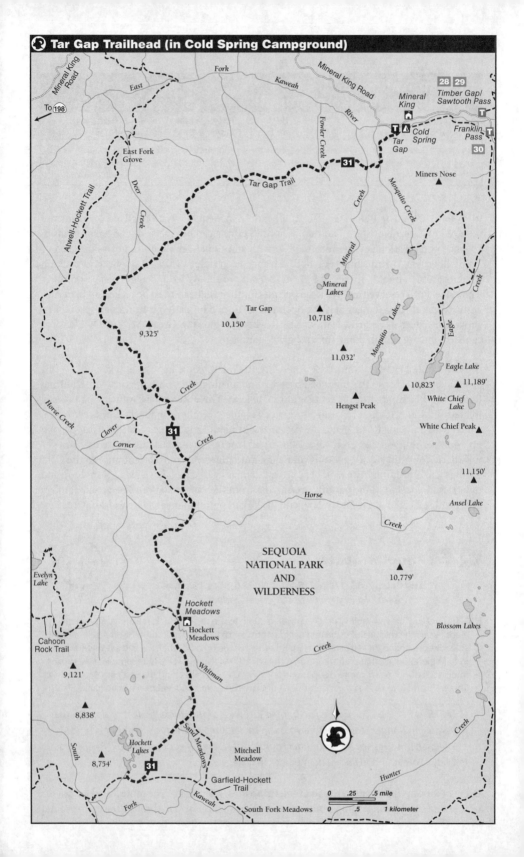

Mineral King
Road

To 198

Fork

East

Kaweah

Mineral King Road

Mineral
King

Fowler Creek

River

28 29
Timber Gap/
Sawtooth Pass

Cold
Spring

Tar
Gap

Franklin
Pass

30

East Fork
Grove

Deer

Creek

31

Tar Gap Trail

Mineral

Creek

Mosquito Creek

Miners Nose ▲

Atwell-Hockett Trail

Mineral
Lakes

Mosquito
Lakes

Eagle

Creek

Tar Gap

10,150'

10,718' ▲

9,325' ▲

11,032' ▲

Eagle Lake

▲ 11,189'

10,823' ▲

White Chief
Lake

Hengst Peak ▲

White Chief Peak ▲

Horse Creek

Creek

31

Clover

Corner

Creek

11,150' ▲

Horse

Creek

Ansel Lake

Evelyn
Lake

SEQUOIA
NATIONAL PARK
AND
WILDERNESS

10,779' ▲

Blossom Lakes

Cahoon
Rock Trail

9,121' ▲

Hockett
Meadows

Hockett
Meadows

Creek

8,838' ▲

Whitman

Hockett
Lakes

Sand Meadows

Mitchell
Meadow

Creek

South

8,754' ▲

31

Garfield-Hockett
Trail

Hunter

Kaweah

South Fork Meadows

Fork

0   .25   .5 mile

0   .5   1 kilometer

to a big placard declaring the start of the Tar Gap Trail. Just behind, the obvious trail heads south up the hill. (There is drinking water available at faucets in the campground.) Immediately after leaving the campground, the trail switchbacks up through steep red fir forest and then begins an ascending traverse into the Mosquito Creek drainage, soon climbing quite steeply alongside the creek.

At 7,930 feet the trail fords Mosquito Creek and crosses a narrow, bouldery rib to Mineral Creek, which it promptly crosses. Both are wades at high flows, quickly transitioning to rock hops as the summer progresses. These are the first of many creek crossings, each draining a separate cirque nestled at the base of the impressively scalloped Hengst Peak ridge. The trail undulates in and out of these drainages, crossing bouldery ribs between each that offer expansive vistas of Conifer Ridge and Paradise Peak across the valley and northeast to Glacier Pass. Next is Fowler Creek, a generally easy step-across and then two unnamed tributaries. Sections have forest cover—mostly red fir and western white pine— while elsewhere the forest has been burned and shrubs, including mountain whitethorn, chinquapin, and chokecherry, cover the slope. Slowly you have better views of the crest to the south, while those northeast are blocked.

About 2.6 miles from the trailhead, the trail bends from west to southwest, crosses a broader, rockier ridge, and then traverses forested slopes, where it reaches the two forks of Deer Creek. At the first creek is the first legal camping area (8,226'; 36.43525°N, 118.65551°W), although usually only the southwestern branch of Deer Creek has water, 0.4 mile beyond the waypoint given. Other campsites can be found on the spur between the two branches.

Beyond the Deer Creek rock-hop crossing, you pass through a dense willow-and-flower jungle with a trickle. The trail continues southwest for another mile before rounding a sharp bend and making a permanent tack toward the south. The trail continues to undulate between ridges and drainages, gaining very little elevation. Rich conifer forests populate the draws, some with magnificently huge red fir. (Only on the lower Atwell Grove Trail do you get to pass through majestic sequoia groves.) At 6.1 miles you round a corner with a view-rich but waterless campsite and hook into a tiny seasonal drainage. Around the next rib is the Clover Creek drainage, offering perennial water, a verdant flower-filled wedge of meadow, and a possibly tricky early-season ford. Another 0.7 mile leads to Corner Creek, an early-summer wade and late-season rock hop. The next 0.5 mile features a modest descent to the junction with the Atwell Trail. Just a few minutes later you reach a broad sand-and-slab shelf, a river terrace above Horse Creek, with many campsites—an ideal place to spend your first night (8,586'; 36.39252°N, 118.65379°W). There was once a wire-and-pulley arrangement suspended between two pines to hang your food, but that has been removed.

DAY 2 (Horse Creek to Hockett Lakes, 3.9 miles): The ford of Horse Creek lies just south of the campsites and can be a thigh-deep wade in early season—it is a much larger drainage than the other creeks you've crossed. After the ford, the path crosses a marshy corridor

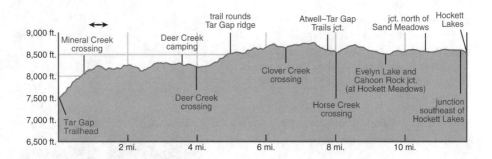

and then continues through a dry red-fir-and-western-white-pine forest, climbing over a moraine crest. Dropping into lusher forest again, you loop first southeast and then south beneath lodgepole pine cover. Quite suddenly you begin walking through young lodgepole pines and arrive at the foot of Hockett Meadows near a junction; right (west) leads to Cahoon Peak and Evelyn Lake, both rewarding side trips, while straight ahead (south) takes you into Hockett Meadows and on to the Hockett Lakes. Following the Evelyn Lake spur just a short distance leads to appealing campsites near Whitman Creek's north bank.

Continuing into Hockett Meadows, after you pass a summer-staffed ranger station the trail jogs slightly west, passing a large lodgepole pine–shaded campsite with a bear box. Standing at the edge of the meadow, you'll enjoy sweeping views of Hengst and White Chief Peaks to the northeast and Vandever Mountain to the east. *Note:* Additional campsites and another bear box are on the east side of Hockett Meadows. To avoid damaging meadow grasses, to reach it, from the ranger station, complete a big clockwise loop around the meadow's periphery.

Unless you linger and explore, you leave Hockett Meadows almost as soon as you reach it, crossing Whitman Creek on a small wooden bridge and climbing onto a shelf that lies just far enough from the river and meadow you don't see them again. The trail traverses through lodgepole pine forest crisscrossed with endless downed logs, evidence of past fires. The lush forest walk continues to a junction at the northeastern corner of Sand Meadows. Here you turn right (west), toward Hockett Lakes, while straight ahead (south) leads to South Fork Meadow.

The trail follows the northwestern edge of Sand Meadows, fording its seasonal inlet creek, crossing a minor ridge, and skirting around the east side of the very flat, marshy basin holding the many Hockett lakes and tarns. The lakes are still out of sight as you approach the next junction, where right (west) is signposted for the Hockett Lakes and left (east) for South Fork Meadow. Ignoring the given mileage (0.7 mile), it is less than 0.2 mile until you step across the Hockett Lakes outlet creek and should turn north to find a campsite (8,539'; 36.35179°N, 118.66756°W). There are reasonably big sandy patches just west of the southernmost lake, with easy access to the shore of the lovely heath-ringed lake. Many of the other lakes are surrounded by marshy vegetation, with less obvious camping opportunities.

A layover day here allows for exploration of this remote corner of Sequoia National Park. Possibilities include a trip to the subalpine Blossom Lakes or the easy summit of Quinn Peak (from Windy Gap). Or maybe you want to move your camp to Hockett Meadows and explore the meadow environs or embark on a trip to Cahoon Rock and Evelyn Lake.

Days 3–4 (Hockett Lakes to Tar Gap Trailhead, 11.8 miles): Retrace your steps. If you have a second car, you may want to contemplate taking the Atwell Trail on the descent; it is almost exactly 1 mile longer. It crosses some giant wildflower corridors beside Corner and Clover Creeks, passes beneath giant sequoias in the Atwell Grove, and crosses the East Fork Kaweah River just downstream of East Fork Kaweah Falls. It also ends with a hot 600-foot climb from the East Fork Kaweah River crossing to the Atwell Mill Campground.

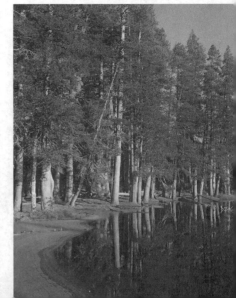

You'll likely find solitude at the Hockett Lakes. Photo by Elizabeth Wenk

CA 190 AND SHERMAN PASS ROAD TRIPS

CA 190 and Sherman Pass Road, in conjunction, offer the Sierra's first road crossing south of CA 120 (Tioga Road) in Yosemite National Park. Spur roads off of these lead to a number of often-forgotten trailheads that launch hikers into two of the southern Sierra's wilderness areas, Golden Trout Wilderness and South Sierra Wilderness, as well as Giant Sequoia National Monument. While the southern Sierra's peaks are muted in comparison to those to the north and lakes are more rare, it is a beautiful landscape of meadows, granite knobs and domes, and, in early summer, splendid wildflower displays. Being at a slightly lower elevation, it is a perfect place for a May–June or September–October hike. Just two trips are included in this book: one departs from the Summit Trailhead in Sequoia National Forest and leads to Maggie Lakes, while the other departs from Blackrock Trailhead on the Inyo National Forest boundary and leads to Redrock Meadows and Jordan Hot Springs.

Trailheads: Summit

Blackrock

Summit Trailhead — 8,276'; 36.21059°N, 118.57798°W

Destination/ GPS Coordinates	Trip Type	Best Season	Pace & Hiking/ Layover Days	Total Mileage	Permit Required
32 Maggie Lakes 36.27589°N 118.62393°W (Upper Maggie Lake)	Out-and-back	Early to late	Leisurely 3/1	19.0	Summit (no quotas)

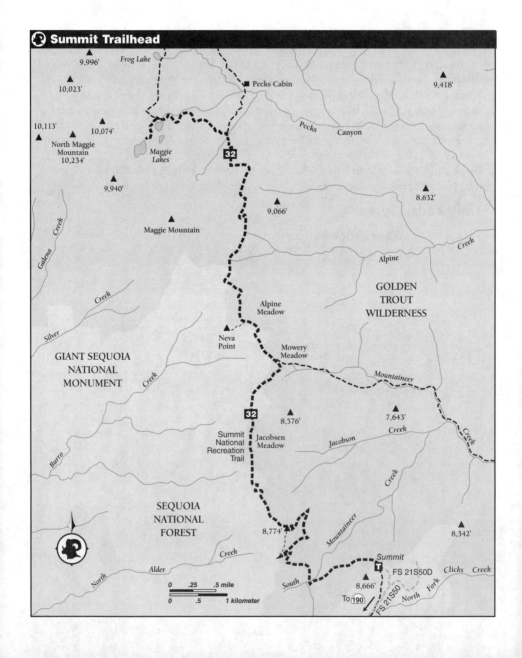

Summit Trailhead

INFORMATION AND PERMITS: This trailhead is in Sequoia National Forest. Permits are required for overnight stays, but there are no quotas. Details on how to reserve permits are available at fs.usda.gov/detail/sequoia/passes-permits. Because there are no quotas, you can simply call ahead to one of the ranger stations or pick up a permit as you drive past. Options are the Western Divide Ranger Station (32588 CA 190, Springville, CA 93265; 559-539-2607) if you're coming from the west or the Kern River Ranger District–Kern Office (11380 Kernville Road, Kernville, CA 93238; 760-376-3781) if you're coming from the south or east. If you plan to use a stove or have a campfire, you must also have a California campfire permit, available from U.S. Forest Service offices or online at preventwildfireca.org/campfire-permit. Bear canisters are not required but are strongly encouraged.

DRIVING DIRECTIONS: From the junction of CA 65 and CA 190 near Porterville, take CA 190 east 40.8 miles, past Camp Nelson to an inconspicuously marked junction with Forest Service Road 21S50. Quaking Aspen Campground is 0.25 mile farther along CA 190—if you reach the campground you've gone too far. Turn left (north) onto FS 21S50, paved for the first 4.5 miles. Thereafter, stay on FS 21S50, now dirt, for an additional 5.4 miles, ignoring both a series of spur roads (FS 20S79 heading right, FS 20S81 heading left, and FS 20S71 heading left) and several intersections with the Summit National Recreation Trail. FS 21S50 ultimately drops steeply and you reach a junction 9.9 miles from CA 190 where FS 21S50 continues right and FS 21S50D climbs to the left; turn onto FS 21S50D and follow it just 0.1 mile to the trailhead.

trip 32   **Maggie Lakes**

> **Trip Data:**   36.27589°N, 118.62393°W (Upper Maggie Lake);
> 19.0 miles; 3/1 days
> **Topos:**   *Camp Nelson, Quinn Peak*

HIGHLIGHTS: Cool, deep fir forest alternates with marvelous meadows on the way to the lovely, peaceful Maggie Lakes, a bit of High Sierra scenery in this largely lakeless southern Sierra landscape. The often-deserted trailhead at the end of a long dirt road gives the sense that this trail has been abandoned, but it is in good condition and a perfect location to find solitude.

HEADS UP! *Maps show a number of trails intersecting Summit National Recreation Trail, but years of neglect have left many of them almost invisible or impassable or both. It's tempting to make this a loop trip by using some of those trails, but that "loop" may be very hard to find and follow.*

HEADS UP! *The 2020 Castle Fire burned from the trailhead to the Maggie Peak ridge just south of the Maggie Lakes, although it is quite likely there are untouched patches of vegetation in the middle of Alpine and Mowery Meadows. The Maggie Lakes themselves have so far escaped the flames. Call Sequoia National Forest to ask about the trail status before taking this hike in 2021 and 2022.*

DAY 1 (Summit Trailhead to Alpine Meadow, 5.2 miles): Head north, briefly through scrub, but soon curving west into moderate to open, mature red fir forest on a gradually descending, dusty trail. Drop to hop across South Fork Mountaineer Creek just below two tributaries that nourish a wonderful hillside meadow. After fording the creek, climb steeply up an east-facing slope, where all the red firs are lichen-clad above the 10-foot mark, the height to which they are standardly snow covered in winter. You reach a saddle, where the main trail makes a sharp right to continue its ascending traverse across the eastern slope, while a use trail departs straight up the ridge, offering a steeper ascent with splendid views and early-summer wildflowers. Turning right to follow the main trail, you loop counter-clockwise to a ridge and follow it west, sidling just north of the summit of Knob 8,774; here the "ridge shortcut" rejoins the main route.

Trending north again, the trail breaks out into the open, following the crest past delicate spring wildflowers and affording marvelous views northeast of the Jacobson Creek drain-age, west down the mountains' intricately folded slopes to the Central Valley and north toward the High Sierra. Continuing nearly along the ridge, the boundary between Giant Sequoia National Monument (to the west) and Golden Trout Wilderness (to the east), the trail switchbacks down through a cool north-facing red fir forest to reach a junction with the little-used Jacobson Trail that descends the Alder Creek drainage to Camp Wishon. Soon thereafter you reach elongate Jacobson Meadow, perched just east of the crest.

Skirting the western edge of seasonally marshy, flowery Jacobson Meadow, you pass a designated "fire-safe" campsite just off the trail. In Sequoia National Forest, this designa-tion indicates you can still have a fire here when certain campfire restrictions are in place; check with a ranger when picking up your permit. Cutting across a minor saddle, the trail descends to Mowery Meadow, passing campsites on the final descent to the meadow and along the meadow's perimeter. From here, another little-used trail descends east down Mountaineer Creek (8,135'; 36.24228°N, 118.59908°W). About 0.1 mile down this trail is a pleasant, fire-safe campsite at the edge of the beautiful meadow.

Still in red fir forest, the trail now climbs more diligently, cresting a broad saddle after 0.5 mile and reaching Alpine Meadow (8,412'; 36.24719°N, 118.60131°W). Here are larger campsites, atop forested ribs down the center of the meadow, many of these "dry islands" offering sites with decomposing camp furniture. The meadow's stream conveniently winds between the first two "islands," providing easy access to water. An added benefit of these campsites is a spur that leads left (west) to Neva Point, offering lovely evening or morning vistas (8,610'; 36.24717°N, 118.60818°W).

DAY 2 (Alpine Meadow to Maggie Lakes, 4.3 miles): From Alpine Meadow's edge, the trail climbs alongside a meadow tentacle back to a ridgecrest, where you reach a junction on the left (west) with the vanished Griswold Trail to Mountain Home State Forest; con-tinuing straight ahead, on the right (east) is lovely Griswold Meadow (unnamed on maps), with a fire-safe campsite. Ahead, the landscape east of the trail was partially burned in the 2015 Cabin Fire and that to the west was very lightly scorched in the 2006 Maggie Fire; fortunately, many trees survived both burns. Continuing across rockier ground, under a mixed canopy of red fir, western white pine, and Jeffrey pine, the trail leads a gradual 500 feet up to Maggie Mountain's northeast shoulder.

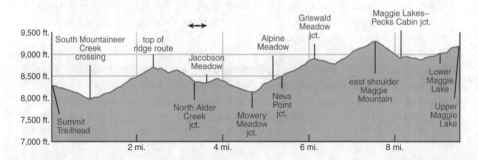

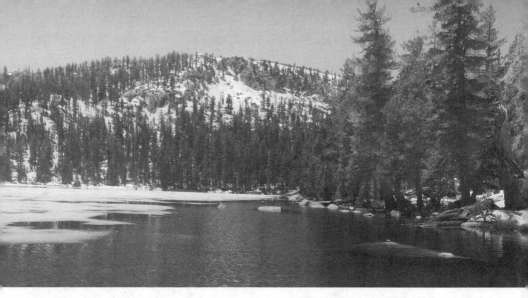

Upper Maggie Lake   Photo by Elizabeth Wenk

MAGGIE MOUNTAIN

Maggie Mountain, 10,022 feet, offers a magnificent view of the southwestern Sierra north to Vandever and Florence Peaks, near Mineral King. There are two straightforward routes to its summit. From where the trail crosses its northeast shoulder you can follow the ridge to the summit, first across an easy sandy ridge and later up the steeper, rockier eastern slopes. Alternately, you can climb from Upper Maggie Lake, heading updrainage and then across a flat shelf to Maggie Mountain's northwestern slopes, that you follow to the summit.

From the shoulder's high point, make a moderate, rocky descent to ford a tributary of Pecks Canyon's creek. Just beyond the ford, there's a signed junction where Summit National Recreation Trail, still your route, branches left (initially west, then northwest) to the Maggie Lakes, while right is signposted for Alpine Meadow. Ahead the trail loops northwest and west, crossing three minor ribs before entering the cirque holding the three Maggie Lakes. This last stretch of trail is rockier and, where the trail becomes faint, you depend upon cairns to identify the route. The forest cover is sparse and the landscape has the classic, open southern Sierra "feel" with foxtail pine growing on rocky ridges. Continuing past small outcrops and across bouldery patches, you reach Lower Maggie Lake's outlet creek. Just beyond is a large campsite with several fire pits and grills (9,029'; 36.27892°N, 118.62084°W). Steep and blocky cliffs rise behind the lake. Fishing at the lakes for golden trout is reportedly excellent.

Lower Maggie Lake has the area's biggest campsites, but your trip is not complete without continuing to the upper lake for at least a look; the middle Maggie Lake is more enclosed without any flat terrain for camping. Continuing along the main trail beyond Lower Maggie Lake, you turn off the trail at the inlet, crossing the creek and following a cairn route south up the ridge to the upper lake (9,185'; 36.27589°N, 118.62393°W). At Upper Maggie, the best campsites are on a ridge, just east of the lake—big, flat, sandy patches that hold many tents. While Lower Maggie is backdropped by steep cliffs, at Upper Maggie you feel more surrounded by the summits, which are set back but taller.

DAY 3 (Maggie Lakes to Summit Trailhead, 9.5 miles): Retrace your steps from Days 1 and 2.

Blackrock Trailhead   8,888'; 36.17583°N, 118.26878°W

Destination/ GPS Coordinates	Trip Type	Best Season	Pace & Hiking/ Layover Days	Total Mileage	Permit Required
33 Redrock Meadows and Jordan Hot Springs 36.27051°N 118.27615°W	Semiloop	Early to Late	Moderate 3/1	18.8	Blackrock (no quotas)

INFORMATION AND PERMITS: This trailhead is in Inyo National Forest. Permits are required for overnight stays, but there are no quotas. Your permit can be picked up at the Blackrock Ranger Station, passed en route to the trailhead. Contact the Kern River Ranger Station at 760-376-3781 with any questions.

DRIVING DIRECTIONS: The route you take to the Black Rock Visitor Information Center (8,068'; 36.09448°N, 118.26452°W) is different if you're driving from eastern (or southern) versus western California. From the east, you want to turn from US 395 onto Sherman Pass Road (also called Nine Mile Canyon Road and Forest Route 22S05) and follow it a very windy 36.9 miles west, passing the Kennedy Meadows Resort en route. From the west, you want to head to the town of Johnsondale along road M50. From there, continue east on Mountain Road 99 for 4.9 miles. Just after you cross the Kern River on the Johnsondale Bridge, turn left onto Sherman Pass Road/FS 22S05 and follow it a very windy 31.7 miles east. The Black Rock Visitor Information Center is a very short distance north along FS 21S44—you can see the ranger station from the junction.

After picking up your permit, continue north on paved Blackrock Road (in part FS 21S44 and later FS 21S03) 8.1 miles to the road-end trailhead. Many spur roads branch off, but this is always the main road and well signposted. There is parking for hikers and equestrians, a one-overnight campground, a pit toilet, and water.

trip 33   Redrock Meadows and Jordan Hot Springs

Trip Data: 36.27051°N, 118.27615°W (Redrock Meadows);
18.8 miles; 3/1 days
Topos: *Casa Vieja Meadows, Kern Peak*

HIGHLIGHTS: Great variations characterize this semiloop: lovely meadows and streams lead to beautiful Redrock Meadows beneath the copper-colored monolith called Indian Head. From there, the descent of Redrock Creek leads through tragic fire devastation to the remote oasis of Jordan Hot Springs. Closing the loop, your ascent of Ninemile Creek is strenuous, but along the second half you are rewarded with beautiful wildflower displays.

DAY 1 (Blackrock Trailhead to Redrock Meadows, 8.8 miles): Under a moderate canopy of red fir and western white pine, head north from the road-end gate on the sandy trail, gradually climbing past the occasional fire-scorched tree. After 0.2 mile, the path enters Golden Trout Wilderness at Blackrock Gap and begins a gradual-to-moderate descent, soon passing a pocket meadow on the right. The trail presently crosses the meadow's seasonal creek, one of the many Ninemile Creek tributaries that coalesce in Casa Vieja Meadows. The trail continues just east of the creek, the red fir yielding to lodgepole pine as you approach the meadow.

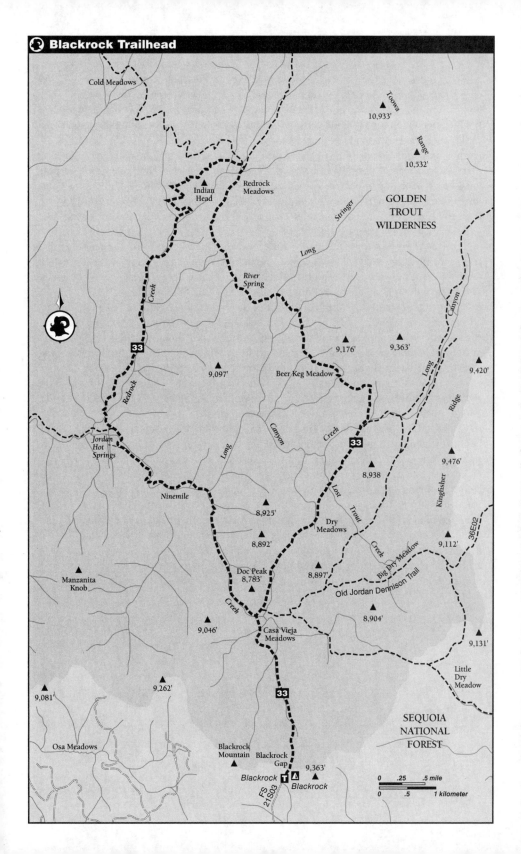

At 1.5 miles, huge Casa Vieja Meadows opens up on the right (north) as the route steps over a pair of Ninemile Creek's tributaries and skirts the western meadow border. It's not long before the trail bends north through cowpies and past an old corral and two more tumbledown buildings to a good view of the meadow, with its weathered buildings, grazing cattle, long fencelines, and excellent seasonal flowers. Nearby are possible campsites on granite sand under lodgepole pine to the west of the trail. Crossing one more seasonal tributary—a long leap or wobbly log crossing—the trail soon reaches Ninemile Creek proper; look for a wobbly log to balance across just downstream. Just beyond is a junction signed for Jordan Hot Springs where the loop part of this trip begins; the trail left (northwest) leads to Jordan Hot Springs, your return route, and right (northeast) to Redrock Meadows (8,301'; 36.20192°N, 118.27329°W).

Take the right fork toward Redrock Meadows and, in 300 feet, pass a junction with a trail that cuts right (east) across Casa Vieja Meadows. You continue straight ahead (north) toward Redrock Meadows, the sandy trail remaining at the lodgepole pine–grass boundary as it traces a dwindling, north-trending arm of Casa Vieja Meadows.

Rising ever so gently, the trail climbs out of the Ninemile Creek drainage and drops to cross a seasonal tributary of Long Canyon Creek and then Lost Trout Creek. Once past the riparian meadow strip, a fast, sandy walk leads through sparse lodgepole pine and past collections of boulders and a delightful bright-white quartz vein, where the ground is strewn with the sharp-angled quartz chunks. Just before you drop to the banks of Long Canyon Creek, you pass a junction where you stay left (north) toward Redrock Meadows, while right (east) leads up the creek corridor into Long Canyon (8,474'). The peripheries of the Long Canyon meadow corridor offer possible campsites.

Crossing Long Canyon Creek on a log, the trail follows a tributary creek due north, beside a sloping meadow lobe. About where the meadow ends, and there is a dilapidated sign marking a generally vanished trail (that diagonals back to Long Canyon), your trail makes a sharp left-hand (west-trending) turn. The trail climbs steeply over a broad ridge before dropping northwest to Beer Keg Meadow, its creek crossed on rocks. There are places to camp on the edges of this beautiful meadow. Onward, the trail undulates through open red fir and Jeffrey pine forest, eventually crossing another pair of Long Canyon Creek tributaries in quick succession; the latter is Long Stringer. The Kern Plateau is famous for its seasonally lush and flowery meadows, and your route is following the most southwestern of the plateau's meadows. Indeed, just a few hundred feet to your left the landscape drops into drier, lower-elevation canyons, the terrain on Days 2 and 3 of the trip.

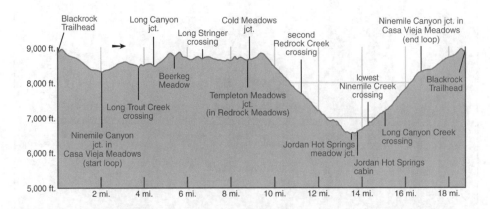

Traverse yet another ridge before descending to the forested nook from which River Spring emerges, its strong flow nourishing a downstream meadow full of corn lilies. On the far side of the next little ridge, at a "trail junction" shown on the USGS 7.5' topo, stay left; the right-hand option is long abandoned. Looking across the landscape you can see that west, generally downslope, much of the landscape has been charred repeatedly, first in the gigantic 2002 McNally Fire and then again in the 2017 Indian Fire, just after your author had done the fieldwork for this update.

It's not long before the trail curves around a decidedly marshy lobe of Redrock Meadows, offering a wonderful view over the meadow toward Indian Head. You then ford a fork of Redrock Creek draining the eastern lobes and quickly reach a trail junction positioned between an old corral downhill and a ruined cabin uphill: the right fork goes northeast toward Templeton Meadows, while the left (west) goes deeper into Redrock Meadows (8,656'; 36.27051°N, 118.27615°W). There are campsites in sandy flats beneath lodgepole pine cover once across the first tributary, with additional sites ahead. Go left at this junction, ford a second tributary, and find another junction where the right fork goes northwest to Cold Meadows; this trip takes the left fork as it curves west over a sandy flat with abundant campsites nearby (for example, 8,718'; 36.27130°N, 118.27806°W). Just northeast of this flat is a large, year-round tributary.

MCNALLY "INCIDENT"

From July 21 to August 29, 2002, a wildfire that began near the Kern River raged, eventually burning 150,670 acres—one of the largest Sierra fires at the time. As is common practice by midsummer, most forest managers had already declared open fires forbidden, even in established campgrounds. Flouting this posted regulation, a mother built a campfire to cook dinner for her kids, and the fire got out of control. . . . You'll see the devastation while descending Redrock Creek. There, the fire burned so hot that it sterilized the soil, consuming tree seeds that might have reforested the region more quickly. Even after 15 years, barely a tree seedling has established. Fire regulations: They're not just advisories. Follow them religiously!

DAY 2 (Redrock Meadows to Jordan Hot Springs, 4.9 miles): Much of this day consists of the sunstruck, 2,300-foot descent to Jordan Hot Springs. Heading southwest, ford Redrock Meadows' final tributary, and follow the track westward across forested flats between the many meadow lobes. As you begin to climb above Redrock Meadows, the trail is so faint at the meadow-forest boundary that there's a sign declaring TRAIL. Then ascend some 200 feet to a saddle behind Indian Head (reportedly Class 3 from here by the easiest route).

You now descend to rejoin Redrock Creek, which dropped down a narrow gorge on the east side of Indian Head. You follow a series of long, sometimes steep switchbacks under sparse, partly scorched forest, with Jeffrey pines providing just sporadic shade. Near the end of the last, very long switchback leg, you pass below a clump of aspens as you near Redrock Creek. The track then turns to parallel the creek downstream, dropping very steeply to its first ford. Once across, the trail clings to the creek bank as far as the next ford, this section still pleasantly shaded.

Once back across the creek—a log crossing or sandy-bottomed wade—the canyon mouth widens, and you enter the area more severely burned by the McNally Fire. Here, the trail climbs away from the creek and wanders through some very flowery spots as it intersects several springs. Along the main creek is a beautiful waterfall that's worth an admiring pause. Nearby are also your very last bits of shade, for ahead there really is barely a mature tree standing. From here to Jordan Hot Springs, not only are all the mature trees dead, but seedlings are, so far, completely absent, for there is no nearby seed source. Instead, prior to the 2017 Indian Fire, this slope was a sea of greenleaf manzanita, mountain whitethorn, and the occasional bit of broad-leaved lotus. These shrubs will have been burned back to ground level but will quickly regrow with a vengeance, always threatening to engulf the trail. Yet another fire, the 2020 Castle Fire, lapped at this area from the west. It appears to have stopped just west of Jordan Hot Springs, but has burned the landscape west to the Kern River.

Your sizzling descent continues. The trail presently rises high above the creek and strays westward away from it, crossing to the far side of a narrow rib. Below, you step across a minor seasonal tributary and angle southeast to cross Redrock Creek for the last time. (*Note:* A junction shown on the USGS 7.5' topo between the tributary and the main creek doesn't exist.) The trail then crosses some runoff channels and enters live forest as it skims the soggy meadow that surrounds Jordan Hot Springs. As you approach the bank of Ninemile Creek, there is a spur trail that leads west to some small campsites and into the meadow (6,541'; 36.22996°N, 118.30117°W). This trail spur continues down Ninemile Creek toward the Kern River. The broad meadow is worth exploring, not just for the springs, but also to admire the extensive white-staining from calcium carbonate deposits; researchers believe such thick deposits exist here because the water picks up minerals as it flows through volcanic rocks upstream.

JORDAN HOT SPRINGS RESORT

For many years before the establishment of Golden Trout Wilderness, concessionaires operated a very rustic hot springs resort here on a U.S. Forest Service lease. While the lodgings consisted of dirt-floored wooden shacks with iron cots (you brought your own sleeping bag), the main lodge building housed a restaurant widely known for its wonderful views and delicious, hearty meals. Rickety bathhouses on the edge of Ninemile Creek sheltered shallow tubs where visitors could relax in the springs' warm waters. By the time the lease last expired, the resort was within the wilderness, and there was no provision for renewing the lease. Consistent with wilderness-management policies, the resort ceased operation in 1990 when the lease expired. The U.S. Forest Service has since removed all but a few of its buildings, keeping only those deemed historically significant (look for their bright metal roofs up on the hillside).

Your route continues southeast on the main (left) fork, crosses Ninemile Creek on a bridge of two flattened logs, and reaches an incense cedar–forested flat with a decaying cabin and packer campsite (6,545'; 36.22895°N, 118.30072°W). The McNally Fire fortunately spared this immediate area, and you'll find several good campsites. The footprints of a few of the old bathhouse tubs from the old Jordan Hot Springs resort, filled with algae-scummed water, still exist downstream on the south bank of Ninemile Creek; follow use trails to find them—on cool mornings, look for steam rising from them. There's reportedly fishing for golden trout in the creek.

DAY 3 (Jordan Hot Springs to Blackrock Trailhead, 5.1 miles): Today's leg consists of the 2,400-foot climb back to the trailhead, much of the elevation gained over the first 3.0 miles. Fortunately, there are repeatedly patches of shade, especially if you get an early start. Leaving the vicinity of the old resort behind, you'll encounter a junction with a signed spur to a public pasture; continue left (southeast) on the main trail. Soon, the trail begins its climb of Ninemile Creek's narrow canyon to Casa Vieja Meadows. Notice the giant, elongate boulder piles—flood deposits dropped here because the canyon's gradient suddenly lessens.

Through a partially burned forest of white fir, ponderosa pine, and incense cedar, the track climbs its first 200 feet over 0.5 mile to reach the next ford of Ninemile Creek (may be difficult in early season, and there are no nearby logs). Once across, resume the moderate ascent, quickly leaving the shaded riparian corridor and ascending a hot, dry slope that is alternately bare soil and carpets of mountain whitethorn, with very few trees surviving. Sections of the trail here can be difficult to discern and elsewhere the trail is objectionably rutted—just keep following the river's northeastern bank upward.

At 0.8 mile above the previous ford, in a thicket of redosier dogwood, the trail fords one of Ninemile Creek's major tributaries, Long Canyon Creek, which you first crossed on Day 1 far upcanyon. This ford may also be difficult in early season. Continuing, the path crosses additional, much smaller, tributaries, as you traverse a marshy area thick with fireweed, meadow rue, streamside bluebell, and thimbleberry. Near here you leave the burn scars behind—finally—and climb under mixed conifer shade.

Before long you reach another ford of Ninemile Creek, requiring a wade at the highest flows, but later transitioning to a rock hop. Above, a couple of switchbacks carry the trail above Ninemile Creek for a while and over more tributaries. Yet another ford soon follows, quite similar to the previous in difficulty. The trail continues winding alongside Ninemile Creek. The showy, seasonal flower gardens along this stretch include lupine, groundsel, meadow rue, ranger's button, Kelley's lily, cinquefoil, asters, and skyrocket, before the trail quite suddenly reaches the green expanse of Casa Vieja Meadows.

On the west edge of Casa Vieja Meadows, you meet your junction from Day 1 and close the loop part of this trip. Turn right (south), find the log over Ninemile Creek, and retrace your steps.

Casa Vieja Meadows   Photo by Elizabeth Wenk

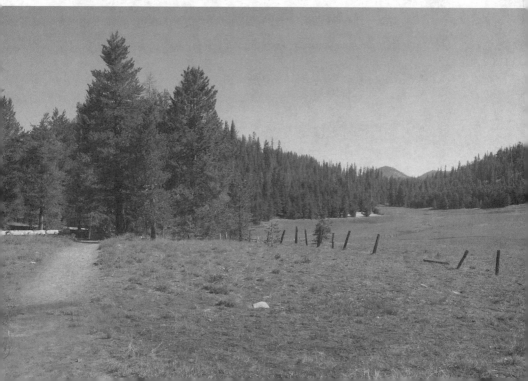

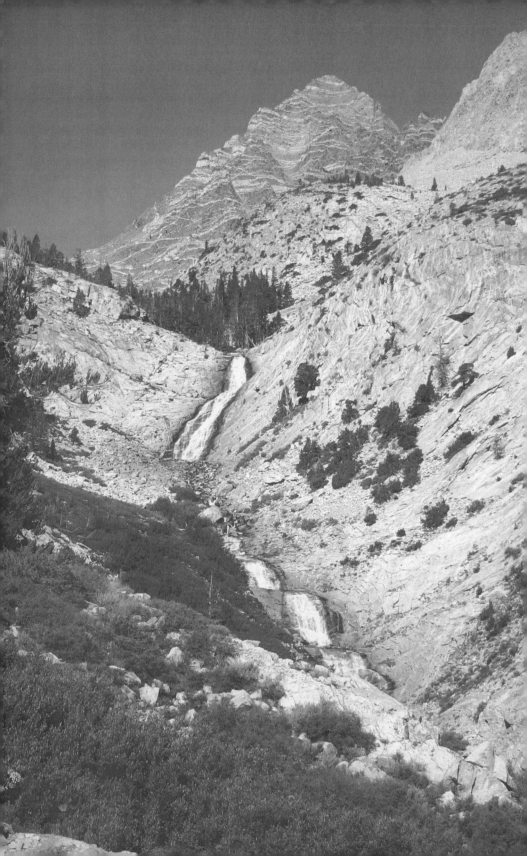

East Side

US 395, which roughly parallels the Sierra's tall eastern escarpment, is the major road from which you take the lesser roads to starting trailheads. These drives start at 4,000–7,000 feet (or more!), they are typically short compared to westside drives, and they are very scenic. A few shuttle trips end at roads not listed below. Small, charming towns along US 395 provide lodging, gas, and stores.

On the east side, you'll enter the Sierra on these roads and highways:

- **Horse Meadow Road** *(just east of Yosemite and south of CA 120)*
- **CA 158** *(the June Lakes Loop)*
- **CA 203** *(through Mammoth Lakes)*
- **McGee Creek Road** *(between Mammoth Lakes and Bishop)*
- **Rock Creek Road** *(also between Mammoth Lakes and Bishop)*
- **Pine Creek Road** *(also between Mammoth Lakes and Bishop)*
- **CA 168 East Side** *(through Bishop)*
- **Glacier Lodge Road** *(through Big Pine)*
- **Taboose Creek Road** *(between Big Pine and Independence)*
- **Division Creek Road** *(also between Big Pine and Independence)*
- **Onion Valley Road** *(through Independence)*
- **Whitney Portal Road** *(through Lone Pine)*
- **Horseshoe Meadows Road** *(also through Lone Pine)*

Falls in Pine Creek Canyon (Trip 53, page 302)   Photo by Mike White

HORSE MEADOW ROAD TRIP

Horse Meadow Road lies one canyon south of Lee Vining Canyon, the busy Tioga Road (CA 120) corridor. Leading only to the Gibbs Lake Trailhead, this valley couldn't be more different—it leads to an equally steep escarpment but is one of the Yosemite area's least visited trailheads.

Trailhead: Gibbs Lake

Steep escarpments rise above Gibbs Lake.   Photo by Elizabeth Wenk

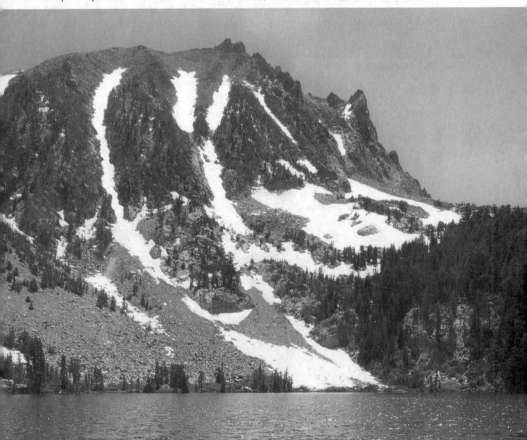

Gibbs Lake Trailhead				7,980'; 37.91976°N, 119.15285°W		
Destination/ GPS Coordinates	Trip Type	Best Season	Pace & Hiking/ Layover Days	Total Mileage	Permit Required	
34 Gibbs Lake 37.90050°N 119.18287°W	Out-and-back	Mid to late	Leisurely 2/1	5.2	Gibbs Lake	

INFORMATION AND PERMITS: This trailhead is in Inyo National Forest. Permits are required for overnight stays and quotas apply. Permits can be reserved up to six months in advance at recreation.gov (60%; $6 permit reservation fee plus $5 per person) or requested in person, first come, first served, a day in advance (40%; free). All permits must be picked up at one of the Inyo National Forest ranger stations, located in Lone Pine (Eastern Sierra Interagency Visitor Center), Bishop, Mammoth Lakes, and Lee Vining (the Mono Basin Scenic Area Visitor Center). If you plan to use a stove or have a campfire, you must also have a California campfire permit, available from a forest service office or online at preventwildfireca.org/campfire-permit. Campfires are prohibited above 10,000 feet. Bear canisters are not required but are strongly encouraged.

DRIVING DIRECTIONS: If you are driving southbound on US 395, from the junction of US 395 and CA 120 just south of Lee Vining, drive 1.3 miles south, then turn right (west)

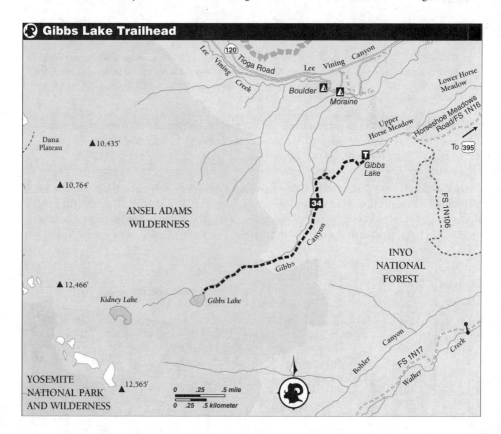

onto Horse Meadows Road/FS 1N16. If you are driving northbound on US 395, this junction is 3.1 miles north of the northern junction of US 395 and CA 158 (June Lakes Loop).

Turn west onto this dirt road and follow it toward the mountains, ignoring a number of intersecting roads departing north and south. After 1.2 miles you reach Lower Horse Meadow and continue west, ignoring two northbound spurs. All vehicles can proceed to the meadow's western end, but the final 1.3 miles to the trailhead require a moderately high-clearance car—currently a station wagon or two-wheel-drive truck/SUV should have no difficulty, but occasionally the steep stretch of road between Lower Horse Meadow and Upper Horse Meadow becomes badly incised and rutted. Then you'll need a high-clearance four-wheel-drive vehicle to get all the way to the trailhead. If you are concerned, stop at the west end of Lower Horse Meadow (7,430'; 37.92479°N, 119.13232°W) where there is a broad pullout and walk the final 1.3 miles to the trailhead (which involves about 525 feet of elevation gain).

Assuming you're still driving, a short steep segment leads to Upper Horse Meadow. Ignoring a tangle of four-wheel-drive tracks departing south, the road continues around the meadow's southern perimeter and soon reaches the trailhead. The drive is a total of 3.4 miles from US 395; the trail begins at the lot's northwest edge, where a locked gate bars vehicles. There are no facilities at the trailhead.

trip 34 Gibbs Lake

see map on p. 207

Trip Data: 37.90050°N, 119.18287°W; 5.2 miles; 2/1 days
Topos: *Mount Dana*

HIGHLIGHTS: The destination of this trip is a little-known lake in Ansel Adams Wilderness on the dramatic east slope of the Sierra, just east of Yosemite. It's a great place to find peace and quiet, and for serious anglers, there is a chance to catch some beautiful golden trout. But it is a stiff walk to the lake, especially if your vehicle can't reach the true trailhead.

HEADS UP! *Don't forget that if your vehicle can't make it to the trailhead and you must park at Lower Horse Meadows, the hike to Gibbs Lake will be 1.3 miles longer (3.9 miles each way) with an additional 525 feet of elevation gain.*

DAY 1 (Gibbs Lake Trailhead to Gibbs Lake, 2.6 miles): From the true trailhead, circumvent the gate and climb steeply up a gully, still following the old road. The trail then jogs north, then west, continuing its steep ascent up a ridge. Enjoying over-the-shoulder views of Mono Lake, you reach the crest of the massive Lee Vining Creek moraine after 0.6 mile

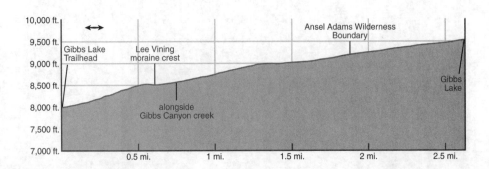

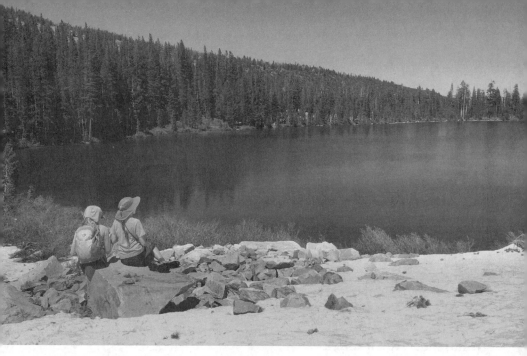

Gazing across Gibbs Lake   Photo by Elizabeth Wenk

(and nearly 550 feet of elevation gain) and breathe a sigh of relief—you've completed the hottest, steepest part of the walk. Dropping slightly, you reach the banks of Gibbs Canyon's creek, a tributary of Lee Vining Creek, near a ruined flume.

The old road now ends and you approximately follow the creek's southeastern bank upstream through mixed conifer forest—white fir, Jeffrey pine, lodgepole pine, juniper, and soon western white pine—just north of the moraine crest. Ahead you garner occasional views to red Mount Dana and darker Mount Gibbs. Some giant curl-leaf mountain mahogany populate the moraine rubble, while strips of stunted aspen fill the gullies. Until about 8,900 feet a subsidiary rib separates the trail corridor from the creek. Soon after it vanishes, you enter cooler streamside lodgepole pine and hemlock forest and proceed upward at a shallower grade. At 1.9 miles you pass the Ansel Adams Wilderness boundary in an expanse of Labrador tea and fragrant red heather. The gradual-to-moderate grade continues until a brief, steep climb just before Gibbs Lake's outlet. There are good campsites along the lake's northern shore (9,535'; 37.90050°N, 119.18287°W) and some sheltered ones to the east of the outlet (a little below the lake).

DAY 2 (Gibbs Lake to Gibbs Lake Trailhead, 2.6 miles): Retrace your steps.

KIDNEY LAKE

Above and west of Gibbs Lake lies brilliantly blue Kidney Lake (10,405'; 37.89778°N, 119.19616°W). Adventurous hikers will find an easy if steep route to Kidney Lake up the forested south side of Gibbs Lake's inlet stream. The expansive views of Mono Lake and the escarpment that encircles the lake (between Mount Dana and Mount Gibbs) are worth the climb. A fishless pothole lake, Kidney Lake lacks an outlet; its "outlet" stream emerges well below the lake, near the base of a long-lasting snowbank. Most of the shore of Kidney Lake is comprised of multicolored lobes of talus (a combination of talus fans and rock glaciers), but some whitebark pines at the east end provide shelter for a Spartan camp.

CA 158 TRIP

CA 158 is the June Lakes Loop Road, looping west of the US 395 corridor past the collection of June Lakes. It also provides access to a selection of dirt roads leading to minor trailheads, including Walker Lake, Parker Lake, and Fern Lake. By far the most-used trailhead along the June Lakes Loop is Rush Creek Trailhead, included in this book. Lying between the busy Yosemite and Mammoth Lake regions, it provides access to a string of reservoirs along Rush Creek (Agnew, Gem, and Waugh Lakes) and to natural lake basins to the north and south of the main Rush Creek corridor.

Trailhead: Rush Creek

Banner Peak sits majestically at the head of Thousand Island Lake.   Photo by Elizabeth Wenk

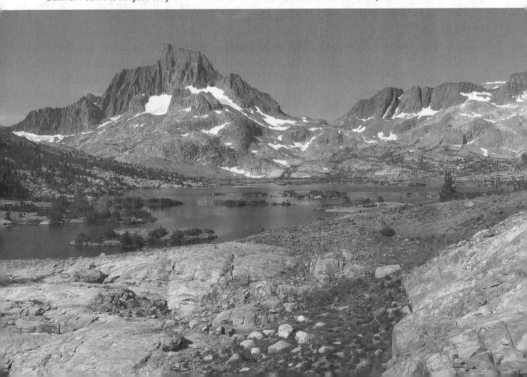

Rush Creek Trailhead

7,240'; 37.78332°N, 119.12813°W

Destination/ GPS Coordinates	Trip Type	Best Season	Pace & Hiking/ Layover Days	Total Mileage	Permit Required
35 Gem, Waugh, and Thousand Island Lakes Loop 37.72851°N 119.17130°W (Thousand Island Lake)	Semiloop	Mid to late	Moderate 3/1	20.1	Rush Creek

INFORMATION AND PERMITS: This trailhead is in Inyo National Forest. Permits are required for overnight stays and quotas apply. Permits can be reserved up to six months in advance at recreation.gov (60%; $6 permit reservation fee plus $5 per person) or requested in person, first come, first served, a day in advance (40%; free). All permits must be picked up at one of the Inyo National Forest ranger stations, located in Lone Pine (Eastern Sierra Interagency Visitor Center), Bishop, Mammoth Lakes, and Lee Vining (the Mono Basin Scenic Area Visitor Center). If you plan to use a stove or have a campfire, you must also have a California campfire permit, available from a forest service office or online at preventwildfireca.org /campfire-permit. Campfires are prohibited throughout most of this region, including at all described campsites. Bear canisters are required in this area. *Note:* In occasional high runoff periods, sections of the trail around Agnew and Gem Lakes have been closed due to concerns about dam safety; hopefully, planned retrofits will prevent this in the future.

DRIVING DIRECTIONS: The Rush Creek Trailhead sits along the June Lakes Loop (CA 158), west of US 395. If you are driving northbound on US 395, turn left onto CA 158 at the June Lake Junction. Follow CA 158 for 7.1 miles, turning left into the Rush Creek Trailhead parking area. It is directly across the street from the Silver Lake Campground. If you are driving southbound on US 395, turn left onto the northern end of the June Lakes Loop, an intersection located just 4.4 miles south of the US 395–CA 120 intersection in Lee Vining. Now follow CA 158 south for 8.7 miles, turning right into the Rush Creek Trailhead parking area. There are toilets at the trailhead.

trip 35 Gem, Waugh, and Thousand Island Lakes Loop

see map on p. 212

Trip Data: 37.72851°N 119.17130°W (Thousand Island Lake); 20.1 miles; 3/1 days

Topos: *Devils Postpile, Koip Peak, Mount Ritter*

HIGHLIGHTS: This delightful semiloop leads up the Rush Creek drainage to the John Muir Trail (JMT), south along the JMT to famous Thousand Island Lake, and back to the trailhead via the near-crest Clark Lakes. Although this trip can be made in a weekend, the unforgettable scenery—from splendid Thousand Island Lake to the intimate little Clark Lakes—warrants a slower pace. The biggest challenge may be deciding in which splendid spot to spend the layover day. The only downside is the initial climb from the trailhead to Agnew Lake—a long hot slog, so get an early start.

HEADS UP! *Camping is prohibited within a quarter mile of Thousand Island Lake's outlet. Bear canisters are required throughout this region.*

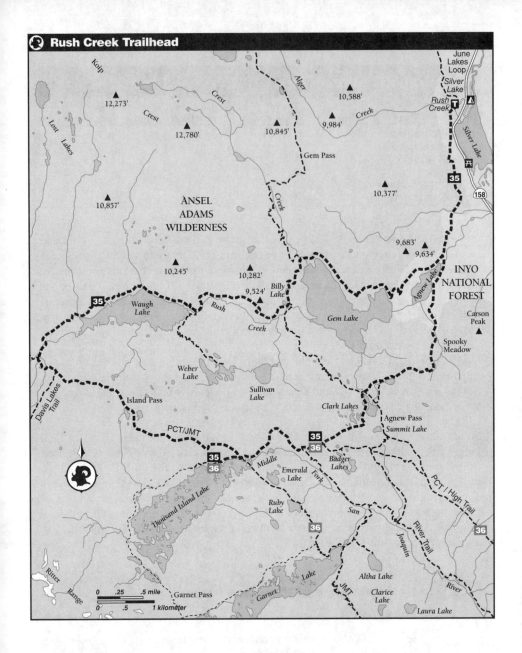

DAY 1 (Rush Creek Trailhead to Waugh Lake, 7.9 miles): Departing southwest from the edge of the parking lot, cross bridges over first the main Alger Creek flow and then a small side channel. Leaving the aspen-lined creek, the route begins a long, steady, shadeless ascent south, quickly passing several use trails that dart downslope toward the Silver Lake Resort. Beyond, the first miles are simply a moderate uphill slog with good views. The trail is rocky and heavily stock traveled.

At a juniper-shaded switchback turn and look for the long, white ribbon of Rush Creek dashing down to the Southern California Edison buildings below (upcoming Agnew, Gem, and Waugh Lakes are dammed for power). Continuing, in places, the trail has been blasted out of the rock; tall, poured-concrete "steps" hold the tread in place. Twice, the trail crosses the tracks of a cable railway (funicular) used to haul personnel and material to the dams on Rush Creek; watch for moving cars and stay off the tracks.

Paralleling the tracks south, you will be pleased to reach a small sign beneath a gigantic juniper (8,477′)—you have now completed the hardest 2.2 miles of the hike. You stay right (southwest) on the main Rush Creek Trail, signposted for Gem Lake, while left (south) leads across Rush Creek to the Clark Lakes, your return route. In a few minutes you pass Agnew Lake's dam. Your steady ascent beneath steep multicolored metamorphic bluffs angles above Agnew Lake's shoreline, crossing some spring-fed seeps colorful with wildflowers and then climbing tight switchbacks that carry you over a ridge just north of Gem Lake's dam.

From a knob above beautiful Gem Lake (9,069′) the track trends down toward the shoreline. Hikers now enjoy a long, undulating stroll along the lake's east and north shores. In one place the trail passes through a corridor delineated by vertically tipped shale beds, channeling you between two rock ribs. Eventually the trail crosses Crest Creek in a tangle of aspens. Just beyond are an abundance of lodgepole-shaded campsites and a junction where you stay left (southwest), while right (north) leads to Gem Pass and the Alger Lakes (Trip 56 in *Sierra North*). Additional campsites can be found on a peninsula extending south into the lake.

Continuing left toward Waugh Lake, you begin ascending away from Gem Lake's shore, climbing over a low notch in a ridge composed of metavolcanic rocks. You then drop slightly to Billy Lake and two small ponds, nestled in a lusher draw. A few more steps lead back to the banks of Rush Creek and a junction; here you stay right (west), toward Waugh Lake, while left (south) leads up to the Clark Lakes. Nearby is a large creekside campsite (where fires are allowed). After crossing a lodgepole pine flat, the trail—and creek—resume their ascent, skirting along the base of outcrops. Soon the creek channel narrows and steepens and you follow switchbacks away from it, crossing a notch where you are suddenly on glacier-polished granite slabs. Descending across broken rock back to creek level, you reach the banks in a very marshy area where the creek broadens and slows; there are two large campsites here. If it is late in the day, you may want to stay here, as there are few tent sites for the next 1.3 miles. Rounding a metamorphic bluff, you climb to another junction, with a lateral that leads left (south) to Weber and Sullivan Lakes; stay right (west).

Continuing to wind up dry slabs dotted with picturesque juniper, the trail soon reaches the dam at the outlet of Waugh Lake. Following Waugh Lake's northern shore, with Mount Davis dominating the western skyline, you amble across exposed slabs; campsites here are poor and few. Only after you cross a seasonal inlet creek and the trail angles from

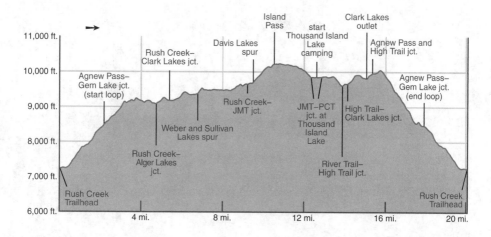

northwest to southwest are there a number of good options in sandy flats and in stands of lodgepole pine. The first sites are near the granite islets toward the west end of the lake (9,481'; 37.75310°N, 119.19603°W; no campfires), with more beyond.

DAY 2 (Waugh Lake to Thousand Island Lake, 4.7 miles): The trail continues through beautiful lodgepole pine to a wet ford of Lost Lakes' outlet. Thereafter you climb steeply away from Waugh Lake. As the grade eases, you cross Rush Creek, a rushing torrent here, on a pair of planed logs. (*Note:* The USGS 7.5' topo map does not show the current trail routing near Rush Creek Forks, the name for this area, where the four forks of Rush Creek combine. It shows the Rush Creek Trail merging with the JMT farther north and individually crossing each of the Rush Creek tributaries once on the JMT.) Once across Rush Creek, the trail traverses a shallow slab knob and descends to ford one of Rush Creek's tributaries, the Davis Lake outlet creek. If water levels make this a wade, stay on the east side of the creek for an extra 0.1 mile (off-trail) and you'll meet the JMT where it crosses the creek itself. Otherwise, cross the creek and just beyond reach the JMT/Pacific Crest Trail (PCT). There are small campsites in this vicinity.

On the JMT, turn left (southeast) toward Island Pass, while right goes northwest to Donohue Pass and into Yosemite. Begin a steady ascent under a continuing forest cover of lodgepole and mountain hemlock. Passing a junction with a faint trail right (south-southwest) to Davis Lakes, climb ahead (left; southeast), crossing the Davis Lakes outlet on a small bridge and angling up through forest and past meadows to Island Pass (10,221'). Just south of this pass, the trail skirts two small lakes (locally called Ham and Eggs Lakes) and then veers eastward. The views from relatively low Island Pass are magnificent and there are many campsites on the broad summit plateau.

Gem Lake   Photo by Elizabeth Wenk

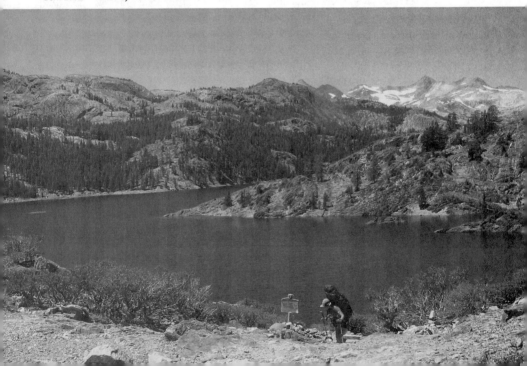

Descending, the trail emerges from dense stands of lodgepole pines and hemlocks (the latter easily identified by their droopy tips) to a dry flower-filled metamorphic slope above Thousand Island Lake.

VIEWS AND GEOLOGY NEAR THOUSAND ISLAND LAKE

Savor the panoramic views from the rocky slopes and notice the striking differences between the predominantly darker rock of the Ritter Range and the lighter granite of the peaks near the Donohue Pass, to the northwest. The dark rocks originate from a catastrophic caldera collapse 100 million years ago; the magma that erupted was some of the same molten rock that formed the plutons deep underground. The volcanic rock was then metamorphosed during subsequent tectonic events that led to the continued formation of the underlying— and somewhat younger—granite. For many a Sierra photographer, the spectacularly jagged dark skyline from Banner Peak southward is one of the Sierra's most revered panoramas.

As the trail switchbacks down to the outlet of Thousand Island Lake, there are classic views across the island-studded waters to the imposing east faces of Banner Peak and Mount Ritter. Just before the outlet, you reach a junction where the PCT and JMT diverge; the JMT continues straight ahead (southeast) to Garnet Lake (Trip 36), while the PCT turns left (east) to traverse slopes east of the headwaters of the Middle Fork San Joaquin River, the so-called High Trail (9,875'; 37.72851°N, 119.17130°W). Departing west (right) from this junction is a use trail that follows Thousand Island Lake's northern shore to numerous scattered campsites. Camping is prohibited within 0.25 mile of Thousand Island Lake's outlet and there are almost no acceptable campsites along the lake's southeast shore, so head west along this trail after reading all the current camping regulations posted at the junction. The campsites get better the farther you go toward the head of the lake, where the scenery is some of the most memorable in the central Sierra, and Lemmon's paintbrush carpets summer's meadows. (The distance given assumes you walk exactly 0.25 mile west of the junction to sites near 9,850'; 37.72789°N, 119.17547°W; no campfires. If you don't camp at Thousand Island Lake, your trip is 0.5 mile shorter.)

DAY 3 (Thousand Island Lake to Rush Creek Trailhead, 7.5 miles): In the morning, return to the junction where the PCT and JMT diverge and take the PCT northeast. Pass several attractive tarns before curving southeast and downhill across a landscape of beautiful dark glacial-polished metavolcanic slabs. Rock spiraea, a small shrub with vibrant pink blooms, stands out brilliantly against this backdrop. Where the nascent Middle Fork San Joaquin River is funneled down a gorge between steep slabs, the trail loops north, descending a separate forested draw. Back near the river, it reaches a junction where the PCT continues straight ahead, while the River Trail branches right (southeast) to follow the Middle Fork San Joaquin toward Agnew Meadows. You stay left (east) on the PCT and after just 0.25 mile meet a second junction, where the PCT (and High Trail) trend right (southeast; Trip 36), toward Agnew Meadows, while you stay left (northeast) on the lesser traveled route toward the Clark Lakes. *Note:* The nearby Badger Lakes offer good campsites.

You cross a lodgepole pine forested shelf and then ascend a steep 200 feet, crossing the Sierra Crest at an unsigned, unnamed pass. Looking back, admire the Middle Fork San Joaquin River's canyon, with the Minarets crowning the far ridge, and Ritter and Banner closer on the right. Directly below are the Badger Lakes.

Descending steeply down a corridor cutting through slabs, you pass a cluster of tarns and two small Clark Lakes, one of which is guarded by a sheer and beautiful rock wall.

Another drop brings you to the west shore of the largest of the Clark Lakes (9,820'), its west end bordered by windswept grass and wild onion. If you want an extra night on the trail, there are a number of good campsites scattered around these lovely lakes. At the outflow of the largest lake, there is a junction, where the left (northwest) branch descends back to Gem Lake and the right (southeast) option, your route, steps across the Clark Lakes outlet creek. You immediately reach a second junction, where right (south) skirts Clark Lakes on their east side and leads up over Agnew Pass and back to the High Trail and thence to Agnew Meadows, while left (northeast), your route, leads to the most northeastern Clark Lake and down to Spooky Meadow and Agnew Lake.

Ascending over volcanic rock—recently deposited volcanic rocks now, not the metavolcanic rocks of the Ritter Range—you reach the final Clark Lake, and yet another junction with a spur that leads back to Agnew Pass; continue straight ahead (left; east), rounding the final lake (9,980') and reaching a small tarn with a good campsite overlooking the valley far below.

Continue climbing, skirting a meadow with views of Gem Lake below and briefly of Mono Lake ahead in the distance; dark Negit Island is prominent. The climb is almost over, and hikers top one last shoulder before descending moderately to a perched meadow. The trail crosses one of Spooky Meadow's inlet streams by a campsite and then recrosses it shortly after beginning a long, steep, loose, rocky descent. This leads to the beautiful meadow and woodland at the foot of Spooky Meadow, nestled in a deep cirque on Carson Peak's west side. Here the grade eases briefly at streamside amid stands of lodgepole pines and mountain hemlocks.

Soon the trail plunges down again, leaving Ansel Adams Wilderness and crossing the stream for the last time as it descends a narrow, rocky canyon. The tread becomes objectionably rocky, as the trail crosses the foot of giant talus fans spilling off Carson Peak's northern spur. Early in this descent there are surprising views of Gem Lake, impossibly blue and barely constrained by its thin, shell-like dam. Below it, Agnew Lake is a long, green pool backed by reddish slopes, across which the Rush Creek Trail that you ascended on Day 1 seems a mere scratch. Tight switchbacks lead to a long traverse across talus slopes that slowly converge with Agnew Lake. You skirt across a bedrock rib and sidle above the lake, following a circuitous route across slabs and between bluffs that leads to a bridge across Rush Creek a little below the dam. Climbing briefly, but steeply, you cross the funicular tracks and meet the Rush Creek Trail. Here, you close the loop part of this trip, turn right (northeast) toward Silver Lake, and retrace the first part of Day 1.

CA 203 TO MINARET SUMMIT ROAD TRIPS

Minaret Summit Road leads from the town of Mammoth Lakes across Minaret Summit to the Middle Fork San Joaquin River valley, the home of famous locales, including Devils Postpile and Reds Meadow. Its trailheads generally lead west to the base of the striking dark-colored Ritter Range. Included in this book are the Agnew Meadows Trailheads, Devils Postpile Trailhead, and Fish Creek (Rainbow Falls) Trailhead. Trails from the first two indeed lead west to lake basins set beneath the steep peaks, justifiably among the Sierra's most famous destinations. The Fish Creek Trail leads south on a shelf above the Middle Fork San Joaquin, connecting to trail networks along Fish Creek and the Silver Divide.

Trailheads: Agnew Meadows
Devils Postpile
Fish Creek

Looking down on Minaret Lake from bluffs to the west (Trip 38, page 229)   Photo by Elizabeth Wenk

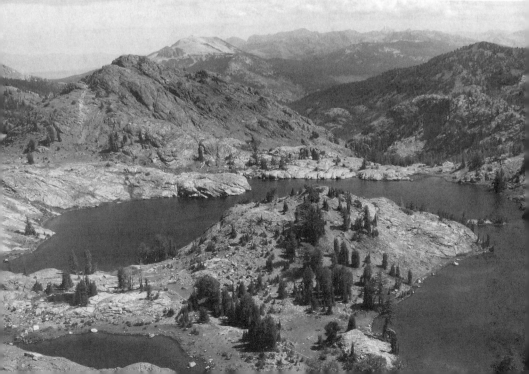

Agnew Meadows Trailheads		8,334'; 37.68282 °N, 119.08471°W (High Trail) or 8,311'; 37.68184°N, 119.08621°W (toward Shadow Creek)			
Destination/ GPS Coordinates	Trip Type	Best Season	Pace & Hiking/ Layover Days	Total Mileage	Permit Required
36 Thousand Island Lake via the High Trail and JMT 37.72851°N 119.17130°W (Thousand Island Lake)	Loop	Mid to late	Moderate 2/1	18.9	High Trail (Shadow Creek in reverse; River Trail for alternate start)
37 Ediza Lake 37.68537°N 119.16862°W	Out-and-back	Mid to late	Moderate 2/1	13.8	Shadow Creek

INFORMATION AND PERMITS: These trailheads are in Inyo National Forest. Permits are required for overnight stays and quotas apply. Permits can be reserved up to six months in advance at recreation.gov (60%; $6 permit reservation fee plus $5 per person) or requested in person, first come, first served, a day in advance (40%; free). All permits must be picked up at one of the Inyo National Forest ranger stations, located in Lone Pine (Eastern Sierra Interagency Visitor Center), Bishop, Mammoth Lakes, and Lee Vining (the Mono Basin Scenic Area Visitor Center). If you plan to use a stove or have a campfire, you must also have a California campfire permit, available from a forest service office or online at preventwildfireca.org/campfire-permit. Campfires are prohibited throughout most of this region, including at all described campsites. Bear canisters are required in this area.

DRIVING DIRECTIONS: From the junction of US 395 and CA 203 (the Mammoth junction), take CA 203 west for 3.7 miles to a major intersection in the town of Mammoth Lakes. Here, straight ahead leads to the Mammoth Lakes Basin while you turn right (north), continuing on CA 203, now also called Minaret Road. Continue 4.2 miles to the main lodge of Mammoth Mountain Ski Area. Here you will have to park your car and take a shuttle bus (fee), unless you arrive before 7 a.m, after 7 p.m., are staying in one of the campgrounds in the Reds Meadow Valley, or are hiking early or late in the season before the shuttle bus is mandatory. To start your trip, take the shuttle bus to the Agnew Meadows stop.

If you have permission to continue to the valley, drive an additional 3.9 miles over Minaret Summit and down the windy road. The turnoff to Agnew Meadows is on the right as the road makes a switchback turn. Turn right here and drive the quarter mile down this dirt road, past a pack station, to the road-end parking lot.

There are two trailheads at Agnew Meadows. The High Trail (Trip 36) departs east from beside a toilet block and water faucet, just after you pass the stables. The road then makes a left-hand bend to the larger road-end parking area. The starting trailhead for the River Trail and Shadow Creek Trail (Trip 37) is on the south edge of this parking lot.

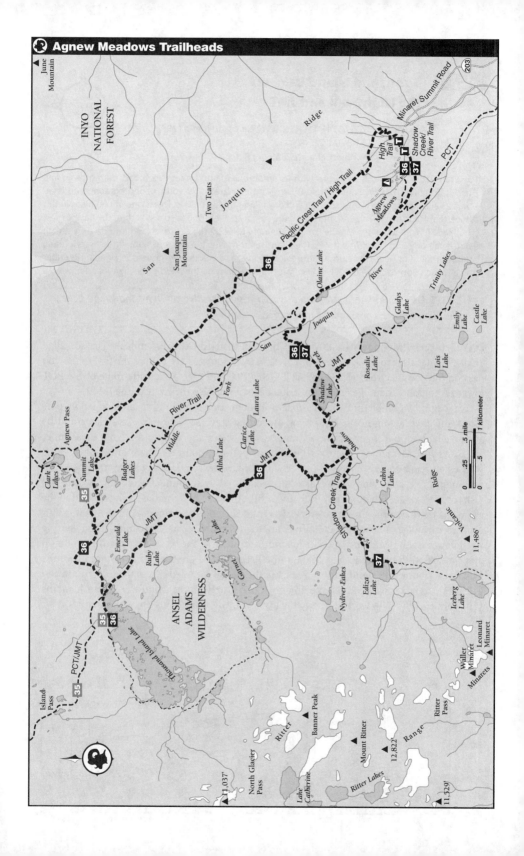

trip 36 Thousand Island Lake via the High Trail and JMT

see map on p. 219

Trip Data: 37.72851°N, 119.17130°W (Thousand Island Lake);
18.9 miles; 2/1 days

Topos: *Mammoth Mountain, Mount Ritter*

HIGHLIGHTS: Thousand Island Lake, with its numerous islands, is set in a broad, barren basin and backdropped by massive Banner Peak. This very popular area is a favorite of photographers and naturalists alike for its superlative scenery and day hiking opportunities. This is one of two hikes in this book that leads here—this variant follows the so-called High Trail (also a stretch of the Pacific Crest Trail [PCT]) high above the Middle Fork San Joaquin River on the approach and returns via a stretch of the famous John Muir Trail (JMT). The High Trail traverses the western slope of the San Joaquin Ridge, a route of near-continuous Ritter Range views and wildflower gardens. A sidebar describes an alternate approach via the "River Trail," ascending alongside the Middle Fork San Joaquin River.

HEADS UP! *Camping is prohibited within a quarter mile of Thousand Island Lake's outlet. Bear canisters are required in this area.*

DAY 1 (Agnew Meadows Trailhead to Thousand Island Lake, 8.4 miles): The so-called High Trail departs from the eastern end of Agnew Meadows, right behind the first toilets you pass on the entrance road (8,334'; 37.68282°N, 119.08471°W). This is the route of the PCT toward Thousand Island Lake and once, long ago, it was also the route of the JMT.

You begin by completing 10 switchbacks through a beautiful red fir and lodgepole pine forest and then swing north on a long, ascending traverse. The next 4.8 miles could be adequately described by the phrase "traverse with views and wildflowers," but these miles are worthy of as many adulatory adjectives as you can conjure. There are endless seeps whose banks are densely covered with bright monkeyflowers, draws that are crammed with mountain mule ears, sandy sagebrush slopes carpeted with countless colorful species, and lush forested glades where delphinium and arnica thrive. The sporadic springs bisecting the slope ensure that some flower color persists until the end of summer. And the views! This route mostly follows a shelf about halfway up the western slope of San Joaquin Ridge, staring straight across the Middle Fork San Joaquin to a shelf to the west (that the JMT follows) and onward to the Ritter Range. Most immediately visible are the serrated summits of the Minarets, Mount Ritter, and Banner Peak, but the glacial rounded ribs in the foreground and the layers of dark-polished metavolcanic rock that rise from the Middle Fork San Joaquin's valley are equally view-worthy. To say the least, you will thoroughly enjoy these miles.

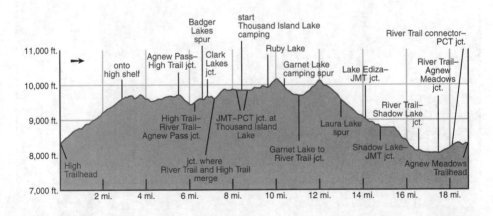

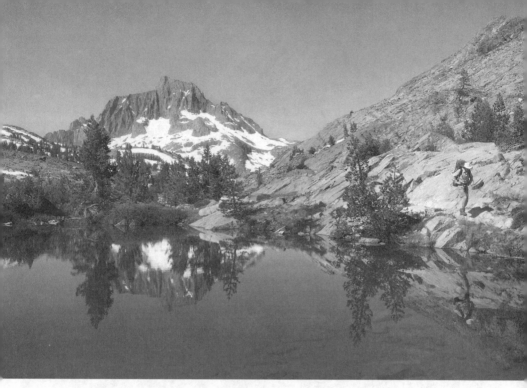

The High Trail approaching Thousand Island Lake　Photo by Elizabeth Wenk

Initially you pass through conifer stands and aspen glades, but with increasing elevation, you transition to an open slope. A little before the 3.0-mile mark, the trail switchbacks a few times as it winds up a minor rib, with volcanic bluffs upslope, the ascent ending on a high shelf. While the rock across the valley is all ancient metamorphosed volcanic rock, you are on volcanic rocks that are geologically young. They are just a few million years old and haven't been buried deep underground; in places you can easily see the depositional layers. The flowers are truly stunning—skyrocket, various paintbrushes, buckwheats, penstemon, and phlox where drier and corn lily meadows, monkshood, larkspur, and orchids along the irrigated corridors. There are occasional flats where you could camp, collecting water from one of the many trickles. After 5.5 miles you reach a junction where you continue left (northwest), while right (north) leads to Agnew Pass. Descending for 0.75 mile, in part through a particularly wet stretch of willows and flowers, you reach a four-way junction, where right (northeast) leads back uphill toward Agnew Pass, left (southeast) descends toward the River Trail, and you continue straight ahead (west) toward Thousand Island Lake.

Now in flat lodgepole pine forest, you continue 0.35 mile to an unsigned spur that leads left (south) to the Badger Lakes (and campsites). Four small tarns sit beside the trail, but the larger, deeper, slab-ringed Badger Lakes lie 0.2 mile to the south. You continue straight (right; west), first through flat lodgepole pine forest and then climbing to a higher shelf where you reach, after 0.3 mile, another junction where right (northeast) trends toward the Clark Lakes (Trip 35) and you stay left (southwest), still on the PCT. The trail now undulates across a dry slope, the lodgepole pine stands broken by bedrock ribs with sandy soils covered in mountain mule ears. In just 0.25 mile you reach another junction, where you continue right (northwest), while the River Trail merges from the left (southeast). This alternate route from Agnew Meadows is 0.7 mile shorter but lacks the striking views that defined your route.

THE RIVER TRAIL

If you wish to take the River Trail on your approach to Thousand Island Lake, you must obtain a wilderness permit for the River Trail rather than the High Trail. The River Trail departs from the south side of the main Agnew Meadows parking area, cutting across a few tiny trickles before curving west around the southern perimeter of often-boggy Agnew Meadows. Staying in the dry conifer forest, the trail bridges a slightly larger creek—the one draining all of Agnew Meadows—and turns northwest to follow a lush forested passageway set between two ribs of rock. At 0.75 mile from the trailhead is a junction where left (south) is the route down the Middle Fork San Joaquin River to Devils Postpile (and the route of the southbound PCT), while you stay right (northwest), on a connector that intersects the River Trail farther upstream.

The trail now makes a gradual descent to the valley below, dropping down a dry sun-struck slope blanketed in pinemat manzanita, sagebrush, and myriad other dry-site shrubs. On the valley floor you meet the riverside trail from Devils Postpile and stay right (north) to follow it upstream. The route is initially one rock rib to the east of the river's course. You skirt the northeast shore of marshy Olaine Lake, set beneath steep bluffs, and then cut through valley-bottom forest to another junction. Here the River Trail, your route, stays right (north-west), approximating the Middle Fork San Joaquin's course upstream, while left (west) leads up to Shadow Lake and Ediza Lake (Trip 37), and is your return route.

The River Trail makes two long switchbacks to climb above the river's steep-walled course, then sidles across a dry slope to reunite with the river in a pleasant lodgepole pine and fir forest upstream. With the Middle Fork San Joaquin River bubbling along on your left, you continue climbing gradually to moderately, enjoying regular splashes of color where side creeks creasing San Joaquin Ridge descend from the east; crimson columbine, corn lilies, monkshood, and Kelley's lily all greet you here. Over the next few miles, there are occasional poor-to-fair camp-sites between the trail and the river, although the terrain is mostly a tad too steep to camp.

Soon after the stream's gradient next increases, the path comes to a signed junction with a spur trail that leads right (north) to Agnew Pass, intersecting the High Trail en route. You stay left (northwest) toward Thousand Island Lake. There is a good campsite nearby. The trail now climbs a steeper, drier slope well above the tumbling river to another flat forested shelf. Here is a junction with a small lateral going left (southwest) across the river and climbing very steeply to Garnet Lake and the JMT. Continue ahead (northwest, right) here.

The next 1.1-mile segment is delightful, with the river and accompanying trail ensconced in a deep valley beneath near-vertical dark metamorphic bluffs. Excepting a few steep uphills, the walking is easy, alternately through forest stands and onto polished slabs; the dark-colored, nongranitic, polished slabs always take the seasoned Sierra hiker by surprise. You pass a few small campsites on shelves above the river and eventually reach the next junction, where you merge back onto the described route. Right (east) is the route the High Trail has followed from Agnew Meadow, while you now turn left (west) to continue to Thousand Island Lake.

The trail comes close to the Middle Fork San Joaquin (and passes a splendid campsite on a shelf above the river), before diverging from the river channel, ascending a forested corridor, then curving left across slabs. Passing several snowmelt tarns, the trail reunites with the river's course, soon reaching the meadow-lined outlet of Thousand Island Lake at a junction with the JMT (9,875'; 37.72851°N, 119.17130°W). Here, right (northwest) leads to Island Pass (Trip 35) and left (southeast) toward Garnet Lake. Departing straight across (west) from this junction is a use trail that follows Thousand Island Lake's northern shore to numerous scattered campsites. Camping is prohibited within 0.25 mile of Thousand Island Lake's outlet and there are almost no acceptable campsites along the lake's southeast shore, so head west along this trail after reading all the current camping regulations posted at the junction. There are excellent campsites near the large peninsula right at the 0.25-mile mark, others after an additional 0.2 miles, and then endless sandy flats among slab once you are about halfway around the lake. Everywhere, the scenery is some of the most memorable in the central Sierra. (The distance given assumes you walk exactly 0.25 mile west of the junction to sites near 9,850'; 37.72789°N, 119.17547°W; no campfires. If you don't camp at Thousand Island Lake, your trip is 0.5 mile shorter.)

CROSS-COUNTRY TO GARNET LAKE

A layover day at Thousand Island Lake would permit an adventurous, part cross-country, looping day hike to Garnet Lake. Follow use trails along Thousand Island Lake's northern and western shores, continuing south to Garnet Pass (10,138'; 37.70642°N, 119.18402°W), the obvious saddle that's the low point on the ridge south of Thousand Island Lake. Then follow Garnet Lake's northern shore back to the JMT; you may lose the use trail as you approach Garnet Lake's western end but will pick it up again as you continue around the lake. Return on the JMT, past Ruby and Emerald Lakes, reversing part of Day 2. The full loop is 7.0 miles.

DAY 2 (Thousand Island Lake to Agnew Meadows Trailhead, 10.5 miles): From your campsite, return to the JMT and turn right (southeast), walk past lakeshore meadows, and cross the bridge over the Thousand Island Lake outlet. Following the JMT south, pass first Emerald Lake (9,885') and its neighboring tarn and then the more strikingly sapphire and picturesque Ruby Lake (9,917'), rimmed to the west by impressive walls; both offer camping. Switchbacking briefly to a shallow saddle, you soon see Garnet Lake below. Rivaling Thousand Island Lake, Garnet Lake is also islet dotted but sits in a slightly more enclosed basin at the base of Banner Peak. Garnet Lake consequently offers fewer campsites, and since there is also a 0.25-mile no-camping zone radiating from its outlet, it is best to follow a use trail along its northern shore in search of legal campsites; depart west at 9,938'; 37.71529°N, 119.15660°W. After this spur junction, the trail winds down between polished slabs to the shore, still walking on the Ritter Range's beautiful dark-colored metavolcanic rock. The trail then traces Garnet Lake's east shore, crossing its outlet on a rickety bridge and passing the near-invisible junction with the lateral from the River Trail, before climbing some 400 feet to a saddle with a seasonal tarn; when there is water about, there are nearby campsites.

Ahead is an 1,100-foot descent, first past a small meadow and through a tiny canyon with mixed lodgepole pine and mountain hemlock cover. At a distinct right-trending bend in the trail, an unmarked and unmaintained trail leads left to Laura Lake (small campsites). Trending southwest, the JMT, your route, drops down a dry, dusty slope of pinemat manzanita and then turns back south into a shaded draw with campsites as long as the adjacent Shadow Creek tributary has water.

As you approach Shadow Creek, you reach a junction where right (northwest) leads to Ediza Lake (Trip 37), while you turn left (east, then northeast), following the JMT down Shadow Creek toward Shadow Lake. Nearby is a flat with another cluster of campsites, your last for many miles, for there is no camping between the creek and the trail along the heavily used Shadow Creek corridor and also no camping at Shadow Lake. Following Shadow Creek's canyon downstream to Shadow Lake, the trail winds through lodgepole forest and across open, slabby knobs of metavolcanic rock beside the fast-flowing stream. A short distance upstream of Shadow Lake, indeed before you see the lake, is a junction where the JMT turns right (south), crossing the creek on a bridge, while your route continues left (northeast) around the lake's forested northern shore. Near Shadow Lake's outlet, take a break on the shoreline to enjoy the view across the lake to Mount Ritter.

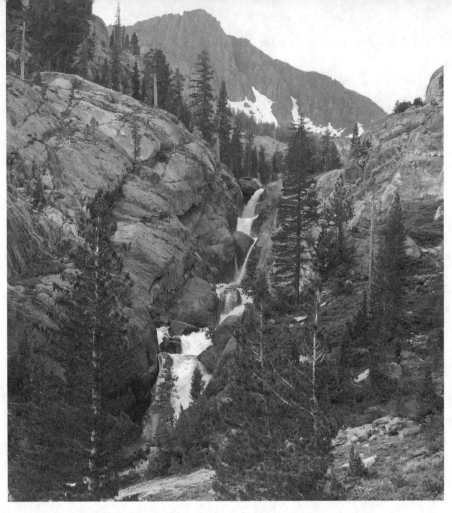

Shadow Creek spills down cascades below Shadow Lake. Photo by Elizabeth Wenk

Beyond the lake, the sunny, rocky, dusty, incredibly scenic trail drops nearly 700 feet alongside the thundering cascades of Shadow Creek as it plunges to join the Middle Fork San Joaquin River below. Once at the base of the dry slope speckled with stately junipers, cross the turbulent river on a stout footbridge, pass a packer campsite, and reach the signed junction with the River Trail (the alternate Day 1 route). Turn right (southeast) here, the trail positioned one rib east of the Middle Fork San Joaquin River. The lush lodgepole pine-forested strip leads past reedy Olaine Lake and across sandy flats, to reach a junction where the River Trail continues right (southeast) toward Devils Postpile and Reds Meadow, while you turn left (east-southeast) to ascend back to Agnew Meadows.

The trail traverses up and across an exposed, sunstruck slope vegetated by sagebrush, pinemat manzanita, and myriad other shrubs that thrive on hot, dry, rocky slopes. The climb ends after 0.6 mile at a junction where right (south) is the route the southbound PCT takes to the river valley, while you stay left (southeast) toward Agnew Meadows, soon reaching a lush forested passageway set between two ribs of rock. Beyond, the trail turns due east to skirt the southern perimeter of often-boggy Agnew Meadows. Cutting across a few tiny trickles, the trail reaches the main Agnew Meadows parking area. From here you can follow a trail across Agnew Meadow's eastern lobe or briefly follow the dirt road back to the High Trailhead where you started your walk.

see map on p. 219

trip 37 **Ediza Lake**

Trip Data: 37.68537°N, 119.16862°W; 13.8 miles; 2/1 days
Topos: *Mammoth Mountain, Mount Ritter*

HIGHLIGHTS: Ediza Lake's alpine scenery and relative ease of access make it one of Inyo National Forest's choice destinations. The environs are so spectacular you will wish for several layover days to explore surrounding peaks and lakes (especially Nydiver, Iceberg, and Cecile), fish, swim, and appreciate the awe that Ansel Adams experienced while photographing this inspiring wilderness now named in his honor. If you're searching for a campsite with more solitude, consider nearby Cabin Lake; there are several campsites before you reach the lake and a lovely one near its outlet.

HEADS UP! *Campfires are prohibited at Ediza Lake and bear canisters are required.*

DAY 1 (Agnew Meadows Trailhead to Ediza Lake's inlet, 6.9 miles): The trail departs from the south side of the parking area, cutting across a few tiny trickles before curving west around the southern perimeter of often-boggy Agnew Meadows. Staying in the dry conifer forest, the trail bridges a slightly larger creek—the one draining all of Agnew Meadows—and turns northwest to follow a lush forested passageway set between two ribs of rock. At 0.75 mile from the trailhead is a junction, where left (south) is the route down the Middle Fork San Joaquin River to Devils Postpile (and the route of the southbound Pacific Crest Trail [PCT]), while you stay right (northwest), on a connector that intersects the River Trail farther upstream.

The trail now makes a gradual descent to the valley below, dropping down a dry sun-struck slope blanketed in pinemat manzanita, sagebrush, and myriad other shrubs that thrive on hot, dry, rocky slopes. On the valley floor you meet the riverside trail from Devils Postpile and stay right (north) to follow it upstream. The route is initially one rock rib to the east of the river's course. You skirt the northeast shore of marshy Olaine Lake, set beneath steep bluffs, and then cut through valley-bottom forest and across sagebrush flats to another junction, where the River Trail continues right (north), while you turn left (west) to ascend Shadow Creek.

Turning left, you pass a campsite beneath aspens and lodgepole pine, and shortly arrive at a bridge over the Middle Fork San Joaquin River. Across the bridge, the trail leaves the river corridor, beginning a sunstruck 700-foot climb up juniper- and sagebrush-studded slopes. Once high above the Middle Fork San Joaquin, the trail turns west onto a shelf high above cascading Shadow Creek; spectacular waterfalls tumble down the deep-set gorge. Slowly the trail and gorge converge, and soon after you admire the beautiful cascades

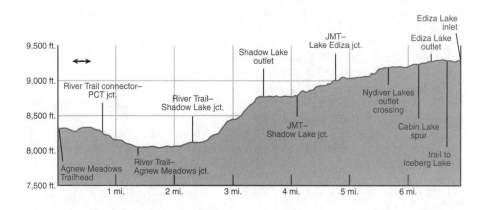

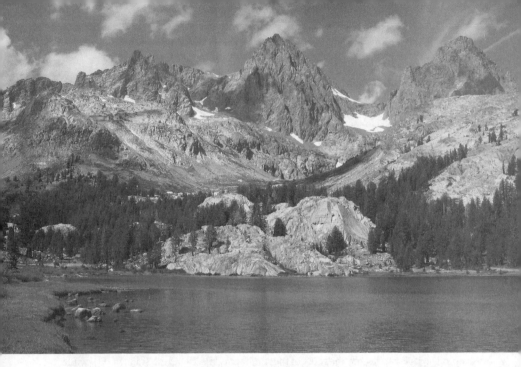

Ediza Lake with Mount Ritter and Banner Peak in the background   Photo by Elizabeth Wenk

from a narrow ledge just above the creek, you pass through a notch in the sublimely polished metavolcanic rocks and arrive at Shadow Lake. Shadow Lake (8,770') is closed to all overnight camping but makes a great lunch spot with views to the Ritter Range. The trail continues southwest along Shadow Lake's north shore, then climbs briefly along Shadow Creek to a junction with the John Muir Trail (JMT). You remain right (west) to follow the northbound JMT up Shadow Creek, while left (southbound), the JMT crosses Shadow Creek on a bridge and continues toward Rosalie Lake.

You follow the JMT for 0.7 mile up Shadow Creek, alternating between lodgepole pine forest and metavolcanic slabs where you're treated to splendid views of the tumbling creek. Camping is prohibited between the trail and the creek all the way to Ediza Lake; the only good choices are right near the next junction, where the JMT turns right (north) toward Thousand Island Lake, while you stay left (west) to continue up Shadow Creek to Ediza Lake.

Parting ways with the JMT, the Shadow Creek Trail first meanders along the edge of broad meadows, looping around several lobes of brilliantly polished dark metavolcanic slab. A steeper, rockier section with showy cascades ensues, before reaching another long, lush lodgepole pine and hemlock flat. The trail crosses the Nydiver Lakes outlet creek on large rock blocks (and a use trail ascends from here to those lakes) and a short distance later fords Shadow Creek at a hairpin bend. The footbridge here was washed out in 2017 and has yet to be replaced (as of 2020), necessitating a chilly, and sometimes tricky, wade. *Note:* Many hikers are currently staying on the creek's northern bank, following use trails the final distance to Ediza Lake, since the shortest (but not easiest) access to legal campsites is along the lake's northern shore anyway.

Continuing on the main trail across the creek, you quickly reach the unsigned junction where the old trail to Cabin Lake departs left (west; 9,231'; 37.68699°N, 119.16160°W), while the Shadow Creek Trail climbs a final step through subalpine stands of lodgepole and mountain hemlock and across outcrops to the outlet of Ediza Lake. The dark, jagged peaks of the Ritter Range jut skyward to the west of the mostly grass-ringed lake. Ediza Lake's legal campsites are in the forest stands along the lake's western side, some in stands of hemlock just 100 feet from the shore and others atop bedrock lumps set farther back. There are no ecologically acceptable campsites along the lake's southern shores. To reach the legal campsites, continue clockwise (south, then west) around the lake, following a well-established trail to the lake's inlet (trip mileage is to here) and then along one of many use trails to your choice of campsite (for example, 9,376'; 37.68403°N, 119.17045°W; no campfires).

Ediza Lake makes a perfect base for exploring the basin above. Particularly fine destinations include the perched Nydiver Lakes (reached either by climbing above Ediza Lake or along the lakes' outlet creek), Cabin Lake (reached by the unsigned old trail, that starts 0.2 mile below Ediza Lake's outlet), and Iceberg and Cecile Lakes (see below). Mountaineers may want to climb Mount Ritter via its southeastern side, a route that requires an ice axe much of the time but is not technically difficult. A use trail leads toward Ritter Pass, and while the top stretch is objectionably steep talus (or snow), there are splendid Minarets views and wildflower gardens to be enjoyed on the first half of the route. The Minarets are renowned for their steep, loose rock and difficult route-finding; they are definitely not recommended locations for exploring if you haven't researched routes in advance and are carrying (and know how to use) mountaineering equipment.

CROSS-COUNTRY SHUTTLE VIA ICEBERG AND CECILE LAKE

Experienced cross-country hikers can turn this trip into a scenic shuttle by returning via Minaret Lake (Trip 38) and exiting at Devils Postpile instead of retracing their steps. Since a shuttle bus leads from Devils Postpile to Agnew Meadows, it is then easy to return to the Agnew Meadows Trailhead, should you have a car there, or the parking area at Mammoth Mountain. The distance from Ediza Lake to Minaret Lake's outlet is just 3 miles, but it is a rough route and, indeed, treacherous if covered with snow. Most people will choose to spend a night at Minaret Lake, continuing down from Minaret Lake to Devils Postpile on the following day.

From the southeast corner of Ediza Lake (9,288'; 37.68361°N, 119.16485°W), follow the obvious trail 0.9 mile to Iceberg Lake's outlet (9,797'). Nearby are numerous small campsites among whitebark pines. The now fainter tread continues across talus above Iceberg Lake's eastern shore and then ascends steeply to Cecile Lake's outlet (10,267'). This stretch may be impassable until late season due to steep, icy slopes, where a slip will carry you straight into Iceberg Lake.

At Cecile Lake, hikers are rewarded with spectacular views of Clyde Minaret, but a meager selection of tiny climbers' bivies as campsites. After following Cecile Lake's northeastern shore, the use trail more or less vanishes. There are many passable cross-country routes, my favorite of which initially stays well north of the Minaret Lake's mapped western inlet stream. From Cecile Lake's easternmost bulge, ascend about 60 feet to a broad saddle from which you have lovely views of Minaret Lake and Minaret Creek's canyon. Proceed first southeast past a tarn, then, as the terrain steepens, cut south down rocky slopes to the aforementioned Minaret Lake inlet stream; depending on your exact route, this can require a little scrambling, so look around to pick a route you're comfortable with. Following the stream toward Minaret Lake, once near the shore you'll pick up a trail that leads around Minaret Lake's northern lobes. From here, follow the description of Trip 38 in reverse: follow the Minaret Lake Trail southeast, along Minaret Creek to reunite with the JMT. Then, turn right and follow the JMT south 1.9 miles, ultimately diverging toward Devils Postpile. You cross the Middle Fork San Joaquin on a stout bridge and then turn north, reaching the trailhead shortly thereafter.

DAY 2 (Ediza Lake to Agnew Meadows Trailhead, 6.9 miles): Retrace your steps.

Devils Postpile Trailhead			7,569'; 37.63000°N, 119.08472°W			
Destination/ GPS Coordinates	Trip Type	Best Season	Pace & Hiking/ Layover Days	Total Mileage	Permit Required	
38 Minaret Lake 37.66213°N 119.15711°W	Out-and-back	Mid to late	Moderate 2/1	14.4	Minaret Lake	
39 King Creek Lakes 37.63365°N 119.14061°W (Superior Lake)	Loop	Mid to late	Moderate 3/1	14.6	Beck Lake (Fern Lake in reverse)	

INFORMATION AND PERMITS: This trailhead is in Inyo National Forest. Permits are required for overnight stays and quotas apply. Permits can be reserved up to six months in advance at recreation.gov (60%; $6 permit reservation fee plus $5 per person) or requested in person, first come, first served, a day in advance (40%; free). All permits must be picked up at one of the Inyo National Forest ranger stations, located in Lone Pine (Eastern Sierra Interagency Visitor Center), Bishop, Mammoth Lakes, and Lee Vining (the Mono Basin Scenic Area Visitor Center). If you plan to use a stove or have a campfire, you must also have a California campfire permit, available from a forest service office or online at preventwildfireca.org/campfire-permit. Campfires are prohibited throughout most of this region, including at all described campsites. Bear canisters are required in this area.

DRIVING DIRECTIONS: From the junction of US 395 and CA 203 (the Mammoth junction), take CA 203 west 3.7 miles to a major intersection in the town of Mammoth Lakes. Here, straight ahead leads to the Mammoth Lakes Basin, while you turn right (north), continuing on CA 203, now also called Minaret Road. Continue 4.2 miles to the main lodge of Mammoth Mountain Ski Area. Here you will have to park your car and take a shuttle bus (fee), unless you arrive before 7 a.m, after 7 p.m., are staying in one of the campgrounds in the Reds Meadow Valley, or are hiking early or late in the season before the shuttle bus is mandatory. To start your trip, take the shuttle bus to the Devils Postpile stop. On your return you will take the shuttle from the trailhead back to the main lodge.

If you have permission to continue to the valley, drive an additional 7.9 miles over Minaret Summit and down the windy road alongside the San Joaquin River. Then turn right toward Devils Postpile, reaching an overnight parking area on your right after 0.3 mile; this is shortly before you reach the road-end campground and ranger station. There are toilets and water near the ranger station.

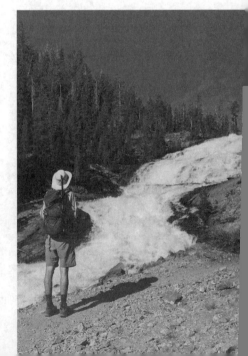

Cascades along Minaret Creek
Photo by Elizabeth Wenk

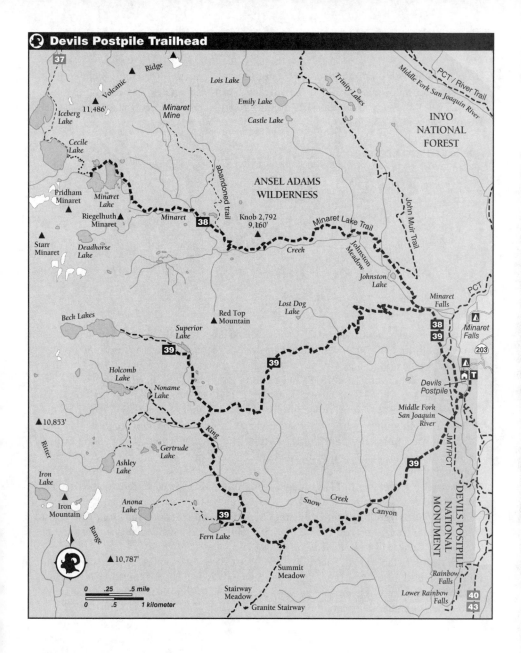

trip 38   **Minaret Lake**

> **Trip Data:** 37.66213°N, 119.15711°W; 14.4 miles; 2/1 days
> **Topos:** *Mammoth Mountain, Mount Ritter*

HIGHLIGHTS: Minaret Lake is a great choice for backpackers who want to get up close to some of the most dramatic scenery in the Sierra. Excursions to Cecile Lake or up Volcanic Ridge provide great extensions for a layover day.

HEADS UP! *Campfires are prohibited at Minaret Lake and bear canisters are required.*

DAY 1 (Devils Postpile Trailhead to Minaret Lake, 7.2 miles): From the Devils Postpile ranger station, follow the broad path 0.2 mile south to a junction. If you've never previously seen Devils Postpile, you should visit it either today or on your return; see the "Devils Postpile Detour" sidebar below.

> **DEVILS POSTPILE DETOUR**
> From the junction after 0.2 mile, go ahead (left; south) a short distance to the base of the eponymous volcanic formation, created when an unusually deep flow of magma accumulated, such that the interior was well insulated and cooled slowly and evenly. As magma cools, it contracts and fractures; just as with a drying mudflat, the cracks create a mosaic of 4-, 5- and 6-side prisms, with hexagonal prisms most common. The tall, slender basalt columns soaring high into the blue mountain skies are a striking sight. From the base of the postpiles, continue south, east, then north along a short trail that loops across the top of the Postpile. Here the glacially polished tops of the hexagonal columns are revealed—a slightly domed, beautifully polished surface of polygons. To continue this trip, return to the first junction and turn left (west) to cross the footbridge.

If you don't take the detour, turn right (west) and cross the Middle Fork San Joaquin on a sturdy footbridge. The trail veers right (north), upstream, reaching the next junction just 200 feet after the bridge; here you turn right (north), signposted for Minaret Falls (and also leading to the John Muir Trail [JMT] and Pacific Crest Trail [PCT] northbound), while left (south) leads toward the King Creek Trail and the JMT/PCT southbound (Trip 39).

Turn right and pass through open forest to a four-way junction where left (south) is the JMT/PCT southbound, right (northeast) is the PCT northbound (and route to Minaret Falls), and you continue straight ahead (northwest) on the JMT northbound. Soon exiting Devils Postpile National Monument, you continue up a dry, open slope with granite outcrops and pumice sand. Many of the tallest trees on this ascent were toppled by the Devils Windstorm in November 2011; although young trees are growing in remarkably rapidly, shade is still a rare commodity. Rising ever farther above the Middle Fork San Joaquin, the trail slowly turns west to parallel Minaret Creek and then reaches a junction, where you continue right (northwest) on the JMT toward Johnston Lake, while left (west) is the trail to the Beck Lakes and Superior Lake (Trip 39).

A few steps farther the JMT fords Minaret Creek. The stout footbridge that spanned the flow was toppled in 2017 and has not yet been replaced (as of 2020), making this a formidable crossing at high flows; it can easily be waist deep and is deceptively fast-flowing—ford with another person under these conditions.

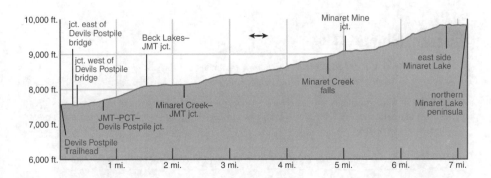

The grasses of Johnston Meadow soon appear on the left, with scattered campsites to either side of the trail. Just past marshy, reedy Johnston Lake (8,100'), you turn left (northwest) onto the trail ascending Minaret Creek, while the JMT continues right (east, then southeast, then north).

Leaving the boggy valley bottom behind, the trail begins ascending through lodgepole pine and red fir. A length of double rock wall indicates your route was once the path of an old mining road. The trail soon climbs onto a rocky rib above the creek—you peer down into the blocky, incised gorge at its slalom course; a knob-top campsite beckons nearby. This steeper step leads to another marshy flat ringed by dense conifer forest with campsites hidden under the trees near the creek. As the trail approaches Knob 2,792 (9,160 feet), the forest thins, then vanishes, and the trail climbs more steeply up broken metavolcanic bedrock. At 4.7 miles is a splendid splaying waterfall, one of the hike's highlights, and your first full Minarets view; there are especially good views of Clyde Minaret, the tallest of the Minarets. Just 0.3 mile later is an unmarked junction, where right (north) is the old trail to Minaret Mine (and across Volcanic Pass to Cabin Lake); parts of the trail to the mine have vanished, but it is an easy route and abundant mining infrastructure and tailings piles to explore may entice you to take this 1.8-mile (each way) detour.

The 0.25 mile beyond this junction is dry and open, but the lodgepole pine and hemlock forest then thickens again, and you are suddenly in a boggy (and often buggy) forest with a carpet of heath species—dwarf bilberry, red mountain heather, and Labrador tea. You continue up, the increasingly rocky slope still interspersed with forested flats but always offering filtered views of the Minarets.

Another rocky ascent, another cluster of forested switchbacks, and the trail abruptly turns north, matching the stream's course. Then transitioning to the alpine, the trail switchbacks up a flower-covered rubbly slope, crosses a series of ephemeral trickles, and reaches Minaret Lake's outlet. Your attention is surely drawn to 12,281-foot Clyde Minaret soaring overhead; even among the rugged Minarets, Clyde is in a class of its own—loftier, sharp-tipped, and undeniably world class, just like its namesake, one of the Sierra's most eminent mountaineers. A copy of *Missing in the Minarets* would make fine reading while lounging on the colorful, polished slabs that ring the lake. As for camping, you'll find small tent sites etched everywhere that is flat—on the slabs and in every stand of trees, but none are large. The biggest sites are on the peninsula that divides the lake's two northern lobes (leave the trail at 9,834'; 37.66213°N, 119.15711°W; no campfires; the distance is marked to here) and on its far-western side, but there are also splendid exposed sites on the bedrock knobs along the lake's eastern shores. The most secluded may be at the various tarns south of and overlooking the lake.

FUN AT MINARET LAKE

There are lots of choices for a layover day at Minaret Lake, although all are off-trail or on use trails. A cross-country route leads from Minaret Lake to Cecile Lake and then onto Iceberg and Ediza Lakes via a rough trail; see the sidebar on page 227 in Trip 37. From the tarn at the northwestern corner of Minaret Lake a straightforward Class 2 route leads north up a gully then northwest up a slope to the high point of Volcanic Ridge (Peak 3,501), from which you'll enjoy truly stupendous views of the Minarets. A detour to Minaret Mine is also intriguing, although perhaps better as a side trip on your hike to or from Minaret Lake, since it branches off more than 2 miles below the lake. Or, explore the lakeshore, or simply enjoy the amazing views right from your camp.

DAY 2 (Minaret Lake to Devils Postpile Trailhead, 7.2 miles): Retrace your steps.

see map on p. 229

trip 39   **King Creek Lakes**

Trip Data: 37.63365°N, 119.14061°W (Superior Lake);
14.6; 3/1 days

Topos: *Mammoth Mountain, Mount Ritter, Cattle Mountain, Crystal Crag*

HIGHLIGHTS: Sitting south of the Ritter Range's more famous attractions—Thousand Island, Garnet, Ediza, and Minaret Lakes—the less-traveled King Creek drainage boasts a half dozen equally spectacular lakes, polished rock, great camping, and—unlike the northern lakes—*solitude*. This is a low-mileage trip with excellent subalpine scenery that you can stretch over as many days as you have available. We recommend starting this loop on the trail to Superior Lake for the shade on the uphill, but you can easily reverse the trip and spend the first night at Fern Lake.

HEADS UP! *On the hike from Devils Postpile to Superior Lake, there's little to no water between Minaret Creek and Superior Lake. Bear canisters are required and campfires are prohibited throughout the upper drainage.*

DAY 1 (Devils Postpile Trailhead to Superior Lake, 6.6 miles): From the Devils Postpile ranger station, follow the broad path 0.2 mile south to a junction. At the junction, turn right (west) and cross the Middle Fork San Joaquin on a sturdy footbridge. The trail veers right (north) upstream, reaching the next junction 200 feet after the bridge. Here you begin the loop portion of this trip, turning right (north), signposted for Minaret Falls (and also leading to the John Muir Trail [JMT] and Pacific Crest Trail [PCT] northbound), while you will return along the trail to the left (south), which heads toward King Creek Trail and the JMT/PCT southbound.

Turn right and pass through open forest to a four-way junction where left (south) is the JMT/PCT southbound, right (northeast) is the PCT northbound (and route to Minaret Falls), and you continue straight ahead (northwest) on the JMT northbound. Soon exiting Devils Postpile National Monument, you continue up a dry, open slope with granite outcrops and pumice sand. Many of the tallest trees on this ascent were toppled by the Devils Windstorm in November 2011; although young trees are growing in remarkably rapidly, shade is still a rare commodity. Rising ever farther above the Middle Fork San Joaquin, the trail slowly turns west to parallel Minaret Creek and then reaches a junction, where you turn left (west) onto the trail to Superior Lake and the Beck Lakes, while the JMT continues right (northwest).

The trail makes an ascending traverse on deep pumice soil beneath dense predominantly hemlock cover, with just filtered views down to Johnston Lake and across to San Joaquin Ridge. The volcanic soil is bare and parched soon after snow melt, but the tree cover provides welcome shade as you switchback upward. Although the slope's gradient eases after about 1.8 miles and the switchbacks cease, the angle of the very well-constructed trail

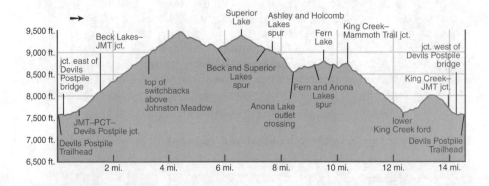

remains remarkably consistent all the way to the top of a minor rib. After a slight descent and traverse above a pocket meadow, the trail cuts across altered-granite talus at the base of Red Top Mountains' southeast-emanating ridge. Walking through open stands of big, mature lodgepole pine, hemlock, and then western white pine, the views west to Iron Mountain and southeast to the Silver Divide start to emerge—a teaser for tomorrow's panoramas. A gentle descent leads to a junction, just beside the old Beck Cabin's ruins, where you turn right (northwest) toward Superior Lake and the Beck Lakes, while left (southwest) leads down the King Creek drainage, tomorrow's route.

The 0.9 mile to Superior Lake is a gradual climb through open lodgepole pine and hemlock, passing small tarns ringed by heath, drier rocky outcrops, and ultimately crossing King Creek just downstream of the lake. There are several good campsites southwest of Superior Lake's outlet, including one on a prominent knob (9,389'; 37.63365°N, 119.14061°W; campfires allowed), and large, seasonally marshy options near the inlet.

Smaller, more austere campsites with bigger views (and fewer bugs) can be found upstream: medium-size sites at about 9,600 feet in the last cluster of taller trees, tiny bivy sites near lower Beck Lake's outlet, or a large site in a hidden flat near the northeastern corner of lower Beck Lake. Beyond Superior Lake the trail is poorly maintained and has been repeatedly obliterated by massive avalanches. The most-used route remains on the south side of King Creek nearly all the way to lower Beck Lake, then crosses the outlet, and continues around the lake's eastern and northern shores. The lake's deep brilliant blue water and some splendid mineral veins on a wall above the outlet are reason enough to continue the additional 0.9 mile upcanyon without your pack.

DAY 2 (Superior Lake to Fern Lake, 2.9 miles): Retrace yesterday's steps back to the junction with the main King Creek Trail, and go right (south-southwest) through crowded trees to immediately meet the junction to Holcomb and Ashley Lakes. Here your route, the main King Creek loop, continues left (southeast), while right leads across King Creek to ascend the Holcomb and Ashley drainage; see the sidebar below for a detour to visit these gems.

HOLCOMB AND ASHLEY LAKES

These lakes are both at least as scenic as Superior Lake and the Beck Lakes, and either a half day's excursion or additional night is warranted to visit this basin—there are plenty of small campsites scattered about the drainage. From the signed junction, ford King Creek and proceed up dry diorite slabs above the Holcomb-Ashley creek. After 0.3 mile, at a cryptic, unmarked junction, the trail to Holcomb Lake trends northwest up slabs, while that to Ashley Lake takes a more due-westerly tack, continuing alongside the drainage. Holcomb Lake's trail continues up a slab rib, then through a gully and around the eastern and northern shores of Noname Lake to reach Holcomb Lake. The best campsites are northwest of the outlet, although there are very few comfortably flat locations that are 100 feet from water (one possibility is at 9,849'; 37.63842°N, 119.15480°W; no campfires). Meanwhile, the fork to Ashley Lake continues pleasantly upward, crossing the Holcomb outlet and continuing not far from the Ashley Lake outlet stream to reach a marshy meadow where you ford the creek. As shown on the USGS 7.5' topo maps, the trail more or less ends here, but a good use trail continues south, following a bedrock rib above the creek's eastern bank. Along the final 0.2 mile to the lake there are campsites to either side of the creek—nothing large, but plenty of legal options for one or two tents. Ashley Lake is set in a stunning location at the base of Iron Mountain. It sits at the border of altered granite and metavolcanic rock, with steep dark cliffs, cascading waterfalls, and a long permanent snowfield leading from the crest nearly to the lake. Clusters of improbably tall, skinny hemlock decorate a lakeside peninsula.

Continuing down the main King Creek Trail, a short distance later you must ford King Creek, a broad, not terribly deep crossing, but one that is dangerous and intimidating at high flows because you are at the top of a waterfall. The trail then zigzags down an enticing rocky slope—the altered granite is brightly colored with prettyfaces and Brewer's aster, and King Creek's gorgeous cascades are foaming to the side. At the base of the slope, the trail vanishes in avalanche debris and flower thickets fringing Anona Lake's outlet; if you head due south across the disturbed area you'll relocate the trail on the far side. The coming 0.75 mile to the Fern Lake junction leads up a draw with pleasant hemlock forest, through a corridor with Fern Lake's meadow-edged outlet, and then to the signed Fern Lake junction; you turn right (west) toward Fern Lake, while left (southeast) is the continuing King Creek loop, tomorrow's route. A 0.25-mile ascent leads to Fern Lake—and a short distance farther to a selection of good campsites in hemlock glades to the northeast of the lake (for example, 8,794'; 37.60833°N, 119.13385°W; no campfires) and in openings along the lake's northern shore. If you fancy a swim, jump in—lower-altitude Fern is one of the warmer lakes in the region.

Solitude seekers might want to set up camp higher up at beautiful Anona Lake (9,107'; 37.61035°N, 119.14762°W; no campfires), accessible via an unmaintained, vanishing trail that continues around Fern's north shore before making a rocky ascent past a tarn, over a saddle, and down into Anona's basin. Anona sits in a broad flower-dotted basin in the shadow of Iron Mountain's southern summit and offers astounding views but meager camping opportunities, for the ground is mostly grass or sharp rock.

DAY 3 (Fern Lake to Devils Postpile Trailhead, 5.1 miles): On your final day, walk back to the main King Creek Trail and turn right (southeast). An undulating traverse through notably marshy vegetation leads 0.5 mile to a junction with the Mammoth Trail; you turn left (northeast) to continue down the King Creek drainage, while right (south) leads past Summit Meadow to the Granite Stairway and ultimately to Clover Meadow in the western Sierra (Trip 69 in Sierra North). After wandering through dense hemlock stands, the trail winds around a granite rib where you're treated to brilliant views back across the King Creek drainage and into Snow Canyon, with Clyde Minaret poking through behind. As the route then switchbacks down an east-facing slope, your attention is drawn to Mammoth Mountain (east), Silver Peak (the granite pyramid to the southeast), and the expanse of burned landscape along the Middle Fork San Joaquin, devastation delivered by the Rainbow Fire back in 1992. Seasonal wildflowers—azure penstemon, mountain pride penstemon, pennyroyal, prettyfaces, stonecrop—provide splashes of color, especially as you cross numerous seeps.

Slowly you drop to King Creek and trade granite soils for pumice, although the granitic bedrock continues to poke through as outcropping ribs. As you approach the creek, the majority of mature trees are missing, again toppled by the 2011 Devils Windstorm. Luckily, unlike following a fire, the younger trees survived and there was no damage to the soil's organic matter, so the forest is regenerating surprisingly quickly. Ahead you ford King Creek, its banks dense thickets of alder. Almost always a broad wade, at high flows it requires caution.

The final 2.2 miles to Devils Postpile are surprisingly hard work. Thanks to the fire and windstorm there is little shade and the trail is entirely sandy pumice. Moreover, although your elevation at the King Creek ford is nearly identical to the trailhead, you have several hundred feet of elevation gain and loss as the trail crosses from the King Creek drainage to the Middle Fork San Joaquin. Eventually you reach a four-way junction with the JMT, where you continue straight ahead (northeast) toward Devils Postpile, while the JMT leads north–south (left–right). A descending traverse offers a good Devils Postpile vista and soon thereafter you reach a junction you'll recognize from Day 1; turn right and retrace your steps to the trailhead.

Fish Creek Trailhead
7,669'; 37.61397°N, 119.07664°W

Destination/ GPS Coordinates	Trip Type	Best Season	Pace & Hiking/ Layover Days	Total Mileage	Permit Required
40 Silver Divide Lakes 37.47178°N 118.97821°W (Peter Pande Lake)	Semiloop	Mid to late	Moderate 6/1	46.6	Fish Creek
43 Iva Bell Hot Springs 37.53343°N 119.02562°W (in reverse of description; see page 257)	Shuttle (public transport option)	Early to late	Moderate 4/1	28.2	Fish Creek (Duck Pass as described)

INFORMATION AND PERMITS: This trailhead is in Inyo National Forest. Permits are required for overnight stays and quotas apply. Permits can be reserved up to six months in advance at recreation.gov (60%; $6 permit reservation fee plus $5 per person) or requested in person, first come, first served, a day in advance (40%; free). All permits must be picked up at one of the Inyo National Forest ranger stations, located in Lone Pine (Eastern Sierra Interagency Visitor Center), Bishop, Mammoth Lakes, and Lee Vining (the Mono Basin Scenic Area Visitor Center). If you plan to use a stove or have a campfire, you must also have a California campfire permit, available from a forest service office or online at preventwildfireca.org/campfire-permit. Campfires are prohibited above 10,000 feet. Bear canisters are required in this area.

Trip 39 follows King Creek for much of its route.   Photo by Elizabeth Wenk

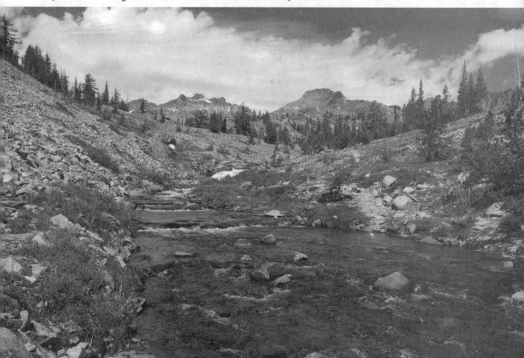

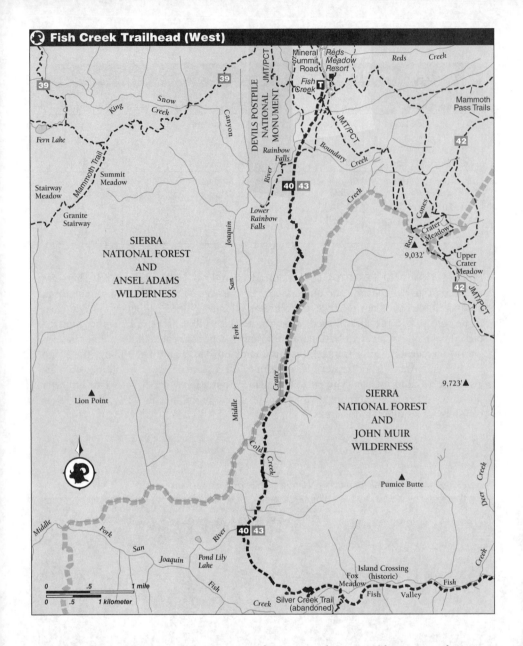

DRIVING DIRECTIONS: From the junction of US 395 and CA 203 (the Mammoth junction), take CA 203 west for 3.7 miles to a major intersection in the town of Mammoth Lakes. Here, straight ahead leads to the Mammoth Lakes Basin while you turn right (north), continuing on CA 203, now also called Minaret Road. Continue 4.2 miles to the main lodge of Mammoth Mountain Ski Area. Here you will have to park your car and take a shuttle bus (fee), unless you arrive before 7 a.m, after 7 p.m., are staying in one of the campgrounds in the Reds Meadow Valley, or are hiking early or late in the season before the shuttle bus is mandatory. To start your trip, take the shuttle bus to the Rainbow Falls stop. On your return you will take the shuttle from the trailhead back to the main lodge. If you have permission to continue to the valley, drive an additional 9.5 miles over Minaret Summit and down the windy road alongside the San Joaquin River. After you've

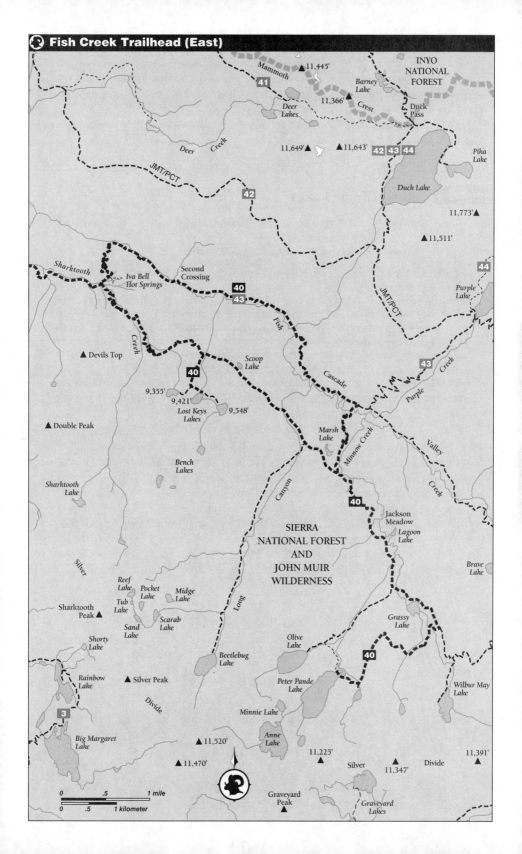

INYO
NATIONAL
FOREST

▲11,445'

41

Barney
Lake

11,366'

Deer
Lakes

Mammoth

Crest

Duck
Pass

Deer   Creek

11,649'▲   ▲11,643'   42 43 44

Pika
Lake

JMT/PCT

42

Duck Lake

11,773'▲

▲11,511'

Sharktooth

Second
Crossing

40

Purple
Lake

Iva Bell
Hot Springs

43

44

Fish

JMT/PCT

Creek

▲ Devils Top

40

Scoop
Lake

Cascade

Creek

43

9,355'

Purple

9,421'

Valley

Lost Keys
Lakes   9,548'

Marsh
Lake

▲ Double Peak

Minnow Creek

Creek

Bench
Lakes

Canyon

Sharktooth
Lake

40

Jackson
Meadow

SIERRA
NATIONAL FOREST
AND
JOHN MUIR
WILDERNESS

Lagoon
Lake

Brave
Lake

Silver

Reef   Pocket
Lake   Lake   Midge
Lake

Tub
Lake

Long

Grassy
Lake

Sharktooth
Peak ▲

Sand   Scarab
Lake   Lake

Shorty
Lake

Olive
Lake

40

Rainbow
Lake   ▲ Silver Peak

Beetlebug
Lake

Peter Pande
Lake

Wilbur May
Lake

3

Divide

Minnie Lake

Big Margaret
Lake

▲11,520'

Anne
Lake

11,225'

11,391'

▲11,470'

11,347'

▲

Silver   Divide   ▲

0   .5   1 mile

0   .5   1 kilometer

Graveyard
Peak
▲

Graveyard
Lakes

passed Devils Postpile and Sotcher Lake, turn right to the Rainbow Falls Trailhead and continue 0.1 mile to the trailhead parking, from which the trail down Fish Creek departs. There are toilets and water at the trailhead.

Note: While popularly known as Rainbow Falls Trailhead, this is also Fish Creek Trailhead. Mercifully for you, the huge summer throngs here are almost all headed for Rainbow Falls.

---

trip 40   ## Silver Divide Lakes

see maps on p. 236–237

> **Trip Data:** 37.47178°N, 118.97821°W (Peter Pande Lake); 46.6 miles; 6/1 days
>
> **Topos:** *Crystal Crag, Bloody Mountain, Graveyard Peak*

HIGHLIGHTS: This scenic trip travels through some lesser-known corners of John Muir Wilderness. After a scenic walk along the Middle Fork San Joaquin River's canyon, you reach the sought-after Iva Bell Hot Springs. This route then leads to the so-called Cascade Valley shelf, providing relatively easy access to five different lake drainages, two of which are included in the described itinerary. You round out the trip by following tumbling Fish Creek through aptly named Cascade Valley. The relatively low elevations and guaranteed water in lakes and major streams mean this is a good loop for a September— or even early October—excursion, when the mosquitos have tapered.

HEADS UP! *The fords of Fish Creek at the base of Minnow Creek and Second Crossing can both be dangerous through June. In addition, the ample water everywhere makes this region a mosquito haven until mid-July.*

DAY 1 (Fish Creek Trailhead to Fox Meadow, 8.3 miles): From the trailhead, take the Fish Creek Trail south, soon stepping across the John Muir Trail (JMT)/Pacific Crest Trail (PCT) and continuing ahead (south). Descending gently beneath scattered Jeffrey pine and white fir, you reach a Y-junction where a trail from Reds Meadow merges from the left; continue due south. At the 0.7-mile mark you reach a second Y-junction with a large information sign about the region's fire ecology; here a trail from Devils Postpile merges from your right and you again continue straight ahead, south. Unless you've gotten an early start, this stretch of trail is crowded with day hikers, all heading toward Rainbow Falls. At the next junction, the Fish Creek Trail again continues straight ahead (left; south), while

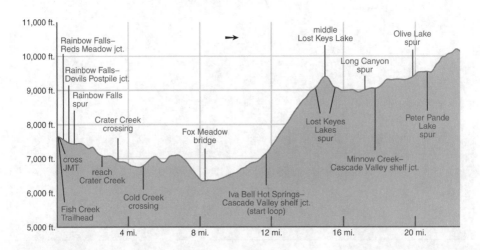

right (west) leads an easy 0.2 mile to the upper Rainbow Falls overlook. It is well worth the detour to the 101-foot cascade if you haven't been here before.

Following the Fish Creek Trail ahead from this intersection, you leave almost everyone else behind as you continue down a much narrower trail and presently enter John Muir Wilderness. You are continuing through terrain that was severely charred by the 1992 lightning-caused Rainbow Fire. Even now, there are only occasional Jeffrey pines emerging from the sea of mountain whitethorn, with magenta-flowered fireweed adding color in the wetter places. It is a shadeless trudge on a hot day, especially because you are walking on dusty pumice–volcanic deposits that have buried the underlying granite. Exactly 2.0 miles into the walk, the trail suddenly drops steeply into an enclosed valley with an intact forest canopy. Here, in a tangle of spring wildflowers and ferns, you meet Crater Creek, tumbling down the eastern wall in a pretty cascade. You are now back on granite and your trail—like Crater Creek—is funneled along a passageway between two polished granite ribs. You pass one campsite near where you cross Crater Creek on a two-log bridge and another as you ford a Crater Creek tributary, also on a two-log bridge. Trending farther west here leads to some outstanding campsites, sandy perches overlooking the Middle Fork San Joaquin River.

Views open up as the track traverses a sloping granite ledge high above the Middle Fork San Joaquin River. The dramatic panorama and the sight of Crater Creek diving spectacularly off the canyon's lip are worth the trip. Turning around, look at the series of granite ribs to the north, each constraining the course of a creek, beautifully illustrating how wide-scale fracture patterns create the fine-scale landscape features you experience on your walk. Soon the trail curves away from the canyon to ford Cold Creek on a flattened log bridge (6,758'); nearby are some more campsites, these under white fir cover. The trail now briefly ascends this creek corridor, yet another trench between granite ribs. Continuing south out of the Cold Creek drainage, the trail traverses spring-irrigated slopes offering a riot of flowers and drops onto a broad ridge (with possible campsites). You walk through a mixed forest, including scattered aspens, white fir, Jeffrey pine, and black oak, emerging at the lip of the Fish Creek canyon.

Now begins a steep, rocky, 500-foot descent down the valley's north wall (watch for rattlesnakes) to meet roaring Fish Creek. Here you cross a bridge spanning Fish Creek (6,353') and reach Fox Meadow. Note that USGS 7.5' topo maps still show an old trail routing, where the trail continues on the north side of Fish Creek to so-called Island Crossing; this route has long been abandoned, so take the bridge across the river. (*Note:* Even more confusing, some

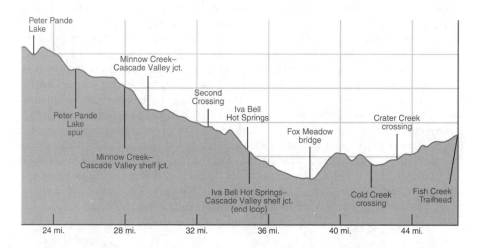

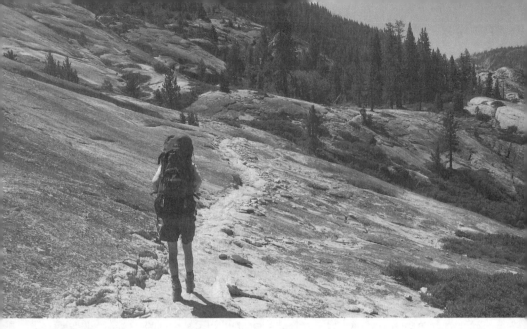

On the Fish Creek Trail   Photo by Elizabeth Wenk

maps incorrectly label the bridge itself as "Island Crossing.") Just left of the trail is a collection of large campsites pleasantly shaded by white fir and incense cedar, with easy access to Fish Creek (6,350'; 37.53381°N, 119.07312°W). Fish Creek offers an unusual fishing opportunity in the High Sierra—the fish here are native, for there are no major falls downstream. Early shepherds gave this drainage its name, thrilled by the easy source of food.

DAY 2 (Fox Meadow to Lost Keys Lakes, 6.7 miles): Today's hike involves the biggest elevation gain of the trip: about 3,000 feet from Fox Meadow to Lost Keys Lakes. Soon after you leave the vicinity of the Fox Meadow bridge, you pass an unsigned, easily missed junction with the abandoned Silver Creek Trail that ascends Silver Creek to the Margaret Lakes Basin—the junction has vanished, but the switchbacks upslope are impressively built and still remarkably intact, with hewn log fences rounding the corners. It is a beautiful route.

The trail loops around the southern boundary of marshy Fox Meadow, and then follows tumbling Fish Creek upstream through the steep-walled, confined glacial-carved valley. You are offered views only where you sporadically exit the conifer canopy. As you meander upward, watch for where Fish Creek descends the valley walls from the north; here is a pleasant campsite. Beyond, you continue up alongside the much-smaller Sharktooth Creek, imposing unfractured walls still rising to the south. Tree cover is more discontinuous for the final 1.4 miles to Iva Bell Hot Springs. In places there are tangles of downed trees, with young saplings growing rapidly in their newfound sunlight. You also cross a series of avalanche zones; in one, nearly all the mature trees have been snapped off 6 feet above the ground, marking the depth of the snowpack when the avalanche tore downslope. Crossing some densely vegetated patches bisected by small creeks, you reach a junction near Iva Bell Hot Springs, where left (northeast) leads back to the Fish Creek drainage and the easiest hot springs access (your return route), while right (southeast) leads up to a shelf high above Cascade Valley and ultimately, as indicated by the junction marker, Goodale Pass; this is today's route to the Lost Keys Lakes. This is a tiny junction with an obscurely placed sign—in case you miss it, if you cross a bridge, you're going the wrong direction, and if you're starting southeast up a steeper hill without crossing a bridge, you're on track.

IVA BELL HOT SPRINGS

Although it's not one of this trip's nightly destinations (but it is the goal of Trip 43), most people who have come this far will want to detour to Iva Bell Hot Springs for at least a break. You have the chance to stop at the springs on Day 2 and again on Day 5, when your route takes you past the easiest access point. And if you want to split Day 2's tough climb, you can add a night at Iva Bell.

It's a magical place in danger of being loved to death. If you decide to camp here, be considerate of other guests and ultraconscientious of your environmental footprint, and absolutely only pick well-used tent sites on compacted bare soil, sand, and rock. There are many rock-lined pools to soak in, offering luxurious bathing at 100°F while imbibing the glorious views west down Fish Creek. To reach the hot springs, cross Sharktooth Creek on a log bridge, follow the trail upslope, and look for an unsigned path near a large campsite beside a tiny tributary creek (about 0.2 mile upstream; 7,174'; 37.53343°N, 119.02562°W). Use trails then lead to many more scattered campsites along the northern periphery of the hot springs, some as far as 200 feet (elevation) upslope. There are also some incense cedar–shaded sites farther downstream and a few on the south side of the marshy expanse, closer to Sharktooth Creek.

According to Peter Browning's *Place Names of the Sierra Nevada* (Wilderness Press), these springs are named for "Iva Bell Clark [who] was born unexpectedly at the springs in July 1936, surprising both parents; Mrs. Clark had thought she had a tumor."

Ignoring the temptation to visit the hot springs until you return on Day 5, begin the loop part of this trip: go right (southeast) toward Lost Keys Lakes. After a brief stint up an open slope, you enter white fir forest beside dashing Sharktooth Creek and climb steeply. Endless switchbacks lead you upward, thankfully mostly under forest cover. Three times you cross a length of boulders, marking the location of an old flood channel. After a 700-foot ascent you cross Sharktooth Creek and immediately resume switchbacking. Along one stretch, nearly all the trees have been blown down, and although the trail has been repaired, it is a rougher tread with tiny zigzags winding between the downed trunks and inverted roots. Climbing higher, a mixture of red and white fir soon provides shade, transitioning to a red fir, lodgepole pine, and hemlock forest by the time the gradient eases.

Near where the trail crosses a tributary creek, the western Lost Keys Lake outlet creek, for the second time, you'll find a pleasant campsite. You are also now on the so-called Cascade Valley shelf. Compared to the steep slopes above and below you, you mostly feel like you're on a shelf as you follow the trail southeast, although it is discontinuous and bisected by multiple drainages.

Rounding a corner, you are suddenly on rolling slabs dotted with lodgepole pine and juniper, with splendid views north and east. A few more steps and you reach the Lost Keys Lakes junction, the signpost currently decorated by a (the?) set of lost keys. Turning right (south) onto this spur trail, you now climb onto a shallow bedrock-and-sand rib and follow it upward. After 0.55 mile, the main trail reaches the central of the three main lakes (9,400'; 37.51588°N, 119.00606°W), with a poorer-quality trail continuing to the eastern lake; both offer lovely lodgepole pine shaded camping beyond their heather-and-blueberry fringe. Rainbow trout are present in both of these lakes. The western lake has limited campsites or views and is a shallower, reedier lake in a more enclosed basin; to reach it, head right about 0.1 mile before reaching the middle lake, cross a shallow saddle, and then hook clockwise down to the lake.

DAY 3 (Lost Keys Lakes to Peter Pande Lake, 7.9 miles): Return to the main trail and turn right (east) to start a gentle ascent toward Minnow Creek. Along the 1.7-mile segment to the Long Canyon junction the trail first traverses open slabs; it is a wonderful feeling to be perched high above the broad valley and simultaneously enjoy views across the valley, to the walls above, and falls below. Beyond, the trail drops to an extensive lodgepole pine and hemlock flat on the shelf holding Scoop Lake and then rises and falls gently to reach the banks of the Long Canyon Creek (with many nearby campsites in lodgepole pine flats alongside the creek). Fording the creek, the trail again traverses open terrain, quickly reaching the junction with the unmaintained (and unsigned) trail up Long Canyon to Beetlebug Lake.

BEETLEBUG LAKE

The 2.8-mile walk up lush Long Canyon leads to Beetlebug Lake, an alternate destination for one of your nights. The trail is narrow and in places indistinct, but the route is straightforward—follow the western side of the valley gently upcanyon to the lake. The final 0.3 mile is steeper as you ascend a headwall clad with stunted hemlock. There are a few campsites in lodgepole pine forest at the north end of Beetlebug Lake, while truly vertical cliffs encircle the rest of the lake, a striking backdrop. Meanwhile, the cluster of lakes around Midge Lake offers fantastic open-slab camping, although reaching it requires some off-trail travel and a stiff climb, best started by leaving the trail and climbing west out of the river valley before the trail begins the final steep ascent to Beetlebug Lake.

Continuing east, more lodgepole pine forest walking leads an easy 0.6 mile past Marsh Lake to a junction with the connector trail leading left (north) down Minnow Creek to Cascade Valley. This is your return route, but for now, continue straight ahead (right; southeast), following the sign for Grassy Lake. Climbing briefly up a slope of lodgepole pine and hemlock, you diverge south from Minnow Creek, before converging with it again at the north end of gigantic sublime Jackson Meadow—a sea of grass and wildflowers set high above the valley floor. The trail skirts southwest around the verdant meadow, staying far from the meandering creek and a collection of shallow oxbow lakes. There are a few abandoned-looking packer camps near the meadow edge, but with a little searching in the fringing forest you will find more intimate options. At 1.8 miles after the last trail junction, you ford Minnow Creek, a broad wade unless you find a log across the flow. Continuing up slabs alongside the creek, you quickly reach a spur trail that leads to lovely Olive Lake.

OLIVE LAKE

The trail up to Olive Lake is infrequently maintained but easy to follow. Although Olive Lake is rather hemmed in by cliffs, you can walk around most of the lake on grassy shores, and there are pleasant lodgepole pine–shaded campsites near the outlet. There are two relatively easy cross-country routes leading from the Olive Lake trail to Peter Pande Lake, described in the sidebar "Routes from Peter Pande Lake to Olive Lake" on page 244.

Onward, you continue left (southeast) on the main trail, passing Grassy Lake (campsites) and looping clockwise around a picturesque, granite-lined meadow at its head. After 0.8 mile, you come to the junction with the signposted spur trail to Peter Pande Lake (9,551'; 37.47838°N, 118.95656°W).

The spur trail to Peter Pande Lake, more so than the other lake-access trails along the Cascade Valley shelf, requires good trail-following skills, for you do not ascend the lake's outlet creek but instead cut up and over several granite ribs, then drop into the lake basin alongside a minor tributary. A trail exists the entire way, and most of it is in good condition, but it is just faint enough that it would be easy to miss some key turns. Begin by looping around the south side of the broad marshy meadow, crossing a sometimes-deep creek (the Wilbur Lake outlet creek), and then cutting across a tongue of lodgepole pine and hemlock forest into the drainage of a second, smaller inlet creek. You ascend alongside this drainage, following a subalpine gully of grass, heath, and stunted hemlocks. At 9,786 feet (37.47412°N, 118.96314°W) the trail turns to the northwest and winds up broken slabs and along lodgepole pine–covered benches. After skirting the edge of a dwarf-bilberry-carpeted stand of lodgepole pine, pay careful attention, for the trail does a near U-turn, suddenly heading south up a shallow sculpted valley between polished granite slabs (10,071'; 37.47754°N, 118.96834°W). Slowly exiting forest cover and crossing open slab, the trail continues up to a lovely flower-dotted meadow and creek crossing (10,138'; 37.46959°N, 118.97319°W). Stepping across the creek, the trail to Peter Pande Lake continues right, heading back downhill into the correct drainage—finally! At this junction, detour just 150 feet south to a magnificent grass-ringed lake offering spectacular views to Graveyard Peak, but limited campsites.

You now descend to Peter Pande on a steeper, rougher section of tread, incised where the trail is co-opted as a spring runoff channel. But you see Peter Pande below and simply pick your way slowly downward to the wide-open basin. Soon you reach the outlet creek, a deep sandy wade at high water levels, while later you cross on big rock blocks. Just beyond you reach fine campsites along the lake's north (9,985'; 37.47178°N, 118.97821°W; no campfires) and northwest shores, with up-close views of Graveyard Peak and the Silver Divide. Sitting on the shores is sublime, admiring the beautiful clear water, the aqua-colored shallows grading to intense blue where deeper. The only downside to the wide-open basin and gigantic lake is that it can be quite windy here.

Looking down on Peter Pande Lake on an excursion to the south   Photo by Elizabeth Wenk

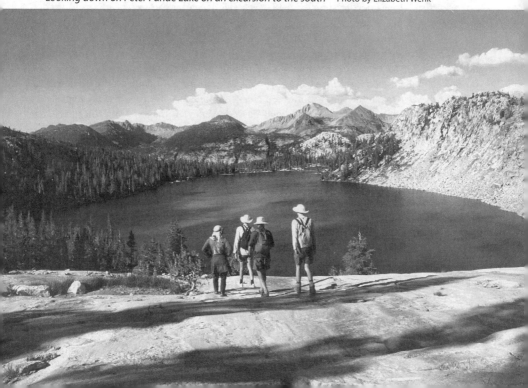

ROUTES FROM PETER PANDE LAKE TO OLIVE LAKE
On a layover day, hike cross-country to Minnie, Anne, and Olive Lakes, taking a use trail around Peter Pande's northwest shore to the inlet stream from Anne and Minnie, then following that stream southwest to Anne Lake. From Anne Lake, go cross-country generally northwest to Minnie Lake and then over the shallow divide between Minnie and Olive Lakes. Descend, still generally northwest, to one pond, then another, and finally veer northeast along the second pond's outlet, Minnow Creek, down to Olive Lake's northwest shore. (This route is a good alternative for strong hikers for Day 4's return trip; from Olive Lake's outlet you can then take the trail 1.4 miles northeast to the main Minnow Creek Trail.) An alternative route toward Olive Lake is to follow the west side of the Peter Pande Lake outlet creek down to Minnow Creek. To do this, follow the broad, nearly flat slabs north from the lake and then down alongside the creek. The terrain looks steep and uninviting, but by always staying a little west of the creek corridor you can safely pick your way down channels between the steep slabs, eventually cutting to the west where the creek plunges into a narrow trench. You reach the spur trail to Olive Lake about 0.25 mile below the lake and turning right can follow the spur alongside Minnow Creek back to the main trail. You can also combine this route with the aforementioned route to Olive Lake to complete a day hike loop from Peter Pande Lake without your overnight pack.

DAY 4 (Peter Pande Lake to Cascade Valley, 6.4 miles): From Peter Pande Lake you either retrace your steps on the main route described or take one of the two alternate routes via Olive Lake back to the Minnow Creek Trail. At that junction, turn left (northwest) and retrace your steps past Jackson Meadow to the junction with the lateral trail that follows Minnow Creek down to Cascade Valley.

Take the connector trail right (north) to reopen the loop part of this trip. After traversing rocky flats alongside the alder-choked creek (with nearby campsites), the trail (and creek) begins a steep descent to meet Fish Creek in aptly named Cascade Valley. It is a cobbly, rocky descent down a steep, narrow trail—unpleasant walking, although for a short distance. At least you have, in places, unbroken views east to Red and White Mountain and north to the waterfalls descending from Purple Lake. Slowly the gradient lessens and you reach the banks of Fish Creek near an old packer's camp, impacted by blowdowns. Here, you have to wade the sandy-bottomed creek—quite deep in early season—and then cross a small meadow to reach the trail down Cascade Valley. At the junction, you turn left (west), signposted for Cascade Valley, while right (east) leads to the JMT/PCT corridor and a spur to Purple Lake. There is a large campsite in the forest just behind the junction (8,378'; 37.51396°N, 118.97309°W). The daily mileage ends here, but there are many other campsites over the coming 2–3 miles or—if you have lots of energy—Iva Bell Hot Springs is an additional 5.6 miles, as described below.

DAY 5 (Cascade Valley to Fox Meadow, 9.0 miles): After traversing a lush lodgepole pine flat, the trail rounds a slab nose and drops beside some beautiful cascades; there is a perfect campsite atop the rocks before you descend. Soon you ford the Duck Lake outlet creek, often a wade (easy), and continue through valley-bottom forest. Between a pair of seasonal tributaries, just downstream of some falls, are more picturesque campsites among aspen groves; the moniker "Cascade Valley" applies equally well to the water cascading over polished slabs along Fish Creek as it does to the valley-wall waterfalls. Continued pleasant forest walking eventually leads to Second Crossing, where you must ford Fish Creek;

there are some acceptable campsites nearby. Fish Creek is now a major river, and this is a very difficult crossing in early summer; even in a below-average precipitation year the water levels can be thigh deep in late June. Fortunately it is broad (i.e., it has less current) and you can place your feet in sandy spots between boulders. If you are unable to ford the creek, your best choice is to retreat to the previous junction, head up to Purple Lake, and then follow the JMT/PCT north to Reds Meadow; nearly the entire route is shown on the maps for this Trip.

A few minutes downstream, the river is suddenly pinched between two rock walls and tumbles spectacularly down its bedrock base. The trail winds beside it across broken slabs. Looking north across the creek, you stare up slopes of dense brush, a monotonous carpet rising all the way to the JMT/PCT corridor. Soon a low gap on the ridge to the south lets you cross over to the Sharktooth Creek drainage; switchbacks first carry you up 150 feet and then back down 600 feet to the lush-green oasis that is Iva Bell Hot Springs.

After visiting the hot springs (see the sidebar on page 241), continue on the main trail to cross Sharktooth Creek on a bridge. At this junction you close the loop part of this trip and turn right (generally west) to retrace your steps 3.4 miles to campsites at the edge of Fox Meadow.

DAY 6 (Island Crossing to Fish Creek Trailhead, 8.3 miles): Retrace the steps of Day 1. Get an early start up the hot, steep switchbacks out of Fish Valley.

Fish Creek   Photo by Elizabeth Wenk

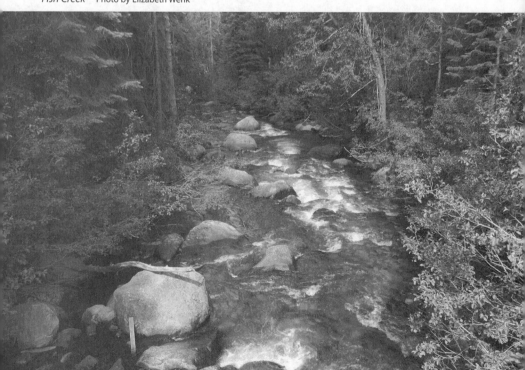

CA 203 TO LAKE MARY ROAD TRIPS

Lake Mary Road leads from the town of Mammoth Lakes into the popular Mammoth Lakes Basin, with its vacation cabins, campgrounds, and giant lakes. From beyond the basin, trails radiate into the surrounding wilderness, including from north to south, Red Cones Trailhead (Horseshoe Lake), Deer Lakes Trailhead (George Lake), and Duck Pass Trailhead. Along all of these trails hikers experience geologic diversity, including young volcanic rocks, old metamorphic rocks, and only small patches of the Sierra's characteristic granite. The trailheads in the Mammoth Lakes Basin are all quite high and the surrounding passes relatively low, making these a good way to access the John Muir Trail and surroundings.

Trailheads: Red Cones

Deer Lakes

Duck Pass

Relaxing walking along the Mammoth Crest with the Ritter Range behind   Photo by Elizabeth Wenk

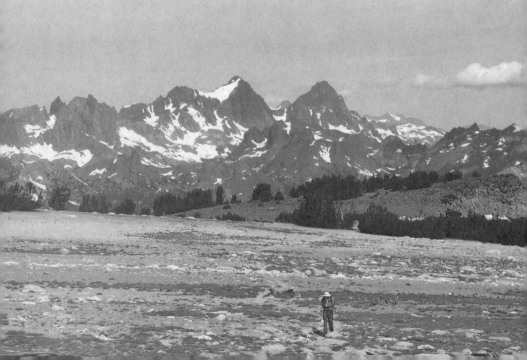

Red Cones Trailhead
9,009'; 37.61299°N, 119.02132°W

Destination/ GPS Coordinates	Trip Type	Best Season	Pace & Hiking/ Layover Days	Total Mileage	Permit Required
42 Upper Crater Meadow 37.58594°N 119.04840°W (in reverse of description; see page 251)	Shuttle (public transport option)	Mid to late	Leisurely 3/0	17.1	Red Cones (Duck Pass as described)

INFORMATION AND PERMITS: This trailhead is in Inyo National Forest. Permits are required for overnight stays and quotas apply. Permits can be reserved up to six months in advance at recreation.gov (60%; $6 permit reservation fee plus $5 per person) or requested in person, first come, first served, a day in advance (40%; free). All permits must be picked up at one of the Inyo National Forest ranger stations, located in Lone Pine (Eastern Sierra Interagency Visitor Center), Bishop, Mammoth Lakes, and Lee Vining (the Mono Basin Scenic Area Visitor Center). If you plan to use a stove or have a campfire, you must also have a California campfire permit, available from a forest service office or online at preventwildfireca.org/campfire-permit. Campfires are prohibited above 10,000 feet and along the Duck Pass Trail corridor. Bear canisters are required in this area.

DRIVING DIRECTIONS: From the junction of US 395 and CA 203 (the Mammoth junction), take CA 203 west 3.7 miles to a major intersection. Here CA 203 turns right, toward Mammoth Mountain, while you continue straight ahead, now on Lake Mary Road. Continue an additional 5.0 miles to the road-end parking area adjacent to Horseshoe Lake.

Deer Lakes Trailhead
9,051'; 37.60355°N, 119.01120°W

Destination/ GPS Coordinates	Trip Type	Best Season	Pace & Hiking/ Layover Days	Total Mileage	Permit Required
41 Deer Lakes 37.56212°N 118.98884°W	Loop	Mid to late	Moderate 2/0	13.1	Deer Lakes

INFORMATION AND PERMITS: This trailhead is in Inyo National Forest. Permits are required for overnight stays and quotas apply. Permits can be reserved up to six months in advance at recreation.gov (60%; $6 permit reservation fee plus $5 per person) or requested in person, first come, first served, a day in advance (40%; free). All permits must be picked up at one of the Inyo National Forest ranger stations, located in Lone Pine (Eastern Sierra Interagency Visitor Center), Bishop, Mammoth Lakes, and Lee Vining (the Mono Basin Scenic Area Visitor Center). If you plan to use a stove or have a campfire, you must also have a California campfire permit, available from a forest service office or online at preventwildfireca.org/campfire-permit. Campfires are prohibited above 10,000 feet and along the Duck Pass Trail corridor. Bear canisters are required in this area.

DRIVING DIRECTIONS: This trailhead is also referred to as the Crystal Lake or Mammoth Crest Trailhead. From the junction of US 395 and CA 203 (the Mammoth junction), take CA 203 west 3.7 miles to a major intersection in the town of Mammoth Lakes. Here

CA 203 turns right, toward Mammoth Mountain, while you continue straight ahead, now on Lake Mary Road. Continue an additional 3.9 miles to a junction just past the Pokenobe Store/Marina; here, turn left onto the Around Lake Mary Road and drive 0.3 mile along the northwest side of Lake Mary. At a T-junction, turn right onto the Lake George Road and continue 0.3 mile to a large parking area. The trailhead departs to the northwest, next to where the Woods Lodge Road continues uphill to vacation homes. There is a toilet on the other side of the lot and water in the adjacent Lake George Campground.

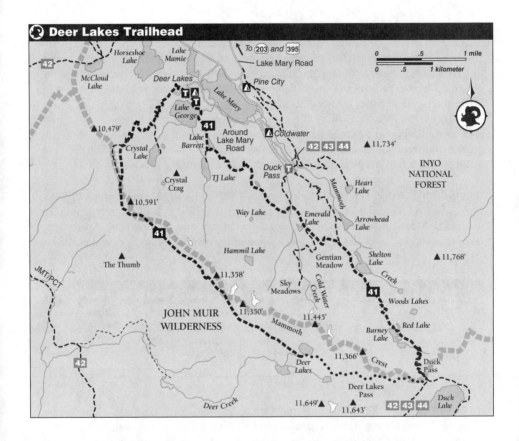

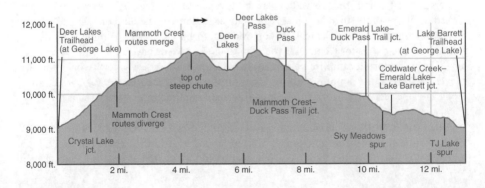

trip 41 **Deer Lakes**

Trip Data: 37.56212°N, 118.98884°W; 13.1 miles; 2/0 days
Topos: *Devils Postpile, Crystal Crag, Bloody Mountain*

HIGHLIGHTS: The Deer Lakes Loop makes an ideal weekend trip or an ambitious day hike. Along the route, hikers encounter both stark alpine and dense forest terrains. The lightly traveled route to Deer Lakes follows the spine of the Mammoth Crest, with expansive views in every direction. The trip is described as a loop; for a shuttle trip, leave a car at the nearby Duck Pass Trailhead (see page 251 for directions) and shave 1.9 miles off the hike.

HEADS UP! *There is no water on the trail before you reach the Deer Lakes basin. Part of this trip on Day 2, from Deer Lakes to Duck Pass, follows an unmaintained use trail. Hikers should be comfortable with route-finding.*

DAY 1 (Deer Lakes Trailhead to Deer Lakes, 5.5 miles): The trail leaves the Lake George parking lot at its north end and heads north, following a route just east of (and below) a road leading to cabins. Slowly arcing west, then southwest, the trail switchbacks diligently upward around the tract of vacation homes. Soon following a forested spur above Lake George, each left-hand switchback affords views down to Lake George and eastward to Red and Gold Mountain, while the right-hand corners lie in hemlock-and-lodgepole pine forest. At a signed junction with the trail left (south) to Crystal Lake (no camping), this trip's route continues right (southwest).

The tree cover slowly thins as the trail works its way up gray and red pumice slopes toward the Mammoth Crest, the views improving step by step. Reaching a denser stand of whitebark pines just past the John Muir Wilderness boundary, the trail descends briefly and passes an unsigned trail junction. Here, right (west) ascends red cinder right to the tip of the Mammoth Crest for fabulous 360-degree views, while the main trail continues left (south) through a gentle swale, the remnant of a crater. After 0.4 mile the trail reaches the Mammoth Crest proper, and the two possible routes reunite at an unsigned junction, where you stay left (south); the crest route would have been 0.1 mile longer and required about 100 feet extra elevation gain.

The excellent views from the crest take in the Ritter Range to the west, the Silver Divide to the south, and between them, to the southwest, the Middle Fork San Joaquin River's canyon converging with Fish Creek's canyon. The rocky-sandy route continues south, and the crest broadens into a moonscape of red and white pumice well decorated with wildflowers in season: woolly sunflowers, Lobb's lupine, and wild buckwheats are particularly abundant. Beneath the veneer of pumice—and sometimes atop it—are granite boulders, reflecting the underlying bedrock, and, with continued ascent, the soil surface transitions to granite sand.

The trail climbs moderately, then steeply, through increasingly dense whitebark pine stands just west of the crestline, offering views down to lush Crater Meadow and briefly touching the crest at the top of a sheer, often snowy chute with dizzying views east. Crossing onto metavolcanic rock, the crest then curves left (eastward) and so does the trail as it descends into the Deer Lakes basin. The trail terminates near the middle (northernmost) Deer Lake (10,669'). Find a campsite near this lake (for example, 10,674'; 37.56212°N, 118.98884°W; no campfires) or along the stream connecting it with the lowest Deer Lake.

DAY 2 (Deer Lakes to Deer Lakes Trailhead via Duck Pass, 7.6 miles, part cross-country): Several indistinct use trails depart south and east from the middle Deer Lake, ultimately converging to follow the Mammoth Crest over gentle, alpine terrain toward

Duck Pass. These trails first ascend the slope due east of the lake and then turn southeast, following sandy slopes just north of the highest Deer Lake (10,887'; sandy campsites to its northwest and northeast). The various use trails are slowly funneled to a short talus chute between steeper bluffs, with a well-worn tread winding up the chute's right side through scree and sand.

After the stiff 200-foot ascent, you are back in delightfully gentle alpine tundra, beguiled by the purple-and-green shaded rock and a lovely broad meadow. A seasonal tarn allows early-season camping nearby. Snaking east across the flats, then southeast up a shallow gully leads to a low saddle, sometimes called "Deer Lakes Pass." From the top of this divide you see Pika Lake, but not the closer landmarks, Duck Lake and the Duck Pass Trail; the unseen trail, your goal, traverses the slope high above Duck Lake's western shore. It is best to intersect the trail just west of Duck Pass (near 10,788'; 37.55838°N, 118.96231°W), but if you trend too far south on the descent (quite easy to do), you'll add just token distance and elevation gain to your route. The best route toward the Duck Pass Trail stays just south of the Mammoth Crest's spine, winding through sandy flats and avoiding dense thickets of whitebark pine krummholz. The use trail is least distinct for the final 0.5 mile to Duck Pass. Once you reach the Duck Pass Trail, turn left (north) and follow it to Duck Pass.

You now take the busy Duck Pass Trail north toward Barney and Skelton Lakes. The sinuous, view-rich descent leads through talus and along ledges atop cliffs as it attempts to avoid long-lasting snow gullies. Tight switchbacks resolve to a descending traverse that leads to Barney Lake (10,210'; campsites to either side of the trail; no campfires). Continuing through pocket meadows, willow thickets, and whitebark pine and lodgepole pine forest, you pass Skelton Lake and reach a junction (9,921'; 37.58022°N, 118.98037°W), where you turn left (west) toward Emerald Lake, while right (straight, north) leads to the Duck Pass Trailhead. Note that the trail to Emerald Lake is not plotted on the USGS 7.5' topo maps and used to be routed farther south—its location is accurately plotted on CalTopo's online maps, but not on the National Map (USGS online map). Alternatively, if you've staged a car at the Duck Pass Trailhead, continue 1.3 miles straight to it.

Turning onto the trail to Emerald Lake, you follow a corridor beside light-colored metamorphic bluffs, enjoying your first views to Ritter and Banner Peaks in many miles. Arcing south then northwest through lodgepole pine, western white pine, and hemlock forest, the trail drops steadily beneath steep cliffs. The trail ultimately follows a draw to Emerald Lake and at the lake's eastern edge reaches a junction, where a faint trail leads left (southwest) to Sky Meadows, while you stay right (northwest). You skirt moraine-dammed Emerald Lake (virtually no camping due to the giant boulders that ring its shore) and proceed through lush conifer forest to a junction, where straight ahead (right, north) leads to the Cold Water Creek Trailhead (at the western end of the Duck Pass Trailhead parking area), while you turn left (west) to cross Cold Water Creek, marked simply as TRAIL.

Cross the creek and bear left (southwest, briefly upstream, then curving northwest), following a well-maintained, obvious trail, that appears on just some published and online maps. The pleasant walk follows a corridor between mossy metavolcanic bluffs (to the west) and mixed conifer forest, passing an elongate tarn and then rolling imperceptibly onto a west-facing slope with broken Crystal Crag and Mammoth Crest views. Switchbacks carry you to sandy-shored Lake Barrett and then a junction where left (south) leads to TJ Lake, while you turn right (north) to continue to Lake Barrett's outlet. Lake George is soon visible ahead, and you drop to the lakeshore on a steep and rocky trail.

At a signed junction with a use trail around Lake George, go right (northeast), cross the outlet stream on a bridge, and skirt the campground on the lake's east shore to the parking lot's south side; your starting trailhead is a few steps away, on the lot's north side.

Duck Pass Trailhead
9,137'; 37.59122°N, 118.98925°

Destination/ GPS Coordinates	Trip Type	Best Season	Pace & Hiking/ Layover Days	Total Mileage	Permit Required
42 Upper Crater Meadow 37.58594°N 119.04840°W	Shuttle (public transport option)	Mid to late	Leisurely 3/0	17.1	Duck Pass *(Red Cones in reverse)*
43 Iva Bell Hot Springs 37.53343°N 119.02562°W	Shuttle (public transport option)	Early to late	Moderate 4/1	28.2	Duck Pass *(Fish Creek in reverse)*
44 Ram Lake and Lake Virginia 37.59122°N 118.98925°W (Ram Lake)	Semiloop	Mid to late	Moderate 4/1	24.8	Duck Pass

INFORMATION AND PERMITS: This trailhead is in Inyo National Forest. Permits are required for overnight stays and quotas apply. Permits can be reserved up to six months in advance at recreation.gov (60%; $6 permit reservation fee plus $5 per person) or requested in person, first come, first served, a day in advance (40%; free). All permits must be picked up at one of the Inyo National Forest ranger stations, located in Lone Pine (Eastern Sierra Interagency Visitor Center), Bishop, Mammoth Lakes, and Lee Vining (the Mono Basin Scenic Area Visitor Center). If you plan to use a stove or have a campfire, you must also have a California campfire permit, available from a forest service office or online at preventwildfireca.org/campfire-permit. Campfires are prohibited above 10,000 feet and along the Duck Pass Trail corridor. Bear canisters are required in this area.

DRIVING DIRECTIONS: From the junction of US 395 and CA 203 (the Mammoth junction), take CA 203 west for 3.7 miles to a major intersection. Here CA 203 turns right, toward Mammoth Mountain, while you continue straight ahead, now on Lake Mary Road. Continue an additional 3.6 miles, past Twin Lakes and to a junction signposted for Lake Mary; turn left here onto the so-called Around Lake Mary Road. Drive 0.6 mile along Lake Mary's eastern shore and then, as the road starts to bend to the right, turn left into Coldwater Campground. Drive 0.7 mile through Coldwater Campground to the Duck Pass Trailhead parking area. There are toilets and a water faucet at the trailhead.

trip 42 ## Upper Crater Meadow

see maps on p. 252–253

Trip Data: 37.58594°N, 119.04840°W; 17.1 miles; 3/0 days
Topos: *Devils Postpile, Bloody Mountain, Crystal Crag*

HIGHLIGHTS: Moderate trails lead through wonderfully varied scenery, including a pair of cinder cones, the Red Cones, one of the eastern Sierra's many fascinating volcanic features. There are some magnificent views—especially from Duck Pass and the Red Cones—but in between much of the hike is simply a pleasant forest walk that is calm, full of birds, and a time to enjoy the forest canopy. The trailheads are only a few miles apart, so this is an easy shuttle to set up, especially since a free shuttle covers most of the distance between trailheads.

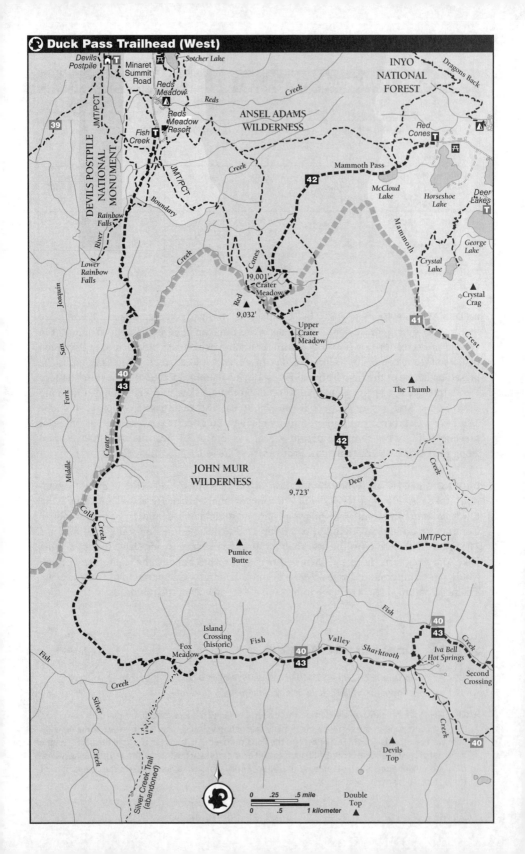

Devils Postpile

Minaret Summit Road

Sotcher Lake

INYO NATIONAL FOREST

Dragons Back

Reds Meadow

Reds

Creek

ANSEL ADAMS WILDERNESS

Red Cones

39

JMT/PCT

Reds Meadow Resort

Fish Creek

Creek

Mammoth Pass

McCloud Lake

Horseshoe Lake

Deer Lakes

DEVILS POSTPILE NATIONAL MONUMENT

JMT/PCT

42

George Lake

Rainbow Falls

Boundary

Mammoth

Crystal Lake

Crystal Crag

River

Creek

19,001

Cones

Crest

Lower Rainbow Falls

Crater Meadow

Red

9,032'

Upper Crater Meadow

41

San Joaquin

40
43

The Thumb

Fork

Crater

42

Middle

JOHN MUIR WILDERNESS

9,723'

Deer

Creek

Cold

Creek

Pumice Butte

JMT/PCT

Fish

Fox Meadow

Island Crossing (historic)

Fish

Valley

Sharktooth

40
43

Creek

Fish

Silver

Creek

40
43

Iva Bell Hot Springs

Second Crossing

Silver Creek Trail (abandoned)

Devils Top

Creek

40

N

| 0 | .25 | .5 mile |
| 0 | .5 | 1 kilometer |

Double Top

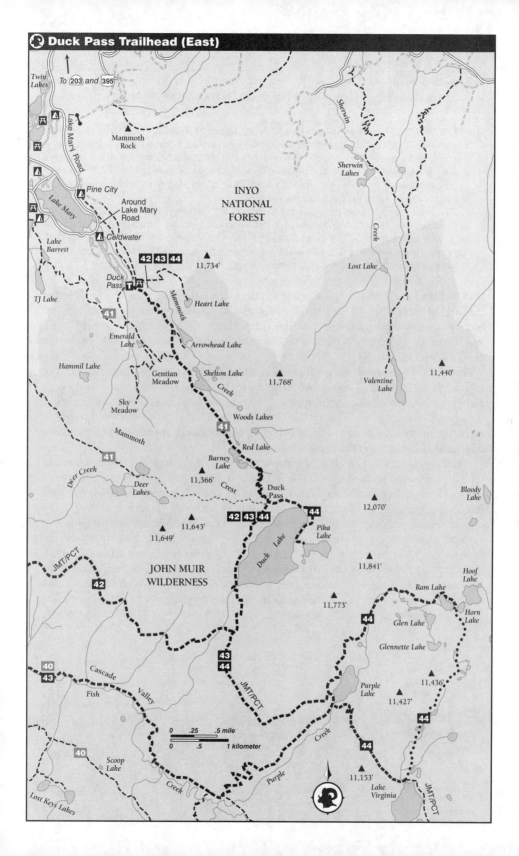

Duck Pass Trailhead (East)

HEADS UP! *After a heavy winter, the Duck Pass Trail may be under snow beyond Skelton Lake well into July; check at the Mammoth Lakes ranger station before setting out.*

SHUTTLE DIRECTIONS: Both trailheads are in the Mammoth Lakes Basin, just 2.7 road miles apart. To reach Horseshoe Lake, the Mammoth Pass (Reds Cone) Trailhead, follow the main trailhead driving directions until you are directed to turn onto the "Around Lake Mary Road." Here, you should instead stay straight, remaining on the Lake Mary Road for an additional 1.4 miles to its end. After leaving a car at Horseshoe Lake, return to the Lake Mary Road–Around Lake Mary Road junction and turn right (south), continuing on to the Duck Pass Trailhead.

In summer, the Lakes Basin Trolley is a free bus service in the Mammoth Lakes Basin. It stops at the Lake Mary Marina (Stop 100; at the entrance to Coldwater Campground, 0.8 mile from the Duck Pass Trailhead) and at Horseshoe Lake (Stop 104), in this order, so you will want to take the shuttle from Horseshoe Lake down to the Riding Stables (Stop 98) and then get onto the next bus up from town to continue back to the Lake Mary Marina and walk the 0.8 mile back to your car.

DAY 1 (Duck Pass Trailhead to Duck Lake's outlet creek, 6.0 miles): From the south end of the parking lot, just behind the toilets, head southeast past an information sign. Then you quickly cross an unmapped streamlet and enter John Muir Wilderness. The dusty Duck Pass Trail climbs gradually to moderately before beginning a series of lazy switchbacks that carry you up a rounded ridge.

After 1.0 mile you reach a marked junction, where you stay right (south, ahead) to Duck Pass, while left (southeast) leads to Arrowhead Lake (just visible below). Climbing through granite outcrops, you pass a small spur west to Emerald Lake at 1.3 miles and then skirt the western shore of lovely Skelton Lake (9,921'). Although there are campsites throughout this drainage, the area is overused; it's better to spend a night acclimating at a frontcountry campground and get over the pass on your first day.

Climbing moderately past alpine meadows, you top a rise overlooking pretty Barney Lake (10,210'; campsites; no campfires). Little Red Lake is visible on the left as the trail crosses Barney Lake's outlet on rocks and skirts the lake's east shore. As you approach the end of the lake, the trail traverses up a dry knob and then begins switchbacking in earnest up steep, rocky slopes. The winding, view-rich ascent leads through talus and along ledges atop cliffs as it attempts to avoid long-lasting snow gullies. You pass wildflower gardens and a perched stand of whitebark pines before surmounting Duck Pass, 3.9 miles from the trailhead (10,803'). From the pass, enjoy the spectacular overlook of huge Duck Lake and its companion to the east, smaller Pika Lake. Just 250 feet later, a spur trail descends left (east) to Duck Lake's northeastern shore; if you wish to have a shorter day, there are campsites 1.1 miles away on the flat-topped knobs just north of Pika Lake (10,537'; 37.55183°N, 118.95517°W; no campfires).

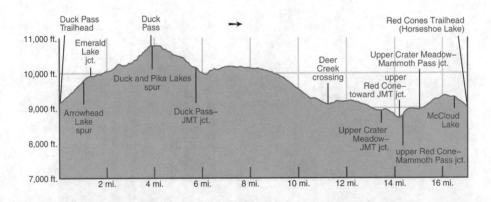

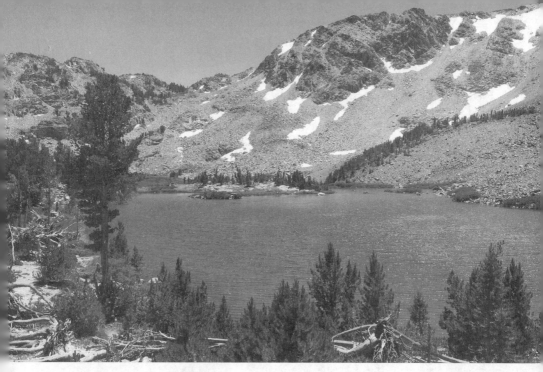

Barney Lake   Photo by Elizabeth Wenk

Otherwise, follow the main tread high above Duck Lake's western shore, in early season hopefully noting the delightful clusters of magenta Sierra primroses. Slowly you descend, intersecting the shoreline just as you reach Duck Lake's outlet. Note that camping is not permitted within 300 feet of the outlet, although there are sites if you continue farther east. You cross the outlet on rock blocks and drop steeply alongside dark, glaciated metavolcanic bluffs and slabs and through lodgepole pine–forested corridors. The descent moderates as you approach the intersection with the John Muir Trail (JMT)/Pacific Crest Trail (PCT).

Turn right (west) onto the northbound JMT and drop to a few small campsites just before the Duck Lake outlet creek ford followed by a too-popular camping area on the bench west of the Duck Lake outlet creek, where there are pleasant, but small, campsites with awe-inspiring views across Cascade Valley to the Silver Divide (9,988'; 37.53846°N, 118.97274°W).

DAY 2 (Duck Lake outlet creek to Upper Crater Meadow, 7.5 miles): Late in the year, or in a dry year, there may be no water between Duck Lake outlet creek and Deer Creek, 5.25 miles away, so fill up water bottles at the Duck Lake outlet creek.

The northbound JMT/PCT leaves the bench and climbs about 200 feet before beginning a long traverse high above Cascade Valley. The trail sidles in and out of several side valleys, minimizing elevation change. Partway along, the footing changes from granitic gravel to pumice—volcanic rock so full of air pockets it floats on water, though here it simply slips and crunches underfoot. Here and there the trees part enough to permit views across Cascade Valley to the Silver Divide, although they are never as good as those you had near Duck Pass and the Duck Lake outlet creek. For long distances, the forest floor is nearly bare. Openings in the forest sport just a few shrubs, most often sagebrush and bush chinquapin. While only lodgepole pines can survive under the dry conditions dictated by the southern exposure, especially in conjunction with coarse, volcanic soils, as you approach Deer Creek, western white pines appear as well.

Eventually the trail veers away from the valley's rim, curves over low knolls, and descends a little to ford Deer Creek; there are well-used campsites just after the creek crossing. Here is also an indistinct and unmarked junction with a lateral up Deer Creek to the Deer Lakes; stay on the JMT/PCT (left, west). The gradually graded trail curves north and climbs along a meadow-bound Deer Creek tributary. You emerge from lodgepole pine cover at a broad sandy saddle, the unlikely drainage divide between the main Middle Fork of the San Joaquin drainage and Fish Creek. Starting gradually downhill, the trail continues past a series of charming pocket meadows, crosses a small fork of Crater Creek and then Crater Creek itself, before skirting to the west of Upper Crater Meadow. The gentle, forested slopes cupping these meadows offer the occasional campsite, although some of the small streams can dry in late summer. A little beyond the northwestern corner of flowery Upper Crater Meadow, you recross Crater Creek on a small bridge and reach a junction (8,922'; 37.58623°N, 119.05150°W). The right fork goes north to Mammoth Pass and Horseshoe Lake, your route, and the left fork is the northbound JMT/PCT to Reds Meadow. Near this junction, leave the trail and search for campsites in the sandy flat just north of Upper Crater Meadow (for example, 8,977'; 37.58594°N, 119.04840°W).

> **REROUTED TRAILS**
>
> The USGS *Crystal Crag* topo shows a junction right in the middle of Upper Crater Meadow. The trail was long ago rerouted to the meadow's western periphery, and the junction you reach is after you start down Crater Creek. However, on a satellite photo—such as Google Earth—you can see still the old trail's scar through the meadow.

DAY 3 (Upper Crater Meadow to Horseshoe Lake, 3.6 miles): From the aforementioned junction, the JMT continues left, while the described route turns right, heading more directly toward the northern Red Cone and Mammoth Pass. Heading right (north) after just 400 feet you reach a second junction, where left (northwest) leads past the upper Red Cone (the route described) while right (northeast) leads you on a higher traverse that bypasses the upper Red Cone. The alternates are almost exactly the same length, but left (west) has better views and the opportunity to summit the cinder cone.

So heading left, your trail leads through unassuming dry forest on dusty soils, dropping slightly to cross two Crater Creek tributaries and reaching another trail junction, where left (west) leads back to the JMT/PCT while you stay right (north and then west), climbing briefly up a steep slope. After just 0.1 mile you reach another junction, where left (west and then north) leads to Reds Meadow and the summit of the upper Red Cone, while your route, toward Mammoth Pass, is right (north). Yes, the trail network here is confusing! Adding to the confusion, you'll come across an old sign declaring you're on the JMT, for it was once routed through here.

Before continuing to Mammoth Pass, a detour up the northern Red Cones is strongly recommended, so head left. You quickly find yourself on a saddle less than 100 feet below the summit and climb west up the red cinders. While Mammoth Mountain, the hulking mass to the north, is 220,000 years old, the Red Cones themselves are just 8,500 years old, most recently erupting about 5,000 years ago. Like all cinder cones, the magma erupted violently out of a central, cylindrical vent; these just happen to be quite small cinder cones. The view from atop is wide ranging and stunning, especially west across the Middle Fork San Joaquin River to the dark, jagged Ritter Range. To the north, beyond Mammoth are, from right to left, San Joaquin Mountain, Parker Peak, and, on the Yosemite boundary, Kuna Peak.

After this detour, you need to retrace your steps 0.2 mile south to the last junction and now head northeast, toward Mammoth Pass and McCloud Lake, the latter misnamed McLead Lake on USGS 7.5' topos. After 0.7 mile, near a noisy spring, the alternative route above Upper Crater Meadow rejoins from the right, and you continue straight ahead (left; north), still through a mixed conifer forest. Soon the route rounds the northern tip of the Mammoth Crest and bends east beneath the steep escarpment.

Go ahead to cross broad, forested, viewless Mammoth Pass, leaving designated wilderness behind. The gradient is so gradual that hikers may not notice the pass. Presently, skirt beautiful McCloud Lake (no camping), tucked picturesquely under the light-colored cliffs of the Mammoth Crest, and reach a junction: left is a different route from Mammoth Pass to Reds Meadow, while you stay right (ahead, east-northeast) to descend to the parking lot at Horseshoe Lake (9,009'; 37.61299°N, 119.02132°W).

> ### HORSESHOE LAKE'S DEAD TREES
> Studies have shown that the trees around the parking lot at Horseshoe Lake died because their roots were suffocated by carbon dioxide seeping up in measurable amounts from some underground source related to the magma body beneath this volcanic area. There are other, similarly caused tree-kill sites here and on Mammoth Mountain. The seepage is small enough that (so far) it poses no threat to people when they're in the open air. Read and heed all warnings here.

trip 43 Iva Bell Hot Springs

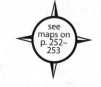

see maps on p. 252–253

Trip Data: 37.53343°N, 119.02562°W (Iva Bell Hot Springs);
28.2 miles; 4/1 days
Topos: *Devils Postpile, Bloody Mountain, Crystal Crag*

HIGHLIGHTS: This trip offers beautiful views along much of the route. Even better are the endless cascading creeks, both those dropping down the surrounding valley walls and in the creek beside you, punctuated by idyllic cold-water pools. But the real treat is one of just a handful of wilderness hot springs in the entire High Sierra. Iva Bell Hot Springs is a magical Shangri-la of a place that is in danger of being loved to death. Tread lightly here.

HEADS UP! *The Duck Pass Trail isn't high, but it holds snow late and has steep drop-offs; check at the Mammoth Lakes ranger station before setting out. The ford of Fish Creek in Cascade Valley ("Second Crossing") is dangerous at high flows. If you want to visit Iva Bell in early season, when these dangers are present, consider doing an out-and-back trip starting at Reds Meadow, the end point. This is also written up as the first 11.8 miles of the description for Trip 40. If you have a dog with you, you are required to have a muzzle for the dog for the return shuttle trip out of Reds Meadow.*

SHUTTLE DIRECTIONS: In the main driving instructions, head to the junction in the center of Mammoth Lakes that is 3.7 miles west of US 395. Here, the trailhead directions point you straight ahead on Lake Mary Road to the Mammoth Lakes Basin. To reach the endpoint, instead turn right (north), continuing on CA 203, now also called Minaret Road. Continue 4.2 miles to the main Mammoth Mountain Ski Area lodge. Here you will have to park your car and take a shuttle bus (fee), unless you arrive before 7 a.m., after 7 p.m., are staying in one of the campgrounds in the Reds Meadow Valley, or are hiking early or late in the season before the shuttle bus is mandatory. On your return you will take the shuttle from the Reds Meadow Store or Rainbow Falls Trailhead to this location. Even if you have permission to continue to the valley, driving a car to the trailhead is only worth it for an out-and-back trip—if you're doing the described point-to-point walk it is best to take the shuttle.

If you have permission to continue to the valley *and* are doing an out-and-back, drive an additional 9.5 miles over Minaret Summit and down the windy road alongside the Middle Fork San Joaquin River. After you've passed Devils Postpile and Sotcher Lake, turn right onto a spur road that leads 0.1 mile to the Rainbow Falls Trailhead (from which the trail down Fish Creek departs; with toilet, water).

Mammoth Lakes has additional shuttle buses that make it easy to do the point-to-point hike with a single car—there are shuttle buses from the Village (located just northwest of the Minaret Road–Lake Mary Road junction) to the Mammoth Mountain Lodge and to the Lake Mary Marina (Stop 100, along the Lakes Basin Trolley), the latter at the entrance to the Coldwater Campground. The only disadvantage is you have to walk the 0.8 mile through Coldwater Campground to the trailhead. When you pick up your wilderness permit, confirm that you are allowed to leave your car overnight in the large Village Parking area along Minaret Road.

DAY 1 (Duck Pass Trailhead to Purple Lake, 8.0 miles): From the south end of the parking lot, just behind the toilets, head southeast past an information sign. Then you quickly cross an unmapped streamlet and enter John Muir Wilderness. The dusty Duck Pass Trail climbs gradually to moderately before beginning a series of lazy switchbacks that carry you up a rounded ridge.

After 1.0 mile you reach a marked junction, where you stay right (south, ahead) to Duck Pass, while left (southeast) leads to Arrowhead Lake (barely visible below). Climbing through granite outcrops, you pass a small spur west to Emerald Lake at 1.3 miles and then skirt the western shore of lovely Skelton Lake (9,921'). Although there are campsites throughout this drainage, the area is overused; it's better to spend a night acclimating at a frontcountry campground and get over the pass on your first day.

Climbing moderately past alpine meadows, you presently top a rise overlooking pretty Barney Lake (10,210'; campsites; no campfires). Little Red Lake is visible on the left as the trail crosses Barney Lake's outlet on rocks and skirts the lake's east shore. As you approach the end of the lake, the trail traverses up a dry knob and then begins switchbacking in earnest up steep, rocky slopes. The winding, view-rich ascent leads through talus and along ledges atop cliffs as it attempts to avoid long-lasting snow gullies. You pass endless wildflower gardens and a perched stand of whitebark pines before surmounting Duck Pass,

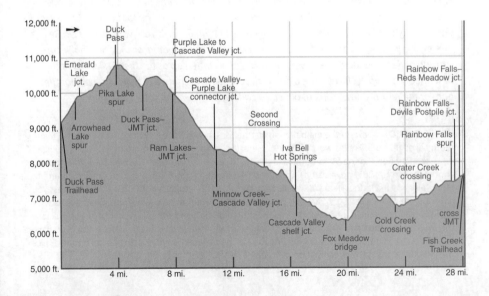

3.9 miles from the trailhead (10,803'). From the pass, enjoy the spectacular overlook of huge Duck Lake and its companion to the east, smaller Pika Lake. Just 250 feet later, a spur trail descends left (east) to Duck Lake's northeastern shore; if you wish to have a shorter day, there are campsites 1.1 miles away on the flat-topped knobs just north of Pika Lake (10,537'; 37.55183°N 118.95517°W; no campfires).

Otherwise, follow the main tread high above Duck Lake's western shore, in early season hopefully noting the delightful clusters of magenta Sierra primroses. Slowly you descend, intersecting the shoreline just as you reach Duck Lake's outlet. Note that no camping is permitted within 300 feet of the outlet, although there are sites if you continue farther east. You cross the outlet on rock blocks and drop steeply alongside dark, glaciated metavolcanic bluffs and slabs and through lodgepole pine–forested corridors. The descent moderates as you approach the intersection with the JMT/PCT, 5.75 miles from the trailhead.

Heading right (west) here leads to an extremely popular camping area along Duck Lake's outlet creek, with pretty, albeit small and often crowded, sites (Trip 42). To continue on the described route, turn left (southeast) and climb out of the basin. Crossing back onto granitic substrate, you begin a waterless, sunstruck traverse high above Cascade Valley that offers astonishing views south to the Silver Divide and east to Mount Abbot on the Sierra Crest.

The trail eventually curves east into Purple Lake's valley and descends to a small junction (9,985'; 37.52898°N, 118.95031°W), where left (north) leads to Ram Lake and campsites along Purple Lake's west shore (for example, 9,970'; 37.53024°N, 118.94979°W; no campfires), while the JMT/PCT continues right (southeast), toward Purple Lake's outlet. Some of the previously popular campsites near this junction were obliterated by the gigantic 2011 Devils Windstorm, but those along Purple Lake's western shore are still mostly intact. A few more steps along the JMT/PCT leads to another junction, where you turn right (south) to descend to Fish Creek in Cascade Valley. There are several more campsites just as you begin your descent, but camping is prohibited within 300 feet of Purple Lake's outlet (9,938').

DAY 2 (Purple Lake to Iva Bell Hot Springs, 8.4 miles): Your 2.7-mile, 1,500-foot descent to Cascade Valley begins with a gradual drop along the northwest side of Purple Creek. For the first mile you are alternating between dry benches and more densely forested lodgepole pine flats, the latter with carpets of wandering fleabane and rings of alpine prickly currant encircling tree trunks. You occasionally pass tangles of downed trees, again dating to the 2011 windstorm. After about a mile, the trail steepens, becoming rockier and drier, and the trail embarks on switchbacks, sometimes under lodgepole pine cover and elsewhere between picturesque gnarled juniper and tall stately Jeffrey pine. Your views south to the Silver Divide and west down Cascade Valley are wonderful, especially of the myriad waterfalls pouring down the precipitous

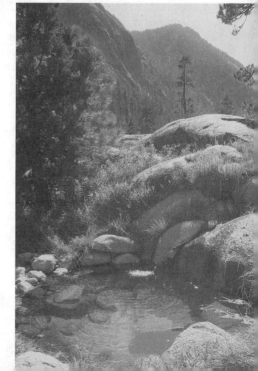

One of the pools at Iva Bell Hot Springs
Photo by Elizabeth Wenk

walls. The well-built trail maintains an almost constant grade, oblivious to the changing angle of the slope. Eventually your views are hidden by conifer cover and a long straight-away ends at a junction with the Cascade Valley Trail and Fish Creek (8,380'), where left (east) leads upstream back to the JMT/PCT corridor and you turn right (west) to descend Cascade Valley toward Iva Bell Hot Springs and Reds Meadow.

After just a few steps you pass a junction with a trail that departs left (south) to ford Fish Creek and ascend Minnow Creek to the shelf south of Cascade Valley (Trip 40); you continue straight, staying on the northeast side of Fish Creek. At the junction, there is a large campsite north of the trail. After traversing a lush lodgepole pine flat, the trail rounds a slab nose and drops more steeply beside some beautiful cascades; there is a perfect campsite atop the rocks before you descend. Soon you ford the Duck Lake outlet creek, often a wade (easy), and continue through valley-bottom forest. Between a pair of seasonal tributaries are more pictur-esque campsites among aspen groves, just downstream of some falls; the moniker "Cascade Valley" applies equally well to the water cascading over polished slabs along Fish Creek as it does to the valley-wall waterfalls. Continued pleasant forest walking eventually leads to Sec-ond Crossing, where you must ford Fish Creek; there are some acceptable campsites nearby. Fish Creek is now a major river, and this is a very difficult crossing in early summer; even in a below-average precipitation year the water levels can be thigh deep in late June. Fortunately, it is broad (i.e., less current) and you can place your feet in sandy spots between boulders.

A few minutes downstream, the river is suddenly pinched between two rock walls and tumbles spectacularly down its bedrock base. The trail winds beside it across broken slabs. You look north across the creek up slopes of dense brush, a monotonous carpet rising all the way to the JMT/PCT corridor. Soon a low gap on the ridge to the south lets you cross over to the Sharktooth Creek drainage; switchbacks first carry you up 150 feet and then back down 600 feet to the lush-green oasis that is Iva Bell Hot Springs.

The previous edition of this book recommended that you camp elsewhere, for this loca-tion is overused; indeed it is, but I can't imagine taking this loop with its prized destination of hot springs and not spending a night here. Instead, be considerate of other guests and ultraconscious of your environmental footprint, and absolutely only pick well-used tent sites on compacted bare soil, sand, and rock. There are many rock-lined pools to soak in, offering luxurious bathing at 100°F while imbibing the glorious views west down Fish Creek. And in early summer, enjoy the prolific giant helleborine, a very showy pink-orange orchid!

To reach the campsites and pools, it is best to leave the trail around 7,174 feet (37.53343°N, 119.02562°W) near the first large campsite you pass. Use trails then lead to many more campsites scattered along the northern periphery of the hot springs, some as far as 200 feet (elevation) upslope. There are also some incense cedar-shaded sites farther downstream and a few on the south side of the marshy expanse, closer to Sharktooth Creek.

CASCADE VALLEY SHELF

Hikers may want to add a few days onto this trip to explore the Minnow Creek area (described in Trip 40). Above and west of Cascade Valley is a broad shelf beneath the summits of the Silver Divide, referred to as the Cascade Valley shelf in this book. Once you've com-pleted the arduous 1,000-foot climb via either the Minnow Creek Trail or the trail ascending Sharktooth Creek, you have easy access to five separate lake basins nestled up to the Silver Divide. Peter Pande Lake is one of the largest and most scenic. Commandeer an old packer's camp in the valley, hide out in a gorgeous high country basin, or fish for legendary trout at Bench Lakes—Minnow Creek and the Cascade Valley shelf is a worthy detour.

DAY 3 (Iva Bell Hot Springs to Cold Creek, 6.9 miles): Leaving Iva Bell Hot Springs, regain the main trail and cross Sharktooth Creek on a log bridge. Just beyond, the route comes to an inconspicuously signed junction: left (south) leads up Sharktooth Creek to the Lost Keys Lakes and Minnow Creek (see the sidebar on page 260 and also Trip 40) and right (west) is the Fish Creek Trail to Fox Meadow and Reds Meadow; turn right. The first half of the 3.4-mile stretch to the Fox Meadow bridge is defined by disturbance. First you cross a series of avalanche zones, where nearly all the mature trees have been snapped off 6 feet above the ground, marking the depth of the snowpack when the avalanche tore downslope. Elsewhere are tangles of downed trees, with young saplings growing rapidly in their newfound sunlight. Meanwhile, the cliffs to the south are imposing, steep, and remarkably unfractured. With all these distractions, you barely notice Fish Creek merging down a narrow, incised gully from the north, except that suddenly the creek to your side is much larger. Nearby is a good campsite. Onward, the valley remains steep walled and confined, but you are increasingly walking beneath conifer shade on the very gradual descent.

As you approach Fox Meadow and the so-called Island Crossing, the trail bends left (south), skirting the massive lobe that is Fox Meadow. Long ago, the trail crossed at Island Crossing, on the meadow's eastern side, but now you continue farther west to a bridge. As the trail trends north again you pass a collection of large campsites pleasantly shaded by white fir and incense cedar, with easy access to Fish Creek (6,350'; 37.53381°N, 119.07312°W). If you dawdled away your morning at Iva Bell Hot Springs, you may want to spend the night here, for it is more than 2 steep miles to your next plausible campsite and farther still to choice ones. Moreover, the next ascent is most pleasant quite early or late in the day. Either way, fill up with water for the stiff climb ahead.

Nearby, an old trail ascends Silver Creek to the Margaret Lakes Basin—the junction has vanished, but the switchbacks upslope are impressively built and still remarkably intact. It is

Admire the magnificent junipers as you drop from Purple Lake to Fish Creek.   Photo by Elizabeth Wenk

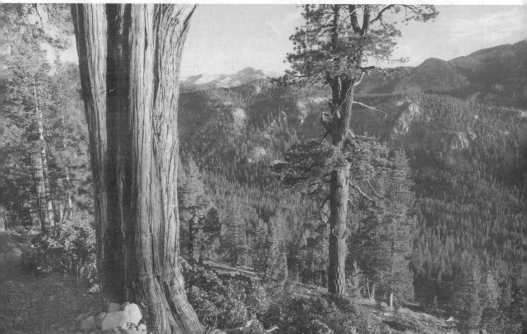

a beautiful route. Onward, you cross a bridge spanning Fish Creek (6,353') and begin your climb toward Reds Meadow.

The trail soon begins switchbacking steeply up the hot, exposed north slope of the canyon—watch for rattlesnakes as you take in expanding views up and down Fish Creek. The route levels off through a mixed forest, including scattered aspen, white fir, Jeffrey pine, and black oak. Rounding the broad county-line ridge, the trail turns north, and now you are looking west, down upon the Middle Fork San Joaquin River. Near here are flat areas where you could camp, provided springs just ahead are flowing. The trail then traverses the spring-irrigated slopes—a riot of color in early summer—and enters an open trough down which Cold Creek is channeled; just beyond the granite rib to the west is an abrupt drop to the valley floor. Tight switchbacks take you into a white fir glade where you cross Cold Creek on a flattened log; just beyond is a cluster of campsites (6,768'; 37.55527°N, 119.08894°W). The day's mileage is marked to here, although there are additional sites in another 0.9 mile.

DAY 4 (Cold Creek to Fish Creek Trailhead, 4.9 miles): Climbing just slightly, you cross expansive granite slabs that, just steps below the trail, angle steeply down to the Middle Fork San Joaquin. The views are fantastic—down into the river gorge and north to the Minarets. The slabs carry you to the Crater Creek drainage, just where it begins its downward plunge. Standing here, you see a series of granite ribs to the north, each constraining the course of a creek, beautifully illustrating how wide-scale fracture patterns create the fine-scale landscape features you experience on your walk. The trail curves northeast tracking Crater Creek's course; tempting broad, sandy, view-rich campsites sit atop the knob to the north, but you need to continue upstream to safely ford Crater Creek and backtrack to them. Onward, you reenter forest cover, cross a Crater Creek tributary on a two-log bridge, and traverse shallow granite slabs back into the Crater Creek drainage.

Soon you cross Crater Creek itself, again on a two-log bridge, and pass another pleasant sandy campsite, your last before the trailhead. You continue up the drainage on dry, sandy slopes, with a rounded granite crest to the west forcing Crater Creek to stay in this high-perched valley. At 2.5 miles from the trailhead, Crater Creek turns east—it is worth leaving the trail for a better look at the falls here—and the trail continues due north, climbing a handful of switchbacks. These carry you to a completely different landscape—the granite is now buried beneath more recent volcanic deposits and you are walking on dusty pumice. Moreover, the landscape was entirely charred by the 1992 lightning-caused Rainbow Fire. Even now, decades later, there are only occasional Jeffrey pine saplings emerging from the sea of mountain whitethorn, with a little fireweed adding color in the dampest places. This shadeless trudge leads to a junction with the spur, left (west), to Rainbow Falls, that leads an easy 0.2 mile to the upper Rainbow Falls overlook. It is well worth the detour to the 101-foot cascade if you haven't been here before.

Now joined by throngs of day-use hikers, you continue north on the ever-broader trail. After 0.15 mile, trend right, while left leads to Devils Postpile. Not long afterward, you finally exit the burned landscape and climb gently beneath scattered Jeffrey pine and white fir. In 0.3 mile you reach another junction, where left leads to the Fish Creek (Rainbow Falls) Trailhead, while right is to Reds Meadow. If you are taking the bus, either works and both destinations are an additional 0.4 mile. Heading to Reds Meadow has the benefit of their café and priority boarding of the buses, but left is the official route—and the only overnight parking. Staying left, you continue through open forest, shortly crossing the JMT/PCT and then reaching the trailhead (7,669'; 37.61397°N, 119.07664°W).

see map on p. 253

trip 44 Ram Lake and Lake Virginia

Trip Data: 37.59122°N, 118.98925°W (Ram Lake);
24.8 miles; 4/1 days
Topos: *Bloody Mountain*

HIGHLIGHTS: Spectacular subalpine terrain is the reward for venturing off the beaten path. This semi-loop takes you to Ram Lake and then onto Lake Virginia on the John Muir Trail (JMT)/Pacific Crest Trail (PCT) corridor via an easy cross-country route. Ram Lake is an infrequently visited spot in a lofty granite basin dotted with sparkling lakes and serene meadows. If you're a strong backpacker looking to explore off-trail, this trip is a good place to start, with just 2.2 cross-country miles.

HEADS UP! *The Duck Pass Trail isn't high, but it holds snow late and has steep drop-offs; check at the Mammoth Lakes ranger station before setting out. The journey from Ram Lake to Lake Virginia is cross-country; route-finding and map-and-compass skills are a must.*

DAY 1 (Duck Pass Trailhead to Pika Lake, 5.0 miles): Follow Trip 43's description 3.9 miles to the summit of Duck Pass. From the pass, enjoy the spectacular overlook of huge Duck Lake and its companion to the east, smaller Pika Lake. Just 250 feet later, take a spur trail left (east), descending steeply down the ruddy metamorphic slopes to Duck Lake's northeastern shore. Your clockwise route leads through marshy meadows and past a giant-boulder alcove that was once a miner's home to reach the creek connecting Duck and Pika Lakes. Ascending the stream corridor, you quickly reach Pika Lake (10,537'; 37.55183°N 118.95517°W) and good campsites sheltered by whitebark pine on flat-topped knobs just north of the lake. Both Pika and Duck Lakes harbor brook and rainbow trout.

DAY 2 (Pika Lake to Ram Lake, 7.8 miles): In the morning, return the 1.1 miles to the main trail below Duck Pass, turn left (south), and follow the tread high above Duck Lake's western shore, hopefully noting the delightful clusters of early season, magenta-hued Sierra primroses. Slowly you descend, intersecting the shoreline just as you reach Duck Lake's outlet. Note that no camping is permitted within 300 feet of the outlet, although there are sites if you continue farther east, an alternative Day 1 destination if you don't want to detour to Pika Lake. You cross the outlet on rock blocks and drop steeply alongside dark, glaciated metavolcanic bluffs and slabs and through lodgepole pine–forested corridors.

The descent moderates as you approach the intersection with the JMT/PCT. Heading right (west) leads to an extremely popular camping area along Duck Lake's outlet creek, with pretty, albeit small and often crowded, sites (Trip 42). To continue on the described route, turn left (southeast) and climb out of the basin. Crossing back onto granitic

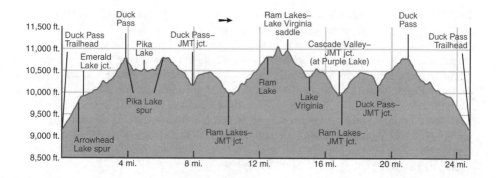

substrate, you begin a waterless sunstruck traverse high above Cascade Valley that offers astonishing views south to the Silver Divide and east to Mount Abbot on the Sierra Crest.

The trail eventually curves east into Purple Lake's valley and descends to a small junction (9,985'; 37.52898°N, 118.95031°W), where left (north) leads to Ram Lake and campsites along Purple Lake's west shore, while the JMT/PCT stays right (southeast), toward Purple Lake's outlet, your return route. Some of the previously popular campsites near this junction were obliterated by the gigantic 2011 Devils Windstorm, but those along Purple Lake's western shore are still mostly intact (9,970'; 37.53024 °N, 118.94979 °W; no campfires). Take the left fork around lovely Purple Lake, where fishing is fair to good for rainbow trout and occasional golden trout. Bearing little resemblance to the route depicted on old USGS 7.5' topos, the trail stays high above Purple Lake's partly timbered shore, crossing a broad-topped ridge, before dropping to the banks of Purple Creek beside a marshy meadow. Following the creek upstream, the river corridor is soon pinched between bluffs to the east and an imposing ridge to the west. Here the river laps at the giant talus fans that have spilled down from the crest separating Purple Creek from Duck and Pika Lakes' basin, and the trail crosses to more amicable terrain on the east bank.

Your ever-fainter trail recrosses the creek in a subalpine meadow and turns to the east. Climbing onward through meadows, up small knobs, and past tarns, you abruptly cross back onto granite. The trail continues along a grassy shelf north of the creek corridor until the landscape steepens and you are funneled up a channel beside the creek. You surmount a granite knob and reach rockbound Ram Lake (10,813'; 37.54423°N, 118.92826°W). Continuing clockwise around Ram Lake, you reach a broad granite-and-sand expanse just east of the lake, which offers spectacular, sparsely visited, sandy campsites near stunted whitebark pine (for example, near 10,790'; 37.54241°N, 118.92497°W; no campfires). From here, you can gaze down upon Ram Lake and its satellites, Horn Lake (also 10,813'; middle lake) and Hoof Lake (yet again 10,813'; farthest east), and up to the jagged Sierra Crest. Continuing farther up the drainage leads to a collection of small tarns and larger Franklin Lake, all offering fishing for golden trout.

GLEN AND GLENNETTE LAKES

If you prefer to visit just Glen and Glennette Lakes, both also with nice camping, although subtly less stunning scenery, and bypass the Ram Lakes altogether, take the following route: where the trail comes close to the river and you ascended the final slope to Ram Lake, you could instead trend due south to intersect the Glen Lake outlet creek and follow it upward over a small rise and past a tarn. Glen Lake (10,675'; 37.54149°N, 118.93124°W) beckons about a half mile beyond. Then walk uphill along the stream connecting the two lakes to find Glennette Lake (10,734').

DAY 3 (Ram Lake to Lake Virginia, 2.2 miles, cross-country): At Ram's southeast shore the trail vanishes, and your route to Lake Virginia is entirely off-trail. This day is a short 2.2 miles but can easily take several hours as you pick your way across the rugged landscape. Standing at the south side of Horn Lake, if you face due south, you'll be staring at a steep granite ridge, but turn your gaze a little to the left (east) and you'll notice a handy sandy ramp angling up the ridge. You need to aim for this ramp and ascend it to gain the ridge. Atop the ridge, just 0.3 mile into your day, you have a good view of what's ahead: nice and easy—albeit high-elevation—cross-country travel. You'll discover that your ramp, aligned with broad-scale fractures in the rock, continues down the south side of the ridge, and you descend easily over firm but rocky footing, aiming for the second lowest of the tarns above Glennette Lake (10,860'; 37.53571°N, 118.92474°W).

Continue cutting south, weaving between the tarns and shallow granite slabs, before cutting to the southwest, possibly picking up a faint use trail, and climbing a measly 120 feet to surmount the saddle separating the Glennette Lake basin from the Lake Virginia basin. Soon you're at the top, enjoying a breathtaking view of the distant Silver Divide peaks and Lake Virginia (10,980'; 37.53162°N, 118.92564°W; 0.9 mile from Ram Lake).

Down the south side, a sinuous corridor between taller bluffs leads to open meadow strips and a small lake, before you are again channeled between low, rounded granite ribs and past more lakelets. If you wish to avoid the crowds found at Lake Virginia, a popular campsite for JMT and PCT hikers, seek out a sandy nook along this descent. Your meandering path traverses low mounds of moraine sediments to reach Lake Virginia's north shore (and the JMT/PCT) (10,357'; 37.51578°N, 118.93491°W). There are many campsites to the northwest on a hill of moraine sediments (for example, 10,372'; 37.51624°N, 118.93546°W; no campfires) and to the southwest at the forest edge; just ensure you do not camp on the fragile meadow turf surrounding the lake.

DAY 4 (Lake Virginia to Duck Pass Trailhead, 9.8 miles): Following the JMT/PCT, you head northwest, climbing up a sandy slope to a fantastic saddle tucked between two steep ridges. To your south, monstrous piles of talus spill across the landscape. This is a rock glacier—there is ice at the center of the rock pile and, just like a glacier, it moves slowly downslope, occasionally dropping boulders down its over-steepened front. You traverse past it on a pleasant sandy tread and then begin a switchbacking descent back into Purple Lake's basin. As you round the south side of the lake, you cross the outlet on a stout bridge, pass a junction with the trail to Cascade Valley (Trip 43), and close your hiking loop at the spur leading to Ram Lake. From here, retrace your steps, skipping the detour to Pika Lake.

Duck Lake   Photo by Elizabeth Wenk

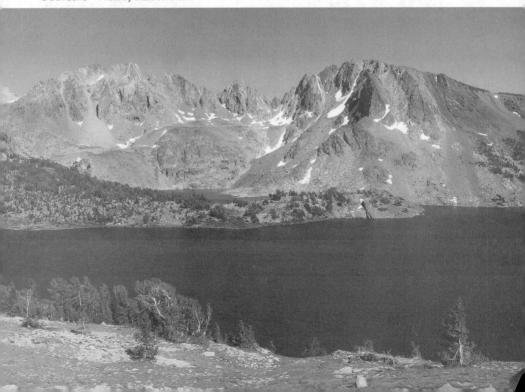

McGEE CREEK ROAD TRIPS

McGee Creek Road accesses one of the eastern Sierra canyons just south of the Mammoth Lakes region. McGee Creek Canyon, like the Convict Creek drainage just to the north, showcases predominately metamorphic rocks, making for colorful valley walls. The narrow, winding McGee Creek Canyon leads to McGee Pass and across to the Fish Creek drainage, where it meets the John Muir Trail (JMT). Relatively straightforward off-trail travel south across the Sierra Crest and Silver Divide allows for some splendid part cross-country trips from here.

Trailhead: McGee Creek

On the west side of McGee Pass above Tully Lake (Trip 48, page 278)   Photo by Elizabeth Wenk

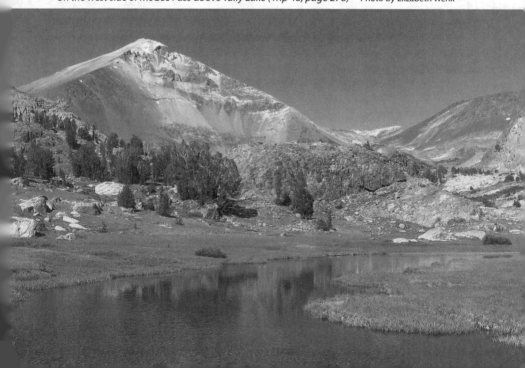

McGee Creek Trailhead
7,872'; 37.55102°N, 118.80254°W

Destination/ GPS Coordinates	Trip Type	Best Season	Pace & Hiking/ Layover Days	Total Mileage	Permit Required
45 Steelhead Lake 37.49978°N 118.81238°W	Out-and-back	Mid to late	Leisurely 2/1	11.6	McGee Pass
46 Pioneer Basin 37.47172°N 118.80347°W	Semiloop	Late	Strenuous, part cross-country 5/1	27.0	McGee Pass
47 Big McGee Lake 37.48851°N 118.84362°W	Out-and-back	Mid to late	Leisurely 2/1	15.0	McGee Pass
48 Rock Creek via the Silver Divide 37.46853°N 118.85401°W (Grinnell Lake)	Shuttle	Mid to late	Strenuous, part cross-country 5/2	31.7	McGee Pass (*Mono Pass in reverse*)

INFORMATION AND PERMITS: This trailhead is in Inyo National Forest. Permits are required for overnight stays and quotas apply. Permits can be reserved up to six months in advance at recreation.gov (60%; $6 permit reservation fee plus $5 per person) or requested in person, first come, first served, a day in advance (40%; free). All permits must be picked up at one of the Inyo National Forest ranger stations, located in Lone Pine (Eastern Sierra Interagency Visitor Center), Bishop, Mammoth Lakes, and Lee Vining (the Mono Basin Scenic Area Visitor Center). If you plan to use a stove or have a campfire, you must also have a California campfire permit, available from a forest service office or online at preventwildfireca.org/campfire-permit. Campfires are prohibited throughout McGee Creek. Bear canisters are strongly recommended in the McGee Creek drainage but required in the Rock Creek area (Trip 48's endpoint).

DRIVING DIRECTIONS: From US 395, 32 miles north of Bishop or 8 miles south of the Mammoth Lakes junction, turn southwest onto McGee Creek Road. Follow the paved road across Crowley Lake Drive, past McGee Creek Campground, and continue on dirt surface past McGee Creek Pack Station to a paved parking loop at the road's end, 3.3 miles from US 395. The trailhead is equipped with vault toilet and horse-loading facilities.

trip 45   ## Steelhead Lake

see map on p. 268

Trip Data: 37.49978°N, 118.81238°W; 11.6 miles; 2/1 days
Topos: *Convict Lake, Mount Abbot*

HIGHLIGHTS: Travelers new to entering the Sierra from its eastern escarpment will discover that the ascent of McGee Creek is fascinating because of the swirling patterns in the highly fractured, red, metamorphic rocks of the canyon wall. An early start is good, as the first few miles' travel up a narrow, essentially shadeless canyon that can be stiflingly hot in the middle of the day. The scenic lakeshore offers splendid campsites and excellent fishing.

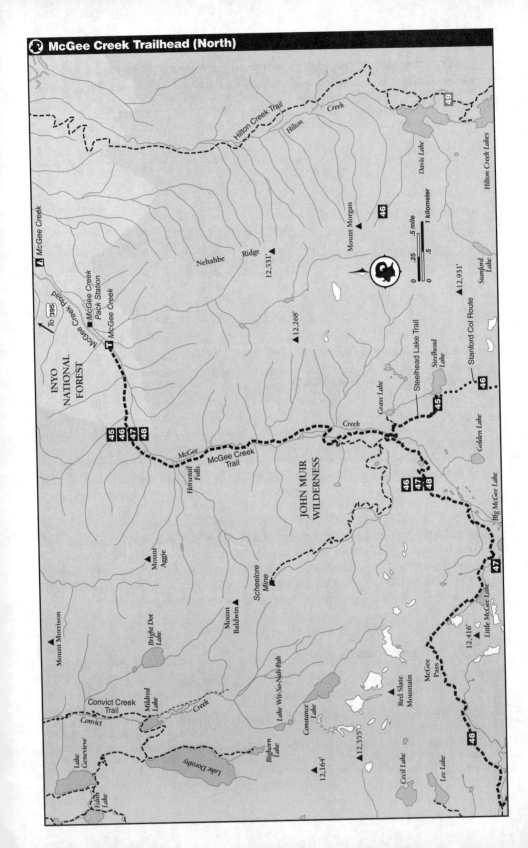

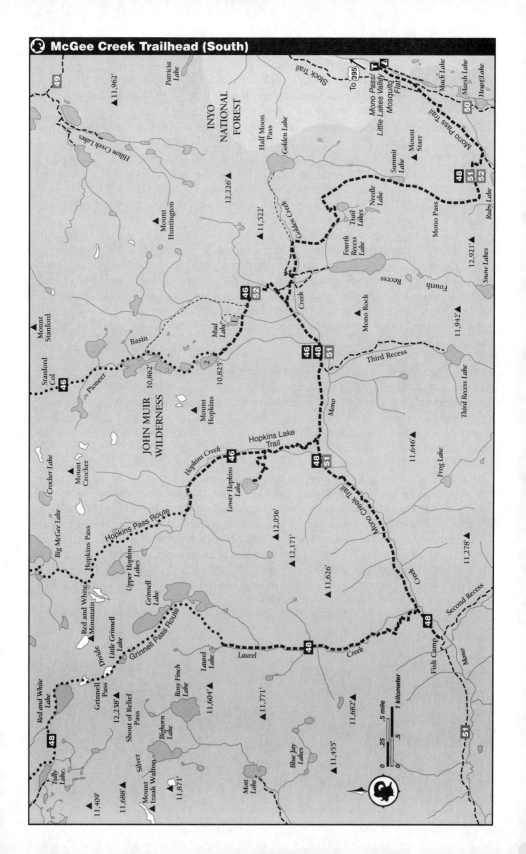

INYO
NATIONAL
FOREST

JOHN MUIR
WILDERNESS

49

50

48
51
52

46
52

46
48
51

46
48
51

48
51

48

43

51

48

Patricia
Lake

▲ 11,962'

Hilton Creek Lakes

Mount
Huntington

12,226' ▲

▲ 11,522'

Half Moon
Pass

Golden Lake

Golden Creek

Fourth
Recess
Lake

Trail
Lakes

Needle
Lake

Summit
Lake

Mount
Starr ▲

Mono Pass

Stock Trail

To 395

Mono Pass/
Little Lakes Valley

Mosquito
Flat

Mono Pass Trail

Mack Lake

Marsh Lake

Heart Lake

Ruby Lake

12,921' ▲

Snow Lakes

11,942' ▲

Fourth Recess

Mono Rock

Third Recess

Third Recess Lake

Mono

Creek

Mount
Stanford ▲

Stanford
Col

Pioneer

Basin

Mud
Lake

10,862'

2

10,825'

Mount
Hopkins ▲

Hopkins Lake
Trail

Hopkins Creek

Lower Hopkins
Lake

▲ 12,056'

▲ 12,171'

▲ 11,626'

11,646' ▲

Frog Lake

11,278' ▲

Mono Creek Trail

Crocker Lake

Mount
Crocker ▲

Big McGee Lake

Hopkins Pass

Hopkins Pass Route

Upper Hopkins
Lakes

Red and White
Mountain ▲

Divide

Grinnell
Lake

Little Grinnell
Lake

Grinnell Pass Route

Laurel
Lake

Laurel

Creek

Fish Camp

Second Recess

Mono

Red and White
Lake

Grinnell
Pass

12,238' ▲

Shout of Relief
Pass

Rosy Finch
Lake

11,604' ▲

▲ 11,771'

▲ 11,682'

▲ 11,455'

Mott
Lake

Blue Jay
Lakes

Tully
Lake

11,409'

11,688' ▲

Mount
Izaak Walton ▲

11,871'

Silver

Bighorn
Lake

0   .25   .5
0   .5   1 kilometer
.5 mile

HEADS UP! *Although Upper McGee Creek Campground doesn't exist anymore, the old access road is now one of the two trails leaving the parking lot—in this case, the wide track that stays near the creek. Don't take it. The trail you need is the dusty, narrower one to the right of the wider track; it heads up the chaparral-clad slopes and is soon well above the creek.*

DAY 1 (McGee Creek Trailhead to Steelhead Lake, 5.8 miles): Leave the parking area near the restrooms and the trailhead signboard; take the narrower, dusty footpath that heads up chaparral-clad slopes and west into McGee Creek's canyon. Ahead to the west, the multi-colored, contorted rock layers composing the canyon walls contrast pleasantly with the open, shrub-covered moraine sediments the trail traverses.

A gradual-to-moderate ascent leads to a crossing of a thin stream trickling downhill from Buzztail Spring and then shortly to the signed John Muir Wilderness boundary. Beyond here, the trail curves slowly southward and proceeds deeper into the gorge of McGee Creek, with improving views of Horsetail Falls spilling down the west wall of the canyon. Seasonal flowers can be spectacular along this stretch in early season. Presently, the trail curves south, and the views are temporarily obscured by a lengthy grove of aspen. Amid the aspen, cross a pair of close streams that overflow the trail, the second of which carries water from the falls.

Eventually, the aspen are left behind, allowing for fine views up the canyon on the way to a ford of McGee Creek. An old section of trail continues up the west bank of the creek for a bit to a stout old bridge that was destroyed in a flood (one wonders how logs of this size were transported this far into the wilderness without mechanized support), replaced, and subsequently damaged again, but is still just usable. The shadeless trail continues along the east side of the creek, climbing to a shelf above a beautiful meadow, where, thanks to some industrious beavers, the stream meanders in sensuous curves.

Another length along a dry, scrubby slope leads to a second bridge, thankfully intact, for a ford here would be tricky. Beyond, the trail curves around a large outcrop past a pair of lodgepole-shaded campsites and passes an obscure junction with an old mining road leading to the Scheelore Mine, the ore from which was used to make tungsten during World War II. The initial stretch of the trail to the mine doubles as a stock route to the McGee Creek Trail for the numerous pack trains that frequent the canyon. Today, only a few mountaineers follow this trail beyond the stock route for access to the south ridge of Mount Baldwin.

Following a sign for McGee Pass, you turn left (southeast) at the junction, cross a tributary on a wood-plank bridge, and proceed through shady forest up the main fork of McGee Creek to a Y-junction, 4.6 miles from the trailhead.

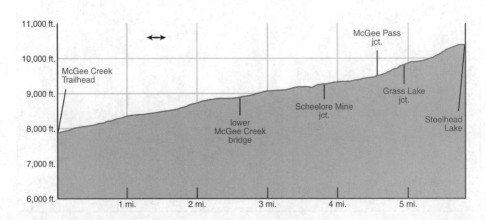

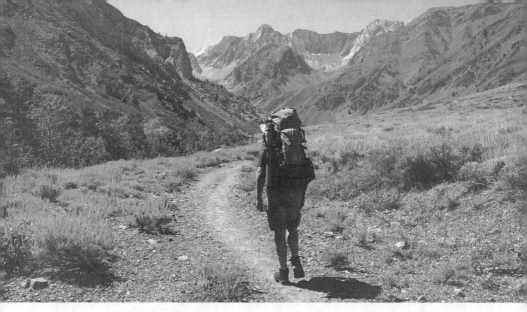

The McGee Creek Trail has little shade in the first few miles, so it's best to start early. Photo by Mike White

At the junction, turn left (south) and ford McGee Creek (difficult in early season) before starting a steep, switchbacking, 460-foot climb up the east wall of the canyon to a junction with the half-mile trail to Grass Lake (9,826'; campsites). Bear right (east-southeast) here on a brief climb, follow and then cross a small brook, wind uphill to where the terrain eases near a couple of tarns, and then descend past good campsites to the northwest shore of picturesque 25-acre Steelhead Lake (10,380'). Look for the best campsites atop the small peninsula above the southwest side of the lake (10,404'; 37.49852°N, 118.81094°W; no campfires).

> **AT STEELHEAD LAKE**
> Views from the lakeshore take in the granite grandeur of Mount Stanford and Mount Crocker to the south and west, and rust-and-buff-colored Mount Baldwin in the north. Anglers will find the fishing for rainbow and brook trout excellent (best in early and late season). The name "Steelhead" is certainly a misnomer for this lake, as the term refers to ocean-going trout. The mistake may be somewhat understandable, as, over the years, rainbow trout from the lake have exhibited pale and faded markings similar in appearance to their silver cousins of coastal waters.

DAY 2 (Steelhead Lake to McGee Creek Trailhead, 5.8 miles): Retrace your steps.

see maps on p. 268– 269

trip 46 **Pioneer Basin**

> **Trip Data:** 37.47172°N, 118.80347°W; 27.0 miles; 5/1 days
> **Topos:** *Convict Lake, Mount Abbot*

HIGHLIGHTS: Pioneer Basin, holding a string of lakes surrounded by alpine meadows and ringed by gray granite peaks, is one of the most scenic spots in the central Sierra. From the basin, visitors have sweeping views across the deep cleft of Mono Creek into the Mono Recesses and to high peaks along the Mono Divide. Backpackers will also sample a stretch of forested Mono Creek, an ascent up the lush canyon of Hopkins Creek, and picturesque Big McGee Lake along this semiloop. This rugged route utilizes two difficult, cross-country crossings of the Sierra Crest: Stanford Col, above Steelhead Lake on the way into the basin, and Hopkins Pass, above Big McGee Lake, on the return to the McGee Creek Trail.

HEADS UP! *Although Upper McGee Creek Campground doesn't exist anymore, the old access road is now one of the two trails leaving the parking lot—in this case, the wide track that stays near the creek. Don't take it. The trail you need is the dusty, narrower one to the right of the wider track; it heads up the chaparral-clad slopes and is soon well above the creek.*

The difficult cross-country sections along this route, especially the climb over talus, loose rock, and scree from Steelhead Lake to Stanford Col, make this a trip for experienced mountaineers only. To take a much easier route to Pioneer Basin, take Trip 52 instead.

DAY 1 (McGee Creek Trailhead to Steelhead Lake, 5.8 miles): Follow Trip 45, Day 1 to Steelhead Lake (10,404'; 37.49852°N, 118.81094°W; no campfires).

DAY 2 (Steelhead Lake to Pioneer Basin, 2.3 miles, cross-country): From the southwest shore of serene Steelhead Lake, head south to ascend the steep and rocky slope just above the lake to gain the more moderately sloping talus field below Stanford Col, the obvious low point at the head of the canyon that becomes visible after the initial climb. Carefully negotiate your way up the talus slope over large, blocky boulders—a climb made perhaps less difficult if solid snowfields allow travel above the jumbled rocks. Without snow, the best way across is to follow the crests of the elongate moraine ribs, where there is slightly more soil formation to hold the boulders in place.

Upon reaching the base of the final slope, a steep, loose collection of scree and rock begins a very steep climb generally south toward the col. Make sure everyone in your party is out of each other's fall line to avoid getting knocked in the head by a stray projectile. A faint use trail exists on a rib just left (east) of the gully. After the 400-foot climb, more secure footing is gained at the col (11,611'; 37.48692°N, 118.80946°W), where an impressive view sweeps across Pioneer Basin toward the rugged peaks of the Mono Divide, a superlative vista that makes the steep and tedious climb seem worthwhile. The view to the north of McGee Creek's multicolored canyon is stunning as well.

With the most difficult part of the entire trip completed, leave the col and easily drop southward down scree slopes toward the upper part of Pioneer Basin. Following the short descent, head generally south cross-country over sandy soil sprinkled with boulders and tiny alpine plants toward Lake 10,862, the largest of the Pioneer Basin Lakes. Along the

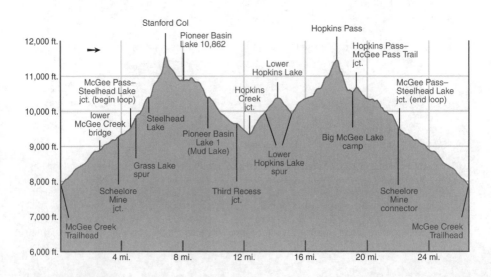

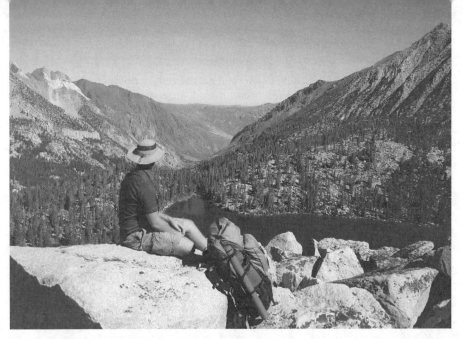

Gazing down McGee Creek Canyon from the route to Stanford Col   Photo by Mike White

way, come alongside and then follow the main branch of the flower-and-meadow-lined creek that drains the basin to the northeast shore of the long, irregularly shaped lake (10,862'). A few windy campsites bordered by dwarf whitebark pines pepper the knoll above the east shore.

Better campsites can be found near the south end of the lake (for example, 10,886'; 37.47172°N, 118.80347°W; no campfires) and around Lake 11,026, but you're more likely to see other backpackers there (along with groups from pack trains) who have accessed the basin via maintained trail over Mono Pass. Pioneer Basin is a fine place to spend additional days exploring the nooks and crannies of the area on easy cross-country romps, or to simply relax and enjoy the panoramic scenery. Although the lakes seem to hold a healthy population of brook and rainbow trout, for some reason, fishing reports seem to be disappointing.

DAY 3 (Pioneer Basin to Lower Hopkins Lake, 6.5 miles): From Lake 10,862, follow a use trail generally south along the lakes on the basin's west side. Ignore a well-trod use trail from Lake 10,862's southeastern peninsula to the basin's east side.

From the southeast shore of the southwesternmost large lake in Pioneer Basin (the almost bathtub-shaped one a little southeast of Mount Hopkins's peak at 10,825'; 37.46046°N, 118.80301°W; also known as Lake 2), maintained trail leaves the idyllic upper basin and drops moderately to steeply away from the lakes into a scattered-to-light forest of lodgepole pines. The rate of descent eases where the trail traverses an open flat harboring the lowest lake, a shallow lake called Mud Lake, and then fords Mud Lake's outlet. Across this flat are good views of the massive hulk of towering Mono Rock and the deep cleft of Fourth Recess.

Heading back into the trees, the descent toward Mono Creek resumes across hillsides carpeted with lush foliage. Approaching the floor of the canyon, step across a brook and head downstream to an unsigned junction with twin laterals to the Mono Creek Trail, one on the left for eastbound hikers and one on the right for westbound hikers. Go right (southwest) and follow the lateral a short distance to an unsigned junction with the Mono Creek Trail (9,913'; 37.44891°N, 118.79260°W).

Turn right (west) at the junction, following the dusty and sometimes rocky Mono Creek Trail through lodgepole pine forest adorned with a lush understory of plants and wildflowers. Make three close crossings of the same tributary stream and continue downstream along Mono Creek on gradually graded trail, hopping across the two streams draining Pioneer Basin and passing Mono Rock on the opposite side of the canyon. Several campsites are spread across the canyon floor, some of which can't be clearly seen from the trail (the ones that can be seen are often within 100 feet of the trail or Mono Creek and are therefore illegal).

Pass by a use trail to a packer's camp and break out of the forest into an open meadow where an unsigned trail heads south across the creek and into Third Recess. Continue downstream on the main trail, generally west, through alternating stands of trees and clearings to a signed Y-junction with the Hopkins Creek Trail.

Turn right (north) to leave the Mono Creek Trail and begin a moderately steep, zigzagging climb up the north wall of the canyon across boulder-studded slopes beneath lodgepole pines to the right of Hopkins Creek. At the top of the switchbacks, climb more moderately through luxuriant vegetation to a ford of the creek and then immediately reach a junction with the trail to Lower Hopkins Lake, a mile from the Mono Creek Trail junction.

Go left (west) at the junction and climb steeply on the winding trail to Lower Hopkins Lake. Eventually, the grade eases, and a short stroll leads past decent campsites to the roughly oval lake (10,367'; 37.45427°N, 118.82686°W; no campfires). A strip of meadow and a smattering of lodgepole pines surround the quiet lake, which has a rugged backdrop of steep granite cliffs. Rainbow and brook trout will tempt anglers.

DAY 4 (Lower Hopkins Lake to Big McGee Lake, 4.9 miles, part cross-country): Retrace your steps to the junction with the Hopkins Creek Trail, turn left (north), and then resume the moderate ascent up the canyon through thickly vegetated meadowlands and scattered

One of the many lakes in Pioneer Basin   Photo by Mike White lodgepole pines. The grade eases as the trail enters a long, flower-filled meadow with views up the canyon toward aptly named Red and White Mountain.

> **MEADOW RUTS**
>
> As these roughly parallel ruts get deeper with repeated use, they fill with water, and then hikers create an adjacent path on higher soil that, over time, will suffer the same fate. Continuing across the meadow, notice several areas where three or more paths have been created by this unfortunate dilemma. This trail desperately needs to be rerouted to higher ground, but a path like the little-used Hopkins Creek Trail is generally a low priority on the U.S. Forest Service's project list.

The tread progressively deteriorates across this meadow, revealing badly constructed sections of trail through soggy areas, which has resulted in parallel ruts in the soil.

Farther up the meadow, the tread periodically disappears, but ducks should help lead the way generally north-northwest toward trailless Hopkins Pass; this route doesn't go to the Upper Hopkins Lakes.

> **UPPER HOPKINS LAKES**
>
> If Upper Hopkins Lakes are the goal, eventually you will have to leave the ducked trail and head west on a faint use trail, or simply strike off cross-country to access these scenic gems. Campsites at the lower lake appear to be more hospitable than ones at the windswept upper lake.

Today's ducked route bypasses the upper lakes and heads straight for Hopkins Pass, going higher into the alpine zone on the way toward the head of the canyon. As the slope becomes rocky and dotted with small, ground-hugging plants, the tread and the ducks completely vanish, but the way to the low point of the broad pass is obvious.

First-timers may reach the edge of Hopkins Pass (11,465'; 37.48003°N, 118.84475°W) and determine there is absolutely no safe way down the far side, where the steep terrain drops precipitously 800 vertical feet to the upper part of McGee Creek's canyon. Fortunately, a large cairn on top of a boulder marks the beginning of a use trail down this slope. Before starting the descent, be sure to take in the colorful view down McGee Creek's canyon out to the White Mountains, and behind Hopkins Creek's canyon.

Exercising extreme caution, follow the use trail generally northwest away from Hopkins Pass on a dicey descent across steep, rocky slopes. Initially, there is no single, defined trail, so you'll have to choose the most suitable path for a secure descent—the set of wider switchbacks appears to be a better choice, as opposed to the short set of switchbacks that zigzag tightly straight down the slope. Eventually, the route becomes less traumatic on the way to a crossing of the outlet that drains the tarn at the head of the canyon. After crossing this outlet, the route continues the descent above the west side of the cascading stream, with picturesque views of the multicolored peaks and ridges making up the upper part of McGee Creek's canyon, as well as the striking waterfall exiting Little McGee Lake. With the drop in elevation, grasses, sedges, clumps of willow, and colorful wildflowers begin to appear, a cheerful sight after the bleak and rocky surroundings above.

Dwarf whitebark pines herald the approach to a bench above Big McGee Lake, which sits in a bowl composed of steep cliffs and high-angle slopes. There are good campsites on top of a cliff on the peninsula on the lake's west side (10,563'; 37.48851°N, 118.84362°W; no campfires). Although widely scattered whitebark pines and mountain hemlocks offer little protection from the wind, these campsites do offer outstanding views of the lake and the upper part of the canyon. Despite limited access to the shoreline, anglers enjoy good fishing for both rainbow and brook trout. Also, there are fair-to-poor campsites on the peninsula that juts southward from the lake's north side; these sites are very popular with those who've come to Big McGee Lake directly from the trailhead on the main McGee Creek Trail.

DAY 5 (Big McGee Lake to McGee Creek Trailhead, 7.5 miles): Pick up a use trail in the vicinity of the peninsula and proceed north through meadowlands up toward the well-defined tread of the McGee Creek Trail. Turn right (east) and follow the trail across a talus slope well above Big McGee Lake before dropping past use trails to the poor-to-fair campsites on the northside peninsula, and then to an area of meadows and slabs just below the lake, where decent campsites are spread along the banks of the outlet.

Hop across a pretty rivulet and descend away from the lake and down the canyon, passing through alternating sections of lodgepole pine forest and verdant, meadow-covered benches. Drop more steeply to a forested junction with an unmaintained trail to Golden Lake and continue a short distance to a small pond just off the trail, known locally as Round Lake, where needy campers could find fair, overused campsites south of the pond.

Proceed on a stiff, switchbacking descent through granite cliffs shaded by hemlocks on a well-engineered section of trail incorporating several granite stairs. The roar of McGee Creek becomes louder on the way to a creekside junction with the Steelhead Lake Trail at the close of the loop. Partway down, a use trail on the left leads west to a packer campsite.

At the junction with the Steelhead Lake Trail, turn left (north, downstream) and retrace Day 1's steps 4.6 miles to the trailhead.

---

trip 47 **Big McGee Lake**

see map on p. 268

> **Trip Data:** 37.48851°N, 118.84362°W; 15.0 miles; 2/1 days
> **Topos:** *Convict Lake, Mount Abbot*

HIGHLIGHTS: In an alpine setting close under the Sierra Crest, Big McGee Lake shares a large granite basin with three other fishable lakes. This beautiful spot nestles below the sheer, colorful walls of 12,816-foot Red and White Mountain, and close to impressive 12,458-foot Mount Crocker.

HEADS UP! *Although Upper McGee Creek Campground doesn't exist anymore, the old access road is now one of the two trails leaving the parking lot—in this case, the wide track that stays near the creek. Don't take it. The trail you need is the dusty, narrower one to the right of the wider track; it heads up the chaparral-clad slopes and is soon well above the creek.*

DAY 1 (McGee Creek Trailhead to Big McGee Lake, 7.5 miles): Leave the parking area near the restrooms and the trailhead signboard; take the narrower, dusty footpath that heads up chaparral-clad slopes and west into McGee Creek's canyon. Ahead to the west, the multicolored, contorted rock layers composing the canyon walls contrast pleasantly with the open, shrub-covered moraine sediments the trail traverses.

A gradual-to-moderate ascent leads to a crossing of a thin stream trickling downhill from Buzztail Spring and then shortly to the signed John Muir Wilderness boundary. Beyond here, the trail curves slowly southward and proceeds deeper into the gorge of McGee Creek, with improving views of Horsetail Falls spilling down the west wall of the canyon. Seasonal flowers can be spectacular along this stretch in early season. Presently, the trail curves south, and the views are temporarily obscured by a lengthy grove of aspen.

Amid the aspen, cross a pair of close streams that overflow the trail, the second of which carries water from the falls.

Eventually, the aspen are left behind, allowing for fine views up the canyon on the way to a ford of McGee Creek. An old section of trail continues up the west bank of the creek for a bit to a stout old bridge that was destroyed in a flood (one wonders how logs of this size were transported this far into the wilderness without mechanized support), replaced, and subsequently damaged again, but is still just usable. The shadeless trail continues along the east side of the creek, climbing to a shelf above a beautiful meadow, where, thanks to some industrious beavers, the stream meanders in sensuous curves.

Another length along a dry, scrubby slope leads to a second bridge, thankfully intact, for a ford here would be tricky. Beyond, the trail curves around a large outcrop past a pair of lodgepole-shaded campsites and passes an obscure junction with an old mining road leading to the Scheelore Mine, the ore from which was used to make tungsten during World War II. The initial stretch of the trail to the mine doubles as a stock route to the McGee Creek Trail for the numerous pack trains that frequent the canyon. Today, only a few mountaineers follow this trail beyond the stock route for access to the south ridge of Mount Baldwin.

Following a sign for McGee Pass, you turn left (southeast) at the junction, cross a tributary on a wood-plank bridge, and proceed through shady forest up the main fork of McGee Creek to a Y-junction, 4.6 miles from the trailhead.

At this junction turn right (southwest), climbing 250 feet to a second junction where the stock trail that split off earlier rejoins the main trail from the right (north). Again stay left (southwest) and begin a moderate ascent that climbs about 450 vertical feet on numerous, short, rocky, hemlock-shaded switchbacks along granite cliffs. As you climb, 12,838-foot Mount Stanford springs into view. Upon reaching the top of the switchbacks, the trail dips into a damp, forested hollow and arrives near a pond, known locally as Round Lake. Fair, overused campsites lie just south of this pond.

Beyond Round Lake, veer north past a verdant meadow and start a switchbacking climb to a series of meadow-covered benches that may become dry by late season and that offer surprisingly few campsites—practically none. The grade eases on these benches, where the trail carefully skirts the flowery meadows.

Reach an area of meadows and slabs below the north end of Big McGee Lake, where several campsites are spread along the banks of the creek. Just beyond and above the lake, use trails lead to fair, but very popular, campsites on the peninsula on Big McGee's north shore.

Above this area, the trail climbs across a lightly forested talus slope to more meadowlands on a bench above McGee Lake's northwest corner. Here a use trail splits away to the left (south; 10,683'; 37.49116°N, 118.84347°W) and accesses good campsites above a cliff on the peninsula that juts into the southwest side of Big McGee Lake (10,563'; 37.48851°N, 118.84362°W; no

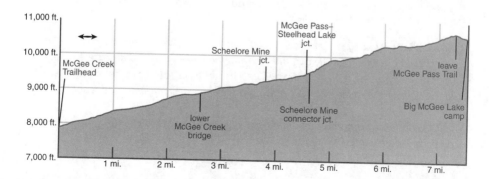

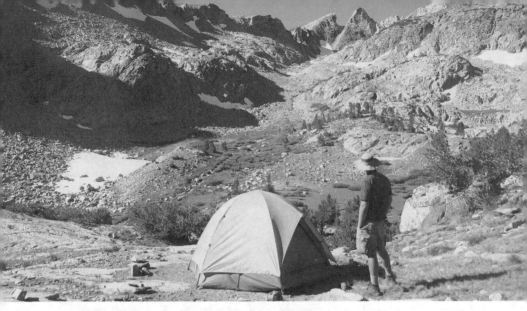

View toward Hopkins Pass from Big McGee Lake   Photo by Mike White

campfires). Although the sparse whitebark pines and mountain hemlocks provide these campsites with little protection from the wind, the view of the aquamarine lake and the upper part of the canyon should more than make up for the potentially breezy conditions.

> **AT BIG MCGEE LAKE**
>
> Although access to the shoreline is somewhat limited by the steep topography around much of the lake, anglers should enjoy good fishing for rainbow and brook trout. If time and inclination allow, anglers can explore the equally attractive fishing at Little McGee Lake (rockbound and campsiteless), Crocker Lake, or picture-book Golden Lake.

DAY 2 (Big McGee Lake to McGee Creek Trailhead, 7.5 miles): Retrace your steps.

see maps on p. 268–269

trip 48   ## Rock Creek via the Silver Divide

> **Trip Data:** 37.46853°N, 118.85401°W (Grinnell Lake); 31.7 miles; 5/2 days
> **Topos:** *Convict Lake, Mount Abbot, Graveyard Peak, Mount Morgan*

HIGHLIGHTS: This rugged route offers excitement and challenge sufficient to satisfy the most jaded appetite. High-country lakes surrounded by rampart-like peaks characterize this colorful route, and the fishing should be good to excellent.

HEADS UP! *Although Upper McGee Creek Campground doesn't exist anymore, the old access road is now one of the two trails leaving the parking lot—in this case, the wide track that stays near the creek. Don't take it. The trail you need is the dusty, narrower one to the right of the wider track; it heads up the chaparral-clad slopes and is soon well above the creek.*

This trip is for experienced mountaineers only. If you're not, trips out of Rock Creek proper are more suitable (Trips 50 and 52).

SHUTTLE DIRECTIONS: From US 395, 25 miles north of Bishop or 15 miles south of the Mammoth Lakes junction with CA 203, turn west on Rock Creek Road at the small community of Tom's Place. Cross Crowley Lake Drive and follow the road past Rock Creek Lake 10.7 miles from US 395. Continue to the Mosquito Flat Trailhead at the end of the road (vault toilets). The road becomes very winding and narrow beyond the Hilton Lakes Trailhead; be prepared to yield to oncoming traffic. There is a small backpackers' campground across bridged Rock Creek from the parking lot, available only for one night before the start of your trip. You must show a valid wilderness permit from the Mosquito Flat Trailhead to demonstrate your eligibility for a campsite.

DAY 1 (McGee Creek Trailhead to Big McGee Lake, 7.5 miles): Follow Trip 47, Day 1 to Big McGee Lake (10,563'; 37.48851°N, 118.84362°W; no campfires).

DAY 2 (Big McGee Lake to Tully Lake, 5.2 miles): Regain the main trail and turn west. From Big McGee Lake, follow the trail across steep meadows, pass above timberline on an exposed climb, and hop across a stream that drains the slopes below Corridor Pass, a pass to the north that leads into the Convict Creek drainage. Pass above Little McGee Lake (rockbound and virtually campsiteless), and then climb steeply up the narrow canyon of the lake's inlet. Continue the ascent with the aid of an occasional switchback up the canyon through broken reddish rock toward 11,909-foot McGee Pass; snow may linger here until late season. Views from the pass across the headwaters of Fish Creek to the Silver Divide are breathtaking.

From the pass, a long, rocky, switchbacking descent ensues, leading nearly 1,000 vertical feet down austere slopes to a large, lovely, meadow-floored basin at the headwaters of Fish Creek. The trail makes a gentle descent on a traverse of this basin, hopping across several seasonal rivulets along the way. Drop past a charming cascade; just beyond, the trail switchbacks distinctly to the right (west) (10,470'; 37.48998°N, 118.88521°W). A use trail departs left (southeast) from here to reach Tully Lake's north shore.

> **FISH CREEK ANGLING**
> Anglers should expect fair-to-good fishing for golden and brook trout. The headwaters of Fish Creek offer many other lakes, meadows, and creeks suitable for layover-day visits. Visitors may wish to try the waters of Red and White Lake, about a mile away over a ridge to the east, with fair-to-good fishing for rainbow trout. Those seeking stream fishing may find smaller rainbow, brook, and some golden trout along meandering Fish Creek.

Turn left (southeast) away from McGee Pass Trail and follow the use trail to the north shore of 10-acre Tully Lake (10,514'; 37.48880°N, 118.88359°W; no campfires). Good campsites may be found in the trees above the lake.

DAY 3 (Tully Lake to Grinnell Lake, 3.0 miles, cross-country): From the east shore of Tully Lake, the route ascends the grassy swale that lies due east of the lake. Upon reaching the outlet from Red and White Lake, the route turns right (southeast) and follows this stream to that lake (large rainbow). Although good campsites are virtually nonexistent, Red and White Lake offers an excellent vantage point from which to enjoy the spectacular and aptly named heights of Red and White Mountain. The saddle, called Grinnell Pass (or Pace Col), is the high point of today's journey and is clearly visible as the low point on the peak's right (west) shoulder. The easiest route to the saddle follows the rocky east shore around the lake. The steepest part of the ascent is over treacherous shale (or snowfields in early to midseason); travelers should proceed slowly and carefully. Carry a rope and use it when necessary, especially when ascending the west side of the pass.

GRINNELL PASS VIEWS

From Grinnell Pass (11,624'; 37.47983°N, 118.86549°W), enjoy a well-deserved and stimulating view of the surrounding terrain. To the north, the immediate, dazzling blue waters of Red and White Lake set off the buff browns and ochre reds of the surrounding rock. Beyond this basin, the meadow-filled cirque forming the headwaters of Fish Creek is a large greensward that contrasts sharply with the austere, red-stained eminence of Red Slate Mountain, and the distant skyline offers sawtooth profiles of the renowned Ritter Range, with the readily identifiable Minarets, and the Mammoth Crest. To the south, the barren, rocky shores of the Grinnell chain of lakes occupy the foreground, and just beyond, the green-sheathed slopes of the Mono Creek watershed drop away, rising in the distance to the Mono Divide.

ALTERNATIVE TO GRINNELL PASS

Grinnell Pass is the Silver Divide crossing that provides the most stunning alpine scenery, but the snow slopes north of the pass may be intimidating in early summer. An alternative cross-country route from the west shore of Tully Lake might be a better choice if you start up Grinnell Pass and are uncomfortable with the exposure. To access this route, stay on the Fish Creek Trail an additional 0.4 mile downcanyon until you reach a signed junction to Tully Lake (10,329'; 37.49079°N, 118.89192°W). Follow this trail 0.5 mile to Tully Lake's southwest shore, then continue southeast updrainage in a nearly straight line, crossing the divide at quite easy Shout of Relief Pass (11,406'; 37.47292°N, 118.87367°W). Continue down tedious but not difficult talus and gravel to large Rosy Finch Lake, briefly follow its northeastern shore, and then climb east up meadow strips and gravelly slopes to another notch, Bighorn Pass (also called Rosy Finch Pass; 11,275'; 37.46594°N, 118.86566°W). The east slopes lead through similar terrain to Laurel Lake. The distance from Tully Lake to Laurel Lake is about 2.8 miles.

As with the ascent to the saddle, descend with care. The sudden, shale-filled drop terminates in a large "rock garden," a jumble of large boulders just above Little Grinnell Lake. The rock-hopping route leads along the east shore of this tiny lake to a long, grassy descent toward the west side of large Grinnell Lake. Midway along this side, where the most prominent peninsula infringes on the long lake, today's cross-country route strikes the distinct fisherman's trail veering southwest down a long swale to tiny Laurel Lake. Several fair campsites near this junction offer excellent views due to their location on a plateau above

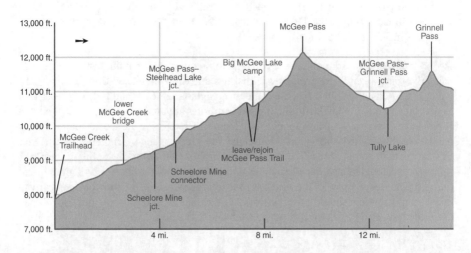

the lake (10,857'; 37.46853°N, 118.85401°W; no campfires). Anglers may find Grinnell Lake to have fair-to-good fishing for brook and rainbow. Other campsites can be found along the meadowed fringe of Laurel Lake (10,300'), about a mile to the southwest, where fishing for brook trout should be excellent.

DAY 4 (Grinnell Lake to Fish Camp, 3.8 miles): The fisherman's trail from Grinnell Lake to Laurel Lake descends southwest via a long, scoop-like swale to the grassy meadows near the headwaters of Laurel Creek. The path, though initially very faint, becomes more distinct along the descent of slender Laurel Creek, which has abundant brook trout.

The gradual descent along the creek becomes somewhat steeper just above the larger meadows. This pleasant, timber-fringed grassland is divided by the serpentine curves of Laurel Creek. The trail across the meadow is hard to follow but can be found again across the creek in the vicinity of campsites at the south end of the meadow. The dense lodgepole cover at the end of the meadow soon gives way to manzanita thickets and occasional clumps of quaking aspen, as the trail reaches the top of switchbacks leading steeply down toward Mono Creek. This unmaintained section of trail is prone to heavy erosion. However, the difficult tread is more than compensated for by the excellent views across the Mono Creek watershed into Second Recess. Particularly impressive are the heights of Mount Gabb and Mount Hilgard, which guard the upper end of that side canyon. A short distance into the steeper descent, the trail crosses to Laurel Creek's western bank (9,697'; 37.43541°N, 118.85646°W).

When the route strikes the Mono Creek Trail, turn right (west) for a gently descending half mile to the campsites at Fish Camp (8,568'; 37.42463°N, 118.85743°W), near the junction with the lateral to Second Recess. Fishing is generally good in Mono Creek for brook and rainbow trout.

DAY 5 (Fish Camp to Mosquito Flat, 12.2 miles): This is a long and strenuous day, so get an early start. From Fish Camp, head upstream and uphill east-northeast on the Mono Creek Trail a half mile back to the junction with the lateral to Grinnell Lakes. Continue ahead (northeast) on the Mono Creek Trail, now a dusty trail through a mixed forest of conifers and quaking aspens. In late season, the groves of aspen lining the creek create an incomparably colorful backdrop to an otherwise monotonous conifer green. Periodic holes on Mono Creek offer good fishing for brook, rainbow, and some golden trout.

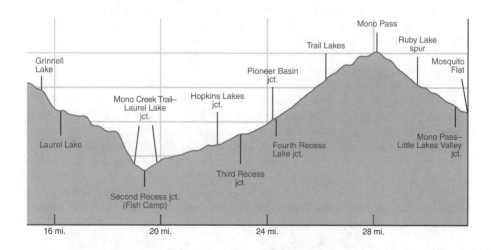

Reach the signed junction with the Hopkins Lake Trail (Trip 46) and continue upstream (ahead, northeast on the Mono Creek Trail) through alternating stands of forest and open clearings to an unsigned junction on the right with the trail into Third Recess. Go ahead (east-northeast) and soon bypass a use trail on the left that leads up to a large packer's camp.

Continuing up the canyon of Mono Creek, the trail passes several shady campsites on the way past the towering ramparts of Mono Rock, which can be seen through periodic breaks in the forest. Proceed through lodgepole pine forest with a thick understory of plants and wildflowers, and after several crossings of side streams, come to an unsigned junction on the left with the lateral to the trail into Pioneer Basin. Shortly, reach a second lateral to the Pioneer Basin Trail (Trips 46 and 52). At both junctions, go ahead (generally east), continuing up Mono Creek.

A short climb along the Mono Creek Trail from the lateral to Pioneer Basin leads to a junction with the trail on the right (southwest and then south) into Fourth Recess (a few campsites). For those who can afford the extra time, beautiful Fourth Recess Lake is well worth a visit. Thousand-foot walls frame the long lake on three sides, and an 800-foot waterfall plunges down the south wall.

From the Fourth Recess junction, continue east up Mono Creek as the trail eventually starts climbing more moderately on dusty and sometimes rocky tread to a junction with an unmapped trail east to Golden Lake (campsites) at a nearby ford of Golden Creek. Here the Mono Creek Trail turns south and begins a stiff climb toward the Trail Lakes, veering southeast after a while. The trail passes just below the lakes, a popular overnight destination for hikers crossing Mono Pass from the east. Along with campsites nestled in clumps of stunted whitebark pines, the Trail Lakes are home to the tiny stone hut of a California snow-survey shelter (no trespassing).

VIEWS FROM THE RIDGE ABOVE THE TRAIL LAKES

Backpackers who take the time to pause here will be treated to a sweeping vista to the northwest of Pioneer Basin over the deep cleft of Mono Creek and bordered by the peaks of Mount Stanford and Mount Crocker. Immediately below are Trail Lakes and Needle Lake (the latter misspelled "Neelle" on the topo).

A steep, switchbacking climb from the Trail Lakes leads to the crest of a ridge. Leave the ridge and traverse a flat before a short climb leads up to austere Summit Lake. Multiple paths lead past the lake, as snow often lingers in this basin and up to Mono Pass well into the season. Continue to Mono Pass (12,060') on the Sierra Crest at the boundary between Sierra and Inyo National Forests. Not only is the pass devoid of views, the stark landscape of shattered and decomposed granite appears lifeless.

WHAT TO SEE AT MONO PASS

Upon close inspection, the ground around Mono Pass soon dispels the impression of lifelessness by revealing an abundance of small, ground-hugging alpine plants. Some of these plants may seem familiar from lower elevations, but the extreme conditions at this elevation tend to dwarf their stature. Vista-starved peak baggers can ascend a Class 2 route of Mount Starr (12,835') to the east for panoramic views. (Note that there are two Mono Passes on the Sierra Crest; the other one is farther north, between Yosemite National Park and Inyo National Forest.)

Leaving Mono Pass, the trail heads south, descending a rock-filled draw before arcing around to the east on a steep, switchbacking drop above Ruby Lake. Views along this descent of Little Lakes Valley and the impressive string of peaks to the west are quite dramatic. About 1.5 miles from the pass, the stiff descent momentarily abates at a junction with the Ruby Lake Trail alongside a verdant meadowland bisected by the lake's outlet.

From the Ruby Lake junction, zigzag down the west wall of the canyon, with fine views of Little Lakes Valley as nearly constant companions. Cross a number of flower-lined, seasonal streams and pass by a picturesque tarn. Nearing the floor of the valley, find a junction with a spur trail to the Rock Creek Pack Station; go right (east and then south) on a switchback. Shortly, reach a junction with the Morgan Pass Trail (Trip 50). Turn left (north) where the trail parallels Rock Creek downstream, descend and exit John Muir Wilderness, and soon arrive at the Mosquito Flat Trailhead parking lot (10,252'; 37.43519°N, 118.74720°W).

Mono Creek Canyon   Photo by Mike White

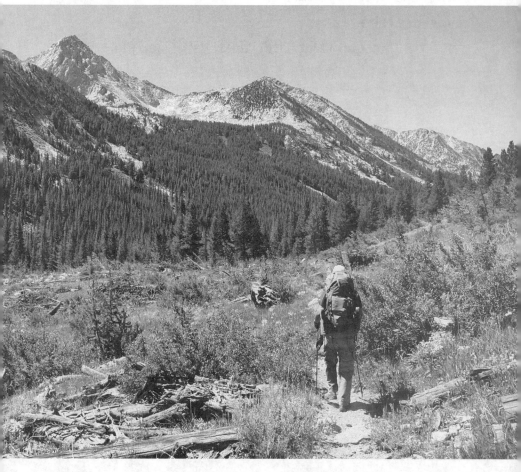

ROCK CREEK ROAD TRIPS

Unlike the canyons to the north, Rock Creek Canyon is predominately granite, characterized by steep glaciated spires and walls. Rock Creek Road leads to Mosquito Flat, which lies above 10,200 feet, making the nearby Little Lakes Valley among the most easily accessed high-elevation valleys in the Sierra. The Mono Pass Trail also departs from Mosquito Flat and makes an easy trans-Sierra passage into Mono Creek drainage, a major tributary of the South Fork San Joaquin River. Meanwhile, Hilton Lakes Trailhead lies about 4 miles before the road's end and offers a long undulating traverse north to the Hilton Creek drainage—another lovely eastside lake basin.

Trailheads: Hilton Lakes

Mosquito Flat (Little Lakes Valley and Mono Pass)

Hilton Lake 3   Photo by Elizabeth Wenk

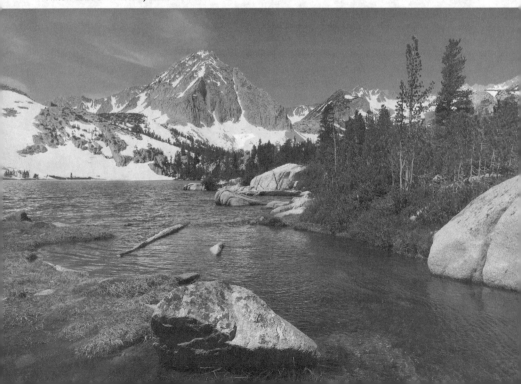

Hilton Lakes Trailhead				9,874'; 37.45494°N, 118.74102°W	
Destination/ GPS Coordinates	Trip Type	Best Season	Pace & Hiking/ Layover Days	Total Mileage	Permit Required
49 Hilton Creek Lakes 37.48260°N 118.76274°W	Out-and-back	Early to late	Leisurely 3/1	13.8	Hilton Lakes

INFORMATION AND PERMITS: This trailhead is in Inyo National Forest. Permits are required for overnight stays and quotas apply. Permits can be reserved up to six months in advance at recreation.gov (60%; $6 permit reservation fee plus $5 per person) or requested in person, first come, first served, a day in advance (40%; free). All permits must be picked up at one of the Inyo National Forest ranger stations, located in Lone Pine (Eastern Sierra Interagency Visitor Center), Bishop, Mammoth Lakes, and Lee Vining (the Mono Basin Scenic Area Visitor Center). If you plan to use a stove or have a campfire, you must also have a California campfire permit, available from a forest service office or online at preventwildfireca.org/campfire-permit. Campfires are prohibited in the Hilton Creek Lakes drainage. Bear canisters are strongly recommended in this area.

DRIVING DIRECTIONS: From US 395 at Tom's Place (14.9 miles south of the junction of US 395 and CA 203 near Mammoth Lakes and 24.1 miles north of the junction of US 395 and CA 168 in Bishop), turn west onto Rock Creek Road/FS 4S12 and continue up it for 9.1 miles to a parking area on the right. The trailhead is a short distance before the parking lot.

trip 49   ## Hilton Creek Lakes

see map on p. 286

Trip Data: 37.48260°N, 118.76274°W (Hilton Lake 4); 13.8 miles; 3/1 days
Topos: *Mount Abbot, Mount Morgan, Convict Lake*

HIGHLIGHTS: With the popular Little Lakes Valley just around the corner, it is easy to bypass the Hilton Creek Lakes. This cluster of lakes offers equally rugged views and good camping, but without the crowds. Hilton Lakes 3 and 4 sit in the upper subalpine, set right at the base of rugged peaks, while Hilton Lake 2 and Davis Lake (aka Hilton Lake 1) lie in more sheltered lodgepole pine forest. All lakes have good fishing and sufficient camping that you should always find solitude. You can complete this trip as an out-and-back (as described) or a thru-hike, ending at the Hilton Creek Trailhead (see the sidebar "Down Hilton Creek" on page 288).

DAY 1 (Hilton Lakes Trailhead to Hilton Lake 4, 5.3 miles): The trail immediately begins a gradual-to-moderate climb up Rock Creek's massive western moraine. The ascending traverse leads across the aspen-covered slopes, crossing wildflower-lined seeps where water oozes through the coarse deposits. Drier, sandier sections are vegetated by shrubs: sagebrush, bitterbrush, mountain snowberry, wax currant, and curl-leaf mountain mahogany. The trail nearly gains the moraine crest and then follows its southern rim northeast, continuing across shrub-covered slopes and through lodgepole pine pockets, crossing a small creek on a plank bridge. Open stretches afford splendid views to the Wheeler Crest, Mount Morgan, Bear Creek Spire, and Mount Abbot. At 1.3 miles, you pass a junction with a rough trail plunging straight down the moraine front to the Rock Creek Resort; you continue left (north). After an additional 0.6 mile, you finally drop off the moraine crest, zigzagging into, then out of a minor drainage.

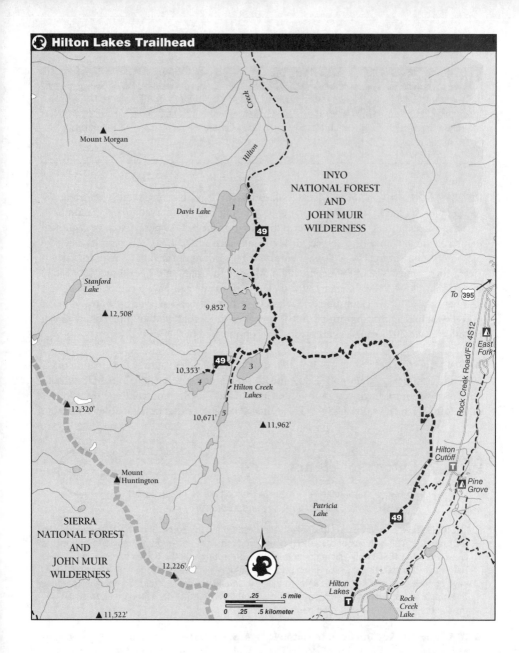

Mount Morgan ▲

Davis Lake

49

1

INYO
NATIONAL FOREST
AND
JOHN MUIR
WILDERNESS

*Stanford
Lake*

▲ 12,508'

9,852'

2

To **395**

Rock Creek Road/FS 4S12

⛺ East
Fork

49

10,353'

4

3

*Hilton Creek
Lakes*

▲ 12,320'

10,671'

5

▲ 11,962'

Mount
Huntington ▲

SIERRA
NATIONAL FOREST
AND
JOHN MUIR
WILDERNESS

12,226' ▲

*Patricia
Lake*

49

Hilton
Cutoff
🚽

Pine
Grove

Hilton
Lakes
🚻

Rock
Creek
Lake

▲ 11,522'

0   .25   .5 mile
0   .25   .5 kilometer

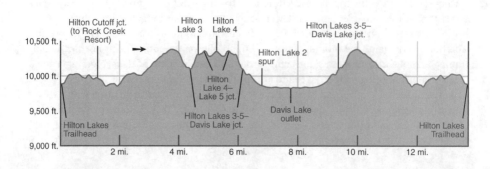

Hilton Cutoff jct.
(to Rock Creek
Resort)

Hilton
Lake 3

Hilton
Lake 4

Hilton Lakes 3-5–
Davis Lake jct.

10,500 ft.

Hilton Lake 2
spur

10,000 ft.

Hilton
Lake 4–
Lake 5 jct.

9,500 ft.

Hilton Lakes
Trailhead

Hilton Lakes 3-5–
Davis Lake jct.

Davis Lake
outlet

Hilton Lakes
Trailhead

9,000 ft.

2 mi.   4 mi.   6 mi.   8 mi.   10 mi.   12 mi.

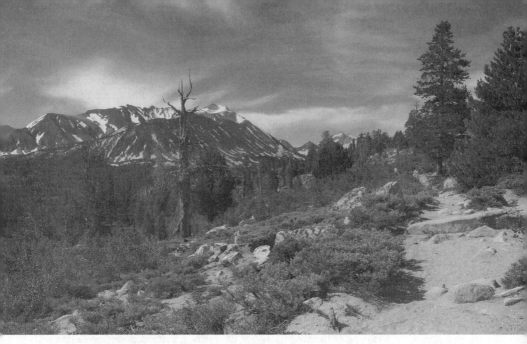

Looking back to Morgan Peak from the Hilton Lakes Trail   Photo by Elizabeth Wenk

You now begin a long, quite flat traverse across the broad eastern flank of the ridge separating the Rock Creek and Hilton Creek drainages. Where a blocked-off old trail departs right, you stay left (north), continuing through open, sandy lodgepole and whitebark pine forest. You cross the top of a willow-covered meadow and then, at 2.7 miles, turn west to begin a more substantial, nearly 400-foot ascent to the top of Hilton Creek's moraine. The trail here was regraded in the early 2010s; the old route is still readily visible, filled with logs to discourage its use and hasten its regeneration.

The trail soon crests the 10,383-foot saddle dividing the drainages and begins a steep 260-foot descent to Hilton Creek. With the views of the southern Mount Morgan now vanishing, you instead enjoy broken glimpses to the northern Mount Morgan and the ridge in front of Mount Stanford and toward the upper Hilton Creek Lakes basin. Your descent ends at a junction, where you turn left (south) toward Hilton Lakes 3–5, while right (north) leads to Hilton Lake 2 and Davis Lake (aka Hilton Lake 1), tomorrow's route. You cross a seasonal stream and almost immediately begin a series of short, steep switchbacks to the upper basin. The ascent levels out at fabulous views northward over Hilton Lake 2 and Davis Lake, and across Long Valley to Glass Mountain. The trail now trends northwest and soon crosses the Hilton Lake 3 outlet stream, navigated on rock blocks.

To either side of this crossing are good campsites (for example, 10,312'; 37.48508°N, 118.75562°W; no campfires; rainbow trout) if you want to stop here and explore the higher lakes without the burden of a pack. Views are magnificent and the sites adequately sheltered by wind-shaped whitebark (and lodgepole) pine. To the west is a prominent ridge extending east from Mount Huntington, although the summit itself is hidden. Mount Huntington and Mount Stanford are named for two of the "railroad barons"; visit Pioneer Basin (Trip 52) to be surrounded by all four of these behemoths, Stanford, Huntington, Hopkins, and Crocker.

To continue to Hilton Lake 4, stay on the main trail and curve briefly southwest along Hilton Lake 3's northwest shore, before veering west up a low ridge offering a fine view of the dashing cascades of Hilton Lake 5's outlet. Atop the ridge is a junction, where left (south) leads up a rib to Hilton Lake 5 (0.5 mile away; very limited camping, but a good day hike; brook trout), while you stay right (northwest) toward Hilton Lake 4. Your 0.5-mile route leads past a tarn and down to a marshy, willow-enclosed meadow where the outlets from Hilton Lake 4 and Hilton Lake 5 merge. You cross Hilton Lake 5's outlet and follow Hilton Lake 4's upward. Lodgepole pine–shaded Hilton Lake 4 offers many excellent campsites to either side of its outlet (10,359'; 37.48260°N, 118.76274°W; no campfires; brook trout). A layover day gives time for a cross-country scramble to the wild, scenic upper lakes, especially those above Hilton Lake 5.

DAY 2 (Hilton Lake 4 to Davis Lake, 2.5 miles): You may well decide that instead of spending a night at Davis Lake, you would prefer to spend a second night at Hilton Lake 3 and then detour the 1.6 miles (each way) to Davis Lake without your pack on the day you hike out, but don't ignore the lower elevation lakes. Sitting in lodgepole pine forest, they have a markedly different feel from the upper, timberline lakes and their own enticing views.

Retrace your steps to the junction between Hilton Lake 2 and Hilton Lake 3. At the junction, instead of turning right (east) toward the trailhead, stay straight ahead (left, north) and continue down through lodgepole pine forest, enjoying the well-built trail. You glimpse Hilton Lake 2 through the trees, then complete a pair of switchbacks down a dry slope and reach the expansive forested flat along its northeastern side, offering campsites just about anywhere you look.

Onward, you pass use trails departing left (westish) to a well-used packer campsite along Hilton Creek halfway between Hilton Lake 2 and Davis Lake and continue north, emerging from tree cover to skirt a seasonally boggy meadow. Davis Lake is now next to you, but still unseen. Resist the temptation to detour toward Davis Lake too early; the good campsites are about halfway along its eastern shore (9,828'; 37.50076°N, 118.75700°W; no campfires) and near the outlet (9,826'; 37.50503°N, 118.75725°W; no campfires). Davis Lake is a lovely big, open lake, offering cross-lake views to cascades from Stanford Lake with Mount Stanford and Mount Morgan rising overhead.

DOWN HILTON CREEK

The description has you returning to the Hilton Lakes Trailhead along the Rock Creek Road. However, from the Davis Lake outlet, you could alternatively walk 5.7 miles downstream to the Hilton Creek Trailhead near Crowley Lake. This all-downhill route is probably easier—although it is hot and exposed—but necessitates a car shuttle. Beyond Davis Lake's outlet, the trail curves east to skirt marshy slopes and meadows, continuing downcanyon right at the base of the sandy moraine slope. The terrain becomes sagebrush scrub and the trail grows sandier as it descends the narrowing canyon, flanked on the west by imposing Mount Morgan and Nevahbe Ridge. At 2.1 miles below the Davis Lake outlet, you ford Hilton Creek (difficult in early season) and pass a series of old roads leading to prospects on Nevahbe Ridge. Now on an old mining road, the route slowly diverges from Hilton Creek, climbing onto the drainage's northern moraine. You pass a junction where an old road leads left (northwest) toward McGee Creek, while you stay right (north) and switchback alongside Hilton Creek through dry sagebrush scrub. These final 2.2 miles offer sweeping views of Crowley Lake, Glass Mountain, the Mono Craters, and surrounding peaks, before arriving at the Hilton Creek Trailhead (7,175'; 37.56450°N, 118.75535°W), located at the northern end of the community of Crowley Lake at the end of Forest Service Road 4S14.

DAY 3 (Davis Lake to Hilton Lakes Trailhead, 6.0 miles): Retrace your steps from Day 2 for 1.6 miles to the junction between Hilton Lake 2 and Hilton Lake 3. Then turn left (east) and retrace your steps from Day 1 an additional 4.4 miles to the Hilton Lakes Trailhead.

Mosquito Flat Trailhead					10,252'; 37.43519°N, 118.74720°W
Destination/ GPS Coordinates	**Trip Type**	**Best Season**	**Pace & Hiking/ Layover Days**	**Total Mileage**	**Permit Required**
50 Little Lakes Valley 37.38981°N 118.75672°W (Gem Lake)	Out-and-back	Mid to late	Leisurely 2/1	7.2	Little Lakes Valley
51 Mono Creek 37.44245°N 118.78614°W (Fourth Recess Lake)	Shuttle	Mid to late	Leisurely 3/2	24.6 (or 19.7 with ferry)	Mono Pass *(Mono Creek [issued by Sierra National Forest] in reverse)*
52 Pioneer Basin 37.46046°N 118.80301°W (Lake 2)	Out-and-back	Mid to late	Moderate 4/2	18.0	Mono Pass
48 Rock Creek *(in reverse of descrip- tion; see page 278)*	Shuttle	Mid to late	Strenuous, part cross- country 5/2	31.7	Mono Pass *(McGee Pass as described)*

INFORMATION AND PERMITS: This trailhead is in Inyo National Forest. Permits are required for overnight stays and quotas apply. Permits can be reserved up to six months in advance at recreation.gov (60%; $6 permit reservation fee plus $5 per person) or requested in person, first come, first served, a day in advance (40%; free). All permits must be picked up at one of the Inyo National Forest ranger stations, located in Lone Pine (Eastern Sierra Interagency Visitor Center), Bishop, Mammoth Lakes, and Lee Vining (the Mono Basin Scenic Area Visitor Center). If you plan to use a stove or have a campfire, you must also have a California campfire permit, available from a forest service office or online at preventwildfireca.org/campfire-permit. Campfires are prohibited above 10,000 feet, including throughout the Little Lakes Valley and Pioneer Basin. Bear canisters are required in the Little Lakes Valley (Trip 50) and strongly recommended in nearby areas.

DRIVING DIRECTIONS: From US 395 at Tom's Place (14.9 miles south of the junction of US 395 and CA 203 near Mammoth Lakes and 24.1 miles north of the junction of US 395 and CA 168 in Bishop), turn west onto Rock Creek Road and drive to its end, about 13 miles upcanyon, at Mosquito Flat.

JOHN MUIR WILDERNESS

SIERRA NATIONAL FOREST

ANSEL ADAMS WILDERNESS

SIERRA NATIONAL FOREST

Laurel Creek

48

▲ 11,682'

Blue Jay Lakes

Fish Camp

Mills Creek

First Recess Lakes

Recess Peak ▲

Divide

12,188' ▲

First

Recess

Mono

▲ 11,221'

51

Creek

Volcanic Knob ▲

Mono

JMT/PCT

Creek

Pocket Meadow

JMT/PCT

Silver Pass Creek

North Fork Mono

Cliffs

8,051' ▲

Quail Meadows

JMT/PCT

Bear Creek Trail

Bear Creek

5

6

7

Vermilion Lake

Vermilion

▲ 11,278'

Feather Lake

8,416' ▲

ferry wharf

Ridge

Arrowhead Lake

51

Shelf Lake

Mono Creek Trail

▲ 9,327'

Upper Graveyard Meadows

Goodale Pass Trail

Graveyard Meadows

Bear Ridge Trail

Bear

4

Graveyard Lakes

▲ 10,228'

Cold Creek

Lake Thomas A. Edison

10,838' ▲

Devils Bathtub

Twin Meadows

4

Bear Ridge

To 168

▲ 11,164'

Mono Creek

4 51

Vermilion Valley Resort (and ferry wharf)

Kaiser Pass Road/FS 5S80

3

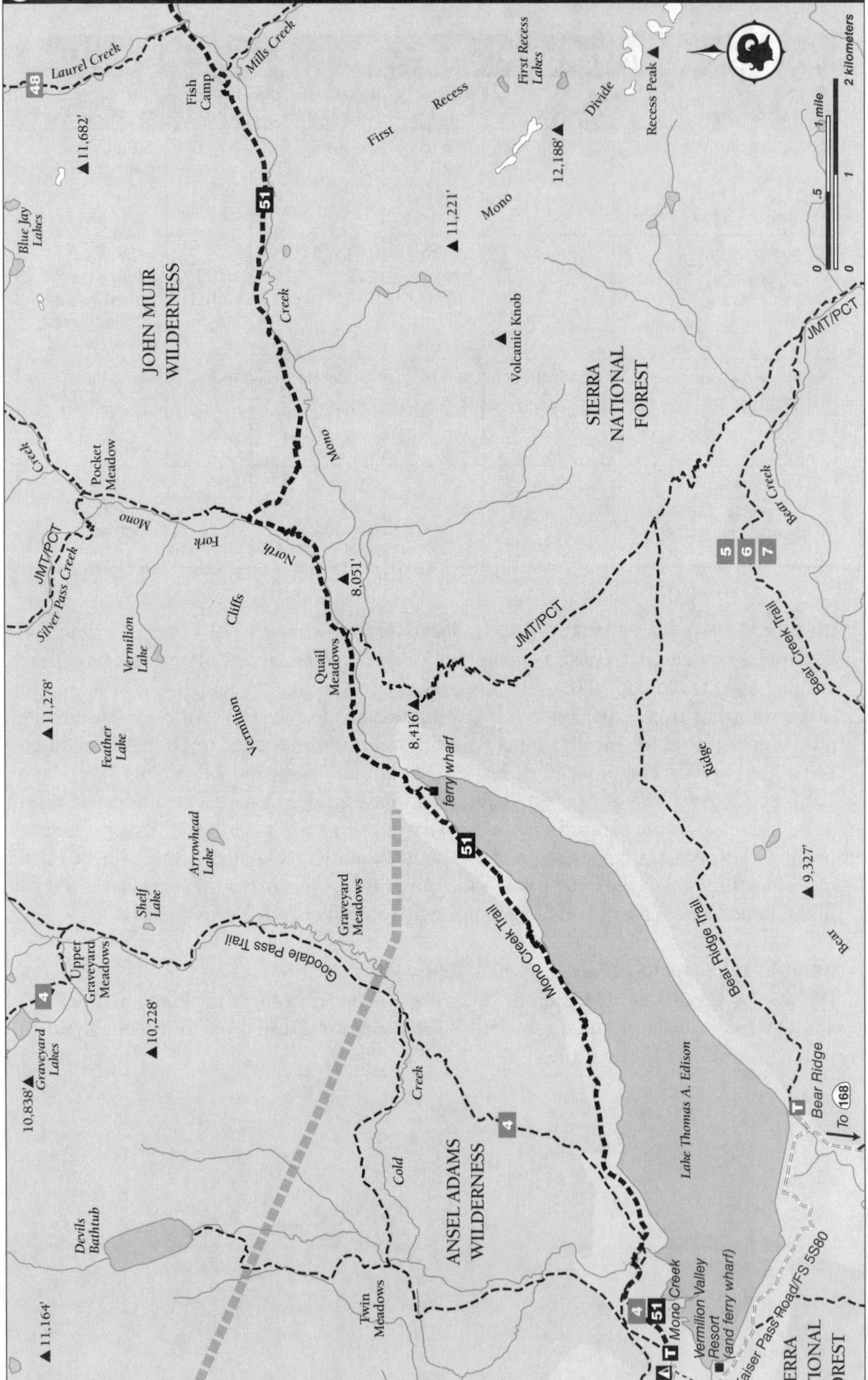

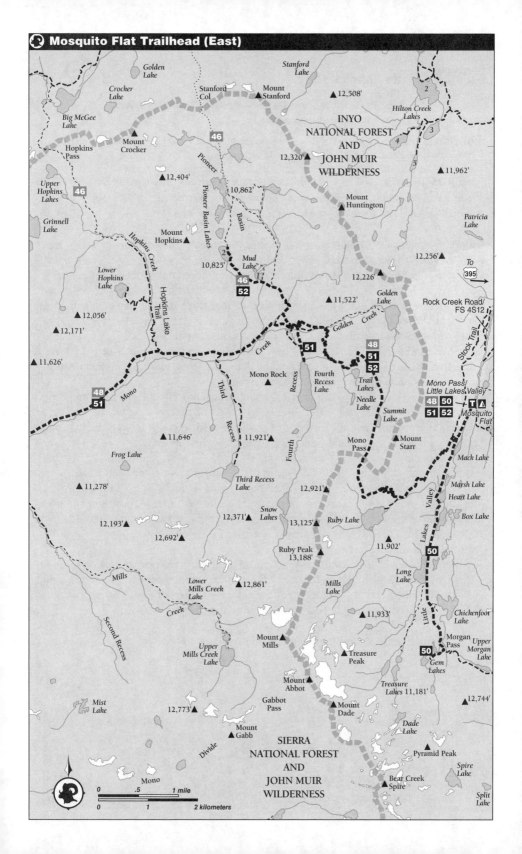

Golden Lake

Crocker Lake

Stanford Lake

Stanford Col

Mount Stanford

▲ 12,508'

Hilton Creek Lakes

Big McGee Lake

Mount Crocker ▲

▲ 12,404'

Pioneer Basin

46

Pioneer Basin Lakes

10,862'

INYO NATIONAL FOREST AND JOHN MUIR WILDERNESS

12,320'▲

▲ 11,962'

Hopkins Pass

Upper Hopkins Lakes

46

Mount Hopkins ▲

Basin

Mount Huntington

Patricia Lake

Grinnell Lake

Hopkins Creek

Hopkins Lake Trail

2

Mud Lake

10,825'

46
52

▲ 11,522'

Golden Lake

12,256'▲

To 395

Lower Hopkins Lake

Creek

Golden Creek

48
51
52

Rock Creek Road/ FS 4S12

▲ 12,056'

12,226'▲

Stock Trail

▲ 12,171'

Third Recess

51

Fourth Recess Lake

Trail Lakes

Mono Pass/ Little Lakes Valley

▲ 11,626'

48
51

Mono

Mono Rock ▲

Recess

Needle Lake

Summit Lake

48 50
51 52

Mosquito Flat

T

▲ 11,646'

11,921'▲

Fourth

Mono Pass

Mount Starr ▲

Mack Lake

Frog Lake

Third Recess Lake

12,921'▲

Marsh Lake

Heart Lake

▲ 11,278'

12,371'▲

Snow Lakes

13,125'▲

Ruby Lake

▲ 11,902'

Box Lake

Long Lake

Lakes

50

12,193'▲

Ruby Peak 13,188'

12,692'▲

Mills

Lower Mills Creek Lake

▲12,861'

Mills Lake

Little

Chickenfoot Lake

▲ 11,933'

Creek

Morgan Pass

Upper Morgan Lake

Second Recess

Upper Mills Creek Lake

Mount Mills ▲

50

Gem Lakes

Mist Lake

12,773'▲

Mount Abbot ▲

Treasure Peak ▲

Treasure Lakes 11,181'

▲12,744'

Gabbot Pass

Mount Dade ▲

Mount Gabb ▲

Dade Lake

Divide

SIERRA NATIONAL FOREST AND JOHN MUIR WILDERNESS

Pyramid Peak

Spire Lake

Mono

Bear Creek Spire ▲

Split Lake

0   .5   1 mile

0   1   2 kilometers

trip 50 **Little Lakes Valley**

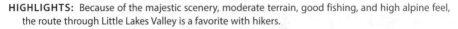

see
map on
p. 291

Trip Data: 37.38981°N, 118.75672°W (Gem Lake); 7.2 miles; 2/1 days
Topos: *Mount Abbot, Mount Morgan*

HIGHLIGHTS: Because of the majestic scenery, moderate terrain, good fishing, and high alpine feel, the route through Little Lakes Valley is a favorite with hikers.

HEADS UP! *Campfires are prohibited. Dogs and goats are prohibited at the valley's south end, including the Treasure Lakes. This area is very heavily used and is perhaps best seen on a day hike. Carefully observe all closures and restoration sites.*

DAY 1 (Mosquito Flat Trailhead to Gem Lakes, 3.6 miles): The wide, rocky-sandy trail starts southwest toward the imposing skyline dominated by soaring Bear Creek Spire. Shortly, the tread enters John Muir Wilderness, climbs a flowered slope, and reaches a junction. Take the left fork, the Morgan Pass Trail, south-southwest. Soon, the route tops a low, rocky ridge just west of Mack Lake, and from this ridge there are fine views of green-clad Little Lakes Valley and the surrounding breathtaking peaks. Flanked by Mount Starr on the right and Mount Morgan on the left, the valley terminates in the soaring heights of Mount Mills, Mount Abbot, Mount Dade, and Bear Creek Spire, all topping out over 13,000 feet. Still-active, although shrinking, glaciers on the slopes of these great peaks are reminders of the enormous forces that shaped this valley eons ago.

Now the trail descends past Marsh Lake and presently fords the stream connecting much higher Ruby Lake with lovely little Heart Lake. Skirt Heart Lake on the west side and then ascend gently past the west side of Box Lake to the east side of aptly named Long Lake. Trace Long Lake's east shore and then climb through a moderately dense forest cover of whitebark pines past a spur trail branching left (east) to Chickenfoot Lake. Dip across a seasonal stream, climb slightly, and dip again to the outlet stream of the Gem Lakes.

Just after a rock-hop ford of Gem Lakes' outlet, reach a junction: left (ahead, east) to Morgan Pass and Morgan Lakes, right (southeast) to the Gem Lakes. Turn right and take this sometimes-faint trail to those lakes, where there are a couple of campsites (10,966'; 37.38981°N, 118.75672°W; no campfires). See the sidebar on the facing page for other campsite options in the Little Lakes Valley.

Alternately, beyond the Gem Lakes junction, on the left is the last switchback on the trail up Morgan Pass, through which the abandoned mining road once reached the tungsten mines in the Pine Creek drainage. There's fair camping at pretty Lower Morgan Lake for those inclined to stay overnight and explore beyond the pass.

DAY 2 (Gem Lakes to Mosquito Flat Trailhead, 3.6 miles): Retrace your steps.

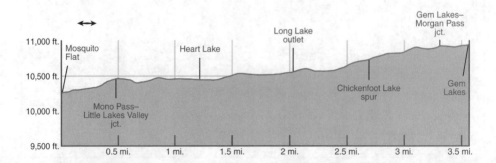

CAMPSITE OPTIONS

You may see less-considerate campers setting up tents directly in view of fellow visitors at illegal or barely legal sites in this area. If you are determined to camp in Little Lakes Valley, head to the more remote campsites away from the trail and the main lakes. (You still may feel like a zoo animal come morning when day hikers and anglers walk through your camp.) Call the ranger station to get updates on any closures.

Here are some suggestions for campsites that are at least the legal distance from water and the main trail. There are doubtless others farther afield, including dry camps. Accessing the more remote campsites east of the trail and the main lakes requires you to cross the connecting streams, which form nascent Rock Creek. These fords may be difficult in early season. Lower Morgan Lake, on the east side of Morgan Pass, also has campsites. (Multiple flat spots within a few yards of each other constitute one campsite with multiple tent sites).

Box Lake: There are a few, fine, sandy campsites off-trail at the north end of Box Lake. The obvious access is via a use trail that makes an abrupt exit hard left (north) off the main trail just where you first glimpse the lake. You'll have to scramble down the shoreline to campsites a little farther down the shore and back into the trees.

Chickenfoot Lake: This lake probably has the most sites, scattered on and between the rocky knolls around the shore. Where the signed spur trail approaches the lakeshore, you'll find a couple of campsites on the right and at least one on the knoll to the left. A use trail branches right from the spur trail well before you reach the lakeshore; this use trail leads past more knolls with additional campsites. Finally, a few remote campsites occupy the lake's northwest peninsula, reached by a rough angler's trail around the west shore of the lake.

Gem Lakes: A couple of campsites are found on the low ridge that rises southeast of the largest Gem Lake, between the inlet and outlet; both sites are above the trail, but the higher one is the better of the two.

Heart Lake: There are three campsites just north of the lake, between the trail and the outlet. Two are in the rocks above the lake and the third is below, at a just barely legal distance from the lakeshore and the inlet from Ruby Lake. Find more campsites nearby on a forested, sandy flat to the west of the inlet from Ruby Lake. The easiest access to those is to continue on the trail across the inlet, take the first use trail on the right, and then hook northward to sheltered and pleasant sites. Finally, a few hard-to-reach, trailless campsites occupy knolls east of Heart Lake.

Long Lake: Highly overused campsites reside on a sandy rise at the lake's north end and across the outlet; these may be the most popular sites in the basin. There are also a couple of trailless campsites high on the rise above the middle of the lake and on the west side. At the south end of the lake, there are three campsites high above the lake; two are on either side of the inlet from Treasure Lakes, and one is near the inlet from the tiny pond high above and well southwest of Long Lake. A faint use trail leads up a dry gully south of Long Lake and west of the main trail, south to a low rise with a campsite, flanked by a wet meadow.

---

trip 51 ## Mono Creek

see maps on p. 290–291

Trip Data: 37.44245°N, 118.78614°W (Fourth Recess Lake); 24.6 or 19.7 (with ferry) miles; 3/2 days

Topos: *Graveyard Peak, Mount Abbot, Mount Morgan*

HIGHLIGHTS: With the starting trailhead above 10,000 feet, this trip is one of the shortest and easiest trans-Sierra backpacks possible. Once you're over Mono Pass, a few hours into your hike, it is (nearly) all downhill, geographically speaking. You are walking beside tumbling Mono Creek for most of the distance, continually impressed by the steep walls rising to either side as you walk the length of this classic U-shaped glacial valley. The hike offers access to several broad lake basins as well as to the famed Mono Recesses, four glacier-sculpted valleys that invite exploration.

HEADS UP! *Taking the ferry across Lake Edison to Vermilion Valley Resort on the final day saves you a not-too-exciting 4.9 miles of walking. For years, the afternoon ferry has left at 4 p.m., but check edisonlake.com/hikers/ferry for details before your trip.*

HEADS UP! *While the hiking distance may be modest, the 253-mile car shuttle, which can take upward of 7 hours (each way) is definitely not short; this hike is probably only worth doing if you have an altruistic family member who will do a drop-off and pick-up. Alternatively, if you don't want to deal with the two-day job of setting up a car shuttle, consider an out-and-back trip, maybe exploring Pioneer Basin (also Trips 46 and 52), Fourth Recess Lake, Third Recess Lake, and Hopkins Basin (also Trip 46) before returning over Mono Pass. Alternatively, you can complete a 41.9-mile hike that leads back via Silver Pass and McGee Pass, outlined in the sidebar "Completing a Loop" on page 297. Other possible passes between McGee Creek/Fish Creek and Mono Creek are described in Trips 46 and 48.*

SHUTTLE DIRECTIONS: From the eastern Sierra, you need to get to Fresno, most efficiently done via Yosemite. From the intersection of CA 180–CA 168 in Fresno, take CA 168 northeast through Clovis and up into the foothills, through the community of Shaver Lake. Continue straight to Huntington Lake, and reach a T-junction near the community of Lakeshore (at Huntington Lake), 67.4 miles from CA 180. Turn right (east) onto Kaiser Pass Road, which soon becomes narrow and twisting. At Kaiser Pass, it becomes even more narrow and twisting before descending past the High Sierra Ranger Station to a Y-junction, 16.7 miles from Huntington Lake. A left turn here heads to the Vermilion Valley Resort and the Lake Edison Trailhead and a right turn goes to Florence Lake. Turn left (still on Kaiser Pass Road/Forest Service Road 5S80) and continue 8.5 miles, driving past Mono Hot Springs, across the base of the Lake Edison Dam, past Vermilion Valley Resort to a junction with FS 6S78. Here, left leads to the pack station, while you should turn right and drive 0.3 mile to the road-end parking lot and hiker campground. *Note:* Once you are 5.5 miles past Huntington Lake, both the Kaiser Pass Road and the Lake Edison Road are very slow and often single lane; expect to drive much of it at just 10 miles per hour.

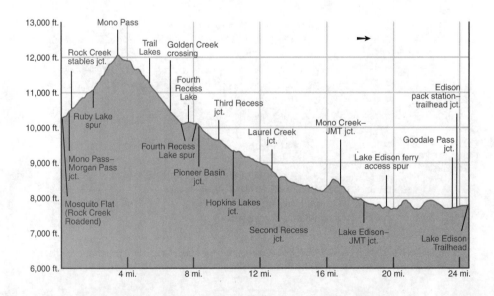

DAY 1 (Mosquito Flat to Fourth Recess Lake, 7.7 miles): Departing from Mosquito Flat, you head southwest alongside Rock Creek on a broad sandy trail, soon climbing through a band of willows, diverging from the creek and arriving at a junction in a sandy flat. Here the main trail to Little Lakes Valley and Morgan Pass continues left (south; Trip 50), while you trend right (southwest) toward Ruby Lake and Mono Pass. After two sandy switchbacks you merge with the trail that has climbed from the pack station and continue left (southwest) on a long ascending traverse. The slope is mostly dry, with the occasional rivulet irrigating clusters of flowers. At 10,865 feet, near a small tarn, the trail is perched atop a high bluff, and you have brilliant views the length of Little Lakes Valley, pyramidal Bear Creek Spire crowning the skyline to the southwest. Beyond, you slowly converge with Ruby Lake's outlet creek and are looking down upon it when you reach a junction with a spur trail that leads to the lake's shores.

Staying right, you begin climbing sandy slopes, your most difficult mile of the trip. Twelve switchbacks lead 500 feet straight up; the trail is well built and evenly graded, but it is a hot, dry climb. At least it is colored by low-growing dry-site flowers such as the wavy-leaf paintbrush and shaggy hawkweed. The views south continue to impress, especially the Sierra Crest, with the summits of Bear Creek Spire, Mount Dade, Mount Abbot, and Mount Mills all rising steeply above the drainage. At the top of these switchbacks you look down upon Ruby Lake one final time as the trail swings northwest, hooking around the cliffs comprising Mount Starr's southern buttress. The trail then sidles into a shallow sandy drainage that leads upward to Mono Pass; note this drainage often still has snow patches in July, but they are not dangerous. Continuous ascent leads upward, mostly in sand, winding through a few outcrops to reach broad, flat Mono Pass (12,073').

Set between two ridges, Ruby Peak to the west and Mount Starr to the right, Mono Pass is hemmed in, offering few views. Continuing north across the sandy expanse, an easy descent leads 0.5 mile to Summit Lake. These slopes seem to be a lifeless moonscape at first glance but host a tremendous diversity of fellfield plants, most reaching only inches above the ground surface. The moist flats near Summit Lake can be yellow with miniature drabas in early July.

Beyond Summit Lake the trail turns northwest to descend to the Trail Lakes. The walking is fast and the views north toward Pioneer Basin (Trip 52) begin to open, only to be cut off again as you drop to the west and zigzag the final distance to the Trail Lakes (11,232'). Passing overused campsites among the highest whitebark pine, the trail continues downward on tight, rocky-sandy switchbacks just above the Trail Lakes' outlet stream. Steepening terrain and bands of bluffs direct the trail north, where it continues toward the banks of Golden Creek, transitioning to more meadowed slopes near the base.

Stepping across the creek, you'll note two trails continuing downstream; the built route is the one that diverges more to the right (north) of the streambank and traverses higher across a moraine. A descending traverse and six quick switchbacks lead to another junction, where left (south) takes you to Fourth Recess Lake and straight ahead (west) is the continuing route down Mono Creek. You turn left and walk an easy 0.5 mile through lodgepole pine forest to this magnificent, giant lake at the mouth of a glorious glacial-carved basin. Camping is limited on this long lake, bounded on three sides by 1,000-foot walls and fed by an 800-foot waterfall, but there some options as you walk along the trail toward the lake's outlet (10,143'; 37.44245°N, 118.78614°W; no campfires).

All four of the numbered recesses are impressive narrow, steep-walled granite basins, with the Fourth Recess the straightest and longest (although not the deepest). Walking around the lake's western shore is easy, but beyond requires creative route-finding. Also admire the rows of steep polished avalanche chutes descending Ruby Peak's western face.

DAY 2 (Fourth Recess Lake to Second Recess, 5.4 miles): Retracing your steps to the main Mono Creek Trail, you turn left (west) and walk just 0.1 mile to reach the next junction, a spur that leads right (north) to Pioneer Basin, a sublime destination if you have a spare day or are doing a shorter out-and-back hike (see also Trip 52). But, ignoring the temptation of alpine lakes and meadows, continue left, passing a selection of unmarked (or barely marked) spurs over the coming half mile; these are all alternative use trails either left (south) to Fourth Recess Lake or right (north) to Pioneer Basin.

The Mono Creek Trail continues down through lodgepole pine forest, alternating between lusher and drier environments. You cross three creeks, each (usually) a rock hop; the latter two drain the two halves of Pioneer Basin, and dense bunches of glossy-leaved clasping arnica decorate their banks. This trail follows the path of one of the American Indians' historic trade routes across the Sierra and was also one of the first routes regularly used by white shepherds and explorers, for it is indeed one of the easiest trans-Sierra passages. After a concerted drop, you then reach a broad flat meadow, where Mono Creek meanders far from the trail. Here you pass a junction with the lateral that leads 1.6 miles to Third Recess Lake (left, south), while you continue straight ahead (right; west) down Mono Creek.

You will now feel like you're deep in a canyon; the walls rise more than 2,000 feet on either side. Remaining well north of the stream corridor, the trail follows the edge of beautifully polished slabs, along which are some lovely campsites, with easy river access and good views of the river, tumbling down the valley's next step. Once water levels are low, pools will tempt you to the banks for a swim. The southern valley wall is striped with avalanche chutes, the slides sporadically leveling the lodgepole pine forest. The next junction you pass leads north (right) to the Hopkins Lakes, another splendid alpine basin (Trip 46). Many layover days are required if you wish to explore all of these side canyons!

A short distance later you cross Hopkins Creek (possibly wet feet). The trail stays well above the valley floor as it crosses the debris from two massive avalanches, dropping back

Ruby Lake   Photo by Elizabeth Wenk

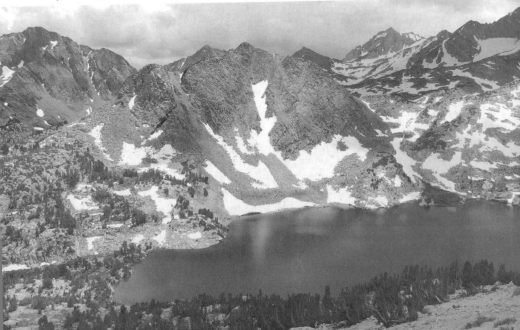

toward the creek just before reaching a big stock camp. Your descent continues, sometimes in meadows, elsewhere on open slopes or through aspen scrub and only briefly in lodgepole pine forests that have been spared by the avalanches. The river is never close, but you can always trend toward it and find a tent site if needed. Eventually you cross Laurel Creek on rocks and logs and just beyond reach the minor unmaintained trail leading up Laurel Creek to Laurel Lake and a selection of popular cross-country routes across to Fish Creek (Trip 48).

One more short descent, here through gorgeous stands of tall white-barked aspens, leads to the signed spur trail ascending the Second Recess to Lower and Upper Mills Creek Lakes and beyond to Gabbot Pass. Nearby is a large stock camp, Fish Camp, a plausible stopping point for the night (8,568'; 37.42463°N, 118.85743°W). While Fish Camp is a convenient area for today's landmark, a large often-dusty campsite doesn't appeal to many backpackers. If that includes you, it is best to camp farther upstream or downstream—or up one of the side drainages.

LAKE BASINS ABOVE MONO CREEK

The Mono Creek Trail offers access to the marvelous Mono Recesses south of Mono Creek and to several beautiful basins north of the creek, Laurel, Hopkins, and Pioneer. The temptation to stray from Mono Creek's valley to visit these many basins is almost irresistible.

In the Fish Camp area, adventurous hikers will want to spend a layover day exploring (or camping in) the Second Recess high country. Follow the trail along the banks of Mills Creek. It can be difficult to follow, but a use trail does lead up to beautiful Lower Mills Creek Lake (10,851'; 37.39969°N, 118.81165°W).

This trip, along with Trips 46, 48, and 52, explores some of these magnificent basins.

DAY 3 (Second Recess to Lake Edison Trailhead, 11.5 miles, or Lake Edison Ferry, 6.6 miles): As you continue, Recess Peak now stands prominently to the southwest. The valley walls become ever steeper and less vegetated. You temporarily diverge from Mono Creek, crossing a wet seep on a wood bridge and then undulating downstream across brushy slopes. You pass the mouth of trailless First Recess and slowly drop back to stream level, in places walking beneath conifer cover, including some magnificent stands of red fir, and elsewhere in whispering aspen glades. Numerous rills descend the walls to either side, providing bursts of color as you intersect them. Pocket meadows are likewise covered in wildflowers.

At 2.6 miles past the Second Recess junction, the trail suddenly begins climbing above Mono Creek, for around the next corner steep bluffs would make continued downstream passage tricky. Instead, the trail switchbacks 300 feet up a dry slope to a polished bedrock bench with stately Jeffrey pine. Absorbing the views, you traverse northwest and then drop just slightly to intersect the John Muir Trail (JMT) along the North Fork Mono Creek.

COMPLETING A LOOP

The most trying part of this hike is the car shuttle, a two-day affair for a three- to four-day hike. An alternative is to complete a near loop, ending at the McGee Pass Trailhead, just a short drive north of Mosquito Flat where you started. To do this, where this route intersects the JMT (at 16.8 miles), turn right (north) and continue along the JMT over Silver Pass to Tully Hole (10.0 miles), then turn right (east) and continue up Fish Creek to the top of McGee Pass (5.9 miles), and down McGee Pass to the McGee Pass Trailhead (9.2 miles), a hike that should take three days. There are good campsites below Silver Pass Lake, near Tully Hole, near Horse Heaven, between 10,800 and 11,000 feet on the west side of McGee Pass, and at various locations on the east side of McGee Pass once you reach Big McGee Lake. See Trip 48 for descriptions of much of this route.

Turn left (west) onto the JMT, switchbacking down broken slabs not far from the creek, beneath towering Jeffrey pine, occasional western juniper, and stands of white fir. Rocky switchbacks lead to a ford of the North Fork of Mono Creek, a flat broad wade at high flows. Just beyond, unseen from the trail, the two forks of Mono Creek converge, and you are now back alongside the main creek. Continuing across a sandy, forested flat you reach a junction, where the JMT continues left (south), crossing Mono Creek on a footbridge, while you stay straight ahead (west), toward Quail Meadows.

The trail continues through Quail Meadows, a lush white fir and lodgepole pine forest (with occasional tiny pocket meadows), not far from the river. Wildflowers are everywhere. Diverging onto slabs where the river is pinched between the Vermilion Cliffs and an unnamed dome to the south, the trail quickly drops past a selection of campsites to a junction where the main Mono Creek Trail continues right (west) to the official Lake Edison Trailhead, while a spur leads left to the ferry landing. Along the spur, you pass another large campsite with a bear box and quickly reach Lake Edison—or often an expansive sand flat that leads to the lake. At times, you have to walk one-third the length of the reservoir before reaching water navigable to the ferry, but getting a ride is still probably worth it!

For those wishing to continue hiking, the Mono Creek Trail leads west across broken slabs and sandy shelves, sometimes close to the water's edge and elsewhere more than 200 feet above it. You have pleasant views south across the reservoir to Bear Ridge. For a long stretch the trail is elevated far above the reservoir among splendid juniper and Jeffrey pine, and then follows a gully back to lake level near a boater's camp (with bear box). After a brief lakeside jaunt the trail climbs again, rising 250 feet beneath white fir and lodgepole pine cover, before beginning a long, hot traverse across open south-facing slopes—morainal deposits with occasional slab outcrops breaking to the surface. (*Note:* the remaining stretch to the trailhead was burned in the 2020 Creek Fire.) Onward through open forest, now white fir and Jeffrey pine, the fairly flat trail reaches a junction where the trail from Goodale Pass merges from the right (Trip 4); continue straight ahead (west). In quick succession you then drop to a bridged crossing of Cold Creek and continue to a junction where the trail to the pack station diverges to the right and you stay left (slightly more to the west). A final 0.6 mile leads through open Jeffrey pine stands to the Lake Edison Trailhead.

see map on p. 291

trip 52   **Pioneer Basin**

Trip Data: 37.46046°N, 118.80301°W; 18.0 miles; 4/2 days
Topo maps: *Mount Abbot, Mount Morgan*

HIGHLIGHTS: It's a tough hike into Pioneer Basin, but the spectacular views along the way and the opportunities for superb day hiking from a scenic base camp in the basin are ample rewards. Amateur botanists will delight in the variety of wildflowers. However, angling is generally poor.

HEADS UP! *Bear canisters are strongly recommended. Campfires are prohibited. Grazing is prohibited. Dogs may be prohibited in parts of this area to protect bighorn sheep; check with Inyo National Forest.*

DAY 1 (Mosquito Flat Trailhead to Trail Lakes, 5.4 miles): Head south and ascend the scenic trail from Mosquito Flat. At the junction with the trail left (south) into Little Lakes Valley (Trip 50), turn right (ahead, south-southwest) for Mono Pass to begin a long climb of Mount Starr's east slope on a sandy trail with increasingly excellent views. Shortly, pass a spur trail coming in on the right from the pack station—an almost invisible junction.

Continuing ahead, the trail intersects seasonal runoff nourishing surprising, seasonal flower gardens. Pass a pretty tarn, and, at almost 2 miles, turn into a swale and reach a junction with a signed lateral to Ruby Lake (campsites), a quarter mile away by turning left (southwest) on this lateral. Near this junction, Ruby Lake's outlet provides the last reliable opportunity for water until Summit Lake, a little beyond Mono Pass.

Bypassing Ruby Lake, take the right fork west and continue relentlessly up, with a view of Ruby Lake below and of the peaks around Little Lakes Valley. Finally, leaving the views behind, the trail turns into a sandy draw that may hold snow until very late in the season. For this reason, there may be multiple tracks between here and the far end of Summit Lake, made by hikers trying to avoid the retreating snow—though there may be no alternative to hiking through it.

At 3.4 miles, arrive at viewless Mono Pass (12,073', though an old sign here says 11,970') and step across the Sierra Crest, from Inyo National Forest into Sierra National Forest, in a stark landscape of shattered granite and decomposed-granite sand. Panoramic views are available by ascending Mount Starr (12,835'; Class 2) to the east.

The trail descends a little toward the shore of Summit Lake, a turquoise oval set in cream-colored rock and gray-brown sand. The trail roughly parallels Summit Lake's outlet before its multiple tracks converge on a flat below the lake to veer northwest. (Don't drop into the meadow around the outlet stream unless you are desperate to find a campsite now.)

Climb a little ridge, possibly through more snow, and begin a switchbacking descent of a dry slope, from which there are breathtaking views over the great glacial canyon of Mono Creek. Especially prominent in these views are Needle Lake—misspelled "Neelle Lake" on the topo—to the west, with the Trail Lakes coming into view below it, and the lowest lake in Pioneer Basin to the northwest, set in a wide, inviting meadow.

Near the Trail Lakes, notice a tiny stone hut that's a California snow survey shelter; no trespassing! The main trail actually swings away from the Trail Lakes (11,200') just before touching their shores, but the smaller lake is on the left as the path comes abreast of them. A rocky plateau a few feet above the larger lake provides several overused campsites (11,230'; 37.44117°N, 118.77570°W; no campfires) among stunted whitebark pines, and there is also a small flat about a tenth of a mile below the lakes, across the trail from the meadow bracketing the lakes' outlet.

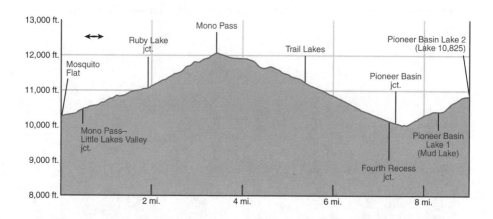

DAY 2 (Trail Lakes to Pioneer Basin Lake 2, 3.6 miles): Return to the main trail to begin a dusty, stony descent of nearly 800 feet to a welcome ford of Golden Creek (10,420'), where a use trail on the north bank turns upstream (east) toward Golden Lake. This trip's route, also on the north bank, turns west and downstream, paralleling Golden Creek and generally staying well above it. The descent eases, though the trail remains deep in dust and full of loose rocks, and the path is soon in moderate forest cover.

The trail presently reaches the signed lateral left (south) to Fourth Recess, a beautiful cirque with a large lake fed by an 800-foot waterfall; it's an enjoyable day hike from Pioneer Basin. Go right (ahead, west) on the Mono Creek Trail and shortly find the signed lateral that goes right (ahead, northwest) to Pioneer Basin. Take this lateral. At first, the lateral avoids climbing straight into Pioneer Basin, instead bobbing over a couple of little ridges. But soon the trail descends to a year-round stream at a junction where a use trail leads left (southwest, downstream) to a few campsites and back toward Mono Creek.

Staying on the lateral, curve right (northeast and upstream) through a moderate forest of lodgepole pines to begin a sometimes steep climb into Pioneer Basin. Ford the stream to ascend rocky switchbacks through patchy forest. The grade eases as the trail approaches the ridgetop east of Lake 1, and the trail soon dips into the meadow around the lake, fording its outlet. This lake (10,404'; 37.45698°N, 118.79519°W; no campfires; called "Mud Lake" by packers) offers the most popular campsites in the basin because they're the easiest to reach and have moderate forest cover. Being the lowest lake, it has the most comfortable temperature for swimming.

However, many more scenic campsites lie above in the upper basin. Continue west on the trail to ford Lake 1's outlet and then begin a moderately steep, stony climb into forest, curving north. Nearing the lower lip of the higher basin, the trees begin to thin, allowing flowers and shrubs to flourish. The grade eases as the path nears the southeast shore of the lowest of the lakes in the upper basin (Lake 2; 10,825'; 37.46046°N, 118.80301°W).

Or, also from Lake 1, a well-beaten trail a little before Lake 1 leads north toward lakes on the basin's east side; this trail isn't on the topo but is on the large USDA/USFS wilderness map.

View-rich campsites may be found on benches around the upper basin's lower lakes. Campsites are fewer the higher you go, but their potential for solitude is much better. Use trails provide straightforward travel to the lower lakes, but reaching the highest lakes takes easy cross-country rambling through gorgeous terrain.

Pioneer Basin is spectacularly ringed by Mount Hopkins, Mount Crocker, Mount Stanford, and Mount Huntington, peaks named for the "Big Four" among California pioneers—hence the basin's name—who were builders of the Central Pacific Railroad.

DAYS 3–4 (Pioneer Basin Lake 2 to Mosquito Flat Trailhead, 9.0 miles): Retrace your steps.

PINE CREEK ROAD TRIPS

Pine Creek Canyon is the northernmost Owens Valley canyon. Compared to the valleys to the north, it has a low valley mouth and particularly tall, steep walls. Moreover, the road leads only to an elevation of 7,400 feet; all trips from this trailhead begin with a steep climb. Three trails leave from the Pine Creek Trailhead—Pine Creek, Morgan Pass (an old mining road), and Gable Lakes Trails—but only the well-used Pine Creek Trail is included in this book. Pine Creek Trail leads through twisted metamorphic rocks to upland granite basins, filled, as always, with gorgeous lakes.

Trailhead: Pine Creek

You can explore Granite Park in Trip 54, page 305.   Photo by Elizabeth Wenk

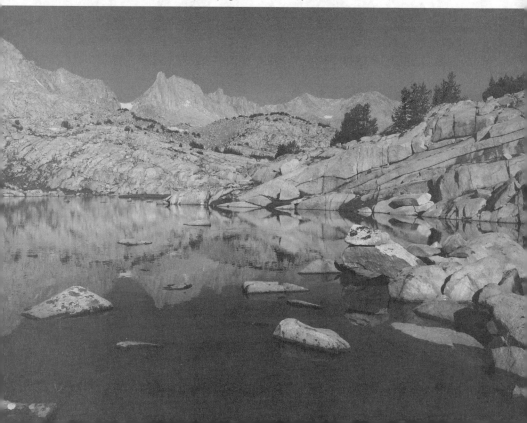

Pine Creek Trailhead

7,420'; 37.36101°N, 118.69220°W

Destination/ GPS Coordinates	Trip Type	Best Season	Pace & Hiking/ Layover Days	Total Mileage	Permit Required
53 Upper Pine Lake 37.34339°N 118.73609°W	Out-and-back	Mid to late	Leisurely 2/2	10.4	Italy Pass or Pine Creek Pass
54 Royce Lakes 37.32356°N 118.76230°W (Royce Lake 11,725)	Semiloop	Mid to late	Moderate, part cross-country 4/1	19.0	Italy Pass
55 L Lake 37.29262°N 118.72432°W	Semiloop	Mid to late	Moderate, part cross-country 3/1	21.3	Pine Creek Pass

INFORMATION AND PERMITS: This trailhead is in Inyo National Forest. Permits are required for overnight stays and quotas apply. Permits can be reserved up to six months in advance at recreation.gov (60%; $6 permit reservation fee plus $5 per person) or requested in person, first come, first served, a day in advance (40%; free). All permits must be picked up at one of the Inyo National Forest ranger stations, located in Lone Pine (Eastern Sierra Interagency Visitor Center), Bishop, Mammoth Lakes, and Lee Vining (the Mono Basin Scenic Area Visitor Center). If you plan to use a stove or have a campfire, you must also have a California campfire permit, available from a forest service office or online at preventwildfireca.org/campfire-permit. Campfires are prohibited above 10,000 feet and throughout the Pine Creek drainage. Bear canisters are strongly recommended in this area.

DRIVING DIRECTIONS: From Bishop, take US 395 northwest 10 miles and turn west onto Pine Creek Road. Drive another 9.4 miles, turning into a signed parking lot next to the Pine Creek Pack Station just before the road crosses Pine Creek and reaches a locked gate.

trip 53 Upper Pine Lake

Trip Data: 37.34339°N, 118.73609°W; 10.4 miles; 2/2 days
Topos: *Mount Tom*

HIGHLIGHTS: The tough, hairpin ascent to Upper Pine Lake offers breathtaking, over-the-shoulder views across Owens Valley to the White Mountains, and the campsite views from the lake's shore to the Sierra Crest make this an outstanding choice for a base camp location on the east side of the Sierra. Anglers should enjoy the chance to ply the waters for the resident trout without much competition from fellow anglers.

HEADS UP! *The trail climbs nearly 3,000 feet in 4.5 miles; don't attempt this strenuous elevation gain unless you're well acclimated and in very good shape. The start of the trip is diabolically steep: You go up 2,000 feet in the first 2.7 miles, mostly on a dusty, shadeless old mining road that has deteriorated in a few places into a rocky jumble.*

DAY 1 (Pine Creek Trailhead to Upper Pine Lake, 5.2 miles): The trailhead is located near the pack station just south of Pine Creek. The dusty, duff trail heads generally southwest

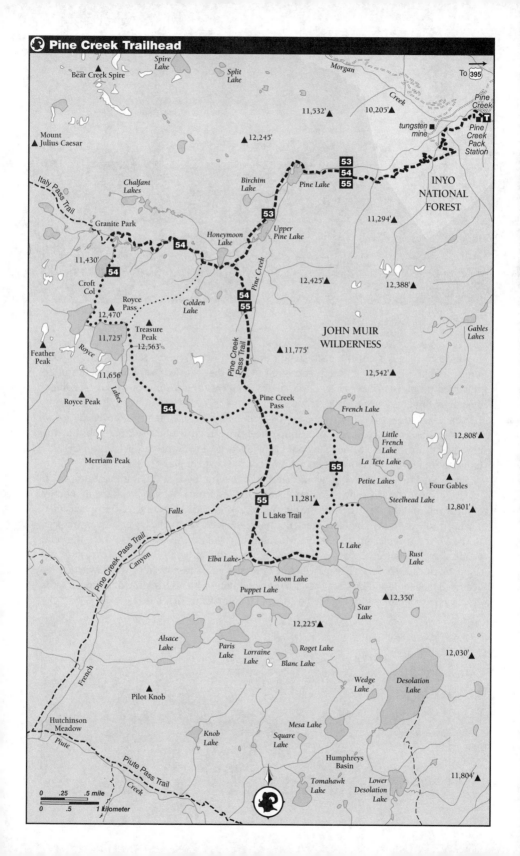

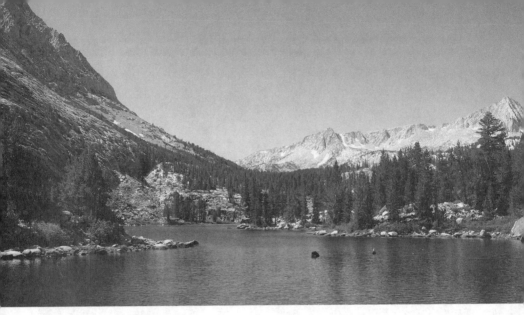

Upper Pine Lake   Photo by Mike White

and ascends steeply from the pack station through a dense, mixed forest of Jeffrey pine, juniper, white fir, quaking aspen, and birch. Along the way, ford several branches of an unnamed tributary of Pine Creek, decorated with plentiful blossoms of wild rose, columbine, tiger lily, and Queen Anne's lace.

About 0.75 mile from the trailhead, the trail emerges from the forest cover and soon after joins the rocky remnants of a four-wheel-drive road leading sharply uphill to the now closed Brownstone Mine. Now out in the open, a view of the defunct Union Carbide tungsten mine will be a constant companion for the next couple of miles.

The slope into Pine Creek canyon is steep and the footing is at times unpleasant, which makes this segment basically a slog-and-pant. Three welcome streams break the monotony of the climb, and the view (despite the ugly road cut that scars Morgan Creek) is spectacular. Gazing northeast down the Pine Creek drainage, you look across the Owens River drainage to the Volcanic Tableland and White Mountain (14,242') on the skyline. Where the road bends sharply left to the now-quiet mine, singletrack trail goes ahead (west) toward the dramatic cascades of Pine Creek, ascending over talus and scree via short, steep switchbacks. Scattered lodgepole and limber pines dot the slope along with a sprinkling of junipers, some of which have left beautiful weathered snags of a dramatic golden hue.

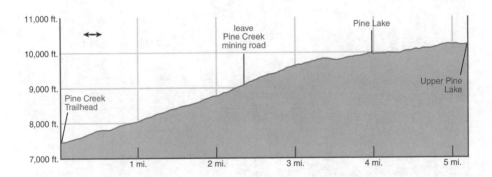

Finally, with the steepest part of the ascent behind, the trail fords another unnamed tributary, switchbacks past a sign at the boundary of John Muir Wilderness, and then loses some of the hard-won elevation on a descent to the south bank of Pine Creek. Here, the creek alternates in cascades, falls, and chutes in a riot of whitewater.

Shortly, arriving at a signed junction with a stock ford, you veer right and cross the creek on a flattened-log bridge, 3.8 miles from the trailhead. Proceed upstream through moderate forest cover of lodgepole pines to the northeast end of Pine Lake (9,942'). The medium-size lake (16 acres) is a popular overnight camping destination for tired backpackers exhausted after the steep climb up the canyon (campsites on the northeast shore). Anglers may wish to tarry along the shore in order to sample the fair fishing for brook trout, but fishing is generally better at Upper Pine Lake.

The trail skirts the rocky northeast side of Pine Lake and ascends through forest to ford the outlet from Birchim Lake. After climbing over a small ridge, the trail parallels the outlet from Upper Pine Lake to arrive at the northwest shore and the first of many conifer-shaded campsites spread around the lake (for example, 10,208'; 37.34339°N, 118.73609°W; no campfires). Anglers will discover good fishing for brook, rainbow, and golden trout.

DAY 2 (Upper Pine Lake to Pine Creek Trailhead, 5.2 miles): Retrace your steps.

---

trip 54   # Royce Lakes

see map on p. 303

    Trip Data: 37.32356°N, 118.76230°W (Royce Lake 2); 19.0 miles; 4/1 days
    Topos: *Mount Tom, Mount Hilgard*

HIGHLIGHTS: A short, straightforward cross-country route leads from the Italy Pass Trail to a chain of stunningly scenic alpine lakes tucked into a rugged basin below a trio of 13,000-foot peaks. Anglers will find the opportunity to fish for a healthy population of golden trout to be quite alluring.

HEADS UP! *The steep climb from the trailhead, along with the cross-country route to Royce Lakes, makes this a trip for experienced backpackers in good condition. Unless you are an expert at staking a tent with rocks, pack a freestanding tent for campsites at Royce Lakes, as the few sandy spots suitable for campsites are on shallow soil that may not hold stakes.*

DAY 1 (Pine Creek Trailhead to Upper Pine Lake, 5.2 miles): Follow Trip 53, Day 1 to Upper Pine Lake (10,208'; 37.34339°N, 118.73609°W; no campfires).

DAY 2 (Upper Pine Lake to Granite Park, 2.3 miles): (For an alternate route to the Royce Lakes that bypasses Granite Park, see the sidebar on page 307.) After skirting the meadows around the north shore of Upper Pine Lake, cross the multibranched inlet stream via a long string of well-placed boulders (may be a wet ford in early season). A moderate ascent leads to the Pine Creek Pass/Honeymoon Lake junction.

Turn right (west), away from the Pine Creek Pass Trail, and follow Italy Pass Trail a short distance to the top of a rise and then quickly to a spur leading right (north) to very popular Honeymoon Lake. At the top of the rise, a use trail provides access to fine though overused campsites on a knoll above the east side of the lake (10,447'; 37.33929°N, 118.74258°W; no campfires) and beneath a grove of pines along the north shore. This lovely lake makes an excellent base camp for side excursions to 40 surrounding lakes in four drainages, or for climbing five nearby peaks that exceed 13,000 feet in elevation. Fishing for a healthy population of brook and rainbow trout is good.

Cross the willow-lined inlet of Honeymoon Lake on a steep but short climb over boulders to the resumption of dirt tread. Then continue climbing to a bench just west of the lake, where overnighters will find seldom-used but excellent campsites. Cross the creek and follow deteriorating tread up the canyon along the north bank of the stream that drains Granite Park through a diminishing forest of lodgepole and then whitebark pines.

Wind up the jumbled valley, passing many lovely diminutive swales and crossing sparkling rivulets. The trail arrives in aptly named Granite Park in a lovely timberline meadow, where the brook trout–filled stream momentarily adopts a lazy course through the verdant grassland. Continue climbing up the drainage on faint tread that continually disappears when crossing bedrock or talus and then reappears in areas of soil.

Reach a large, irregularly shaped tarn (11,355'; 37.34141°N, 118.76112°W; no campfires) and search for Spartan campsites tucked into small pockets of soil scattered around the basin. The extraordinary scenery and high probability of solitude will more than make up for the lack of highly developed campsites. The short day of backpacking allows plenty of time to explore the nooks and crannies of remarkable Granite Park. Italy Pass is visible on the ridgeline to the west; the tread to the pass becomes increasingly faint.

DAY 3 (Granite Park to Royce Lakes, 2.0 miles, cross-country): From the tarn, head south cross-country toward Lake 11,430, 0.35 mile north-northwest of Peak 12,470. Pass the lake on the east and leave the sublime surroundings of Granite Park on an increasingly steep climb over talus toward Croft Col, the obvious notch just west of Peak 12,470. At Croft Col (11,851'; 37.33256°N, 118.76919°W), the uppermost Royce Lake pops into view, nestled in an austere, rockbound, above-timberline basin towered over by Feather Peak. At these lofty heights, fingers of snow cling to the peak's shady crevices throughout the summer. Immediately striking is the crystal clarity of the lake's water and the aquamarine hue. Although the Royce Lakes are quite deep, thanks to the water's clarity, golden trout may be seen patrolling the shallower waters near the shore. Anglers will surely be tempted by the presence of this notable species.

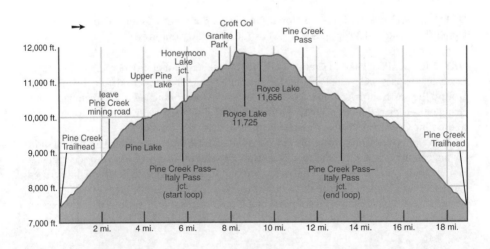

Drop shortly to the lakeshore by carefully negotiating blocky talus and proceed around the lower slopes of Peak 12,470 toward Lake 11,725, the largest of the Royce Lakes. Pass along the north shore to the northeast tip of Lake 11,725. Although much of the shoreline is a jumble of talus, there are a couple of Spartan campsites on small patches of sand above the northeast shore.

From Lake 11,725, you must negotiate a steep slope of talus in order to head south toward the lower lakes. Beyond this minor obstacle, the way becomes much easier and traces of a use trail can be found toward the south end of the lake. All the while, the looming summits of Feather, Royce, and Merriam Peaks dwarf the mere mortals who pass below them. In between Lake 11,725 and the next lower lake, a few sandy campsites bordered by small patches of ground-hugging vegetation offer overnight sanctuary amid the dramatic scenery (11,726'; 37.32356°N, 118.76230°W; no campfires).

ALTERNATE ROUTE TO ROYCE LAKES

You can get to the Royce Lakes from Honeymoon Lake (without going to Granite Park): On the bench above Honeymoon Lake, leave the Italy Pass Trail immediately before fording the creek draining Granite Park and start climbing on a ducked route over granite slabs toward "Royce Pass," the obvious low point directly right (west) of Treasure Peak (12,563'). Through scattered pines, proceed along a ridge just to the left of a stream and then drop off the ridge around 10,385 feet onto a grassy ramp. Continue climbing toward the pass through open terrain covered with granite boulders and slabs and small pockets of meadow watered by trickling rivulets. Curve slightly around the base of Treasure Peak and then proceed directly to Royce Pass (11,771'; 37.33016°N, 118.76117°W). At the pass, Lake 11,725, largest of the Royce Lakes, bursts into view immediately below the towering northeast faces of 13,240-foot Feather and 13,280-foot Royce Peaks. Descend to the lake and pick up the route described above.

DAY 4 (Royce Lakes to Pine Creek Trailhead, 9.5 miles, part cross-country): Continuing the cross-country leg, head south around the shoreline of the smallest of the lakes and continue toward Lake 11,656, where the previously narrow basin widens eastward. In the shadow of Merriam Peak, leave Lake 11,656 near its midpoint and head east over open, rock-and-sand slopes to the top of a rise. Here, a sweeping vista unfolds of a horseshoe of peaks, including the dark, imposing hulk of 13,986-foot Mount Humphreys in the southeast and the row of peaks forming the Glacier Divide to the south. A bevy of lakes on benches above French Canyon also springs into view (Trip 55).

From the rise, descend an easy slope toward the ponds in the next drainage and cross spongy meadows just below the uppermost pond. Climb the sandy and rocky slope above the ponds to an even more impressive view of the surrounding peaks and lakes. Drop down to a large, flat area on a bench overlooking French Canyon and then descend more steeply toward the small tarns near Pine Creek Pass. Pick your way down slabs and past rock humps and boulders through a smattering of whitebark pines to the south side of a tarn and then swing around the tarn to intersect the trail just below Pine Creek Pass (11,142'; 37.31765°N, 118.73602°W), the end of the cross-country section.

Now on the Pine Creek Pass Trail, head north across the pass's gentle terrain past the smaller of the two tarns, and then follow a steeper, winding descent on difficult tread down Pine Creek's boulder-studded canyon. Pass through a drift fence, descend to ford the creek, and then wind down across a talus slope. Beyond the talus, a growing number of whitebark pines, along with clumps of shoulder-high willows, a bevy of wildflowers, and meadows lining the stream soften the previously stark surroundings.

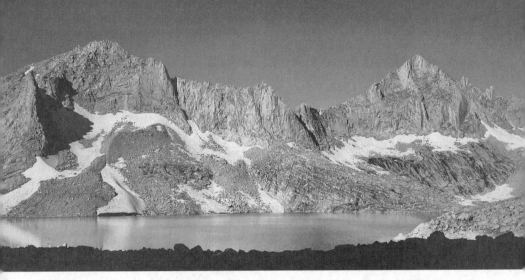

One of the Royce Lakes with Royce and Feather Peaks in the background   Photo by Mike White

Continue downstream along the west bank to a good-size pond and cross the outlet. Gently graded trail moves away from the creek, passing through a scattered forest of lodgepole and whitebark pines, before a steep, dusty descent leads to the Pine Creek Pass/Italy Pass junction.

From the junction, turn right (northeast) and retrace your steps 5.75 miles to the trailhead. (Breaking the one long day into two shorter ones is made easy thanks to the many camping opportunities along the way.)

see
map on
p. 303

trip 55   L Lake

Trip Data: 37.29262°N, 118.72432°W; 21.3 miles; 3/1 days
Topos: *Mount Abbot, Mount Tom*

HIGHLIGHTS: This trip samples picturesque alpine scenery near the lightly used lakes above French Canyon on a semiloop requiring minimal cross-country skills.

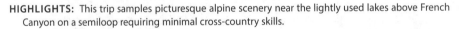

HEADS UP! *Although the navigation along the cross-country section of this trip is straightforward, backpackers will have to negotiate a difficult stretch of talus between Steelhead and French Lakes.*

DAY 1 (Pine Creek Trailhead to Upper Pine Lake, 5.2 miles): Follow Trip 53, Day 1 to Upper Pine Lake (10,208'; 37.34339°N, 118.73609°W; no campfires).

DAY 2 (Upper Pine Lake to L Lake, 5.1 miles): Pass meadows at the north end of Upper Pine Lake, make a long boulder hop of the multibranched inlet, and climb moderately to the junction of the Pine Creek Pass and Italy Pass Trails.

Turn left (south) and begin a steady, gradual climb toward Pine Creek Pass. Originally a Mono Indian trading route, this route over the pass has been in use by humans for nearly 500 years. The moderate forest cover of lodgepole and then whitebark pines thins as the trail climbs past a good-size pond to the right. Tiny, emerald green, subalpine meadows break the long granite slabs, and wildflower fanciers will find clumps of color from wallflower, shooting star, penstemon, lupine, primrose, and columbine.

The trail draws alongside a tumbling creek, the headwaters of Pine Creek, and ascends a long swale between steep granite walls. A final, rocky climb leads through a drift fence and up to a level area harboring two tarns before reaching Pine Creek Pass (11,142'; 37.31765°N, 118.73602°W) on the Sierra Crest.

Descending from the pass through a rocky meadow, views open up of Elba Lake to the south, of Pilot Knob and the Glacier Divide to the southwest, and of Merriam and Royce Peaks to the west. The trail skirts above a boggy meadow, crosses the outlet stream, and proceeds downhill across slopes covered predominantly by lush grasses, sedges, small plants, and wildflowers. Continue through the meadowlands of French Canyon to a Y-junction with the trail to L Lake (10,664'; 37.30504°N, 118.73510°W), 1.0 mile from the pass.

Turn right (south) and follow a moderate climb across flower-filled slopes over a trio of rivulets for 0.6 mile to the Moon Lake–Elba Lake junction. Turn right (south) and follow the trail to Elba Lake, enjoying improving views of the dramatic waterfall spilling out of the Royce Lakes and down the north wall of French Canyon, along with the impressive ridge of spires known as the Pinnacles. Soon, you arrive at the northeast shore of island-dotted Elba Lake.

LIFE IN THE "MOONSCAPE"

Typical of these high, montane lakes, at first glance, Elba seems virtually devoid of life, and first-time visitors often describe the terrain as "moon country," but those who come to know and love this landscape soon discover the beauty that hides close beneath the near-sterile veneer. Spots of green between the tumbled talus blocks indicate grassy tundra patches or clumps of willow, and occasionally the weathered landscape is broken by a dwarfed lodgepole or whitebark pine. Steady, silent scrutiny will usually discover movement indicating animal life. A bird is usually the first to be detected, oftentimes a rosy finch or a hummingbird. Four-footed movement among the rocks is most likely from a cony (pika) or marmot, or possibly a bushy-tailed wood rat. Anglers will soon find life, as Elba Lake has a good population of golden and golden hybrids.

From Elba, ascend alongside the inlet stream steadily to a small pond and pick up the use trail that leads to larger Moon Lake (10,998'). Fair campsites can be found on the southeast side. Fishing for golden trout is excellent.

Continue on trail along the north side of Moon Lake and then over a hill toward the southwest end of L Lake, where the path dead-ends near good campsites on a knoll above the outlet (11,117'; 37.29262°N, 118.72432°W; no campfires).

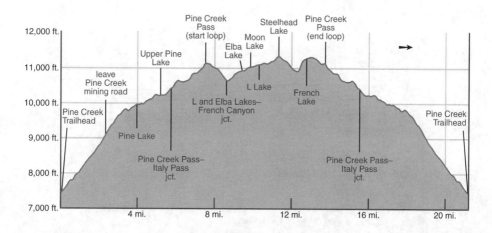

DAY 3 (L Lake to Pine Creek Trailhead, 11.0 miles, part cross-country): From the southwest end of L Lake, follow an easy cross-county course across open, sandy-and-rocky slopes west of the lake toward the north shore. Then, make a steady climb, generally northeast, away from the lake and toward the crest of a ridge directly east of Peak 11,281. Before gaining the top of the ridge, veer east and follow the north side of Steelhead Lake's outlet on a short climb to the northwest shore of the 11,361-foot lake. One of the larger lakes in the area, Steelhead sits majestically in a basin below the rugged, rock-strewn slopes of Four Gables.

From the shore of Steelhead Lake, retrace your steps briefly back down the outlet and climb up to the crest of the ridge east of Peak 11,281. Before continuing, take some time to plot the route to French Lake, selecting a course that attempts to minimize the amount of talus crossed en route. Drop off the ridge and descend generally northwest toward a small pond in the bottom of the canyon. Pass around the pond and begin an angling ascent up the far hillside to the southwest shore of French Lake (11,255'). Spartan campsites can be found on a rise just above the outlet (11,285'; 37.31404°N, 118.72387°W; no campfires).

Leaving French Lake, the object of the next cross-country part of the journey is to reach hidden Pine Creek Pass without losing a great deal of elevation along the way. The elevation difference between the lake and the pass is a mere 100 feet, but the pass is out of sight around a hill and across uneven terrain, which makes achieving this goal something of a challenge. Traverse as best you can, contouring generally west across the hillside toward the pass. Rounding the hill, the pass eventually comes into view, allowing you to set your bearings.

Once at Pine Creek Pass (11,142'; 37.31765°N, 118.73602°W), take the Pine Creek Pass Trail generally north and retrace your steps. (Breaking the one long day into two shorter ones is made easy thanks to the many camping opportunities along the way.)

Hiking along the shore of Elba Lake   Photo by Mike White

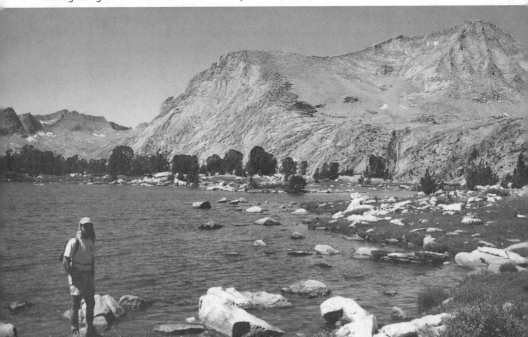

CA 168 EAST SIDE TRIPS

The eastern stretch of CA 168 climbs west from Bishop. Just here the Sierra Crest jogs to the east and Bishop Creek's tributaries spread out to fill the broad slopes created by the crest's eastward curve. Unlike canyons to the north and south, the lower reaches of Bishop Creek are not steep, and three roads climb to well above 9,000 feet, easing access to subalpine and alpine elevations. North Lake Trailhead lies on North Fork Bishop Creek and is the trailhead for both the Piute Pass and Lamarck Lakes Trails. Sabrina Lake Trailhead is along Middle Fork Bishop Creek, with trails leading to the Lake Sabrina basin. Finally, Bishop Pass Trailhead (at South Lake) is along South Fork Bishop Creek and climbs to Bishop Pass. All of these trails, and their many spurs, lead to worthwhile eastside cirque lakes, but only the Bishop Pass and Piute Pass Trails cross the Sierra Crest. While the passes exiting the Lake Sabrina basin are all steep, requiring mountaineering skills, a use trail climbs to Lamarck Col, beyond the Lamarck Lakes, and provides a perfect off-trail adventure for strong backpackers.

Trailheads: North Lake

Sabrina Lake

Tyee Lakes

Bishop Pass (at South Lake)

North Lake Trailhead

9,364'; 37.22731°N, 118.62746°W

Destination/ GPS Coordinates	Trip Type	Best Season	Pace & Hiking/ Layover Days	Total Mileage	Permit Required
56 Humphreys Basin 37.24345°N 118.71506°W (Upper Golden Trout Lake)	Out-and-back	Mid to late	Moderate 2/2	14.4	Piute Pass
57 Lamarck Lakes 37.21764°N 118.64013°W	Out-and-back	Mid to late	Leisurely 2/0	5.0	Lamarck Lakes
58 Darwin Lakes 37.18739°N 118.68783°W	Out-and-back	Mid to late	Moderate, part cross-country 3/1	14.0	Lamarck Lakes
59 Evolution Basin via Lamarck Col 37.17215°N 118.70030°W (Evolution Lake)	Loop	Mid to late	Moderate, part cross-country 6/1	39.0	Lamarck Lakes
67 South Lake to North Lake (in reverse of description; see page 350)	Shuttle (public transport option)	Mid to late	Moderate 8/1	55.0	Piute Pass (Bishop Pass– South Lake as described)

INFORMATION AND PERMITS: This trailhead is in Inyo National Forest. Permits are required for overnight stays and quotas apply. Permits can be reserved up to six months in advance at recreation.gov (60%; $6 permit reservation fee plus $5 per person) or requested in person, first come, first served, a day in advance (40%; free). All permits must be picked up at one of the Inyo National Forest ranger stations, located in Lone Pine (Eastern Sierra Interagency Visitor Center), Bishop, Mammoth Lakes, and Lee Vining (the Mono Basin Scenic Area Visitor Center). If you plan to use a stove or have a campfire, you must also have a California campfire permit, available from a forest service office or online at preventwildfireca.org/campfire-permit. Campfires are prohibited above 10,000 feet. Bear canisters are strongly recommended in this area.

DRIVING DIRECTIONS: In the town of Bishop, turn west from US 395 onto West Line Street (CA 168 East Side). Drive 18 miles southwest past the signed junction with South Lake Road and almost to Lake Sabrina. At the signed junction with dirt North Lake Road, turn right, cross the creek on a bridge, and continue 2 airy miles past little North Lake to a junction with the signed spur road to the pack station. Turn right here, pass the pack station's entrance, and shortly find the overnighters' parking lot. Alas, this lot is 0.6 mile from the true trailhead, which is farther up the road at the west end of North Lake Campground. Drop all the packs and most of the party at the true trailhead, and then designate someone to drive the car back to the overnight parking lot and then walk back up the road.

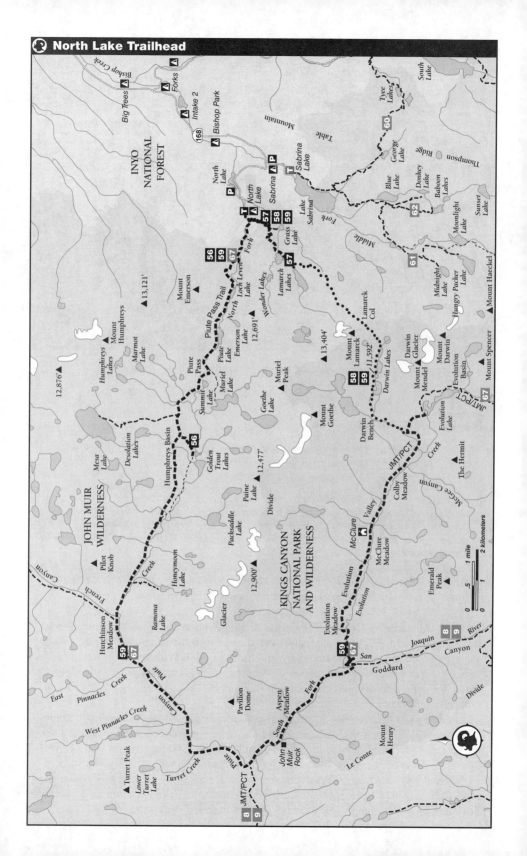

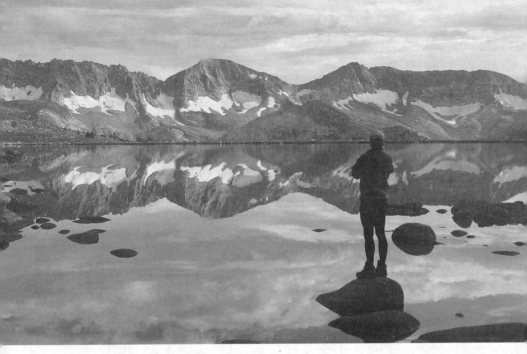

Gazing at the Glacier Divide from Mesa Lake in Humphreys Basin   Photo by Mike White

see map on p. 313

trip 56   Humphreys Basin

Trip Data: 37.24345°N, 118.71506°W (Upper Golden Lake);
14.4 miles; 2/2 days
Topos: *Mount Darwin, Mount Tom*

HIGHLIGHTS: Humphreys Basin offers fine cross-country hiking to, and fishing in, dozens of lakes. Peak baggers have a bevy of summits from which to choose, ranging from difficult Mount Humphreys—Class 4 by the easiest route—to gentle, unnamed knobs. A base camp in Humphreys Basin provides the gateway to countless high-country delights. Going only as far as Loch Leven or Piute Lake makes a great weekender.

HEADS UP! *Because you'll be away from a maintained trail, be prepared for cross-country travel, ranging from easy off-trail to enjoyable but demanding bouldering.*

DAY 1 (North Lake Trailhead to Humphreys Basin, 7.2 miles): From the trailhead, go west and almost immediately reach a junction with the trail to Lamarck Lakes (Trips 57–59); go ahead (west) on the Piute Pass Trail. Soon entering John Muir Wilderness, the trail ascends gently along slopes dotted with patches of meadow, aspen groves, and stands of lodgepole pines. A wealth of wildflowers covers these meadows in season, including paintbrush, columbine, tiger lily, spiraea, and penstemon.

After a pair of fords of North Fork Bishop Creek (on log bridges), the climb becomes moderate. As you climb, the aspen are left behind, the lodgepole become sparse, and some limber pine join the thinning forest. Flat-topped Peak 12,691 on the south and 13,118-foot Mount Emerson on the north flank the glaciated canyon. The trail switchbacks up a headwall with views of Loch Leven's cascading outlet and then follows gently graded trail to the lake (10,700'), where picnic spots are scattered around the shoreline. A campsite is off-trail near the west end. Fishing is fair for brook, brown, and rainbow trout.

Beyond Loch Leven, the trail ascends moderately again through a sparse cover of lodge-pole and whitebark pines, winding among large, rounded boulders, and skirting a pair of small lakes. Eventually, the climb abates, and the trail crosses a bench to Piute Lake's shore (brook and rainbow). Overused, wind-prone campsites are on the north side of the lake near the trail (10,985'; 37.23644°N, 118.66856°W; no campfires). (Solitude seekers can scramble cross-country southeast up a fairly steep, rocky slope to less used sites at granite-bound Emerson Lake.)

From Piute Lake, follow the trail northwest toward timberline, ascending granite slabs, passing through meadowlands sliced by refreshing brooks, and skirting tiny ponds. Sooner than expected, a final traverse leads to Piute Pass (11,423').

VIEWS FROM PIUTE PASS

Views from this aerie abound. Immediately below and to the west is the wide expanse of scenic, lake-dotted Humphreys Basin. In the southwest, the rugged Glacier Divide towers over the basin forming the northern boundary of Kings Canyon National Park. To the north is the dramatic summit of Mount Humphreys—at 13,986 feet, the highest peak this far north in the Sierra. To the west lie Pilot Knob and the deep cleft of South Fork San Joaquin River.

From the pass, the rocky-dusty trail passes well above Summit Lake along the treeless edge of the great cirque of Humphreys Basin. Below to the south, the headwaters of Piute Creek spill ribbonlike down the basin, forming a lake here and a pond there. Hidden from sight above and to the north lie Marmot Lake and the Humphreys Lakes, whose outlets the trail crosses where they nourish trailside patches of willows, shooting stars, and sneeze-weed. Small, high campsites with panoramic views cling to the open slopes between the trail and these remote lakes. When searching for a campsite, seek a location well away from the main trail, as those close to the trail have become greatly overused.

Near a point where the Piute Pass Trail is above and north of a small lake with a green island, the route meets the unsigned but highly visible use trail heading north to the Desolation Lakes (11,164'; 37.24812°N, 118.70217°W). Those intrigued by the Desolation Lakes' reputation for fishing and who are fond of treeless, open camps will find some decent campsites above Lower Desolation Lake (11,221'; 37.25805°N, 118.71088°W; no campfires) and on the wind-raked flats among the great white boulders surrounding aptly named Desolation Lake (11,375'; golden trout).

The Piute Pass Trail continues descending to the cascading outlet of the Desolation Lakes—the last reliable water source before Hutchinson Meadow during dry years, although sometimes even it dries up. (If you missed the use trail to the Desolation Lakes, follow their outlet from here northward.) Below, the Golden Trout Lakes gleam down in

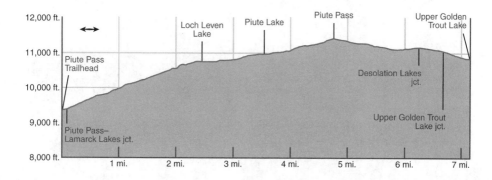

the cirque bottom. If headed for the good campsites on the knolls around Upper Golden Trout Lake (10,846'; 37.24345°N, 118.71506°W; no campfires), descend about 0.5 mile south. There, small whitebark pines shelter little flats overlooking the water, which gracefully mirrors the Glacier Divide. These sites offer fine views northeast to Mount Humphreys and west to Pilot Knob as well. Lower Golden Trout Lake is closed to camping within 500 feet of the shoreline. Campsites in Humphreys Basin make fine base camps for exploring the area's wonders.

DAY 2 (Humphreys Basin to North Lake Trailhead, 7.2 miles): Retrace your steps.

trip 57   Lamarck Lakes

see map on p. 313

Trip Data: 37.21764°N, 118.64013°W; 5.0 miles; 2/0 days
Topos: *Mount Darwin*

HIGHLIGHTS: This short trail leads to two attractive lakes and an optional cross-country tour of the seldom visited but highly scenic Wonder Lakes.

HEADS UP! *While the 2.5-mile distance to the lakes is short, the elevation gain of 1,700 feet makes this hike no easy trek.*

DAY 1 (North Lake Trailhead to Upper Lamarck Lake, 2.5 miles): From the trailhead, almost immediately find the junction with the Piute Pass Trail (Trip 56); for this trip, turn left (south) on the Lamarck Lakes Trail. Cross three bridges over branches of North Fork Bishop Creek and make a moderately steep, switchbacking climb through aspens, lodgepole pines, and limber pines to a junction with a 0.2-mile lateral to aptly named Grass Lake, 1 mile from the start of the trail. As the season progresses, Grass Lake, down in a deep hole, usually becomes less of a lake and more of a meadow.

Go right (west) at the junction and continue climbing toward the Lamarck Lakes. Switchbacks resume as the trail becomes steep and rocky near some exposed cliffs, where the open terrain allows good views of Grass and North Lakes until they become obscured by the return of light forest. Beyond another set of switchbacks, pass a small pond and soon spy Lower Lamarck Lake (10,667'; 37.21764°N, 118.64013°W; no campfires). Make a short drop to ford the outlet and find the east shore of the 10,662-foot lake, 1.9 miles from the campground.

Lower Lamarck Lake is quite scenic, cradled below granite cliffs and backdropped by the pyramidal summit of Peak 12,153. Well-used, limber pine–shaded campsites near the

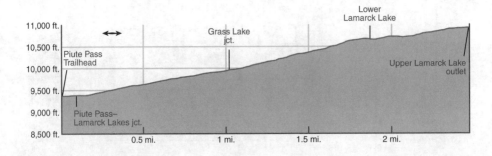

outlet will tempt late-starting backpackers, although clearings above the northeast shore may offer more privacy. Anglers can test their skill on a resident population of brook and rainbow trout. Easy cross-country travel from Lower Lamarck Lake leads into the lovely backcountry and more-remote campsites around the Wonder Lakes.

Continue up the trail from the lower lake through the rock-strewn wash of Lamarck Creek. Following a series of short switchbacks, the trail drops to ford the creek and then follows the northwest bank through diminutive meadows dotted with pines. At 2.7 miles, reach the outlet of Upper Lamarck Lake (10,918').

Tucked into a narrow, steep-walled canyon of rock, austere Upper Lamarck Lake is much longer than its lower counterpart. The stark surroundings create an inhospitable ambiance in comparison to the pine-shaded shores of Lower Lamarck Lake. Find campsites amid a copse of stunted pines clinging tenuously to a low rise above the southeast shore, or near some small tarns east of the lake (for example, 10,936'; 37.21227°N, 118.64537°W; no campfires). The upper lake also harbors brook and rainbow trout.

DAY 2 (Upper Lamarck Lake to North Lake Trailhead, 2.5 miles): Retrace your steps.

Lower Lamarck Lake   Photo by Mike White

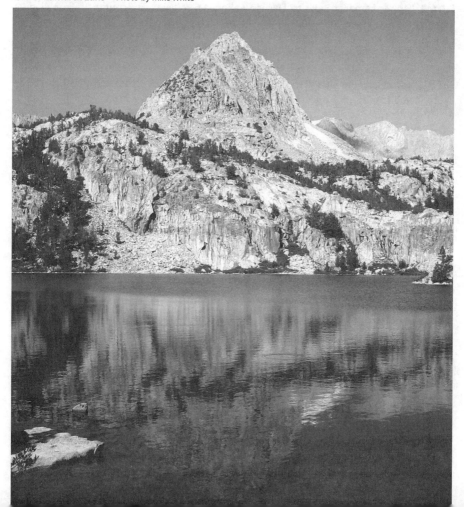

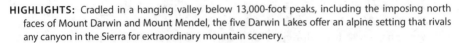

trip 58 Darwin Lakes

see map on p. 313

Trip Data: 37.18739°N, 118.68783°W; 14.0 miles; 3/1 days
Topos: *Mount Darwin*

HIGHLIGHTS: Cradled in a hanging valley below 13,000-foot peaks, including the imposing north faces of Mount Darwin and Mount Mendel, the five Darwin Lakes offer an alpine setting that rivals any canyon in the Sierra for extraordinary mountain scenery.

HEADS UP! *The route to 12,290-foot Lamarck Col is physically challenging, gaining 3,600 feet in 5 miles; attempt this only if you are well acclimated. A short but steep ascent over a snowfield may be necessary to gain the col, and the cross-country route on the west side follows a steep descent over interminable blocky talus all the way to the lakes. Avoid crossing Lamarck Col when thunderstorms are possible.*

DAY 1 (North Lake Trailhead to Upper Lamarck Lake, 2.5 miles): Follow Trip 57, Day 1 to Lower Lamarck Lake (10,667'; 37.21764°N, 118.64013°W; no campfires) or Upper Lamarck Lake (10,936'; 37.21227°N, 118.64537°W; no campfires).

DAY 2 (Upper Lamarck Lake to Darwin Lakes, 4.6 miles, cross-country): From Upper Lamarck Lake, retrace your steps down the trail several hundred yards to a use trail that crosses Lamarck Creek and then heads southeast up a rise. Take that path past a small pond to a gurgling rivulet bisecting a meadow. Climb along this watercourse to a crossing and then follow a ducked route on a serpentine ascent of a boulder- and rock-strewn hillside. Nearing the crest, fine views open up of Grass Lake, Lamarck Lakes, North Lake, Lake Sabrina, and the Owens Valley, backdropped by the White Mountains.

The grade eases as the path follows the left-hand side of the ridge through widely scattered pines to a lush hillside well watered by seasonal brooks. Beyond this verdant oasis, the path zigzags more steeply across an arid hillside and then follows an ascending traverse before a stiff climb leads into a sloping valley below the Sierra Crest. Head up this valley toward the perennial snowfield just below the col. While crossing the snowfield may be straightforward under normal conditions and there is usually a deep trench etched by previous hikers across the snow, some parties might feel more comfortable ascending this potential obstacle with the aid of ice axes. Upon surmounting the snowfield, a very short rock scramble leads to 12,920-foot Lamarck Col (37.19037°N, 118.66755°W), 5.6 miles

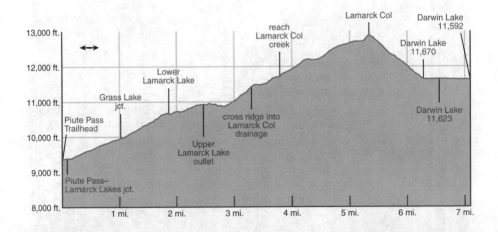

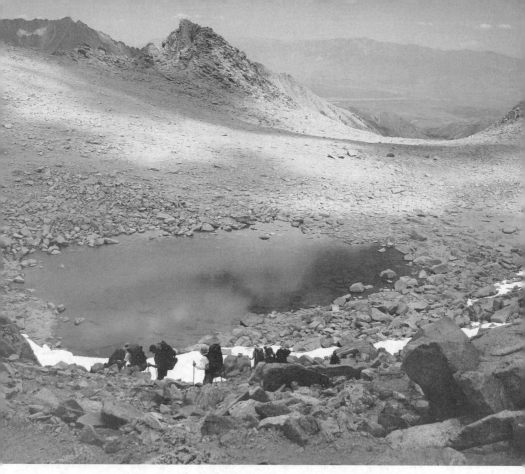

Hikers descend a permanent snowfield on the east side of Lamarck Col.   Photo by Mike White

from the trailhead (or 5.1 miles if you bypassed Upper Lamarck Lake). This lofty aerie offers an impressive view of Mount Darwin and Mount Mendel, Darwin Glacier, Darwin Lakes, and the deep cleft of Evolution Valley beyond Darwin Bench.

From the col, you will be forced to pick your way down a trailless, boulder- and talus-filled slope. Although the way to the lakes is clear and route-finding is not particularly difficult, the actual descent can be quite tedious while carrying a full backpack, especially following the tiring climb to the col. The going becomes easier when you reach a faint use trail running along the north shore of the lakes. There is a short but quite cumbersome section where the trail crosses giant talus blocks along the shore of the second-highest lake (the first lake you reach), but otherwise walking along the shores of the lakes is straight-forward. Proceed along this path to Lake 11,592, 7 miles from the trailhead, where a few decent campsites are scattered above the shoreline (11,623'; 37.18739°N, 118.68783°W; no campfires). There are also good campsites at Darwin Bench, another 1.2 miles down-canyon, with open views toward Evolution Valley (for example, 11,281'; 37.18538°N, 118.70279°W; no campfires). Darwin Bench, Evolution Basin, or the giant lakes southeast of Mt. Goethe are good locations to explore on your layover day.

DAY 3 (Darwin Lakes to North Lake Trailhead, 6.9 miles, part cross-country): Retrace your steps to the car, skipping the 0.2-mile detour to Upper Lamarck Lake.

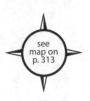
see map on p. 313

trip 59   Evolution Basin via Lamarck Col

Trip Data: 37.17215°N, 118.70030°W (Evolution Lake);
39.0 miles; 6/1 days

Topos: *Mount Darwin, Mount Henry, Mount Hilgard, Mount Tom*

HIGHLIGHTS: Backpackers with off-trail skills can sample some of the High Sierra's most spectacular scenery on a mostly on-trail loop that visits such highlights as Darwin Canyon, Evolution Valley, Hutchinson Meadow, and Humphreys Basin.

HEADS UP! *The route to 12,920-foot Lamarck Col is physically challenging, gaining 3,600 feet in 5 miles; attempt it only if you are well acclimated. A short but steep ascent over a snowfield may be necessary to gain the col, and the cross-country route on the other side follows a steep descent over interminable blocky talus all the way to the lakes. Avoid the crossing of Lamarck Col when thunderstorms are possible.*

DAY 1 (North Lake Trailhead to Upper Lamarck Lake, 2.5 miles): Follow Trip 57, Day 1 to Lower Lamarck Lake (10,667'; 37.21764°N, 118.64013°W; no campfires) or Upper Lamarck Lake (10,936'; 37.21227°N, 118.64537°W; no campfires).

DAY 2 (Upper Lamarck Lake to Evolution Lake, 7.8 miles, part cross-country): Follow Trip 57, Day 2 for 4.9 miles to Darwin Lake 11,592. There are a few decent campsites scattered above the shoreline (for example, 11,623'; 37.18739°N, 118.68783°W; no campfires), but today's description continues into Evolution Basin.

Continue along the faint use trail as it parallels Darwin Creek toward lovely, tarn-dotted Darwin Bench. After the stark surroundings of Darwin Canyon, the alpine gardens of Darwin Bench combined with the stunning vistas across Evolution Valley create a picture-perfect scene. Eventually, you must bid farewell to lovely meadowlands of Darwin Bench and follow a use trail on a descent to the well-trod John Muir Trail (JMT) and coincident Pacific Crest Trail (PCT). The goal is to meet the JMT near the top of a set of switchbacks climbing out of Evolution Valley (10,637'; 37.17730°N, 118.70757°W).

Once at the wide and well-maintained JMT, turn left (southeast) and stroll an easy 0.8 mile southeast to Evolution Lake. Splendidly scenic, although popular, campsites can be found near the small peninsula on the northwest shore (10,871'; 37.17215°N, 118.70030°W;

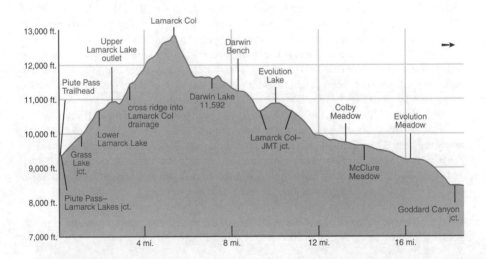

no campfires). While the dramatic scenery continues up the basin past Evolution Lake, campsites are at a premium and they become increasingly marginal the closer you get to Muir Pass. With an abundance of incredible scenery, spending additional layover days in Evolution Basin would be quite enjoyable.

DAY 3 (Evolution Lake to Goddard Canyon Trail Junction, 8.2 miles): Retrace your steps 0.8 mile to where the cross-country route from Darwin Lakes intersected the JMT.

From there, go ahead on the JMT into a thickening forest of lodgepole pines. A zigzagging descent leads down the headwall of Evolution Valley, with periodic views through gaps in the trees of the deep cleft. Hop across a pair of flower-lined streams spilling across the trail and continue toward the floor of the canyon, passing below a thundering waterfall on Darwin Creek, and soon come to a crossing of this raucous stream.

Gradually graded trail winds down the valley through stands of scattered pines, across small pockets of meadow, and beside granite slabs and boulders to Colby Meadow. Campsites shaded by lodgepole pines near the fringe of the meadow will lure overnighters to this pastoral haven, where good views of the valley, the winding creek, and the surrounding peaks abound. Fishing in nearby Evolution Creek is reported to be decent for golden trout.

Continue the gentle descent downstream amid light forest, crossing a couple of streams on the way to McClure Meadow, the largest and probably most popular of Evolution Valley's meadows. Numerous campsites are spread around the edge of the meadow, some with fine views of the lazy creek sinuously coursing through the verdant clearing. The McClure Meadow Ranger Station (9,652'; 37.18800°N, 118.74289°W), a summer home for the seasonal ranger who patrols the area, is found on a low rise just north of the trail.

Past the cabin, the gently graded trail continues to the end of the meadow. Away from McClure Meadow, the creek picks up speed again, and, over the next couple of miles, the trail travels in and out of lodgepole pine forest and crosses a trio of streams draining the north side of Glacier Divide. Breaks in the forest allow fine views of the surroundings, including a prominent avalanche swath and a picturesque waterfall below Emerald Peak. Near the far end of Evolution Valley, skirt Evolution Meadow, passing by several lodgepole-shaded campsites, on the way to a crossing of a twin-channeled stream. From there, the trail curves south to ford Evolution Creek beyond the west end of Evolution Meadow, where the creek is wide and relatively slow moving. Follow the trail across the meadow toward the creek and then wade

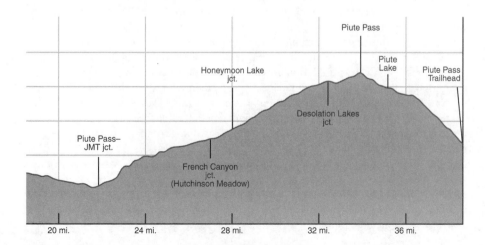

across (may be difficult in early season). Pick up the trail again on the south bank and curve through campsites before continuing downstream.

Back on the JMT, a stretch of nearly level trail along the south bank leads to a steep descent, where the creek suddenly begins a raucous plunge, tumbling over slabs and careening through boulders on the way to its convergence with South Fork San Joaquin River. Initially, the trail seems to match the fall of the plunging creek on a zigzagging drop across the exposed west wall of the canyon, with good views of the gorge and the river below. Nearing the floor of the canyon, enter the welcome shade of a mixed forest of aspens, lodgepole pines, and incense cedars, and arrive at a wood bridge spanning South Fork San Joaquin River. On the far side of the bridge is a junction with the Goddard Canyon Trail (8,487'; 37.19281°N, 118.79504°W), 7.4 miles from where the cross-country route from Darwin Bench intersected the JMT. Find good campsites on either side of the bridge (for example, 8,484'; 37.19243°N, 118.79452°W).

DAY 4 (Goddard Canyon Trail Junction to Hutchinson Meadow, 8.7 miles): Go north on the JMT from the junction, following the course of the river through mixed forest to a crossing of the stream draining the canyon east of Mount Henry. A mixed bag of vegetation greets travelers over the next mile as they wander in and out of scattered forest and across open slopes covered with sagebrush, currant, and an assortment of wildflowers, including lupine, paintbrush, penstemon, pennyroyal, cinquefoil, and mariposa lily.

Just before another bridge across the river, a short spur trail leads above the south bank to good campsites shaded by a dense grove of pines. Downstream from the bridge, the canyon narrows to a slim gorge that powerfully propels the river through a rocky chasm. Walk alongside the raging waters to a more placid stretch of the river about a mile past the bridge. Just past the crossing of a side stream, arrive at Aspen Meadow, which is more an aspen-covered flat than a bona fide meadow. A few infrequently used campsites are nearby.

Past the meadow, continue downstream through mostly open, rocky terrain, following the trail bending past John Muir Rock. Veer away from the river and hike through widely scattered conifers to a lightly forested flat harboring a number of decent campsites. Just before reaching a steel bridge spanning Piute Creek, a sign indicates your imminent departure from Kings Canyon National Park.

Across the bridge is a junction with the Piute Pass Trail (8,082'; 37.22511°N, 118.83350°W), 3.6 miles from the Goddard Canyon Trail junction. Turn right (north) on rocky trail climbing and then descending briefly to Piute Creek, which may provide the last easily accessible water late in the year until West Pinnacles Creek. The trail keeps to the west side and well above the briskly flowing creek as it ascends moderately and then steeply across a granite nose before reaching a ford of multibranched Turret Creek.

Follow switchbacks across hot, chaparral-covered slopes rewarding hikers with excellent views of highly fractured Pavilion Dome and the surrounding, unnamed domes composing the west end of Glacier Divide. The trail then swings east through a narrowing canyon; crosses a couple of gullies on log bridges; fords tiny West Pinnacles Creek; pursues a steep, rocky course; and then enters moderate lodgepole forest cover on the way to the easy ford of East Pinnacles Creek. Views of the cascading tributary stream are frequent along this section of trail.

From the ford, the trail ascends gently to beautiful Hutchinson Meadow, where there are excellent campsites near the Pine Creek Pass Trail junction (for example, 9,497'; 37.26691°N, 118.78049°W). Fishing for golden and brook trout is reported to be good to excellent. The lovely meadow setting provides fine views of several granite peaks to the east and northwest, including Pilot Knob.

DAY 5 (Hutchinson Meadow to Humphreys Basin, 5.4 miles): Walk through Hutchinson Meadow, going ahead (east) at the junction with the trail into French Canyon and crossing the braided distributaries of French Canyon's creek. Hike along Piute Creek through subalpine gardens and groves of shady lodgepole pine forest. The green meadowlands are rife with color from a wide array of seasonal wildflowers, including paintbrush, shooting star, fleabane, swamp onion, red mountain heather, buttercup, cinquefoil, penstemon, buckwheat, yarrow, senecio, and Douglas phlox. Labrador tea, lemon willow, and alpine willow shrubs complement the verdant grasses and flowers.

Eventually, the climb through Piute Canyon leads through progressively thinning forest into the stunningly beautiful environs of expansive Humphreys Basin, bordered by Glacier Divide to the south and towered over by the Sierra Crest to the east, with 13,986-foot Mount Humphreys the dominant peak to the northeast.

The Piute Pass Trail continues to ascend to the cascading outlet of Desolation Lakes. Below, the Golden Trout Lakes gleam down in the cirque bottom. If headed for campsites on the knolls around Upper Golden Trout Lake (10,846'; 37.24345°N, 118.71506°W; no campfires), about a half mile south depending on the route, leave the main trail hereabouts and find little flats on the knolls around that lake. Lower Golden Trout Lake is closed to camping within 500 feet of the shoreline. Campsites in Humphreys Basin make fine base camps for exploring the area's wonders.

Farther up the Piute Pass Trail is the unsigned but highly visible use trail that heads north to the Desolation Lakes. Those intrigued by the Desolation Lakes' reputation for fishing and those fond of treeless, open camps will find some decent campsites above Lower Desolation Lake (11,200') and on the wind-raked flats among the great white boulders surrounding aptly named Desolation Lake (11,375'), where anglers can ply the waters in search of golden trout. When searching for a campsite, seek a location well away from the trail, as those close to the trail have become greatly overused. Extra layover days could easily be spent exploring the various nooks and crannies of Humphreys Basin—use trails or cross-country routes provide easy access to many of the area's lakes. (The daily mileage is to the Desolation Lakes junction at 11,164'; 37.24812°N, 118.70217°W.)

DAY 6 (Humphreys Basin to North Lake Trailhead, 6.4 miles): Follow Trip 67, Day 8 over Piute Pass to North Lake Campground (9,364'; 37.22731°N, 118.62746°W). There is no parking there, so at least one member in your group must continue 0.6 mile down the road and then left to the parking area (9,279'; 37.23053°N, 118.61867°W).

Sunset at Evolution Lake   Photo by Mike White

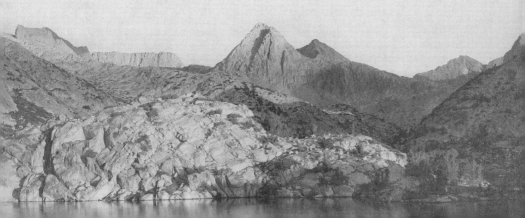

Sabrina Lake Trailhead
9,077'; 37.21363°N, 118.61007°W)

Destination/ GPS Coordinates	Trip Type	Best Season	Pace & Hiking/ Layover Days	Total Mileage	Permit Required
60 Tyee Lakes 37.18161°N 118.57782°W (Tyee Lake 3)	Shuttle (public transport option)	Mid to late	Moderate 2/0	8.1	George Lake (Tyee Lakes in reverse)
61 Midnight Lake 37.16760°N 118.64545°W	Out-and-back	Mid to late	Moderate 2/2	11.8	Sabrina Lake
62 Baboon Lakes 37.17006°N 118.62337°W	Out-and-back	Mid to late	Moderate, part cross-country 2/1	9.4	Sabrina Lake

INFORMATION AND PERMITS: This trailhead is in Inyo National Forest. Permits are required for overnight stays and quotas apply. Permits can be reserved up to six months in advance at recreation.gov (60%; $6 permit reservation fee plus $5 per person) or requested in person, first come, first served, a day in advance (40%; free). All permits must be picked up at one of the Inyo National Forest ranger stations, located in Lone Pine (Eastern Sierra Interagency Visitor Center), Bishop, Mammoth Lakes, and Lee Vining (the Mono Basin Scenic Area Visitor Center). Campfires are prohibited above 10,000 feet, which includes all campsites described for this trailhead. Bear canisters are strongly recommended in this area.

DRIVING DIRECTIONS: In the town of Bishop, turn west from US 395 onto West Line Street (CA 168 East Side). Drive 18 miles southwest to the backpackers' parking, just east of (below) the junction with the road to North Lake. You may want to drop off packs and most of your party at the actual trailhead, a half mile farther up this road on the left (about 300 feet below Lake Sabrina's dam), and then have one of the party park the car and walk back to the trailhead. The apparent mismatch that the Sabrina Lake Trailhead departs from Lake Sabrina is "correct"—the lake is officially "Lake Sabrina" while the trailhead is called "Sabrina Lake Trailhead" at both recreation.gov and on the Inyo National Forest website.

trip 60 Tyee Lakes

Trip Data: 37.18161°N, 118.57782°W (Tyee Lake 3); 8.1 miles; 2/0 days
Topos: Mount Thompson

HIGHLIGHTS: After a night at George Lake, which sees few visitors, this short, steep trail climbs over Table Mountain, enjoying splendid, far-ranging views and carpets of alpine wildflowers. Then it descends through the small and charming Tyee Lakes, an alternate location to spend the night. Sturdy hikers can complete this route as a day hike.

SHUTTLE DIRECTIONS: From the Lake Sabrina Trailhead, drive 3.7 miles back down CA 168 to the South Lake Road junction. Turn onto South Lake Road and drive up it for 4.9 miles to the Tyee Lakes Trailhead parking area, a broad pullout on the west side of the road.

If you have only a single car, the Eastern Sierra Transit Shuttle provides a way to shuttle between the trailheads. See estransit.com/routes-schedule/community-routes/bishop-creek-shuttle for the current schedule.

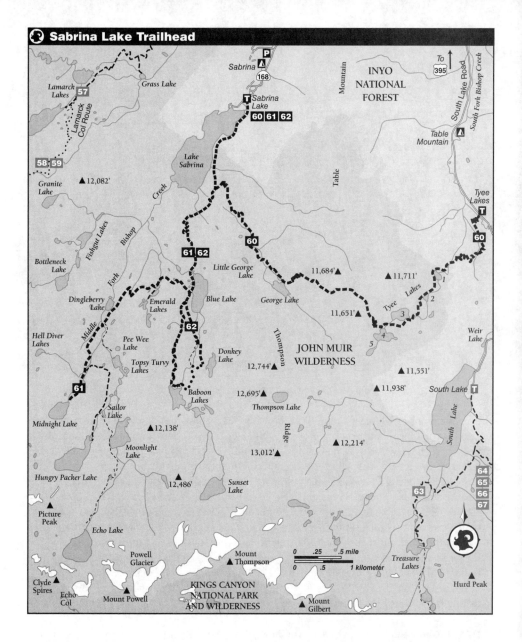

DAY 1 (Sabrina Lake Trailhead to George Lake, 3.1 miles): From the trailhead, the well-used Sabrina Basin Trail climbs generally south above Sabrina Dam and begins a long traverse of the slope above the blue expanses of Lake Sabrina. The route is initially through lush greenery and over small streams, but it soon strikes out across the dry, sunny hillside above the lake. Here, there is only a sparse cover of aspen, juniper, various pines, and mountain mahogany.

The trail undulates gently until about halfway along the lake, then ascends steadily across an open talus slope to a junction where the trail to George and Tyee Lakes branches left (east), heading uphill, while the main Sabrina Basin Trail continues right (south; 9,420′; 37.19981°N, 118.61674°W). Turn onto the George Lake Trail and follow its switchbacks up an open, exposed hillside for more than a half mile before reaching welcome

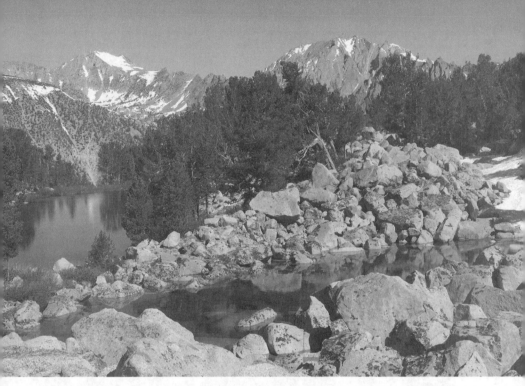

View to the Sierra Crest from near George Lake   Photo by Elizabeth Wenk

denser clumps of whitebark pine. Take a breather and enjoy the expansive views over the Lake Sabrina basin and south and west to the Sierra Crest. You continue to climb quite steeply up the dry, rocky slope beside the tumbling creek, ultimately climbing 1,000 feet over 1.0 mile, a very steep clip for a Sierra trail. Then the gradient abruptly eases and you are walking through pleasant lodgepole pine forest beside the now meadow-bound and meandering creek as you ascend this glacier-carved valley nestled between the imposing escarpments of Table Mountain and Thompson Ridge. You soon cross the George Lake outlet stream on a small footbridge, skirt the southern periphery of a larger meadow, and recross the creek on rocks. Then the trail veers right (southeast); climbs to the side of a sloping, willowed meadow; rises another sandy 100 vertical feet; and suddenly arrives at George Lake (10,737′; 37.18577°N, 118.60271°W; no campfires). There are fine campsites near the trail on the northeast side of the lake beneath scattered whitebark pines, and fishing is good for brook trout.

DAY 2 (George Lake to Tyee Lakes Trailhead, 5.0 miles): Before reaching the east end of George Lake, the trail turns left (northeast) to ascend slopes of granite sand dotted with whitebark pine. Twelve tight switchbacks positioned in a broad gully between cliff bands carry you up 500 feet in just under 0.5 mile, a similar gradient to your ascent above Lake Sabrina. As you climb, your views west keep improving, although Thompson Ridge blocks those to the south. After a brief respite, another 0.5-mile ascent leads to the top of Table Mountain; the nearly flat mesa is a surreal change in topography after the rugged climb. This broad plateau, extending nearly 4 miles to the north, is an unglaciated landform, just as is Coyote Ridge, the next crest to the east. On both of these ridges there exists an unusually great diversity of tundra plants, for the bedrock was not scoured clear of soil during the Pleistocene glaciations. A botanist will readily find 50 species in these seemingly barren sands—especially near the seeps with year-round water. Alpine lewisia, condensed phlox,

Nuttall's sandwort, pygmy fleabane daisy, Peirson's serpentweed, Sierra arnica, whorled penstemon, and peak saxifrage are just a few that you might see. The trail becomes nearly level before reaching its high point (11,589'; 37.18470°N, 118.59155°W). From here, your westward views, from north to south, include Mount Humphreys, Merriam Peak, Royce Peak, Mount Emerson, Mount Lamarck, and Mount Darwin, while to the south you see Mount Agassiz, Mount Sill, and North Palisade.

From the broad sandy plateau, you are then funneled toward the shallow drainage that bisects Table Mountain. Where the little valley narrows and steepens, a trail becomes obvious on the right side of the creek. This tiny water-table-fed trickle usually persists all summer, irrigating a corn lily meadow in the broad swale. Just before the creek drops into a gorge, there is a beautiful lunch spot beside the stream with a commanding view of the largest Tyee Lake. Once the slope's gradient increases, the trail begins switchbacking down through sand and gravel; in places parallel trails may exist, for this trail is infrequently maintained and hikers easily etch alternate routes in the soft substrate—stick to the main trail.

Soon the winding route reaches the uppermost trailside Tyee Lake (Lake 4; 11,015'), with some just-acceptable campsites on its northern side; most of the terrain is a little sloping. Climbing ever so slightly, the trail crosses the outlet stream and descends to the next lake (Lake 3; 10,914')—notice how glaciers etched out a series of bedrock basins, each holding one of the Tyee Lakes behind a bedrock dam. Beside the outlet of Lake 3 are some good campsites near a very picturesque, rock-dotted pond (10,918'; 37.18161°N, 118.57782°W; no campfires).

Beyond these campsites, the path again winds downcanyon. A set of switchbacks takes you to small, shallow, partly reed-filled Lake 2 (10,612'), with just a few small tent sites on a rocky knob on its eastern side. Descending the next cluster of switchbacks, you suddenly enter more continuous lodgepole pine forest and drop to the willow-encapsulated shores of Lake 1 (10,325'). The willow thickets block access to the shores, but soon after you leave the lake there are some good campsites between the trail and the outlet stream.

Now past the lakes, your moderate descent continues through increasingly dense forest. In a half mile, the trail fords the creek again (via a log) and then switchbacks down in a generally eastward direction, crossing another stream soon after. The descent continues on dusty switchbacks down an often-steep hillside, ducking in and out of forest cover and then back between low bluffs. You finally cross a bridge over the South Fork Bishop Creek to the Tyee Lakes Trailhead (9,057'; 37.19590°N, 118.56477°W) on the South Lake Road. For reference, you are 2.2 miles downhill of the South Lake parking area.

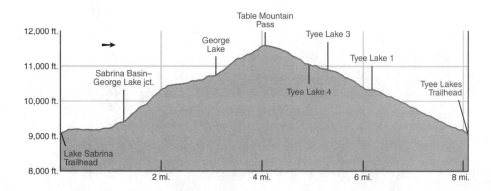

see
map on
p. 325

trip 61 **Midnight Lake**

Trip Data: 37.16760°N, 118.64545°W; 11.8 miles; 2/2 days
Topos: *Mount Thompson, Mount Darwin*

HIGHLIGHTS: The lakes at the head of the Middle Fork Bishop Creek drainage, colloquially considered part of the Lake Sabrina basin, are the eastern Sierra at its finest. A moderate walk with less than 2,000 feet of elevation gain takes you to a timberline wonderland of granite slabs and endless lakes (with brook and/or rainbow trout) ringed by craggy, evocative summits. Meadow strips host a rainbow of diminutive wildflowers and trickles of water criss-cross the landscape.

DAY 1 (Sabrina Lake Trailhead to Midnight Lake, 5.9 miles): After a brief set of switchbacks, the trail flattens, contouring across mostly open, sandy slopes just above Lake Sabrina. About 0.75 mile into the hike, the trail executes a pair of short switchbacks and begins a traversing ascent, with the mountain mahogany scrub and conifers (many dead) soon yielding to bare slopes. At 1.25 miles from the trailhead you meet a junction with a trail that leads steeply uphill (east, left) to George and Tyee Lakes (Trip 60).

You stay right (southwest), on the main track, and quickly ford George Lake's vigorous outlet; you can usually balance across on rocks. Beyond, you begin ascending moderate-to-steep switchbacks beneath whitebark pine cover, step across a tiny seasonal channel, and surmount a glacial-polished slab ridge with splendid views the length of Lake Sabrina. After winding a stretch up the ridge, the trail curves south, gradually converging with a ravine. Crossing the gully, the trail completes a set of tight zigzags among talus blocks and soon approaches the north end of Blue Lake. After passing spurs to campsites along the lake's northeastern shore, the trail makes a short descent to Blue Lake's outlet, 2.9 miles from the trailhead and crossed on a log jam (10,395').

Now the trail winds through granite outcrops on the lake's west side, passing a selection of beautiful shoreline slabs perfect for a break as well as sandy campsites beneath scattered whitebark pines. About midway along the lake is a trail junction (10,414'; 37.18433°N, 118.62163°W), where you turn right (northwest) toward Dingleberry and Midnight Lakes, while left (south) leads to Donkey and Baboon Lakes (Trip 62).

Your trail heads northwest, following forested strips between rounded slab ribs, winding slightly upward as required by the topography, and then crossing the top of a steep talus slope onto a narrow granite ledge. You then rock-hop across the Emerald Lakes' outlet creek and skirt the northwestern border of the lowest of the reedy Emerald Lakes. Where the trail curves west to cross the next rounded granite rib, you could continue up to the higher Emerald Lakes and campsites. The main route snakes south and west across granite slabs, following convenient fracture-delineated corridors, to Dingleberry Lake, ultimately angling down to the lake's southeastern corner. On slabs just south of the lake you'll find abundant

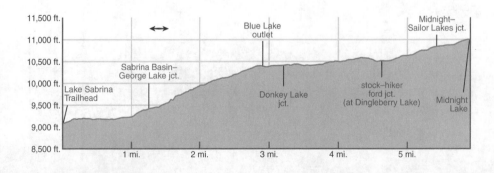

campsites, although Dingleberry Lake has grassy shores and consequently a healthy (and hungry) early-season mosquito population. The view is stunning: pyramidal-shaped Picture Peak stands behind unseen Hungry Packer Lake, while Clyde Spires and Mount Haeckel, on the Sierra Crest, stick out to either side.

Just past Dingleberry Lake you reach a minor junction, where hikers are directed right (west) to ford the Middle Fork Bishop Creek on blocky rocks, while stock users head left to a broad sandy crossing (10,520'; 37.18071°N, 118.63773°W). *Note:* If you wish to visit little Pee Wee Lake or islet-dotted Topsy Turvy Lake in their barren talus basin, it is best to stay on the north side of the creek; you'll soon pick up a use trail that continues up the creek bank to these lakes. Across the creek, the stock and foot routes rejoin and you soon step across a minor tributary and follow its banks southward through alpine turf and across slabs, before trending a little southeast back to the main Middle Fork Bishop Creek corridor. Soon, the trail bypasses an unsigned spur trail, an old route toward Pee Wee Lake. You continue straight ahead (south-southwest) on the main trail, climbing back up slab ribs. Now in the upper basin, the beautiful polished, bright white granite slab ribs scattered with glacial erratics (stray boulders) are ubiquitous and whitebark pine cover is retreating. A few moderate switchbacks and streamside ascent lead to a signed trail junction, now 5.4 miles from the trailhead, where you go right (southwest) up a side canyon to Midnight Lake, while left continues up the main Middle Fork Bishop Creek drainage to Hungry Packer (1.25 miles distant; another basin-enclosed lake with a few campsites), Sailor Lake (0.9 mile distant; excellent campsites on broad granite slabs), and Moonlight Lake (1.3 miles distant, in part off-trail; gorgeous jewel-blue lake, but limited campsites). Almost immediately, the trail fords—on rocks and logs—the outflow creek from the Hell Diver Lakes, sitting far above you in their own barren granite basin. Beyond, the path comes to a tarn and then climbs easily over granite shelves and quickly reaches Midnight

Midnight Lake   Photo by Elizabeth Wenk

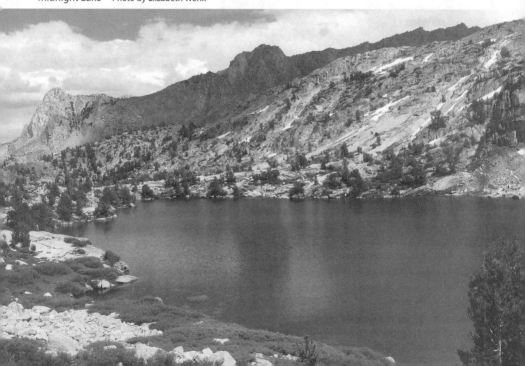

Lake, a brook trout fishery (10,988'; 37.16760°N, 118.64545°W; no campfires). The lake lies at treeline in a granite bowl with sheer sides stretching upward to the Sierra Crest, famous Mount Darwin guarding its head. A mountain stream tumbles down a grass-edged course to the lake's western shore. Just below the outlet are deep, inviting pools. Excellent camping possibilities begin at the aforementioned tarn and continue among the whitebark pines to the lake's outlet. One or more layover days to explore the other lakes in the upper basin are strongly recommended. You could contentedly spend two additional days here, camping at other lakes or exploring for the day, perhaps even following a use trail as far as sublime Echo Lake, harboring rainbow trout.

"DRUNKEN SAILOR LAKE"

Peter Browning's book *Place Names of the Sierra Nevada* (Wilderness Press) is a wonderful source of information on this subject, and the following information comes from it. Browning writes that Art and John Schober ran a pack station on Bishop Creek, stocked the lakes, and mined in the eastern Sierra in the 1930s and 1940s. They were also responsible for most of the colorful names in this basin. As reported by Art Schober's wife: "There was an old sailor who hung out around the Lake Sabrina lodge. When the packers went up to this little lake [Sailor Lake] to stock it with fish, they found the sailor there sleeping off the effects of too much drink." Sailor Lake was labeled "Drunken Sailor Lake" on the 1983 7.5' quad, but before and since then, it has been simply Sailor Lake. John Schober named Baboon Lakes for a group of Civilian Conservation Corps boys he saw there, looking "like a bunch of baboons" as they were waving their arms and going over the rocks. John also named Hungry Packer Lake, this time for an episode in the 1930s when he and his party, while stocking this lake and Midnight Lake, were caught by nightfall here and "had to spend the night without blankets or food." Guess for whom the Schober Lakes are named.

DAY 2 (Midnight Lake to Sabrina Lake Trailhead, 5.9 miles): Retrace your steps.

---

trip 62   **Baboon Lakes**

see map on p. 325

    Trip Data: 37.17006°N, 118.62337°W; 9.4 miles; 2/1 days
    Topos: *Mount Thompson, Mount Darwin*

HIGHLIGHTS: The vast majority of visitors to the Lake Sabrina basin head to Hungry Packer, Moonlight, and Midnight Lakes in the western part of the basin, leaving the Baboon Lakes perfect for those seeking solitude. There is only a use trail for the final stretch to Baboon Lakes, making this hike a perfect introduction to cross-country travel for confident trail hikers who want to explore farther afield.

HEADS UP! *This trip requires some cross-country travel. There is only day-use parking at the trailhead itself; overnight hikers must park their cars 0.5 mile down the Lake Sabrina Road in long pullouts on either side of the road.*

DAY 1 (Sabrina Lake Trailhead to Baboon Lakes, 4.6 miles, part cross-country): After a brief set of switchbacks, the trail flattens, contouring across mostly open, sandy slopes just above Lake Sabrina. At 0.75 mile into the hike, the trail executes a pair of short switchbacks and begins a traversing ascent, with the mountain mahogany scrub and conifers (many dead) soon yielding to bare slopes. At 1.25 miles from the trailhead you meet a trail that leads steeply uphill (east, left) to George and Tyee Lakes (Trip 60).

You stay right (southwest), on the main track, and quickly ford George Lake's vigorous outlet; you can usually balance across on rocks. Beyond, you begin ascending moderate-to-steep switchbacks beneath whitebark pine cover, step across a tiny seasonal channel, and surmount a glacial-polished slab ridge with splendid views the length of Lake Sabrina. After winding a stretch up the ridge, the trail curves south, gradually converging with a ravine. Crossing the gully, the trail completes a set of tight zigzags among talus blocks and soon approaches the north end of Blue Lake. After passing spurs to campsites along the lake's northeastern shore, the trail makes a short descent to Blue Lake's outlet, 2.9 miles from the trailhead and crossed on a log jam (10,395').

Now the trail winds through granite outcrops on the lake's west side, passing a selection of beautiful shoreline slabs perfect for a break and sandy campsites beneath scattered whitebark pines. About midway along the lake is a trail junction (10,414'; 37.18433°N, 118.62163°W), where right (northwest) leads to Dingleberry and Moonlight Lakes (Trip 61), while this trip continues straight ahead (left; south), signposted for Donkey Lake. Diverging slightly from the lakeshore, continue just another 0.15 mile through granite-slab and forested terrain, to reach a signless post and some cryptic lines of rock. Here, left (south-southeast) leads to Donkey Lake (also with campsites) and right (south-southwest) is the most direct route to the Baboon Lakes—although you could go either direction and indeed the trip is described as a loop beyond this point, returning via the other trail.

Past this junction the tread is narrow, basically a use trail, winding up sparsely forested slopes. At about 10,800 feet the surrounding terrain steepens and you continue along grassy benches and through corridors constrained by granite bluffs, now high above the valley. At about 11,060 feet is the first place the trail becomes indistinct (37.17357°N, 118.62477°W). Here you need to cut more to the southeast (left), away from the cliff face you have been following and round a slight rib, before merging onto a second shelf. Finally, a short downhill leads to the lovely Baboon Lakes, set beneath steep Thompson Ridge.

The lowest Baboon Lake is the largest, but just upstream are two more lakes and a clutch of tarns. And for the true adventurer—maybe without a pack on your layover day—turquoise-watered Sunset Lake lies another mile up the drainage. The best-used campsites are along lower Baboon Lake's northern shore (11,005'; 37.17006°N, 118.62337°W; no campfires), with some additional options tucked among whitebark pines just southeast of the log-jammed outlet.

DAY 2 (Baboon Lakes to Sabrina Lake Trailhead, 4.8 miles, part cross-country): From the lowest Baboon Lake you can return to Lake Sabrina the way you came—this is the easiest option—or take a slightly longer and more rugged route that leads past Donkey Lake. For

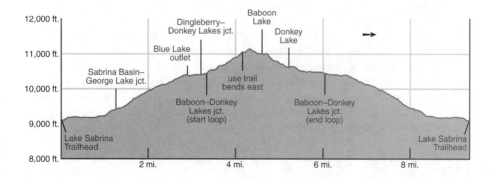

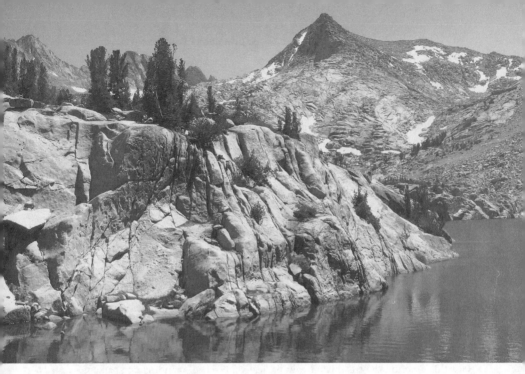

Baboon Lake   Photo by Elizabeth Wenk

the second option, cross to the east side of the outlet on an impressive log jam and then turn right (southeast) and follow a sandy passageway over a shallow rib, landing one gully east of the outlet creek. A minimal use trail descends this chute, snaking between willows. Where there is a break in the slabs to the west (left), head farther left and follow a shallower corridor that leads back to the Baboon Lakes outlet creek; you should now be on a fairly obvious use trail again.

Just as you reach the creek (10,712'; 37.17294°N, 118.62093°W) you are faced with a minor trail junction and a choice—crossing the creek and continuing along the left (west) bank is the most direct route back to Blue Lake (and the trailhead), while a sharp right (east) leads back away from the creek to Donkey Lake. Head right, unless you're in a hurry. After climbing just briefly, you descend a shallow slope, wending along sandy strips between polished slab outcrops. Near a small tarn—and to its north—the terrain is quite flat, suitable for camping (for example, 10,652'; 37.17431°N, 118.61869°W; no campfires). Just beyond, you spy Donkey Lake, lying in a basin beneath steep Thompson Ridge, with giant talus fans spilling into the lake. Aficionados of lake swimming will find a 15-foot jump into very deep (and cold) water.

Near the aforementioned tarn (just west of Donkey Lake) you should pick up a better-built trail—it leads gradually back toward the Baboon Lakes outlet creek, crossing it on a pair of logs on the north side of a marshy lodgepole pine flat. Just across is an indistinct junction (10,518'; 37.17655°N, 118.62001°W), where left leads back toward the Baboon Lakes, while you take a sharp right, climb a few steps, and then begin a long, mostly descending traverse back toward Blue Lake. At 1.6 miles into your day—although you've likely spent many hours on your explorations—you reach the junction with the unsigned post and lines of rocks and now continue north (right), retracing your steps from Day 1 to Blue Lake and onto the Sabrina Lake Trailhead.

Tyee Lakes Trailhead
9,057'; 37.19590°N, 118.56477°W

Destination/ GPS Coordinates	Trip Type	Best Season	Pace & Hiking/ Layover Days	Total Mileage	Permit Required
60 Tyee Lakes (in reverse of description, see page 324)	Shuttle (public transport option)	Mid to late	Moderate 2/0	8.1	Tyee Lakes (George Lake as described)

INFORMATION AND PERMITS: This trailhead is in Inyo National Forest. Permits are required for overnight stays and quotas apply. Permits can be reserved up to six months in advance at recreation.gov (60%; $6 permit reservation fee plus $5 per person) or requested in person, first come, first served, a day in advance (40%; free). All permits must be picked up at one of the Inyo National Forest ranger stations, located in Lone Pine (Eastern Sierra Interagency Visitor Center), Bishop, Mammoth Lakes, and Lee Vining (the Mono Basin Scenic Area Visitor Center). Campfires are prohibited above 10,000 feet, which includes all campsites described for this trailhead. Bear canisters are strongly recommended in this area.

DRIVING DIRECTIONS: In the town of Bishop, from the junction of US 395 (Main Street) and CA 168 (West Line Street), turn west onto CA 168. Drive 15 miles to the signed junction with South Lake Road. Turn left onto South Lake Road and drive an additional 4.9 miles to the Tyee Lakes Trailhead parking area, a broad pullout on the west side of the road.

Bishop Pass Trailhead (at South Lake)
9,825'; 37.16934°N, 118.56580°W

Destination/ GPS Coordinates	Trip Type	Best Season	Pace & Hiking/ Layover Days	Total Mileage	Permit Required
63 Treasure Lakes 37.14522°N 118.57544°W	Out-and-back	Mid to late	Leisurely 2/1	5.8	Treasure Lakes
64 Chocolate Lakes 37.14841°N 118.54932°W	Semiloop	Mid to late	Leisurely 2/0	6.8	Bishop Pass– South Lake
65 Dusy Basin 37.10369°N 118.55158°W (Lake 11,347)	Out-and-back	Mid to late	Moderate 2/1	14.0	Bishop Pass– South Lake
66 Palisade Basin 37.08201°N 118.50601°W (Glacier Creek Lake 11,673)	Semiloop	Mid to late	Strenuous 6/2	37.4	Bishop Pass– South Lake
67 South Lake to North Lake 37.11205°N 118.67093°W (Muir Pass)	Shuttle (public transport option)	Mid to late	Moderate 8/1	55.0	Bishop Pass– South Lake (Piute Pass in reverse)

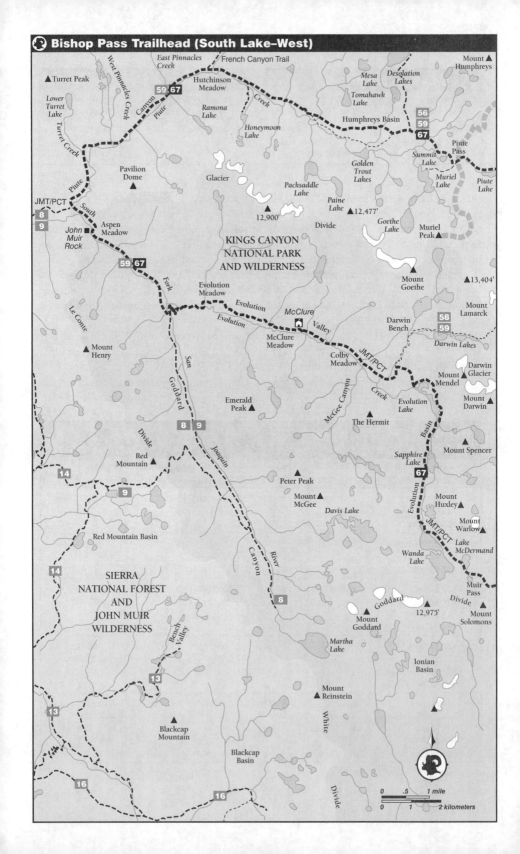

Mount Humphreys

Turret Peak

West Pinnacles Creek

East Pinnacles Creek

French Canyon Trail

Mesa Lake

Desolation Lakes

Lower Turret Lake

59 67

Hutchinson Meadow

Tomahawk Lake

Ramona Lake

Creek

Humphreys Basin

56
59
67

Turret Creek

Piute

Canyon

Honeymoon Lake

Summit Lake

Piute Pass

Pavilion Dome

Glacier

Packsaddle Lake

Golden Trout Lakes

Muriel Lake

Piute Lake

Paine Lake

▲12,477'

Goethe Lake

Muriel Peak ▲

JMT/PCT

8
9

Piute

South

Divide

Fork

John Muir Rock

Aspen Meadow

59 67

KINGS CANYON
NATIONAL PARK
AND WILDERNESS

12,900'

Mount Goethe

▲13,404'

Le Conte

Evolution Meadow

Evolution

Evolution

McClure

Valley

Darwin Bench

58
59

Mount Lamarck

Darwin Lakes

Mount Henry

San

Goddard

McClure Meadow

Colby Meadow

Creek

JMT/PCT

Mount Mendel

Darwin Glacier

Emerald Peak ▲

McGee Canyon

Evolution Lake

Mount Darwin ▲

Divide

8 9

The Hermit

Basin

Mount Spencer

Red Mountain ▲

Joaquin

Sapphire Lake

14

9

Peter Peak ▲

67

Mount Huxley ▲

Red Mountain Basin

Mount McGee ▲

Davis Lake

Evolution

Mount Warlow ▲

JMT/PCT

Lake McDermand

Canyon

River

Wanda Lake

14

SIERRA
NATIONAL FOREST
AND
JOHN MUIR
WILDERNESS

Bench Valley

8

Goddard

12,975'

Muir Pass

Divide

Mount Solomons

Mount Goddard ▲

13

Martha Lake

Ionian Basin

13

Mount Reinstein ▲

Blackcap Mountain ▲

White

Blackcap Basin

16

Divide

16

0   .5   1 mile
0   1   2 kilometers

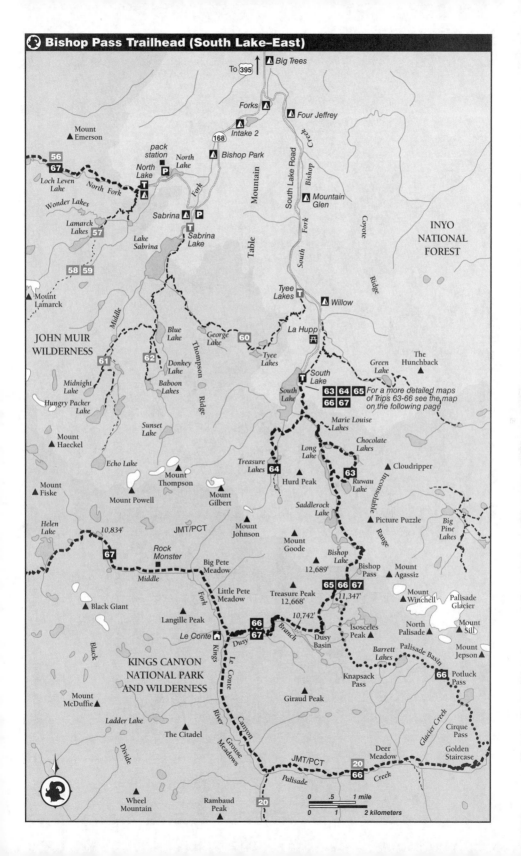

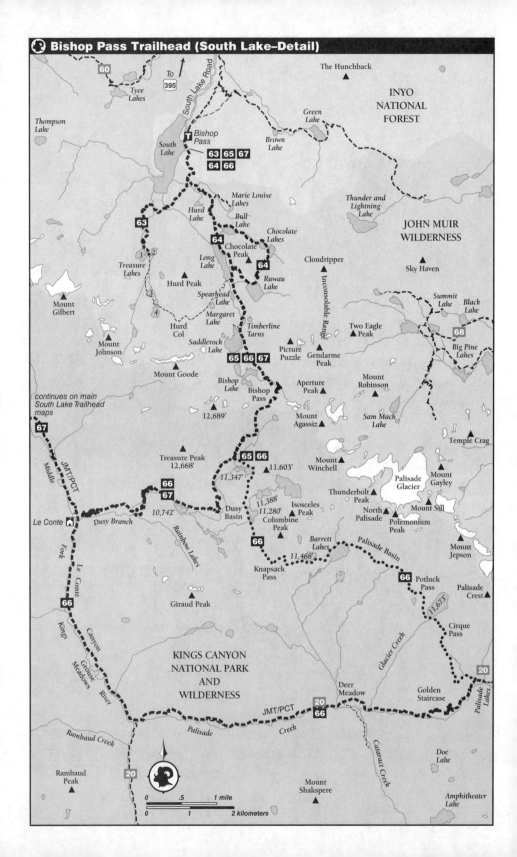

INFORMATION AND PERMITS: This trailhead is in Inyo National Forest. Permits are required for overnight stays and quotas apply. Permits can be reserved up to six months in advance at recreation.gov (60%; $6 permit reservation fee plus $5 per person) or requested in person, first come, first served, a day in advance (40%; free). All permits must be picked up at one of the Inyo National Forest ranger stations, located in Lone Pine (Eastern Sierra Interagency Visitor Center), Bishop, Mammoth Lakes, and Lee Vining (the Mono Basin Scenic Area Visitor Center). If you plan to use a stove or have a campfire, you must also have a California campfire permit, available from a forest service office or online at preventwildfireca.org/campfire-permit. Campfires are prohibited above 10,400 feet in Inyo National Forest (east of the Sierra Crest) and above 10,000 feet in Kings Canyon National Park (west of the Sierra Crest). Bear canisters are required east of Bishop Pass (Trips 63 and 64) and in Dusy Basin (Trip 65 and part of Trips 66 and 67).

DRIVING DIRECTIONS: In the town of Bishop, from the junction of US 395 (Main Street) and CA 168 (West Line Street), take CA 168 west. Drive 15 miles to the signed junction with South Lake Road. Turn left onto South Lake Road and drive an additional 7.1 miles to the road-end parking area above South Lake (a reservoir). Note that some parking spots are day use only. If the overnight parking spots are full, a common midsummer occurrence, you must park 1.3 miles down South Lake Road (just below the pack station), in extensive roadside pullouts, and then walk up the road to the trailhead. The trailhead is adjacent to a large information sign, just east of the restrooms.

trip 63   Treasure Lakes

see maps on p. 335–336

> **Trip Data:** 37.14522°N, 118.57544°W (lowest Treasure Lake);
> 5.8 miles; 2/1 days
> **Topos:** *Mount Thompson*

HIGHLIGHTS: Few trips offer so much High Sierra beauty for so little effort. Not only is there a wealth of dramatic scenery, there's also good camping and fishing. This trip also makes a good day hike.

DAY 1 (Bishop Pass Trailhead at South Lake to lowest Treasure Lake, 2.9 miles): Starting just left of the information sign, the trail crosses an unmapped creeklet and meets the trail climbing from the pack station; turn right here, heading south. The trail descends slightly toward South Lake and then immediately begins a steady climb up the sandy slope rising from the shore with splendid views across the lake. Soon out of sight of the lake, you wind upward, through pocket meadows and conifer stands.

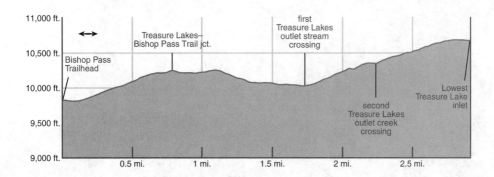

The trail presently reaches a junction where you turn right (southwest) onto the trail signposted for Treasure Lakes, while the main Bishop Pass Trail continues left (southeast; Trips 64–67). Dropping down a sandy slope, the trail crosses a flower-lined tributary creek on a small plank bridge, ascends briefly, then continues a gentle descent through open lodgepole and whitebark pine forest that offers filtered views to Hurd Peak and Thompson Ridge. Continuing its westward traverse, the trail soon crosses the South Fork Bishop Creek on a more substantial bridge, steps across a seasonal tributary, and mounts a minor rib to reach the Treasure Lakes drainage.

You briefly parallel the Treasure Lakes' outlet stream downward, enjoying the dense shade and carpet of Labrador tea, then cross the creek on a planed two-log bridge. Beyond, the trail quickly begins to switchback up, channeled between broken granite bluffs. Roseroot, mountain pride penstemon, fireweed, and Sierra arnica color the otherwise gray, gravelly slopes as you zigzag diligently upward, surmounting many a big step. Slowly the fractured rock transitions to smoother granite slabs dotted with glacial erratic boulders and you cross the Treasure Lakes outflow on another planed-log bridge. Surrounded by steep granite cirques, the views from here are stupendous. The glaciers readily plucked out chunks of the fractured rock, creating the magnificently steep walls that surround you: Hurd Peak sits to the southeast and Gilbert Peak to the southwest. Passing a clutch of heath-ringed tarns, the trail embarks on another series of switchbacks to reach the lowest Treasure Lake (10,668'; Lake 1). Most campsites near this lake do not abide by Leave No Trace tenets, for they are too close to water or on vegetation; instead, seek out the sites on the knob to the east (for example, 10,693'; 37.14704°N, 118.57567°W; no campfires). This lake, the largest in the Treasure Lakes basin (12 acres), affords fair-to-good fishing for golden-rainbow hybrids. There are additional campsites at fishless Lake 11,159 (Lake 3); see the sidebar on the facing page. The listed mileage ends where you ford the lowest lake's inlet stream—usually a wade.

Treasure Lake 1   Photo by Elizabeth Wenk

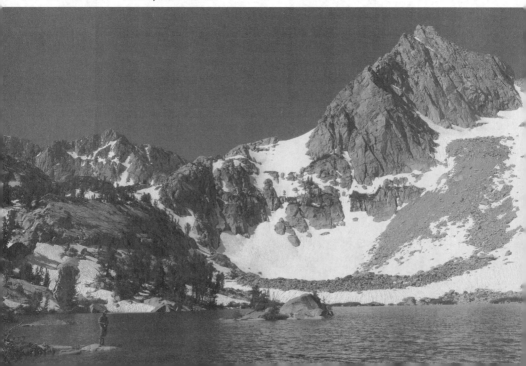

DAY 2 (lowest Treasure Lake to Bishop Pass Trailhead at South Lake, 2.9 miles): Retrace your steps.

CROSS-COUNTRY SEMILOOP

Adventurous hikers can make a semiloop of this trip by adding a cross-country segment and returning on the main Bishop Pass Trail. This option adds 2.7 miles and many hours to Day 2. After fording the creek separating Lake 1 and Lake 2, a use trail leads up a bedrock rib and then alongside Lake 2's inlet stream. The trail becomes fainter and disappears in stretches; aim for Lake 3 (11,159'), where you'll stumble upon a large collection of splendid sandy campsites among whitebark pines (for example, 11,192'; 37.13843°N, 118.57628°W; no campfires). The use trail proceeds around the western shore of this lake and the next one upstream, then cuts across the outlet of Lake 11,175 (Lake 4) and begins climbing the rocky, sandy slope to Hurd Col (11,731'; 37.13253°N, 118.56867°W).

While a passable use trail exists up the western slope to this saddle, the eastern side of Hurd Col is steeper and rockier and mostly lacks a worn tread; you descend slabs and work your way down narrow gullies between steeper bluffs to reach Margaret Lake. Overall, from the saddle, descend north-northeast about 300 feet and then veer over to a little stream, paralleling it momentarily beside a short waterfall. From there, work almost directly down to Margaret Lake's northwest side (10,968'; 37.13535°N, 118.55988°W) to find a use trail that leads northeast to the southernmost point of Long Lake. Ford the inlet, go east past campsites, and meet the Bishop Pass Trail; turn left (north) on it. Return to the trailhead, staying on the Bishop Pass Trail at all junctions (Trip 65 for a description in reverse). It is 2.0 miles to the Treasure Lakes–Bishop Pass Trail junction, then an additional 0.8 mile to the trailhead.

---

trip 64 **Chocolate Lakes**

see maps on p. 335–336

Trip Data: 37.14841°N, 118.54932°W (Lowest Chocolate Lake); 6.8 miles; 2/0 days

Topos: *Mount Thompson*

HIGHLIGHTS: Like Trip 63 to the Treasure Lakes, this trip offers abundant, dramatic High Sierra scenery for relatively little effort and can be done as a day hike. The lakes are named for the striking peak just west of them, Chocolate Peak, which looks from the north like a chocolate sundae, and can easily be ascended from the midpoint of the hike for far-reaching views. The trail is rough between the upper Chocolate Lake and Ruwau Lake, but not difficult to follow.

DAY 1 (Bishop Pass Trailhead at South Lake to Lower Chocolate Lake, 2.5 miles): Starting just left of the information sign, the trail crosses an unmapped creeklet and meets the trail climbing from the pack station; turn right here, heading south. The trail descends slightly toward South Lake and then immediately begins a steady climb up the sandy slope rising from the shore with splendid views across the lake. Soon out of sight of the lake, you wind upward, through pocket meadows and conifer stands. At the signed junction to the Treasure Lakes, 0.8 mile into your walk, turn left (southeast), while right (southwest) leads to the Treasure Lakes (Trip 63). You switchback upward beneath lodgepole pine cover, cross a stream on a small footbridge, and reach a trail junction where you stay right (south), while left (northeast) is a minor lateral to the Marie Louise Lakes.

Onward, you climb tight switchbacks tucked beneath bluffs and ascend a shallow gully to a trail junction where the Bishop Pass Trail continues straight ahead (right; south), while you turn left (east), signposted for the Chocolate Lakes. You drop into an incised gully and then climb beside blocky outcrops, quickly reaching scenic Bull Lake (10,778'), set beneath the north face of Chocolate Peak and with excellent views west to Hurd Peak. There are scattered small campsites beneath whitebark pines and fishing for brook and rainbow trout. Continuing, skirt Bull Lake's shoreline to its flowery inlet stream and then climb beside its bubbling course, ascending into the narrow valley between Chocolate Peak and the rugged Inconsolable Range. Over-the-shoulder views are also splendid.

The best campsites at the lowest Chocolate Lake are to the northwest of the outlet under tall whitebark pines (10,991'; 37.14841°N, 118.54932°W; no campfires), easily missed as the trail bypasses the outlet on the far side of a shallow ridge. This lake and its two higher companions support a brook trout fishery. There is also a selection of small campsites nestled beneath stunted, many-trunked whitebark pines at the middle lake (11,065'), but the highest lake (11,074'), which sits in an enclosed basin right at the foot of the Inconsolable Range, has no campsites.

DAY 2 (Lowest Chocolate Lake to Bishop Pass Trailhead at South Lake, 4.3 miles): From the lowest Chocolate Lake, the trail continues across broken slab and small, red metamorphic talus, stepping across the creek and looping clockwise around the middle lake. Along its northern shore are campsites with good lake access. The trail is increasingly faint as it cuts toward the upper Chocolate Lake, fording the interconnecting stream in a thicket of willows. The track is more like a use trail as it rounds the upper lake's west side, becoming yet rougher as it climbs steeply toward a saddle on Chocolate Peak's southeast shoulder. Through here the track is braided, repeatedly splitting and merging as people have tried to find a marginally better route; it matters little—just stay right (west) of the meadow strip and climb up and across the sandy slope, where snow can linger into midseason.

The saddle (11,371'; 37.14314°N, 118.54647°W) itself offers decent views, but from the summit of Chocolate Peak the panorama is truly striking. To reach the peak, 0.25 mile distant and with a 300-foot elevation gain, climb up the ridge in a northwesterly direction; the going is always easy—Class 1—with a use trail in parts. Views of the Inconsolable Range, especially the range's high point, rugged, 13,525-foot Cloudripper, are breathtaking, as are the views across the entire South Fork Bishop Creek basin to Bishop Pass.

From the saddle, a rough trail heads down toward Ruwau Lake. Less than 100 feet below the pass the trail seems to vanish in a tongue of talus (11,327'; 37.14240°N, 118.54667°W)— here the trail has actually taken a sharp right (west-trending) turn, and with a moment's search you will quickly pick up the route again as it traverses and then switchbacks down the south slope of Chocolate Peak to pretty Ruwau Lake (11,044'), set at the base of steep cliffs dropping from Picture Puzzle Peak. Ruwau Lake offers only a few tiny one-tent campsites near the outlet. Skirt the lake's north side before descending again, very steeply at the

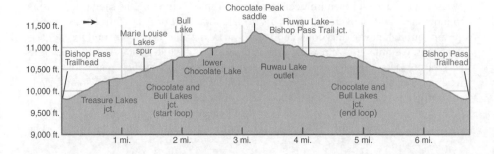

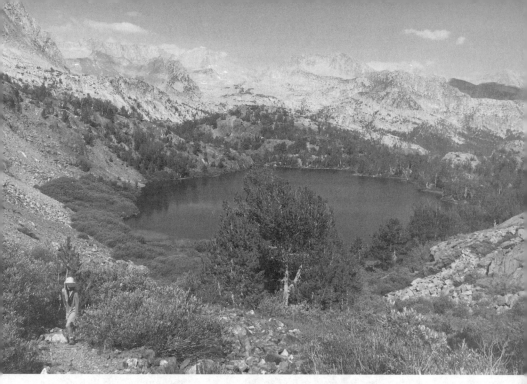

Climbing above Bull Lake toward the Chocolate Lakes   Photo by Elizabeth Wenk

end, to meet the Bishop Pass Trail at beautiful Long Lake (10,763'). Skirting the western base of Chocolate Peak, you first pass a selection of small campsites and the trail then undulates just feet from the lake's east side, soon crossing the Bull Lake outlet creek on big rock blocks. Taking one last backward view to Bishop Pass, the trail climbs just briefly and then drops back to the junction signposted for the Chocolate Lakes, closing the semiloop. Staying left (north), retrace your steps.

trip 65   **Dusy Basin**

see maps on p. 335–336

    Trip Data: 37.10369°N, 118.55158°W (Lake 11,347); 14.0 miles; 2/1 days
       Topos: *Mount Thompson, North Palisade*

HIGHLIGHTS: Ascend the spectacular drainage of the South Fork Bishop Creek on the popular Bishop Pass Trail to enter Kings Canyon National Park and find the high, granite slab country of Dusy Basin and its wonderland of alpine lakes, ponds, streams, and soaring peaks.

DAY 1 (Bishop Pass Trailhead at South Lake to Dusy Basin, 7.0 miles): Starting just left of the information sign, the trail crosses an unmapped creeklet and meets the trail climbing from the pack station; turn right here, heading south. The trail descends slightly toward South Lake and then immediately begins a steady climb up a sandy slope rising above the shore with splendid views across the lake. You wind upward, through pocket meadows and conifer stands, soon out of sight of the lake. At a signed junction 0.8 mile into your walk, turn left (southeast), while right (southwest) leads to the Treasure Lakes (Trip 63). You switchback upward beneath lodgepole pine cover, cross a stream on a small footbridge, and presently reach a trail junction, where you stay right (south), while left (northeast) is a minor lateral to the Marie Louise Lakes.

Onward, you climb tight switchbacks tucked beneath bluffs and ascend a shallow gully to a junction signed for the Chocolate Lakes (left, east; Trip 64). You stay straight ahead (right; south) on the Bishop Pass Trail, which soon levels off at the islet-dotted north end of Long Lake, populated by rainbow, brook, and brown trout. Here you are treated to your first views of the upper basin, most notably Mount Goode's imposing north face. After crossing one of the lake's inlets on big rock blocks, the route first undulates just feet from the lake's east side and then diverges a little from the shore, skirting the base of marble-streaked Chocolate Peak. Here, to either side of the trail, you pass some campsites and soon reach a small trail that leads left (east) to Ruwau Lake. Continue ahead (right; south) on the Bishop Pass Trail to ford Ruwau's outlet, on rocks, and then arrive at well-used campsites on the knolls above Long Lake's southern tip. Fisherman may also want to try their luck along the stream connecting Spearhead and Long Lakes.

Your continued ascent leads up and across a steep talus slope above Spearhead Lake to reach the basin's upper lakes. You first pass the Timberline Tarns, their charm and small campsites mostly hidden from the trail, cross South Fork Bishop Creek on rocks (sometimes a wade), and then climb beside the bubbling creek to reach spectacular Saddlerock Lake (11,128'). Here you'll find scenic, well-used campsites to the northwest of the outlet and bigger, less view-rich options near the lake's northernmost lobe. There is fishing for brook trout. Stepping across South Fork Bishop Creek on a bridge, you proceed around Saddlerock Lake, walk the length of daintily flowered subalpine meadows, and before long meet the unmarked fisherman's spur trail that leads right (southwest) to Bishop Lake (11,240'; exposed campsites among whitebark pines and brook trout).

Beyond Bishop Lake, the trail fords one of that lake's inlets, again on large rock blocks, passes the final timberline whitebark pines, and continues southeast up a shallow rib beneath the imposing cliffs of the Inconsolable Range. Ahead, the trail was rerouted in the early 2010s, for in 2009 giant boulders rolled down the active rock glacier in front of you, obliterating part of the trail. The colossal tongue of rock, more easily visualized on a satellite photo than from the trail, has ice at its center and like a true glacier moves slowly downhill, sometimes shedding rocks down its over-steepened front. Once past the rock glacier you ascend a series of well-engineered, moderate switchbacks at the head of this breathtaking cirque basin. Breather stops offer unforgettable views north across the basin you've just traversed. Once atop the headwall, the ascent moderates and you continue a final 0.3 mile to Bishop Pass (11,977'). Since the pass is broad, views from the pass itself aren't memorable except of Mount Agassiz to the east; you had your best views north before you reached the pass and those to the south improve as you continue.

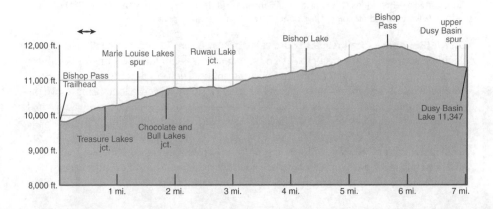

From the pass, the trail cuts west across the alpine tundra, then descends southward on a sandy slope at the base of Peak 12,668, colloquially Treasure Peak. Dusy Basin's lakes are initially hidden by the basin's topography, but as you round the end of the ridge, the trail's orientation shifts to southwest and you enjoy increasingly expansive views over Dusy Basin, its lakes and its encircling peaks. No longer finding the basin barren and dry, you continue down rock-bench systems, your descending traverse interspersed with switchbacks.

Stay alert for an unmarked junction beside a small tarn (11,369'; 37.10481°N, 118.55368°W) with a use trail that cuts southeast across Dusy Basin to the basin's highest big lakes. Take this trail and you'll quite quickly cross a creeklet and approach the basin's northernmost large lake (11,347'; 37.10379°N, 118.55160°W; no campfires; golden and brook trout). Staying a short distance above the lake, follow the trail about 500 feet beyond the creeklet to reach a large campsite on sand and slab with far-reaching views. Other fair campsites can be found at the west end of the lake and to the southwest, along the outlet stream. Whatever site you choose, just be sure to be 100 feet from water and not camped on any vegetation. A very sparse cover of gnarled whitebark pines dots the granite landscape on all sides, and the fractures in the granite have become grassy, heather-lined pockets. The setting at this upper lake is incomparable: The Palisades fill the northeastern skyline, while the southeastern horizon is defined by aptly named Isosceles Peak, more massive Columbine Peak, and Knapsack Pass. Giraud Peak towers in the south, catching the sunrise. What a fitting location to be named for Frank Dusy, a photographer turned shepherd who was one of the first white explorers to reach this basin.

If you want to explore Dusy Basin further—either to find an alternate campsite or on your layover day—continue clockwise around Lake 11,347. At the east end of the lake, follow a ramp up and south to cross the southern end of the ridge that is topped by Peak 11,603 and reach the next shelf, this one harboring the splendid chain of eastern lakes (with golden and brook trout) that encircles Isoceles Peak. Trip 66 describes more distant destinations,

Camping in lower Dusy Basin near Lake 10,742   Photo by Elizabeth Wenk

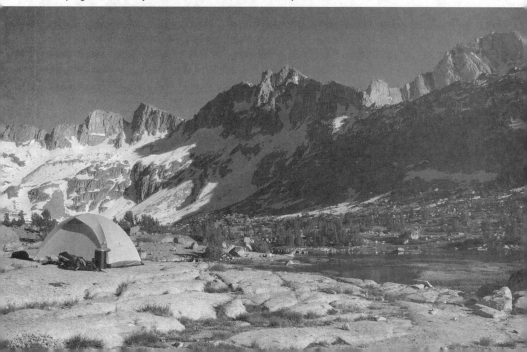

including the Barrett Lakes in the Palisades Basin. Alternatively, if you seek more cover, stay on the main trail and descend another 1.8 miles to Lake 10,742 at the northwestern end of a lower chain of lakes (golden trout); the chain extends southeastward for about a mile from there, and there are ample campsites under slightly denser tree cover, some near the trail (for example, 10,760'; 37.09464°N, 118.56458°W; no campfires) and others farther upstream.

DAY 2 (Dusy Basin to Bishop Pass Trailhead at South Lake, 7.0 miles): Retrace your steps.

see
maps on
p. 335–
336

trip 66 Palisade Basin

> **Trip Data:** 37.08201°N, 118.50601°W (Glacier Creek Lake 11,673);
> 37.4 miles; 6/2 days
> **Topos:** *Mount Thompson, North Palisade, Split Mountain.*

HIGHLIGHTS: The Palisade peaks are justifiably some of the Sierra's most famous summits, and this semiloop takes strong, adventurous hikers past their southern flanks on a well-traveled cross-country route through splendid Palisade Basin. The challenging hike also leads to other famous High Sierra locales along and near the John Muir Trail: the incomparable views of Dusy Basin, the Golden Staircase, and Le Conte Canyon are more than ample rewards for the demands of reaching these landmarks.

HEADS UP! *This strenuous trip is only for backpackers experienced in cross-country navigation with map and compass (and perhaps carrying a GPS unit as well). It is also recommended that you are well acclimated to high altitudes and experienced in carrying a full pack over Class 2 terrain. The cross-country part crosses three trailless passes, with short stretches of easy Class 3 on Cirque Pass. If you find the approach from Dusy Basin to Knapsack Pass at the limit of your ability, consider an out-and-back trip to the Bartlett Lake instead of continuing over Potluck Pass and Cirque Pass, as both these passes are technically more challenging than Knapsack Pass.*

DAY 1 (Bishop Pass Trailhead at South Lake to Dusy Basin, 7.0 miles): Follow Trip 65, Day 1 to Dusy Basin Lake 11,347 (11,347'; 37.10379°N, 118.55160°W; no campfires).

DAY 2 (Dusy Basin to Glacier Creek Lake 11,673, 5.6 miles, cross-country): You can cross into Palisade Basin via any one of three climbers' passes: Knapsack Pass, Isoceles Pass (12,088'; Class 3 on the west side; the saddle between Columbine Peak and Isosceles Peak), and Thunderbolt Pass (12,374'; Class 2, with tedious talus near the top; the notch just southwest of Thunderbolt Peak). The route we describe here uses Knapsack Pass (11,696'), the prominent saddle just south of Columbine Peak that provides the easiest access between Dusy and Palisade Basins.

Hikers likewise have a choice of cross-country routes through Dusy Basin to the base of Knapsack Pass. All aim for the top of a marshy area at about 11,245 feet (very approximately at 37.08963°N, 118.54846°W). Two of the options require that you first descend lower into Dusy Basin and then reascend to Knapsack Pass. These routes are popular with hikers completing the Sierra High Route (Roper's Route), since they are coming up from Le Conte Canyon, but are out of your way. The third option is the most scenic and shortest, and requires the least extra elevation gain, but has a slightly longer use trail section through Dusy Basin—it is the option described here.

Continue around Lake 11,347 to its northeastern corner and turn south, traversing up and across ramps on the slope to its east. You top out at about 11,460 feet (37.09947°N, 118.54990°W) beside a tarn and drop down a spur to the lakelets downstream of Lake 11,388. Crossing another minor saddle deposits you on the shores of Lake 11,280. Although the use trail comes and goes, the terrain through here is not difficult—with careful route-finding you can walk entirely through sandy corridors and across low angle slab. You skirt Lake 11,280's western shore; there are some splendid but small campsites among whitebark pines near the lake's outlet with perfect views to Isoceles Peak, an alternative first night's destination. About 0.2 mile beyond the outlet you reach the top of the aforementioned marshy area.

From here the route winds through some large boulders and then traverses up and across talus slopes. A faint pad or cairns appear from time to time, indicating you're on route. The talus leads to a willow-clad shelf beneath bluffs and then onto fractured slabs that lead south-southeast toward Knapsack Pass. Once on bedrock (about 0.25 mile, in a straight line, from the pass) the trail, of course, disappears, but continuing a south-southeasterly traverse lets you step from one broken slab-ramp to the next without finding yourself in cliffy terrain. Finally, easier, lower-angle slabs lead the final stretch to the pass (11,696'; 37.08367°N, 118.54366°W). Impossible as it may seem, there are recorded visits to Palisade Basin via this pass with stock!

THE VIEW FROM KNAPSACK PASS

To the west you stare across Dusy Basin into the headwaters of the Middle Fork Kings and a ring of peaks: the massive Black Giant, pointed Mount Warlow and Mount Fiske, and farther north, the flatter-topped Mount Powell, and Mount Thompson. Turning to the east you gaze into Palisade Basin and the Palisade Peaks. Your view takes in the Sierra's northern seven summits that exceed 14,000 feet: Thunderbolt Peak, Starlight (North Palisade's northern satellite summit), North Palisade, Polemonium Peak, Mount Sill, Middle Palisade, and Split Mountain. These peaks look, as one climber expressed it, "like mountain peaks are supposed to look." Precipitous faces composed of relatively unfractured rock, spires, couloirs, buttresses, and glaciers (on the crest's northeastern side) combine to make this crest one of the finer mountaineering areas in the Sierra Nevada. From this vantage point, the vast expanse of Palisade Basin appears totally barren of life except for an isolated whitebark pine stretching toward the deep blue sky and small patches of grass.

The secret to descending from Knapsack Pass into Palisade Basin is to keep to the left at first, even climbing a little; you'll notice on the elevation profile for this trip that Knapsack Pass is not the high point. You only begin descending moderately to steeply over talus and down a gully after about 0.2 mile. Once you've dropped about 300 feet, follow your choice of ledge systems to the westernmost large Barrett Lake (Lake 11,468). After passing around the south end of this slab-bound lake (there are some excellent sandy campsites near its southeastern corner if you want a less strenuous day; 11,484'; 37.08431°N, 118.53295°W; no campfires), the route climbs east up slab and grass benches to a broad bedrock rib (more campsites) that overlooks the largest lake of the chain (Lake 11,523) and descends to follow a use track around its north side. From this lake, the dark, sheer pinnacled cliffs of the southwest face of North Palisade dominate the skyline. Beyond the lake, your route continues southeast, climbing just north of the lake's eastern inlet stream over increasingly steep slabs and past several tiny, rockbound lakelets to the saddle just northeast of Point 12,005. Keeping to the left, traverse into the shallow bowl west of Potluck Pass, and pass a small pond (several sandy campsites just to its west). Continuing, ascend splendid slabs to Potluck Pass (12,149'; 37.07964°N, 118.50833°W). Along with the continuing views of the Palisades, this vantage point also looks south across the Palisade Creek watershed to Amphitheater Lake. To the southwest, the terrain is an endless sea of peaks.

The descent from Potluck Pass requires careful route-finding or you'll end up trading straightforward Class 2 slabs and ramps for vertical cliffs. From the pass, locate a ramp that leads south (right) and down. It segues to a series of shorter shelves among bluffs that you work your way down. As soon as possible, head toward a slope of scree and sand; here you'll pick up a use trail that carries you to flatter terrain. (*Note:* If there are lingering snowfields, a less exposed alternative is to continue northeast to a point 0.2 mile farther up the ridge [12,358'; 37.08201°N, 118.50601°W] and then zigzag down a different collection of sloping slab shelves where the snow vanishes earlier.)

Where the descent levels out, a little upstream of a triangular lake, cross sand, meadows, and easy talus, and then ascend gently up slab to the bedrock rib separating the two branches of Glacier Creek. Follow the rib nearly due south until you are directly above the outlet of large Lake 11,673 and then wind down slabs to its outlet. As you approach the lake, you pass a selection of small sandy campsites on knobs overlooking the water (for example, 11,727'; 37.07321°N, 118.50408°W; no campfires) and there are others just below the lake along the outlet (fishing for golden trout). Grassy sections around the sandy-bottomed lake provide a foothold for colorful alpine wildflowers, including yellow Coville's columbine and dainty white mountain heather.

DAY 3 (Glacier Creek Lake 11,673 to Deer Meadow, 5.3 miles, part cross-country): After fording Lake 11,673's outlet—Glacier Creek—ascend steep granite ledges up the slope to the southeast to Cirque Pass (12,095'; 37.07100°N, 118.50001°W). Cirque Pass is the most technical of the three climbers' passes on this route; it is rated an easy Class 3, indicating you'll need hands for sections—although I'll wager most people have already used their hands for balance or scrambling on Knapsack and Potluck Passes. You zigzag up steep slab benches, taking care to find safe places to scramble to the next ledge above. Accept that you may take some dead ends—it is much better to backtrack slightly and find a safer way through this labyrinth of interconnected shelves than to attempt an exposed scramble with a full pack. The ascent is relatively short, however, and views from this saddle are more expansive than

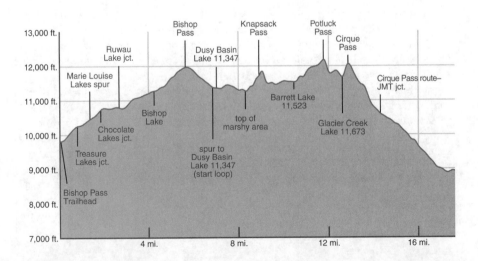

on the previous passes: to the south are endless peaks in the Middle Fork Kings and South Fork Kings drainage; to the west is the Black Divide with Devils Crags, Wheel Mountain, and Mount McDuffie; to the north is North Palisade and its neighbors; and to the east you admire Middle Palisade, flanked by Norman Clyde Peak and Disappointment Peak.

The descent from Cirque Pass is the final leg to the John Muir Trail (JMT), and easier than the ascent to the pass. You zigzag down ledges and benches, forging a technically easy route through steep slab. Snowfields may remain on the upper slopes into July; if snow is present, be especially careful stepping onto or off snow banks, for there are often unseen air pockets alongside steeper rock faces, and you don't want to break through a veneer of snow and slip into a hole. Overall, the best route stays just west of the middle of the drainage. Soon after the terrain moderates, you reach a pair of lakelets (with small campsites) and continue nearly due south across sand and meadows, slowly diverging about 700 feet west of the creek. Where the terrain next steps steeply down, it is essential to be these 700 feet west of the drainage; the route beside the creek is Class 3, with exposed bluffs separated by wet grass strips. Your route will still require a little scrambling but minimal exposure, leading you to the southwest end of an elongate tarn (10,835'; 37.06003°N, 118.49595°W). Follow the tarn north back to the drainage and then follow the creek through easy meadowed terrain to reach the JMT (and coincident PCT). You intersect this famous route about 0.15 mile west of Lower Palisade Lake's outlet. If you want to make this day shorter, there are abundant, albeit busy, campsites near the lake's outlet (10,609'; 37.06019°N, 118.48812°W; no campfires).

However, today's leg, as described, continues 3.4 miles west along the JMT. Turning right, you begin by descending beside bubbling Palisade Creek, walking down corridors above the incised river. With a trail underfoot and correspondingly easier footing, you can better enjoy the wildflowers, such as the magenta mountain pride growing in cracks in the rock. After 0.7 mile, just as you're walking down a splendid polished slab rib, the valley drops out beneath you and you can look down nearly 1,500 feet to Deer Meadow. This, the Golden Staircase, was the last section of the JMT to be constructed, completed in 1938. Impressively built walls form the foundation for the approximately 50 switchbacks that make for a steep decline down a much steeper headwall. Great trail-building skill was required to engineer this route; notice how tight switchbacks take you down one gully and then lead you seamlessly to the next passable gully, as you slowly work yourself down the

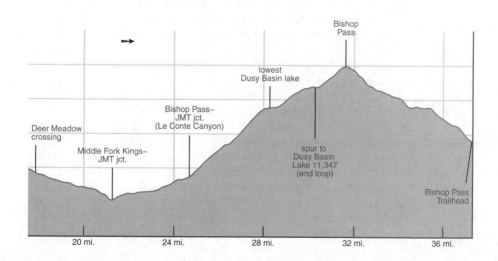

steep face at a nearly unchanging grade. For stretches, the trail is dry and rocky, while elsewhere, small seeps provide water and nourish colorful flowers. Look at tumbling Palisade Creek, taking the direct route to Deer Meadow, and west to Devils Crags, the dark, jagged mass of pinnacles at the southern end of the Black Divide.

At the base of this long descent, you cross a series of brush-covered rockslides and talus fans and abruptly enter dense forest cover, a mixture of red fir and lodgepole pine, where you'll find a series of pleasant streamside campsites. After another 0.5 mile, the trail turns north to ford the many channels of Glacier Creek, the outflow of Lake 11,673, where you camped last night; rocks and logs almost always allow you to cross with dry feet. Then exiting forest cover, the trail again trends west, now crossing a slope of endless flowers and scrubby aspen, irrigated by upslope springs. You reenter drier lodgepole pine forest and quickly spy a use trail that leads southeast to numerous well-used campsites, the "Deer Meadow" camping area (8,860'; 37.05614°N, 118.52551°W). It is a pleasant location to camp, but "meadow" has been a misnomer for this lodgepole pine forest for many decades already.

DAY 4 (Deer Meadow to Le Conte Canyon, 6.8 miles): Continue westward on the JMT, soon fording the unnamed, multibranched outlet of Palisade Basin; logs are generally present across all the channels. Look south across Palisade Creek to Cataract Creek's showy cascades—a rough trail, an alternative crossing into the South Fork Kings drainage before the JMT was completed, once ascended alongside them, but now only vestiges remain. Along the coming 3.0 miles, most trees were burned during the 2002 lightning-started Palisade Fire. For nearly 15 years following the fire, blackened logs and dead trees continually reminded you of the fire's destruction, but now, nearly all the burned snags have toppled and the logs have vanished beneath brush. Moreover, enough adult trees survived and young trees have regrown that if you didn't know a fire had passed through here, you might think the valley bottom was open because of rocky soils or avalanches; it is wonderful to see nature regenerating. And there are still some beautiful streamside campsites beneath stands of surviving trees. Continuing down Palisade Creek's canyon, forever hemmed in by a pair of imposing walls, you slowly reach the confluence with the Middle Fork Kings. Just before you reach the low point, note on your left the remains of a bridge that once crossed Palisade Creek; lacking a bridge, the continued route to Simpson Meadow (Trip 20) can be impassable at high flows. Beyond the current trail junction, you reach a big, lovely campsite beneath towering red fir, Jeffrey pine, and lodgepole pine.

The trail then turns north to ascend Le Conte Canyon alongside the Middle Fork Kings. Over the first 0.6 mile, the trail thrice steps steeply up open, broken slabs beside impressive cascades, the ascents broken by sandier flats. You then approach idyllic Grouse Meadow, where the Middle Fork's emerald-colored water loops lazily through a broad, deep channel, and western blueberry bushes provide a tasty sample for late-summer hikers. There is a selection of lodgepole pine–shaded campsites to either side of the trail through here. Continuing upstream, you pass through forested sections, while elsewhere you walk across open, scrubby slopes, the result of recurrent avalanches or rockslides that prevent a conifer forest from establishing. Scrubby aspen and chinquapin are particularly common in the disturbed areas. Soon you are staring west at the Citadel's glacier-carved profile and Ladder Falls, and farther upcanyon your gaze is drawn to steep-fronted Langille Peak. There are scattered, small tent sites throughout your ascent, but once the gradient declines for the final 0.5 mile to the Bishop Pass Trail junction you'll pass a selection of bigger campsites (for example, 8,719'; 37.09321°N, 118.59408°W). There are additional, unseen sites across the river and a short distance up the Bishop Pass Trail. The trail crosses the Dusy Branch creek via a substantial steel footbridge and soon meets the Bishop Pass Trail. Turning left

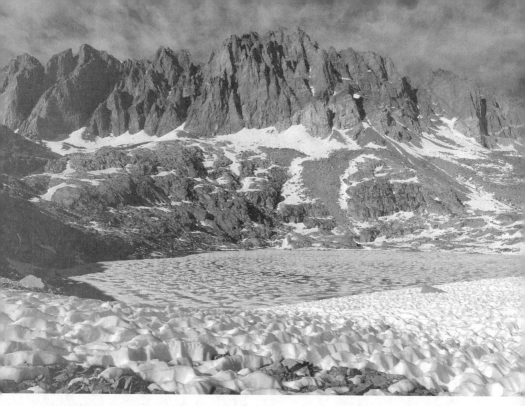

North Palisade rises skyward behind Barrett Lake 11,523.   Photo by Elizabeth Wenk

(west) at this four-way junction leads to the Le Conte Ranger Station (emergency services when a ranger is present), the JMT continues straight ahead (north), and you turn right (east) to climb back to Dusy Basin.

DAY 5 (Le Conte Canyon to lower Dusy Basin, 3.8 miles): This trip turns right (east) onto the Bishop Pass Trail and begins a steep, switchbacking ascent of the east canyon wall. The coming 3.25 miles are hard work; you climb 2,000 feet with only an occasional pause. The rocky zigzags quickly lead you from the valley floor to splendid water-and-glacier polished slab, down which flows the Dusy Branch. After pausing for the requisite photo op, you continue up the next sequence of switchbacks, ogling at Langille Peak's magnificent profile and the rugged junipers that cling to the rocky soils. The ascent moderates slightly in a broad lodgepole pine–cloaked valley, where you'll find some pleasant forested campsites. This is a good stopping point if you want to complete Days 4–6 across two days instead of three. After a scrubbier stretch, the trail turns southeast to cross the Dusy Branch; a trivial crossing most of the time, this can be a deep ford at peak flows. Beyond, the switchbacks resume, partially under lodgepole pine cover and elsewhere on broken slab benches. As you approach steeper bluffs, the trail is channeled back toward the Dusy Branch, offering stunning views of its upper sparkling waterfalls fringed by water-loving flowers: fireweed, rein orchids, Kelley's lilies, shooting stars. The trail recrosses the Dusy Branch on a stout bridge with excellent waterfall views and proceeds up again, slowly rolling over the lip of the valley into Dusy Basin. Be sure to look back into the Middle Fork one final time, imagining it filled with ice to beyond your current altitude—and indeed to above the summit of Langille Peak.

As the trail next approaches the Dusy Branch, you trade westward views for eastward ones, admiring Dusy Basin's surrounding peaks for the first time in several days. The meadow-and-slab-fringed trail leads alongside the calmly flowing Dusy Branch to Lake

10,742, the lowest in Dusy Basin's lower chain of lakes. Both near this lake and slightly upstream are pleasant campsites (for example, 10,760'; 37.09464°N, 118.56458°W; no campfires), more sheltered than those in the upper basin if bad weather threatens. Alternatively you may choose to continue to the campsite you stayed at on Day 1 or even continue across Bishop Pass to Bishop Lake or Saddlerock Lake for the final night.

DAY 6 (lower Dusy Basin to Bishop Pass Trailhead at South Lake, 8.9 miles): Upward bound, the trail works its way remarkably circuitously through the broken granite slab, wiggling endlessly up sandy channels between polished slabs. The upcanyon views are truly phenomenal: from left to right you admire massive two-toned Mount Agassiz (its view-rich summit is accessible via a long but straightforward climb from Bishop Pass, if you have spare time on your hike out), striped Mount Winchell, jagged Thunderbolt Peak, sharp-tipped Isosceles Peak, broad-flanked Columbine Peak, and the impressive, steep, unnamed ridge to the southeast of Knapsack Pass. As dictated by the terrain, the trail eventually swings north, following a fork of the Dusy Branch north, back toward Lake 11,347, where you spent your first night. While there are good campsites in the lower part of Dusy Basin and near this upper lake, there are remarkably few options in between—the terrain is either sloping or grassy.

Once back at the junction that led through upper Dusy Basin to Knapsack Pass, reverse the steps of Day 1 to the trailhead.

see maps on p. 334–336

trip 67   **South Lake to North Lake**

> **Trip Data:**   37.11205°N, 118.67093°W (Muir Pass); 55.0 miles; 8/1 days
> **Topos:**   *Mount Abbot; Mount Thompson, North Palisade, Mount Goddard, Mount Darwin, Mount Hilgard, Mount Tom, Mount Henry*

HIGHLIGHTS: This trip is one of two quintessential High Sierra on-trail loop hikes; the other is the Rae Lakes Loop (Trip 22). In between two crossings of the Sierra Crest, it visits beautiful and famous Dusy Basin, Le Conte Canyon, Evolution Basin, Evolution Valley, and Piute Creek. This trip's trailheads—both out of Bishop—are close enough together that it's relatively easy to set up the shuttle, and, if you have only a single vehicle, a bus can currently be used to complete most of the shuttle.

SHUTTLE DIRECTIONS: From the South Lake parking area, drive the 7.1 miles back to the CA 168 junction. Now turn left, uphill, and drive an additional 3.0 miles south along CA 168, passing the community of Aspendell partway. At the signed junction, turn right onto dirt North Lake Road, cross the creek on a bridge, and continue 1.6 miles. Then turn right toward the pack station and trailhead parking, located 0.2 mile down the spur road. Alas, this parking area is not the trailhead—to reach that, at the junction with the spur road, continue an additional 0.4 mile along the main North Lake Road. You'll find the trailhead adjacent to toilets within the North Lake Campground, but there is no parking here.

If you have only a single car, the Eastern Sierra Transit Shuttle covers most of the distance between the trailheads; you only have to walk the 2.0 miles along the North Lake Road. See estransit .com/routes-schedule/community-routes/bishop-creek-shuttle for the current schedule.

DAY 1 (Bishop Pass Trailhead at South Lake to Dusy Basin, 6.9 miles): Follow Trip 65, Day 1 to Dusy Basin Lake 11,347 (11,347'; 37.10379°N, 118.55160°W; no campfires). (The mileage is to the use trail junction, excluding the final 0.1 mile to the campsite.)

> **VIEWS THROUGH DUSY BASIN**
> Occasional clumps of the flaky-barked, five-needled whitebark pine dot the glacially scoured basin, and impressive Mount Agassiz, Mount Winchell, and pinnacled Thunderbolt Peak dominate the far eastern skyline. Steep-fronted Isoceles Peak and more massive Columbine Peak mark Dusy Basin's southeastern boundary. Look for the prominent gap of Knapsack Pass, just south of Columbine Peak. To the south and southwest, a meandering crest of unnamed, dramatic peaks mostly block your views to Giraud Peak's dark, vertical north face.

DAY 2 (Dusy Basin to Big Pete Meadow, 7.2 miles): Onward, the main trail diverges from Dusy Basin's largest lakes, continuing its descent southwest, then south over smooth granite slabs and through sand to avoid the basin's delicate dry tundra, meadows, and stream verges.

Once the terrain permits, the trail swings westward above the lowest lakes of Dusy Basin, Lake 10,742 and the chain above it. Near here are many good campsites, more protected than those in the upper basin (for example, 10,760'; 37.09464°N, 118.56458°W; no campfires). Passing Lake 10,742, the trail continues beside the meadow-lined Dusy Branch and soon begins a series of steady switchbacks along its north side. Colorful wildflowers along this descent include giant red paintbrush, corn lilies, coyote mint, lupine, penstemon, fragrant shooting star, and some yellow Coville's columbine. Just below a waterfall, a wooden bridge leads to the creek's south side. Enjoying the ongoing views of the glacier-carved U-shaped Middle Fork Kings River canyon, zigzag downhill, and, on the far side of the valley, notice the major peaks of the Black Divide, foregrounded by lighter-colored granitic summits, the Citadel and Langille Peak.

As the trail descends, the initially sparse cover of stunted whitebarks transitions to other tree species, including juniper on exposed knobs, aspen in avalanche chutes, western white pine on deeper-soiled slopes, and lodgepole pine on flat shelves. The trail recrosses Dusy Branch on a forested bench, continues along a series of little shelves with campsites, and then makes the final 1.5-mile switchbacking descent to Le Conte Canyon, in places gazing upon the sparkling creek as it dashes down 700 feet of unbroken granite.

At the foot of the descent you reach a signed junction with the John Muir Trail (JMT) (8,752'). From this same point, a spur trail heads west (straight; riverward) to a summer ranger cabin; you can find emergency help here if the ranger is in. There are campsites scattered along the JMT corridor just to the south.

This trip turns right (north) onto the famous trail and ascends gradually over forest duff through moderate-to-dense stands of lodgepole, providing pleasant walking conditions. You soon approach largish Little Pete Meadow, named for sheepherder "Little" Pierre Giraud, offering well-used campsites along its perimeter and fishing for rainbow, golden, and brook trout. The Middle Fork Kings meanders through the meadow, narrow sinuous oxbow lakes depicting the river's old course. Ahead the trail emerges from forest cover and climbs a juniper-speckled slope on sand and rock. There are phenomenal views westward to the steep, glacier-polished face of Langille Peak; fracture patterns determine where giant vertical blocks were plucked by glaciers or have subsequently fallen from the upper walls, while talus fans show the accumulation of fallen rock since the glaciers retreated. The view north includes spurs radiating off Mount Powell and Mount Thompson. Where the gradient eases in a lodgepole pine flat, a spur trail departs left (west, riverward) toward the south end of unseen Big Pete Meadow and some large off-the-trail campsites. If you continue north on the trail, after 0.2 mile it bends left (west) itself, leading to busier trailside campsites just north of Big Pete Meadow (9,246'; 37.11260°N, 118.60683°W).

DAY 3 (Big Pete Meadow to Wanda Lake, 8.3 miles): This is a long, strenuous day on, in sections, rough trail with a 2,750-foot elevation gain—there are few camping options for the last miles over Muir Pass, so if you want to make this day shorter, your best choice is to extend your previous day a little, by staying in one of the campsites described ahead.

Leaving the Big Pete Meadow environs, the trail crosses (on logs) the stream draining the southern slopes of Mount Powell, Mount Thompson, and Mount Gilbert and passes additional campsites. Westward, you have a broken view through upper Le Conte Canyon toward the darker rock of the Black Divide. For the next mile the gradient is moderate and the walking pleasant, as the trail traverses the toes of old talus fan deposited by avalanches and debris flows, approximately following the river's path.

At 0.9 mile past the aforementioned crossing, to the left of the trail, is a John Muir Trail fixture, the Rock Monster. Daring souls can climb behind the monster's teeth for a photo op (or camp nearby). As you approach the Rock Monster, the rock on the trailbed suddenly has sharp, fractured edges; the talus fan you are now crossing is from more recent rockfall. The rock is bigger and more angular, and soil has yet to fill many of the cracks; the Rock Monster is simply the largest, most intact piece of talus to come tumbling down this chute. As you cross talus fan upon talus fan ahead, you'll certainly notice that some offer more pleasant walking substrate than others. Aspen scrub, the first tree to colonize areas after disturbance, grows densely on the alluvial fans, while less frequently disturbed pockets of soil offer a partial forest cover of lodgepole, western white pine, and, in the most shaded alcoves, hemlock. The dashing cascades of the Middle Fork Kings River offer visual relief on this steep, rugged, sunny ascent. You slowly climb far above the deep river gorge to avoid steep, polished slabs. To navigate through one section, called Barrier Rock, the trail had to be blasted into the canyon's sheer granite wall.

Where the gradient next eases, there are campsites south of the trail (10,335'; 37.11434°N, 118.63712°W; no campfires; Starr's Camp) and more on the next shelf up (around 10,480'). Departing west from the trail offers more choices. All these sites have splendid views of the vertical dark-colored rock comprising the Black Giant, a peak intimidating from this angle, but an easy climb from Helen Lake. Notice how the lake basins before you are still on granite—the geologic contact is right at the base of the cliffs. Winding upward, past endless trickles and wildflower gardens, leads to campsites on a whitebark pine–shaded shelf east of the trail (10,812'; 37.12162°N, 118.64148°W; no campfires); these are the final campsites for a while. Around the corner you reach a large lake at 10,834 feet where camping is prohibited.

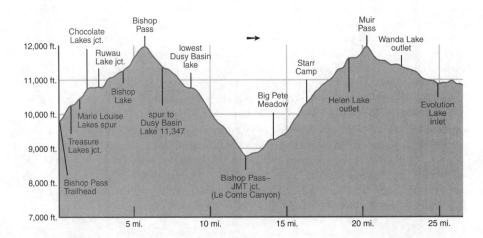

After crossing Lake 10,834's multichanneled inlet, you have a steady, zigzagging climb over sand and rock to the next meadowed shelf. Walking across alpine tundra and stepping over a tributary stream, you soon reach a much smaller shelf with sparse whitebark cover and tiny timberline campsites and beyond reach a round talus-bound lake (10,480'). Cross the cascading creek and follow the trail through a meadow filled with dense patches of mountaineer shooting stars interspersed with cobble-paved waterways. Above, the infant Middle Fork Kings River is confined to an enticing little gorge, paved with dark metamorphic rock, the trail winding through ever-more-rugged terrain as it ascends the terminal shoulder of the Black Divide. This stretch can remain snowbound well into summer. As you approach Helen Lake, if you turn around, you have a vista back to the Palisades peaks and also to Giraud and Langille Peaks.

At Helen Lake's outlet, the trail crosses back to the south side of the stream and follows the lakeshore southwest. Here, near the contact between granite and metamorphic rock, you'll find broken rocks in colorful reds, yellows, blacks, and whites, but few campsites, for the metamorphic rocks decompose to angular cobble, not pleasant sand. Only at Helen Lake's southwestern corner, back on granite, are there a few better camping options—although continuing on to Evolution Basin is recommended. You are now staring at the western face of the Black Giant, an easy off-trail ascent from the saddle south of Lake 11,939 if you're keen for the challenge. Staying on the trail, soon you ascend the final switchbacks to Muir Pass, across either a well-trodden path in late-lasting snow or up a sandy slope.

VIEWS FROM MUIR PASS

From this pass, the views are magnificent. The darker crags to the north and south relieve the intense whites of the lighter granite farther to the east. Situated in a gigantic rock bowl to the west, Wanda Lake's emerald-blue waters contrast sharply with the white hue of the low bedrock rib to its immediate west, which on the south side merges into the darker rock of the Goddard Divide.

Atop Muir Pass (11,971') is a stone hut, built in 1930 in memory of John Muir. It was intended to provide emergency shelter during storms, but it is, like the entire John Muir Trail, overloved, and camping in—or near—it is now prohibited. George Frederick Schwarz, an early Sierra Club supporter, provided the $5,810.48 to build it. The descent from the pass is moderate to gradual, first across sand and then over fragmented rock, leveling out as the trail passes the south end of talus-bound Lake McDermand. Climbing ever

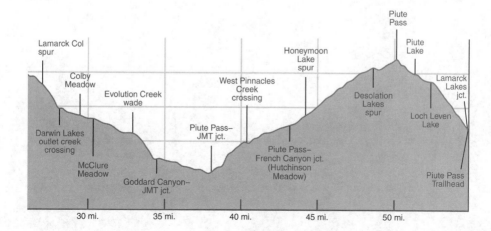

so slightly, the trail then descends toward Wanda Lake, skirting its east side. Once halfway around the lake, you have unforgettable views of uppermost Evolution Basin—a green stripe of grass; the grading blue waters of Wanda Lake; a low, rounded white-granite rib; the stark, steep, dark face of pyramidal Mount Goddard; and (usually) the brilliant blue skies of the alpine Sierra. These superlative views continue until you arrive at the barren campsites near the lake's outlet (11,426'; 37.12860°N, 118.69733°W; no campfires). The expansive views from these campsites include Mount Goddard and the Goddard Divide to the south and the Evolution peaks, Mount Warlow, Mount Huxley, Mount Spencer, Mount Darwin, and Mount Mendel, to the north and east. Note that these campsites are small and exposed, and the alpine tundra in which they are located is exceedingly fragile; you must take the utmost care not to camp (or walk) on the diminutive tundra species that grow here. There are many more campsites near Sapphire Lake—ahead—if the ones here are occupied.

DAY 4 (Wanda Lake to Colby Meadow, 7.1 miles): Just below Wanda Lake, the trail crosses multibranched Evolution Creek and begins a long moderate descent toward Sapphire Lake. You soon pass Lake 11,293, to which you could detour east in search of small campsites. On your descent you trade your upper basin views of the Goddard Divide for better views of the core Evolution peaks, Mount Darwin and Mount Mendel, whose steep, broken walls rise vertically before you. Note the steep avalanche chutes that decorate their western face and the trimline that marks the level to which the valley was once filled with ice. The trail reaches the creek bank near the outlet of stunning Sapphire Lake (10,966'; trout); a stop on the slabs near the outlet is nearly mandatory—here you will find absolutely perfect examples of glacial polish and chatter marks, the curved grooves left as a glacier dragged rocks along its base. The best campsites are on the east side of the lake.

Wanda Lake   Photo by Elizabeth Wenk

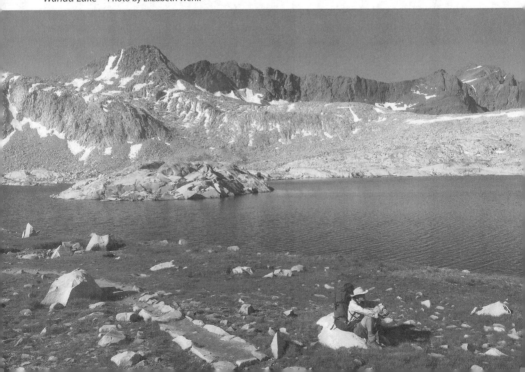

Onward, you cross sandy flower-filled corridors between rounded slabs, then drop an easy 100 feet to the next glacial step, this one filled by Evolution Lake (10,852'). You cross its inlet on a long line of giant rock blocks, placed a big step apart. The trail now stays high above Evolution Lake's meadowed shoreline until it reaches the lake's north end, where there are a few campsites among the first stunted whitebark pines.

"EVOLUTION" RAMBLING

A layover day in Evolution Basin allows time to explore the glorious lakes on Darwin Bench or ascend one of the easiest of the basin's peaks, Mount Spencer. In July 1895, Theodore Solomons, the visionary of the John Muir Trail, named the first six peaks of the Evolution Range after the most prominent figures in the new field of evolutionary biology: Darwin, Fiske, Haeckel, Huxley, Spencer, and Wallace, along with Evolution Lake.

Just where the trail turns to the right, leaving Evolution Basin, you should briefly detour to one of Evolution Basin's best hidden features, Slissate Falls (a historic name), where Evolution Creek tumbles 250 feet down smooth granite slabs toward Evolution Valley. This waterfall is absolutely hidden from the trail—you must walk over to the creek to see it plunging downward. Back on track, you walk to the northern tip of Evolution Basin and then sidle a bit farther northwest, to where an easy-to-follow use trail heads to Darwin Bench, the Darwin Lakes, and Lamarck Col (Trips 58 and 59). Thereafter the trail swings south and west as it switchbacks down to Evolution Valley, following sandy ramps between steeper outcrops, the timberline whitebark stands transitioning to the subalpine expanses of lodgepole pine by the time you reach the base. The views down Evolution Valley and south to the McGee Lakes drainage and the Hermit, the unmissable sharp arête due south, are wonderful. At the base of the grade, you pass a small campsite on open slabs and shortly ford the multibranched stream that drains Darwin Canyon—while not difficult, it is potentially cumbersome. Ahead, your route is largely within dry lodgepole forest with occasional excursions to the edge of meadows or onto granite slabs. The next good camping choices are when you reach Colby Meadow (9,740'; 37.18425°N, 118.73101°W; golden trout in Evolution Creek). Here you will find both large sites beneath lodgepole pine cover and more open choices in openings between slabs. The views from the meadow edge are superlative.

Hikers with energy left may want to continue to campsites at McClure or Evolution Meadow, as described in the first part of Day 5.

DAY 5 (Colby Meadow to Piute Creek Bridge, 8.5 miles): From Colby Meadow, the route continues westward, quickly reaching McClure Meadow with its many overused campsites—both human and stock travelers have taken a heavy toll on the environment here. The trail skims the meadow's edge, again offering views to immerse yourself in. Near the northwest end of McClure Meadow you step across a creeklet and soon pass a spur to a ranger station; emergency services are available here when there is a ranger on duty.

Below McClure Meadow, the path makes a moderate-to-steady descent that fords several tributaries draining the Glacier Divide, the banks fringed with wildflowers—swamp onion, crimson columbine, and Kelley's lilies are some of the showiest. The pleasant but unassuming walk through lodgepole pine forest leads to Evolution Meadow, the final Evolution Valley meadow. If you are hiking under high water conditions, it is wise to leave the JMT at the eastern end of Evolution Meadow, where the trail jogs right; the main crossing of Evolution Creek is dangerous under these conditions and an alternative crossing exists toward the middle of Evolution Meadow. It is similarly deep to the main crossing (and takes you through the fragile meadow environment), but there are no rapids downstream. Assuming you continue along the JMT, you presently reach the creek crossing—always a wade.

Within minutes you reach the head of switchbacks that drop to the South Fork San Joaquin River. Looking west, enjoy excellent views of the cascades streaming down Mount Henry and the falls and cascades along Evolution Creek. The first cascades the trail passes are still on granite with its characteristic rounded pools, but as the gradient increases you cross onto metamorphic rock and the stream assumes an incised, straight course, just like what you're staring at across the valley. Indeed, the entire headwaters of the South Fork San Joaquin River, Goddard Canyon, are in metamorphic rocks; take Trip 8 or 9 to see its wonders. Much of the descent is on a rocky slope, but you drop into lodgepole pine forest as the grade eases.

At the bottom, the trail hooks left and follows the creek south past a collection of nice campsites. Just beyond these campsites, the trail crosses a footbridge and reaches a junction where the Goddard Canyon/Hell for Sure Pass Trail branches left (south; Trips 8 and 9), while the JMT, your route, turns right (north).

You traipse downstream through relatively moist lodgepole forest, quickly reaching a creek crossing (easy, but sometimes a wade) and eventually emerging from tree cover at a handsome bridge. Just before the bridge, you pass a use trail that heads north to a large camping area. Goddard Canyon's steep-walled gorge of fractured metamorphic rocks is strikingly different from the smooth granite slabs in Evolution Valley and Evolution Basin—it is splendid to experience the rapid change in landforms. You continue downstream, taking in the impressive canyon walls and the turbulent waters of the South Fork of the San Joaquin River. Common species on the dry slopes you are traversing include western eupatorium, ocean spray, granite gilia, and Bridge's penstemon. Beyond you pass through Aspen Meadow, a forest with limited camping, and resume traversing the sunny southwest, canyon wall. Where a steep knob pinches the canyon and the trail is channeled onto talus, you pass the John Muir Rock, a large boulder into which MUIR TRAIL 1917 is carved; this is worth a stop. Continuing above the rolling, tumbling river, you shortly reach shallower slopes dotted with Jeffrey pine and juniper. There are many campsites for the coming 0.5 mile to the bridge across Piute Creek, but as this is a popular destination, it is wise to take the first site you find (for example, 8,078'; 37.22490°N, 118.83248°W).

DAY 6 (Piute Creek Bridge to Hutchinson Meadow, 5.2 miles): The Piute Bridge is the Kings Canyon boundary, and once across it, you are in John Muir Wilderness (Sierra National Forest). Just past the bridge you reach a junction where the JMT continues left (west) to Blayney Meadows and over Selden Pass, while you turn right (north) to ascend toward Piute Pass. The trail heads up a sunstruck southeast-facing slope above the churning river, guarded over by steep imposing walls. There is just a sparse cover of shrubs and the occasional dot of shade from a Jeffrey pine or juniper whose roots have found purchase in the rocky soils. With some big steps to surmount and a rocky trail, this is slow going. Note the contrast between the dark-colored metamorphic rock comprising the valley walls and the granite river rock that has been transported from far upstream.

After 1.4 miles you cross Turret Creek and proceed across a giant vegetated talus fan, the outflow of Turret Creek over eons of floods. You've now crossed onto granite, but the trail is still rocky, scrubby, and devoid of shade. The river remains far below you as you cross first slabs, then a forested corridor in a narrow stretch of canyon, and arrive at the next talus outwash fan, this one bisected by West Pinnacles Creek. After this possibly wet ford, you descend toward river level for the first time, where you should take a break on the glorious polished slabs, enjoying the spectacle of whitewater cascades early season or taking a dip when the runoff has subsided. Where the river curves to the south (right) is the first plausible, nearly flat campsite since the JMT. Slowly the canyon walls part a little more, and the valley bottom is broader. Hidden on shelves at the tops of the steep walls are delightful lake basins. As you approach East Pinnacles Creek, 4.2 miles from the Piute Bridge, there are, for the first time, good campsites in lodgepole pine flats. The final mile to Hutchinson Meadow is gentler and more shaded, although the trail also crosses both open sandy terraces and then pocket meadows as it reaches a junction, where left (northeast) is the trail up French Canyon to Pine Creek Pass, while you stay right (southeast) toward Piute Pass. There are excellent campsites nearby and golden and brook trout are in the creek (9,497'; 37.26691°N, 118.78049°W). You've completed 5.2 miles today, and if you choose to complete a few extra miles, maybe deciding to split Days 6–8 over two days, you will find many additional campsites en route to Piute Pass. Note also that you start to diverge from Piute Creek after 2.1 miles and in late summer the side creeks might run dry, necessitating a detour to find water.

DAY 7 (Hutchinson Meadow to Humphreys Basin, 5.4 miles): From the Hutchinson Meadow junction you continue east (right), crossing at least five braided distributaries of French Canyon Creek; most are a rock hop by midseason, but possibly a cobbly wade in early summer. The trail leads gradually upward through lodgepole pine forest, sometimes creekside, elsewhere farther to the north. Pocket meadows offer a burst of color—shooting stars, swamp onions, and buttercups—while sandier stretches are more delicately tinted with spreading phlox and alpine flames. Under the lodgepole pine grow one-sided wintergreen, western Labrador tea, and wandering fleabane.

After 1.0 mile you pass a lateral to the Honeymoon Lakes (and large campsites beside the river) and continue upward. In places the creek bank is forested, and elsewhere there are beautiful slab benches; both environments offer some nice campsites. You have good downcanyon views to the Pinnacles, but those to the ridges to either side are still blocked by the lower canyon walls. Slowly the valley's gradient increases and the forest cover thins, and by the time you cross the outlet creek from Tomahawk Lake around 10,340 feet you feel like you're walking across slab and through meadow patches at least half the time. Around here you begin to diverge from the river; an old trail routing toward Lower Golden Trout Lake was long ago abandoned to preserve the fragile timberline turf. Similarly, camping is prohibited within 500 feet of the lake, although there are some good campsites on knolls outside this exclusion zone.

By the time you cross Desolation Lake's outlet creek (11,000'), there are just scattered stunted trees about, and soon you are truly in the alpine, rambling across enormous Humphreys Basin, a wonderland of slabs, sand, and lakes that extends to either side of the trail. Next, you pass an unsigned, but highly visible, spur trail toward the Desolation Lakes (11,164'; 37.24812°N, 118.70217°W at junction); from here you have magnificent views of the Glacier Divide to the south and the Sierra Crest to the east, with 13,986-foot Mount Humphreys the dominant peak to the northeast. Those intrigued by the Desolation Lakes' reputation for fishing for golden trout and those fond of treeless, open camps will find some decent campsites above Lower Desolation Lake (11,221'; 37.25805°N, 118.71088°W; no campfires) and on the wind-raked flats among the great white boulders surrounding aptly named Desolation Lake (11,375'). Muriel Lake, sitting in the broad basin to the south and best accessed from near Piute Pass, also offers good campsites. Overall, Humphreys Basin is worth a multiday stay—but probably another time, starting from North Lake, when you haven't carried your food for 48 miles (Trip 56). When searching for a campsite,

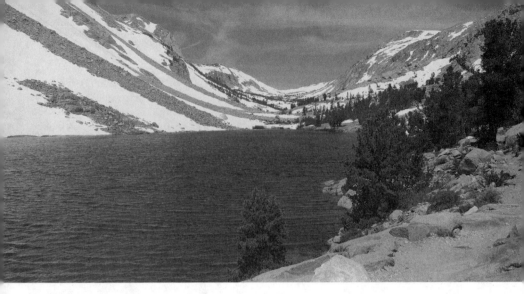

Loch Leven Lake   Photo by Elizabeth Wenk

seek a location well away from the trail, as those close to the trail have become grotesquely overused. The daily mileage is up to the aforementioned junction, but you may well choose to walk an additional half mile off the main route to find a perfect campsite.

DAY 8 (Humphreys Basin to North Lake Trailhead, 6.4 miles): Beyond the Desolation Lake junction, the main trail turns southeast and climbs across a steeper slope above Summit Lake. Rounding the lake's northern and eastern sides, you soon reach view-rich Piute Pass (11,423'). Just 50 feet before the pass is an unmarked but distinct use trail heading southwest, which leads to Muriel Lake and its beautiful, but exposed, small, sandy campsites. Descending from Piute Pass, the trail passes diminutive tarns, staying on broken slab to the north of the marshy drainage. You presently reach the northeast shore of Piute Lake, offering fishing for brook trout and numerous small campsites tucked beneath whitebark pines. Leaving Piute Lake, the path skirts some small, unnamed lakes, these with both rainbow and brook trout. Continuing a relatively gentle drop across slabs, you reach the next step, an elongate meadow corridor leading past more unnamed lakelets to Loch Leven Lake; the best camping opportunities are at its western end, and this lake hosts brook, brown, and rainbow trout.

Talus fans and slabs constrain the route as the trail traces the northern shore to the outlet. Now begins a steeper descent across a headwall, the trail following an undulating ledge, with bluffs above and below dictating the route. Crossing a side trickle, you begin a long descending traverse below the Piute Crags, enjoying the view of the North Fork Bishop Creek cascading below Loch Leven Lake and then tracing a green line far below you. Resolving into switchbacks, the trail drops down the increasingly red talus into more continuous tree cover. Switchbacks continue down to the canyon floor, passing a few small campsites where you wind down a granite knob. Your final mile to the trailhead is a pleasant walk through lodgepole pine and aspen forest, colored by tall wildflowers in season. You ford the North Fork Bishop Creek twice, both times on log bridges, and then switchback beside the gurgling creek. You reach a junction where the lateral to Lamarck Lakes leads right (south), while you continue straight ahead (left; east), soon reaching the trailhead in the North Lake Campground beside the toilet block (9,364'; 37.22731°N, 118.62746°W). There is no parking here, so at least one member in your group must continue 0.6 mile down the road and then left to the parking area (9,279'; 37.23053°N, 118.61867°W).

GLACIER LODGE ROAD TRIPS

Glacier Lodge Road climbs to Big Pine Creek Trailhead, where trails depart up the North and South Forks of Big Pine Creek. These trails lead to the eastern base of the Palisades, the Sierra's premier mountaineering locale. Six summits rise above 14,000 feet, and the Sierra's largest glacier, Palisade Glacier, fills the broad cirque beneath North Palisade. The well-built trails lead to rugged basins, as attractive to hikers seeking views as they are to climbers seeking adventure. Neither trail crosses the Sierra Crest—the Palisade escarpment is so steep that only difficult cross-country routes lead to the western Sierra.

Trailhead: Big Pine Creek

A storm approaches over the Palisades.   Photo by Elizabeth Wenk

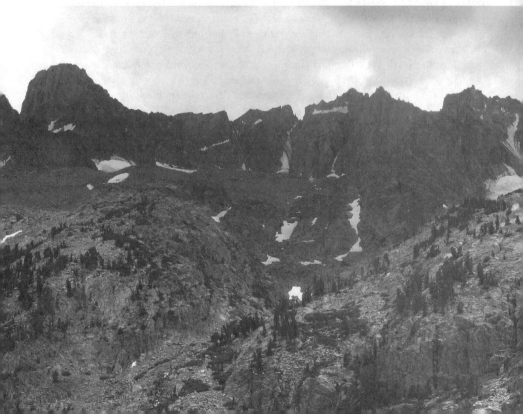

Big Pine Creek Trailhead   7,833'; 37.12526°N, 118.43759°W

Destination/ GPS Coordinates	Trip Type	Best Season	Pace & Hiking/ Layover Days	Total Mileage	Permit Required
68 Big Pine Lakes 37.12922°N 118.50260°W (Fourth Lake)	Semiloop	Mid to late	Moderate 3/2	12.2	North Fork Big Pine Creek
69 Brainerd Lake 37.09187°N 118.45751°W	Out-and-back	Mid to late	Moderate 2/1	9.2	South Fork Big Pine Creek

INFORMATION AND PERMITS: This trailhead is in Inyo National Forest. Permits are required for overnight stays and quotas apply. Permits can be reserved up to six months in advance at recreation.gov (60%; $6 permit reservation fee plus $5 per person) or requested in person, first come, first served, a day in advance (40%; free). All permits must be picked up at one of the Inyo National Forest ranger stations, located in Lone Pine (Eastern Sierra Interagency Visitor Center), Bishop, Mammoth Lakes, and Lee Vining (the Mono Basin Scenic Area Visitor Center). If you plan to use a stove or have a campfire, you must also have a California campfire permit, available from a forest service office or online at preventwild fireca.org/campfire-permit. Campfires are prohibited above approximately 9,600 feet along North Fork Big Pine Creek and above approximately 8,600 feet along South Fork Big Pine Creek, including at all the described campsites. Bear canisters are required in this area.

DRIVING DIRECTIONS: From US 395 in Big Pine, turn west on Crocker Street, which becomes Glacier Lodge Road as it exits town. The true trailhead is at the road's end at 10.5 miles, but the parking there is only for day users. The overnight parking area is 0.8 mile back down the road on the north side. There is a trail that climbs directly from the parking area into the North Fork Big Pine Canyon; it makes a 1.1-mile ascending traverse up a shadeless south-facing slope, joining the route of Trip 68 at the 0.8-mile mark. It is therefore considerably shorter than following the road to the true trailhead but not a pleasant way to start your excursion. For Trip 69 to Brainerd Lake, this trail leads the wrong direction. For both trips it is recommended that you drop your party and all your packs at the road's end and then elect one person to drive the car back to overnight parking and walk back to the trailhead along the road.

° trip 68   Big Pine Lakes

    Trip Data: 37.12922°N, 118.50260°W (Fourth Lake);
                        12.2 miles, plus extra to other lakes; 3/2 days
      Topos: *Split Mountain, Coyote Flat, Mount Thompson, North Palisade*

HIGHLIGHTS: The North Fork Big Pine Creek is a sought-after destination by mountaineers, with the Palisades offering some of the Sierra's most famous alpine ice couloirs and rock climbs. Hikers flock here as well to absorb the rugged alpine scenery from the shores of one of the 10 beautiful lakes, many a gorgeous milky color from the influx of glacial sediment. A layover day allows an adventurous side trip to the Sierra's largest glacier, the Palisade Glacier, and up-close views of the aptly named Palisades.

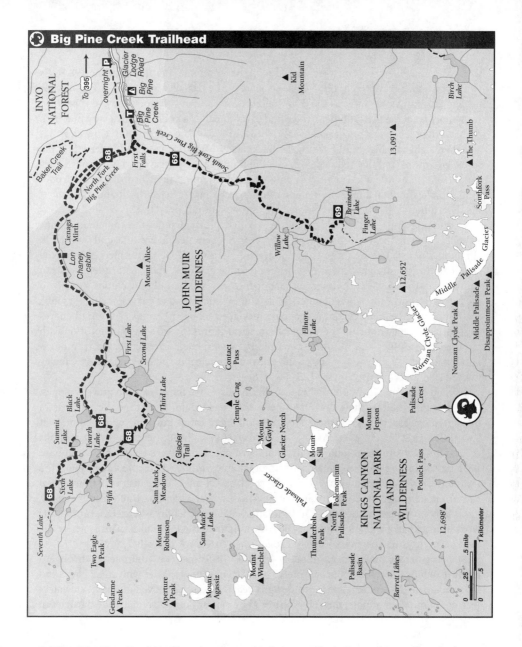

DAY 1 (Big Pine Creek Trailhead to Second Lake, 4.7 miles): From the road's end, skirt a gate and walk along a creekside road past summer cabins. After 0.2 mile, the road—and the creek—turns right. Just beyond, the road leads to the driveway of a final cabin, while the continuing upcanyon trail abruptly veers left (north-northwest) and becomes singletrack. This track switchbacks above the cabins to a bridge over First Falls on the North Fork Big Pine Creek and after a few steps reaches a junction, where you turn right (north-northwest) to climb alongside the North Fork Big Pine Creek, while left (southwest) continues up the South Fork Big Pine Creek drainage (Trip 69).

You switchback up the steep slope beneath tall Jeffrey pines, the vegetation becoming lusher where the trail straightens out at the top of First Falls. Passing through a thicket of wild roses and alders, you intersect an old road, never rebuilt after floods in the 1980s. As you turn right (north) to continue upslope, stare at the passageway you've just exited, for no sign currently marks this as the trail—and on your return you won't want to miss it.

A short jaunt leads to another bridge and just thereafter a confusing five-way junction. A sharp right leads to a small picnic area, the old First Falls Campground. Up a short bit and then right is a high trail back to the backpackers' parking area. To the far left is the so-called Lower Trail that follows alongside Big Pine Creek upstream and is signposted NF BIG PINE. Up a little and then left is an alternative route up the North Fork, the Upper Trail, which is about 0.2 mile shorter and offers better views of Second Falls, but is sunnier; the description leads you up the Lower Trail and down the Upper Trail.

Continuing your creekside journey for 0.6 flat, pleasant mile, the trail then begins switchbacking up the dry, brushy slope of bitterbrush, greenleaf manzanita, and sagebrush, climbing 200 feet to reach a four-way junction. Here the Upper Trail merges from the right (southeast), straight across (east) leads up to Baker Creek, and you turn left (west) to continue up the North Fork drainage. The open rocky-sandy trail now climbs steadily to the top of Second Falls, where it enters John Muir Wilderness and curves northwest along the rollicking creek. Jeffrey and lodgepole pines grow along the banks as the trail curves west toward Cienaga Mirth, "merry marsh" in Spanish. It is indeed a pleasant location with streamside campsites and lush forest colored by wintergreen, arrowleaf ragwort, monkshood, and Kelley's lily. Soon you pass a handsome stone cabin, built by actor Lon Chaney in the 1920s and now used by the U.S. Forest Service.

Beyond Cienaga Mirth, the trail repeatedly climbs above the creek onto gravelly slopes, traverses spring-fed gardens, and then meets the creek again. Each time the trail passes through lodgepole pine forest near the creek, there are campsites—one good option is at 9,613'; 37.13122°N, 118.47321°W; 3.5 miles from the trailhead. Beyond, the trail climbs around a rocky knob and follows a dry slope just above the river's banks. Here you have your first stunning views upcanyon to unforgettable, immense Temple Crag. Soon, the trail steps across the small Black Lake outlet creek and climbs a slope lush with flowers and aspen, the tall magenta-flowered fireweed particularly striking. The trail ascends steeply, but briefly, crosses the outlet a second time, and reaches a junction, where right (northeast) leads to Black Lake and left (southwest) to the numbered Big Pine Lakes. This is where the loop part of this trip begins, and you head left, signposted for Lakes 1–7.

Stepping across the Black Lake outlet creek a third time, you continue up through a mixture of lodgepole and whitebark pines. The terrain is now rockier with small bluffs and more boulders. Ascending, you quite abruptly reach the slopes above First Lake, staring at its stupendous aqua waters, the color bestowed by glacial flour, extremely fine particles of

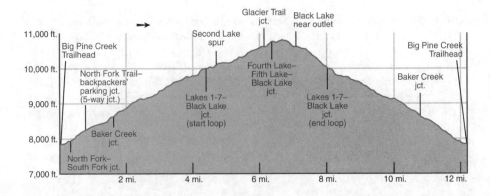

silt—"flour"—ground by glaciers. These particles are so fine they remain suspended in the water column, coloring the lakes. Being closer to the glacier, Second Lake and, especially, Third Lake are even milkier in color. Only Lakes 1–3 have this color, for Lakes 4–7 are on the north side of the drainage, not receiving runoff from the Palisade Glacier.

From First Lake upward, every last plausibly flat bit of ground has been appropriated as a tent site. Excepting some sites around Fourth Lake, the campsites are all small—the rugged beauty of this canyon is, after all, its unceasingly steep terrain. Around First and Second Lakes there are probably more than 30 "campsites," but many are awkwardly positioned high above water and certainly most are out of sight of the trail. The largest campsites are on a forest flat near the stream between First and Second Lakes; head left on a spur at 10,088'; 37.12645°N, 118.48618°W. You'll also find some old mining equipment in this direction.

DAY 2 (Second Lake outlet to Fourth Lake, 1.7 miles, plus extra to other lakes): Ahead are six additional lakes with campsites—read below to decide which you'd like to make your base for further exploration. You may wind up at Third, Fourth, Fifth, Sixth, Summit, or Black Lake, or somewhere in between! The mileage is calculated to the junction near the southwestern corner of Fourth Lake, but most likely your distance will be a little greater. Continue up the main trail around Second Lake to Third Lake. The trail remains high above the water as it curves around Second Lake; only a few tiny campsites cling to the steep slopes that lead down to the shore. Across the lake looms Temple Crag, a fascinating, formidable, convoluted peak. Take a moment to stare south at the near-vertical dark face of Temple Crag and the light-colored granite rubble heap that is Mount Alice; the geologic boundary is stark, and the contrasting piles of talus can be traced upslope to aptly named Contact Pass.

As the path leaves Second Lake behind, hikers can hear the roar of Third Lake's outlet making its final fall into Second Lake. Between Second and Third Lakes, the trail winds along benches between the creek and imposing granite faces. At one point, the trail travels high above the creek on a rock causeway. Beyond Third Lake, the trail climbs onward on long switchbacks. Few people camp here, for the creek now sits in a less aesthetic willow-choked channel beneath steep bluffs. As the switchbacks end, the trail parallels a lovely meadow, crosses Fourth Lake's outlet, and reaches a junction with a trail leading left (southwest) toward the Palisade Glacier (signed GLACIER TRAIL; 10,641').

GLACIER TRAIL

The Glacier Trail climbs steeply 0.8 mile to Sam Mack Meadow (with a very few tiny tent spots beneath whitebark pines) and then onward for another 1.0 mile to the base of the giant terminal moraine left by the retreating glacier. The downcanyon views from the bluffs below the moraine are splendid, but a fair bit of effort and talus hopping is required to surmount the moraine and obtain unbroken views of the Palisade Peaks themselves. This is a good excursion, however, if you have a full spare day for adventuring.

The main route described continues right (north), signposted for Fourth Lake, and after 0.25 mile reaches a four-way junction (10,775'; 37.12922°N, 118.50260°W). The official trip mileage is given to this point, but you're almost certain to extend your trip farther. From here, left (northwest) leads 0.25 mile to Fifth Lake and straight ahead (north) leads 0.1 mile to Fourth Lake, 0.6 mile to Summit Lake, or 1.3 mile to Sixth Lake. Right (east) leads 0.75 mile to Black Lake, the continued route of the loop. Each of these lakes is worth visiting, for each offers unique views of the basin and has a remarkably different feel. From a base near Fourth Lake or Fifth Lake you could contentedly spend the rest of the day exploring upward with just a day pack. Here are the options:

Fifth Lake: Set below Mount Robinson and Two Eagle Peak, this lake has perhaps the loveliest setting but limited camping. There are a few beat-out sites at its outlet, crowded between the trail and the stream, and others across the outlet on a shallow knob near some seasonal tarns. The trail continues along the east shore, soon petering out. From here, a spur trail leads right (east) to a saddle where a use trail takes off to Fourth Lake, and there are campsites on this saddle (10,827'; 37.13116°N, 118.50606°W; no campfires). From the outlet you have splendid views from Temple Crag to North Palisade.

Fourth Lake: Fourth Lake is less stark than most of the basin's lakes, ringed by forest and with grassy shores. It correspondingly has the most sheltered camping, with the best selection of campsites along its southern and western edges. The largest is on a forested knob about halfway along the western side (10.786'; 37.13091°N, 118.50381°W; no campfires). Just past this, the use trail from the saddle above Fifth Lake joins in a meadowy draw. Continuing, just before the trail crosses Fourth Lake's major inlet, a use trail leads left and upstream (generally north) along the base of a low ridge to some small campsites. Across the inlet, the trail quickly climbs to a large, well-used camping area on the right (south) that was once the site of a walk-in lodge built in the 1920s and demolished after the area became part of John Muir Wilderness. It is now a gigantic packer campsite. If this is unoccupied it offers superlative views of the Palisade peaks—you are finally high enough on the north canyon wall to look directly at their jagged profiles.

Sixth Lake: Continuing farther along the trail north from Fourth Lake, you quickly reach a junction (10,905'; 37.13374°N, 118.50302°W) with a weather-beaten sign proclaiming the left (north) spur leads to LAKES 6, 7; the alternative right-hand (east) trail heads to Summit Lake. Onward to Sixth Lake, the trail climbs up a dry slope and skirts a beautiful little meadow with an idyllic pond and stream, bringing it to the foot of massive talus fans pouring off Sky Haven. The meadow is cupped by low ridges, on which you may find campsites quieter than those at Fourth Lake. Staying just off the rubble, the trail turns to the northwest, crosses a minor ridge, a second little drainage, and then ascends a second, slightly larger ridge.

Finishing this roller-coaster route, you now see Sixth Lake below you, the most remote and therefore peaceful lake in this busy area. Descending briefly on the narrow trail, you soon reach pleasant lodgepole pine–shaded campsites just above the lake's northern tip. The steep cliffs of Mount Robinson and Temple Crag dominate the view here while the main Palisade peaks are now hidden behind Mount Robinson. The trail leads to near Sixth Lake's inlet, but the most expansive campsites are actually near the outlet (11,111'; 37.13487°N, 118.50942°W; no campfires). These can be reached by following the lake's northeast shoreline across awkward talus slopes or by dropping directly to the outlet from the previously described ridge. If you choose the latter, to avoid steep terrain, leave the trail before dropping toward Sixth Lake and follow the ridge that lies northeast of the lake for nearly 0.2 mile before descending to lake level. From Sixth Lake's inlet, Seventh Lake lies a farther 0.25 mile to the west, across a marshy expanse of grass and willow; it offers no camping, and the route to it is cumbersome and damaging to the meadow environment, really only a detour to consider if you're continuing to the head of the canyon for more exploring.

Summit Lake: From the aforementioned junction above Fourth Lake, you have just an additional 0.2 mile to reach Summit Lake. Go ahead on the rocky-sandy path, passing a little spring-fed garden and climbing 100 feet to top a ridge among stunted trees. A 30-foot drop leads to the shores of Summit Lake and its few small campsites. As you reach the shore, the track abruptly grows very faint and rocky as it wanders up the northeast side of this rocky bowl to a ridgetop overlooking Black Lake, 330 feet below. It is worth detouring to the ridge just southwest of Summit Lake, for excellent Palisade views.

DAY 3 (Fourth Lake to Big Pine Creek Trailhead, 5.8 miles, plus extra to other lakes): Return to the junction between the trails from Third, Fourth, Fifth, and Black Lakes, and resume the loop part of this trip by going northeast toward Black Lake. The trail crosses Fourth Lake's outlet before ascending a low ridge and then making a short descent to Black Lake's south shore. Black Lake offers a few campsites on the far side of its outlet under dense lodgepole pine cover and a much more enclosed feel.

Continuing downward, the path crosses a trickle and soon leaves forest for a scrubby slope high above the North Fork Big Pine Creek. Black Lake's outlet runs under the rocks where the trail goes through rockfall, then the trail briefly follows the outlet. This slope boasts some fine wildflowers and spectacular views. Soon the track drops down the exposed slope on rocky-dusty, moderate-to-steep switchbacks where you are sandwiched between tall mountain mahogany shrubs. After a long-seeming 0.9 mile, the trail reaches the junction where you originally turned west toward First Lake. Here you end the loop part of this trip, turn left (east), and retrace your steps toward the trailhead.

However, on your return, at the four-way junction below Second Falls, stay straight ahead on the slightly shorter Upper Trail. And where you reach the "confusing five-way junction" near the old First Fall Campground, you might choose to traverse directly to the backpackers' parking lot on the high trail, a distance of 1.1 mile from this junction.

Temple Crag, Mount Gayley, and Mount Sill behind Summit Lake   Photo by Elizabeth Wenk

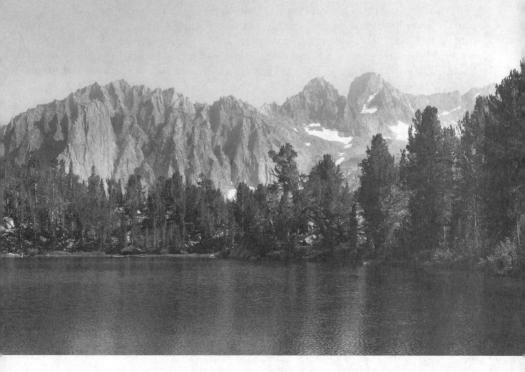

see
map on
p. 361

trip 69   Brainerd Lake

Trip Data: 37.09187°N, 118.45751°W; 9.2 miles; 2/1 days
Topos: *Split Mountain*

HIGHLIGHTS: The rugged South Fork Big Pine Creek canyon offers solitude—in stark contrast to the adjoining, over-crowded North Fork. However, lacking are large campsites and a well-graded trail (in places), but a small group will be delighted with the views of the central Palisade peaks. A layover day—or half day, before you hike out—is strongly recommended to ascend an additional half mile (on a use trail) to Finger Lake, a deep, brilliantly blue lake captured in a narrow trench right at the base of Middle Palisade.

HEADS UP! *This trip is not recommended for beginners and large parties, for Brainerd Lake has mostly very small campsites. Do not take the trail from the backpackers' parking lot; it goes far out of your way. Instead, walk up the road to the day-use parking lot.*

DAY 1 (Big Pine Creek Trailhead to Brainerd Lake, 4.6 miles):   From the road's end, skirt a gate and walk along a creekside road past summer cabins. After 0.2 mile, the road—and the creek—turns right. Just beyond, the road leads to the driveway of a final cabin, while the continuing upcanyon trail abruptly veers left (north-northwest) and becomes singletrack. This track switchbacks above the cabins to a bridge over First Falls on North Fork Big Pine Creek and after a few steps reaches a junction, where your trail up the South Fork Big Pine Creek continues ahead (left, southwest), while right (north) leads up along the North Fork Big Pine Creek (Trip 68).

The trail traverses brushy slopes at the foot of Mount Alice, far above the broad rocky floodplain through which the South Fork cuts a winding green stripe. You have little shade but fine views up the creek toward distant Middle Palisade and Norman Clyde Peak. Shortly the trail crosses the old road coming down from North Fork Big Pine Creek and continues upward. Wildflowers along this leg are seasonally magnificent, with desert paintbrush, Bridge's penstemon, western eupatorium, and sulfur buckwheat especially showy. In late summer the wax currants are laden with sometimes-tasty red berries.

With continued ascent, there are more boulders for the trail to weave between and the trail slowly converges with the creek drainage, its banks choked by willow and alder. At 1.6 miles from the trailhead, the trail dives into the alder thicket to ford the South Fork. In some years there is a stout log across the considerable flow, but in other years it is missing, most recently absent in 2018; this is at least the second time it has disappeared over the preceding 15 years. The safest place to wade is about 50 feet upstream of the main crossing, although if you alder-and-talus bash about 500 feet up the north bank you may find a collection of spindly alder logs to cross on. During spring and early-summer runoff, the

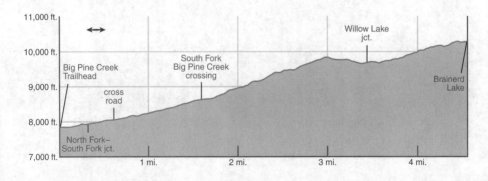

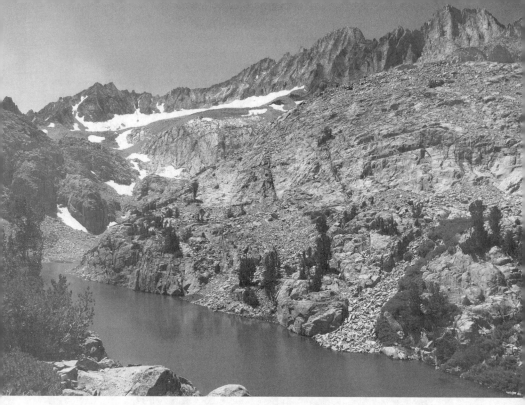

Finger Lake, with Middle Palisade and Norman Clyde Peak in the background   Photo by Elizabeth Wenk

upper option may be the only safe choice. Before leaving the creek, top up on water, for many dry switchbacks lie ahead.

Continuing west around the base of a gigantic vegetated talus fan, use trails from the various plausible crossing points converge. This broad plain provides good views of the channeled South Fork plunging down in showy cascades and has a spectacular display of tall white-flowered poison angelica in midsummer. Soon the gravelly trail cuts up the fan and then when it reaches the base of small bluffs begins switchbacking diligently, but pleasantly, to their right (west). Passing through a gorgeous stand of limber pine, the trail reaches the base of an amazing vertical headwall colored by chartreuse lichen and seeping water from its base, hosting colorful wildflower gardens. This wall is also the guardian of the limber pine stand, for it protects the trees from avalanches that regularly tear down most of the canyon's slopes.

Beyond, the trail crosses a talus slope, slower going with cobble and boulders to contend with—and moreover, it can hold late snow, so take care! The tread then winds up broken slabs to a bedrock rib high above the South Fork and follows a shallow trough south. Cresting a temporary high point, stop and admire the views from the Thumb, on the far left, to Mount Sill, the steep arête on the right. Middle Palisade sits proudly in the center, boasting its scalloped face of avalanche chutes.

Descending slightly down a spring-fed slope where the trail is narrow and often muddy, you spy Willow Lake below, little more than a broadening of the meandering river channel. Climbing again, you pass a minor junction (9,679'; 37.09819°N, 118.45738°W) that leads to acceptable campsites north of Willow Lake. The use trail to Willow Lake begins as a well-beaten track but soon becomes very hard to follow with few cairns for help.

Continuing, you step across a seasonal creeklet and then cross the Brainerd Lake outlet creek on a two-log bridge. Dense lodgepole pine forest soon leads to a steep winding climb up a rocky rib beside the tumbling, noisy Finger Lake outlet creek. Two hundred feet higher the trail turns left (southeast) and passes a dark-watered tarn, choked with tree frog tadpoles and fat, lazy, satiated garter snakes in midsummer. Your meandering trail now works its way across a small drainage, around multiple bluffs and over broken slabs, finally passing through a notch and curving right along a corridor that leads to Brainerd Lake (10,286'; 37.09187°N, 118.45751°W). The lake is guarded over by a tall, sheer headwall, all but obliterating the Palisade views, although you do have splendid downcanyon views to Mount Alice and toward Temple Crag.

First-time visitors may be puzzled by the lack of campsites at this point. The biggest campsite is to the northeast of the lake, hidden within a stand of lodgepole and whitebark pines—and yet the only campsite at Brainerd Lake with satisfying views to Middle Palisade and Norman Clyde (10,288'; 37.09182°N, 118.45602°W; no campfires). There are also many single tent sites in sandy nooks between slabs near the outlet and on the bluffs just west and southwest of the lake's outlet.

FINGER LAKE

A trip to Brainerd Lake is not complete without an excursion to Finger Lake, lying 0.5 mile to the southwest. A use trail—rough and hard to find in places—leads southwest up the bedrock rib just west of Brainerd Lake. Where the slabs transition to small-size talus the use trail becomes more prominent, leading you up a chute to easy slab walking and Finger Lake's outlet (10,814'; 37.08908°N, 118.46119°W). There are a small number of climbers' bivies nestled among whitebark pines nearby. Finger Lake is surreal—a deep lake grading from aqua in the shallows to a brilliant cerulean at the center. The truly adventurous can continue up the bedrock ridge just east of the lake, for ongoing panoramas in all directions, and offering the possibility of looping back to Brainerd Lake along its inlet or down the slope to its east.

DAY 2 (Brainerd Lake to Big Pine Creek Trailhead, 4.6 miles): Retrace your steps.

TABOOSE CREEK ROAD TRIP

Taboose Creek Road leads to the Taboose Pass Trailhead, one of the eastern Sierra's five trailheads between Big Pine and Lone Pine that requires a 6,000-foot climb to surmount the Sierra Crest. The canyon is steep, rugged, and narrow, and the well-built trail also maintains a steep grade to the summit, as it leads hikers from the desert to the alpine. Across Taboose Pass is the South Fork Kings River.

Trailhead: Taboose Pass

Near the summit of Taboose Pass   Photo by Elizabeth Wenk

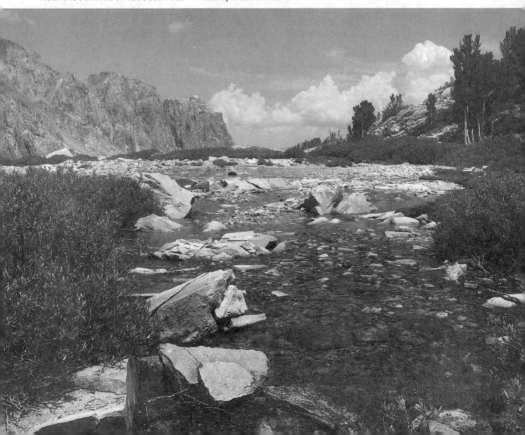

Taboose Pass Trailhead   5,424'; 37.00957°N, 118.32736°W

Destination/ GPS Coordinates	Trip Type	Best Season	Pace & Hiking/ Layover Days	Total Mileage	Permit Required
70 Bench Lake and Woods Lake Basin 36.95153°N 118.46369°W (Bench Lake)	Shuttle	Mid to late	Strenuous 5/1	33.4	Taboose Pass (Sawmill Pass in reverse)

INFORMATION AND PERMITS: This trailhead is in Inyo National Forest. Permits are required for overnight stays and quotas apply. Permits can be reserved up to six months in advance at recreation.gov (60%; $6 permit reservation fee plus $5 per person) or requested in person, first come, first served, a day in advance (40%; free). All permits must be picked up at one of the Inyo National Forest ranger stations, located in Lone Pine (Eastern Sierra Interagency Visitor Center), Bishop, Mammoth Lakes, and Lee Vining (the Mono Basin Scenic Area Visitor Center). If you plan to use a stove or have a campfire while on national forest lands, you must also have a California campfire permit, available from a forest service office or online at preventwildfireca.org/campfire-permit. Campfires are prohibited along the entire Taboose Creek corridor, above 10,400 feet along the Sawmill Pass corridor, and above 10,000 feet in Kings Canyon National Park (west of the Sierra Crest). Bear canisters are required along the Taboose Pass Trail and in Kings Canyon National Park south of Pinchot Pass (including in the Woods Lake basin) and strongly recommended elsewhere.

DRIVING DIRECTIONS: From the junction of US 395 and Crocker Street in the center of Big Pine, drive 12.2 miles south on US 395 to Aberdeen Station Road. This junction is 14.3 miles north of the intersection of US 395 and Market Street in Independence. Turn west onto paved Aberdeen Station Road, signposted for Taboose Creek as well. After 1.2 miles go straight at a four-way junction with Tinemaha Road. Your road is now named Taboose Creek Road/ FS 11S04 and becomes a narrow dirt road. After an additional 0.5 mile, bear right; you are still driving on the most prominent of the dirt road options. Stay right at a Y after 1.9 miles and continue straight to the trailhead, a total of 5.7 miles from US 395. This should be a two-wheel-drive road, but occasionally washouts necessitate vehicles with more clearance.

trip 70   Bench Lake and Woods Lake Basin

see maps on p. 372– 373

Trip Data: 36.95153°N 118.46369°W (Bench Lake); 33.4 miles; 5/1 days

Topos: Aberdeen, Mount Pinchot, Fish Springs

HIGHLIGHTS: There are five trails in the eastern Sierra that require a 6,000-foot climb to reach the crest: Taboose, Sawmill, Baxter, and Shepherd Passes, and Trail Crest, on the Mount Whitney Trail. Of these, Taboose, Sawmill, and Baxter are known as the "hard three," all ascending at a fairly continuous 1,000 feet per mile from the desert to the alpine. This trip leads you over two of them, Taboose Pass on the way up and Sawmill Pass to descend, the two linked by a lovely stretch of the John Muir Trail (JMT) over Pinchot Pass. This is a hard trip, your steep admission price to gems like Bench Lake and the Woods Lake basin. If you don't want to bother with a car shuttle, retrace your steps to the Taboose Pass Trailhead, perhaps detouring north along the JMT to Upper Basin (Trip 20) instead of heading to the Woods Lake basin.

SHUTTLE DIRECTIONS: From the junction of US 395 and Crocker Street in the center of Big Pine, drive 18.0 miles south to Black Rock Springs Road, an additional 5.8 miles south of the Taboose Creek turnoff. This junction is 8.5 miles north of the intersection of US 395 and Market Street in Independence. Turn west onto the dirt Black Rock Springs Road. Go west 0.8 mile to a junction with paved Tinemaha Road. Turn right and continue 1.2 miles. Then turn left onto Division Creek Road and follow it 2.0 miles to the trailhead.

HEADS UP! *Only strong hikers in top condition should undertake the long, hot ascent to Taboose Pass.*

DAY 1 (Taboose Pass Trailhead to second Taboose Creek crossing, 4.7 miles): Today is a long, steep, hot climb—a very early or late start is recommended. The elevation profile shows the trail climbing at a remarkably consistent 1,000 feet per mile, becoming just slightly steeper for the second half of the climb. If you are in shape to climb 1,000 feet an hour, leaving late afternoon can be a good choice: you could climb to the first good campsite, just 3.7 miles into the walk (and a little under 3,000 feet up) and then be staged to complete the other half of the ascent to Taboose Pass in the early-morning cool on Day 2.

With a trailhead at just 5,424 feet, you are starting not far above the Owens Valley floor and distinctly feel like you're walking through the desert as you start up the alluvial fan spilling from the mouth of Taboose Creek. After briefly walking just outside the riparian corridor, the trail diverges from Taboose Creek, and the enlivening strip of green remains out of reach until the canyon narrows 1.2 miles into your walk. Beyond, you are never far from this water source, although the trail is routed through the dry sagebrush scrub above the creek's northern bank. Bitterbrush, sagebrush, sulfur buckwheat, mountain whitethorn, and early summer wildflowers line the trail. Upcanyon, you are staring straight at the red cliffs dropping from Goodale Mountain's northern satellite. Up and up the sandy tread leads deeper into the steep-walled canyon. Several times the trail leads closer to creek level and then higher again to avoid talus fans or small landslides. Just the occasional white fir provides a shady break spot until you drop to cross Taboose Creek in a thicket of alder and dogwood, 3.4 miles from the trailhead (8,014'). *(Note:* the miles up to this crossing were, in part, burned during the 2019 Taboose Fire, leading to a 2020 trail closure. Presumably there is now even less shade along these first miles.)

A few switchbacks lead up the southern bank, now under glorious white fir cover. These lead quickly to a mountain mahogany–covered bench with several campsites (8,298'; 36.99219°N, 118.37202°W). You now truly feel like you've left the desert behind—it is still dry and hot, but you are surrounded by mid-elevation shrubs, chinquapin, and tall mountain mahogany on a north-facing slope. The climb continues past big cliffs and across sporadic drainage gullies, filled with angular rubble from thunderstorm-triggered debris flows; you pass a particularly impressive one just below 8,800 feet. An upcanyon waterfall becomes ever more prominent; the second creek crossing, the first night's destination, lies at its base. As you approach it, the previously pleasantly sandy tread is increasingly replaced by cobble, as the ubiquitous talus fans stretch more regularly to the canyon bottom. Just before crossing the creek there are two small tent sites beside the trail (9,154'; 36.98963°N, 118.38499°W). If these are occupied it is another 0.5-mile and 500-foot ascent to the next ones.

DAY 2 (second Taboose Creek crossing to Bench Lake, 7.0 miles): Stepping across the bouldery creek, you complete 10 switchbacks straight up the north wall of the increasingly stark, steep canyon, with ever-less-vegetated talus slopes. These switchbacks lead to the banks of a tiny seasonal drainage, a pleasant location among fireweed and willows. Onward, the terrain flattens a tad and there is another cluster of small campsites beneath

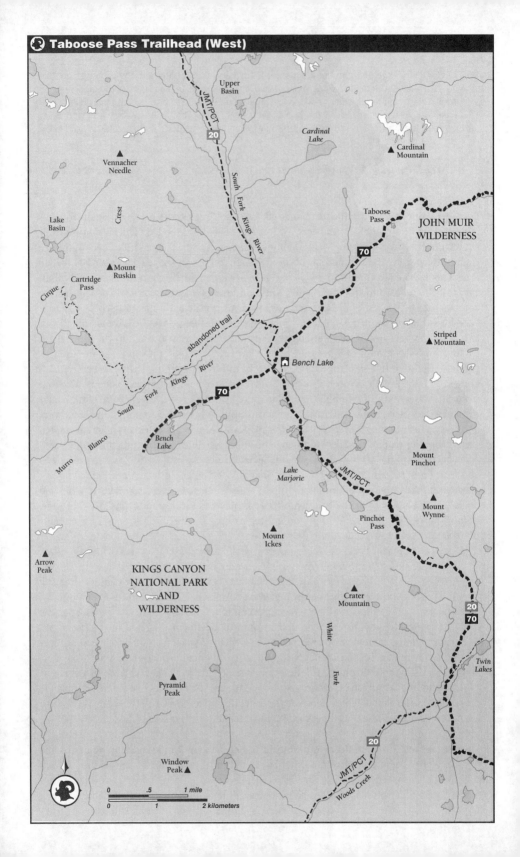

Upper
Basin

JMT/PCT
20

Cardinal
Lake

Cardinal
Mountain

Vennacher
Needle

Taboose
Pass

JOHN MUIR
WILDERNESS

Crest

Lake
Basin

70

Mount Ruskin

Cirque

Cartridge
Pass

abandoned trail

South Fork Kings River

Striped
Mountain

Bench Lake

River

Kings

70

Fork

South

Bench
Lake

Blanco

Mount
Pinchot

Murro

Lake
Marjorie

JMT/PCT

Arrow
Peak

Mount
Wynne

Mount
Ickes

Pinchot
Pass

KINGS CANYON
NATIONAL PARK
AND
WILDERNESS

Crater
Mountain

20
70

White

Pyramid
Peak

Fork

Twin
Lakes

20

Window
Peak

JMT/PCT

Woods Creek

0   .5   1 mile
0   1   2 kilometers

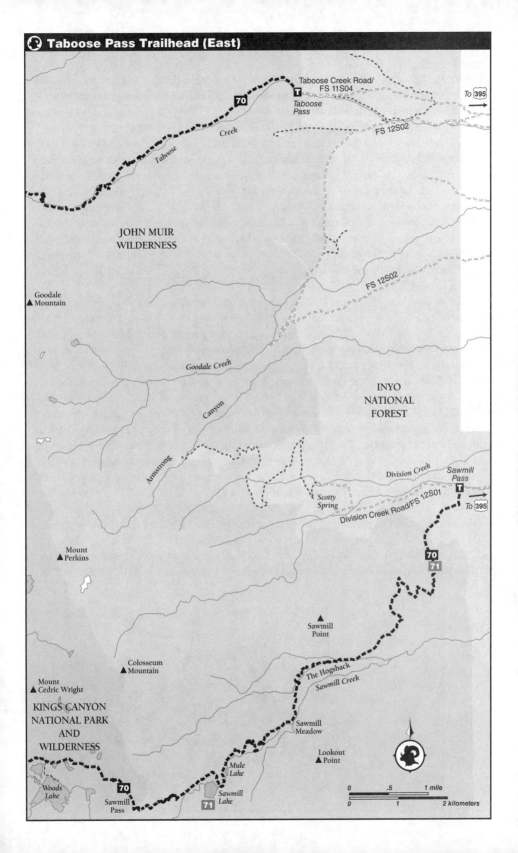

JOHN MUIR WILDERNESS

INYO NATIONAL FOREST

KINGS CANYON NATIONAL PARK AND WILDERNESS

Taboose Creek Road/ FS 11S04

To 395

Taboose Pass

Taboose **70**

FS 12S02

Creek

Taboose

Goodale ▲ Mountain

Goodale Creek

Canyon

FS 12S02

Armstrong

Division Creek

Sawmill Pass

Scotty Spring

Division Creek Road/FS 12S01

To 395

Mount ▲ Perkins

70
71

Sawmill ▲ Point

Colosseum ▲ Mountain

Mount ▲ Cedric Wright

The Hogsback

Sawmill Creek

Sawmill Meadow

Lookout ▲ Point

Mule Lake

Sawmill Lake

Woods Lake

Sawmill Pass **70**

71

0   .5   1 mile

0   1   2 kilometers

limber pines. The following 1.5 miles are almost entirely across cobble and are hard on your feet, but you will gain an appreciation for the trail underfoot if you look at the canyon on Google Earth before your trip and realize that you are skirting the base of about six talus fans and then zigzagging up a seventh. You'll see that the trail follows the best possible path, hugging the slightly less rocky creek drainage until cliffs and steeper terrain force the trail to switchback straight up the seventh talus fan. Luckily, through July there are ample alpine flowers to cheer you upward—magenta Sierra primrose, glossy yellow-petaled alpine gold, red mountain heather, coyote mint, and tiny species of buckwheats and paintbrushes. Atop this fan, the trail trends west again, and you walk past willow thickets and along grassy creek banks, step across the creek's broad shallow flow, and soon reach the most delightful bowl of tarns. Here, the surrounding slab is crisscrossed by dark-colored rock dikes, part of the Independence Dike swarm. Sadly, the terrain is too lumpy to offer good camping. Gaining a little additional elevation, you reach Taboose Pass (11,419') and stare west to Bench Lake, Arrow Peak, and down the South Fork Kings River canyon.

The western side of Taboose Pass could not be more different from its eastern half—you are now in a wide sandy tundra basin, walking gently downslope. This pass was used by the Paiute Indians for centuries, for these open uplands were popular summer hunting grounds. As a creek starts to coalesce in the middle of the expanse, you will find possible sandy campsites, exposed and windy but with brilliant views. The majestically carved Mount Ruskin is now visible north of the South Fork Kings. Ahead, the trail has been rerouted to the south to skirt a marshy meadow, but other trails persist; at an elevation of 11,100 feet (36.97899°N, 118.42132°W), make sure you turn south (left), continuing just beneath a band of whitebark pines. The sandy trail leads onward, past more small campsites and eventually along a bench high above the drainage. You jump across a gushing creek, the outflow of three big lakes hidden at the base of Striped Mountain (with campsites). Slowly the timberline whitebark pine krummholz transitions to a taller-statured lodgepole pine forest, and then you meet the JMT. Here you turn left (south), toward Pinchot Pass, while right leads north to Mather Pass and Upper Basin (Trip 20). You step across a robust little creek and just 400 feet later reach a second signed junction, where you turn right (west) toward Bench Lake, while the JMT continues left (south), tomorrow's route. If you do not wish to carry your pack the extra 1.7 miles to Bench Lake's shores, there are also campsites just a short distance ahead along the JMT or just to the southeast in stands of trees north of a lake. You could establish camp

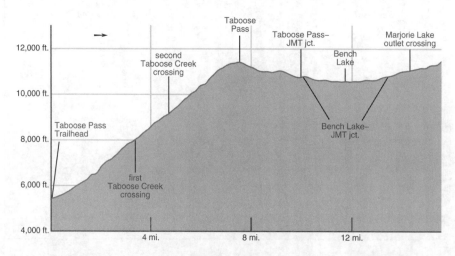

nearby and walk to Bench Lake without your pack. Some years, a white canvas tent to your east marks a summer ranger cabin, with emergency services if the ranger is present.

Onward to Bench Lake, you head west through unassuming lodgepole pine forest on a narrower trail. At first you are traversing wet meadows and then later transition to drier forest stands interspersed with polished slabs. Your views are mostly broken by the trees, but you are just steps from the edge of a shelf, which drops dramatically to the South Fork Kings River. Passing a cluster of tarns, you cross the broad, shallow Bench Lake outlet and approach the iconic lake. For its absolutely clear waters and splendid setting amid granite peaks and spurs, this sparkling jewel has few peers in the High Sierra. There are many campsites around it and the one you select should meet two criteria: make sure you are 100 feet from water and positioned somewhere you can easily stumble out at sunrise to photograph Arrow Peak reflected in the still dawn waters of Bench Lake (for example, 10,570'; 36.95132°N, 118.46298°W; no campfires).

DAY 3 (Bench Lake to Woods Lake, 10.3 miles): Today is a longer day by distance but much more moderately graded. You could easily split with a night near Lake Marjorie or on the south side of Pinchot Pass. Or perhaps enjoy a rest day at Bench Lake and continue once you're rejuvenated.

Returning to the JMT, you turn south (right) and find yourself on a distinctly busier route. You pass a use trail that leads east to the sometimes-staffed Bench Lake ranger tent and continue upslope along an eroded moraine remnant. Small campsites exist on sandy, slightly forested knobs to the side of most of the next several tarns you pass. You cross a number of small creeks on rock blocks, the largest of them the Lake Marjorie outlet creek. Heading west (right) here leads to campsites alongside the two lakelets downstream of Lake Marjorie, tucked beneath whitebark pines. Climbing gradually on polished granite slabs, you skirt the larger of these lakes and then giant, deep Marjorie, staring up at the angular cliffs and talus piles spilling into its waters from the west. Zigzagging upward, past a few final campsites, you look down upon two more talus-bound lakes and soon a third. Your upward climb leads across rills and past endless well-irrigated alpine wildflower gardens. A giant tongue of red talus, a rock glacier, occupies a sheltered cirque to the west. Nearly devoid of talus or cobble, the JMT carries you south to Pinchot Pass, ultimately squiggling up tight switchbacks to surmount the final blocky headwall (12,132').

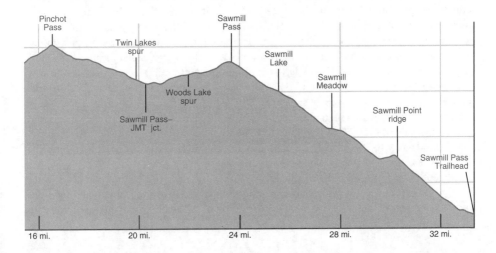

From the summit, you have a brilliant view north to steep granite peaks, with the dark tip of distant Mount Goddard just visible. Farther northeast are the rugged Palisades. To the south are giant Colosseum Peak and cliffier Mount Cedric Wright, behind which the Woods Lake basin sits. While the pass is on granodiorite, the summit of Mount Wynne rising just to your east, as well as Mount Pinchot to the northeast and Crater Mountain to the southwest, are composed of ancient metamorphic rocks. The small patches of white in the otherwise red rock are bits of marble, the remains of ancient sea creatures.

You navigate switchbacks down the south side of the craggy headwall and then cross flower-strewn alpine meadows, stepping across streamlets. Once you are past the uppermost meadows, the JMT curves east to traverse above an enchanting series of ponds and lakes. The trail once followed the meadow corridor downstream but has been rerouted to protect the fragile alpine turf. You continue winding south beneath Mount Perkins, reaching your first trailside campsite beside a small tarn on a ridge with lodgepole pines. Below sit the Twin Lakes and behind them Mount Cedric Wright. Descending more steeply, you approach the Twin Lakes outlet and good campsites, but it is best to continue a little farther and camp off the heavily impacted JMT. After another 0.5 mile, you reach the signed junction with the Sawmill Pass trail and turn left (south), off the JMT.

You quickly step across the Twin Lakes outflow (sometimes wet feet) and pass a small lodgepole pine–shaded campsite. Then begins a long traverse south beneath Mount Cedric Wright with spectacular views unfolding west down Woods Creek's canyon, majestic, steep Mount Clarence King piercing the skyline to the southwest. You are mostly crossing open slopes, with just scattered pockets of lodgepole pines in flats, whitebark pines on knobs, and foxtail pines on dry slopes; the trees each have their preferred habitat. In places, this is a narrow, rough trail, alternating with sections showing recent trail work. Trending south and then east you reach the broad Woods Lake basin, with a dozen lakes and countless tarns and lakelets sprawling between polished slabs; cutting off the trail just after the second trailside lake (10,759'; 36.89159°N, 118.38527°W) leads to possible campsites on knobs near the northern tip of Woods Lake (10,767'; 36.88917°N, 118.38448°W; no campfires). There are, overall, relatively few legal campsites in this basin, for steep, convoluted topography means there are limited flat ridgetops, while endless tarns and marshy meadows fill the hollows between the ribs.

DAY 4 (Woods Lake to Sawmill Meadow, 5.7 miles): Today begins with a 1.7-mile uphill to Sawmill Pass, first skirting endless seasonal tarns beyond Woods Lake. Some of the quite deep pothole lakes drain completely in drought years—the bedrock here is fractured metamorphic rock, not impervious granite slab, and the water vanishes downward. You continue across subalpine plains of gravel and sand, passing the last lodgepole pines and watching the whitebark pines diminish in size. Multicolored metamorphic talus fans descend off Colosseum Peak. Slowly the trail curves south, climbing switchbacks to the broad vegetated plain that leads to Sawmill Pass. This unglaciated expanse hosts some unusual tundra plants, especially since it is irrigated by late snowbanks and the plants are nurtured by nutrient-rich metamorphic soils. Sawmill Pass lacks much of a view however, sitting in a trough (11,327'). Like Taboose Pass, abundant American Indian artifacts have been found along the Sawmill Pass corridor, indicating this passage has been used for centuries to cross into the upper Woods Creek drainage.

Abruptly dropping over the northeastern side of the pass you begin your downward plunge, gravelly and sandy switchbacks snaking along dry shelves and through passageways between steeper metamorphic bluffs. The surrounding walls seem to expand rapidly as you descend to the drainage of narrow, rugged Sawmill Canyon. Fortunately, unlike Taboose, the valley floor is just broad enough that you avoid the talus fans, walking on a sandier tread. You eventually reach a delightful little pond, its willow-clad inlet full of birdlife, and soon see Sawmill Lake below. As you approach Sawmill Lake, you alternately walk through foxtail and whitebark and lodgepole pines, again each established only in its preferred habitat. There are a number of small campsites at Sawmill Lake, especially along the bench you traverse east of the lake (for example, 10,031'; 36.88682°N, 118.34511°W).

You drop one more step to sometimes dry Mule Lake (no campsites) and continue north of the creek through scattered trees. At about 9,500 feet the trail passes a sandy, Jeffrey-shaded flat, where there are a few poor tent sites, and then briefly brushes the creek. The zigzags continue down the steep gravel-and-sand tread, staying northwest of the creek, sometimes through stands of Jeffrey pine and even red fir, an eastern Sierra rarity, and elsewhere onto slopes burned in a 2005 fire. The knee-knocking descent finally pauses in Sawmill Meadow, boggy and lush green in early season but drying considerably as the months progress. There are a few campsites at the meadow's western end and better ones near the outlet in a mixed stand of burned and surviving conifers (8,373'; 36.89784°N, 118.32797°W).

DAY 5 (Sawmill Meadow to Sawmill Pass Trailhead, 5.7 miles): A descending traverse across burned slopes now leads 0.5 mile to the top of a peculiar triangular ridge, the Hogsback. This is a moraine from the most recent glacial maximum, although it has been somewhat reshaped by the two forks of Sawmill Creek that flow down opposite sides of it. From atop the Hogsback, you may also notice a more eroded linear feature farther north, the remnants of an older moraine.

Atop the Hogsback, you leave the main Sawmill Creek drainage and descend toward the sometimes-dry northern fork of Sawmill Creek, sandwiched between the two aforementioned

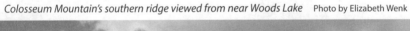

Colosseum Mountain's southern ridge viewed from near Woods Lake　Photo by Elizabeth Wenk

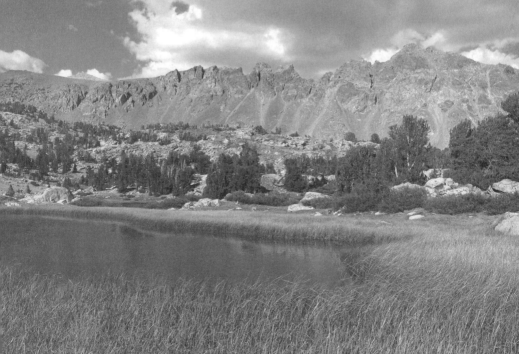

moraines. You cross the creek in a pleasant white fir grove and switchback down the creek's northern bank with just scattered Jeffrey pines and occasional black oaks providing shade. The creek corridor keeps its color after the surrounding sandy soils are parched, most welcome in midsummer. Just below 7,500 feet you pass an intriguing basalt flow and cross the creek twice more, your last water before the trailhead. Nearby, a careful look at the lower end of the Hogsback may reveal the remains of the Blackrock sawmill and flume (dating from the 1860s), after which Sawmill Creek and Sawmill Pass are named.

The trail now begins a long traverse out of the Sawmill Creek drainage, frustratingly even climbing slightly toward the end to bypass cliffs. Look across the canyon at the steep, fractured granite walls in the lower part of Sawmill Canyon that have eroded into imposing triangular cliff faces. Eventually you round a corner, a ridge extending off Sawmill Point, and can see the trail winding its way down to the Owens Valley, the trailhead visible far below.

The remaining 3.1 miles are increasingly hot with not a single plant tall enough to provide shade. However, it is all downhill, and the trail is delightfully sandy, perfect for a descent. You have views of the Big Pine volcanic field to the north. The lava field is spotted with reddish cinder cones and black lava flows that erupted from the west side of Owens Valley. Mormon tea, sagebrush, rabbitbrush, and cacti keep you company as you switchback down the next 1,400 feet. Thereafter you begin a long northward traverse, ultimately crossing a corner of red cinders and then dropping to a giant alluvial fan, debris carried down Spook Canyon and Division Creek by countless storms. This fan is beautiful in spring, with a plethora of desert shrubs and herbs in bloom, including indigobush, yellow and white buckwheat, and bright blue giant woollystar, but only gray-green leaves remain by mid-June. Finally, crossing just above a tongue of lava and some dry washes, you reach the small parking area (4,607'; 36.93891°N, 118.29029°W).

DIVISION CREEK ROAD TRIP

Division Creek Road leads to the Sawmill Pass Trailhead, one of the Sierra's five trailheads between Big Pine and Lone Pine that requires a 6,000-foot climb to surmount the Sierra Crest. Sawmill Pass Trailhead is also the eastern Sierra's lowest, at just 4,607 feet. The trail accesses the Sawmill Creek drainage, one canyon to the south, but steep topography at Sawmill Creek's base necessitates that the trail start alongside Division Creek, only crossing into the Sawmill Creek drainage several thousand feet higher. The trail then leads across the Sierra Crest to the headwaters of Woods Creek, a major South Fork Kings tributary.

Trailhead: Sawmill Pass

The verdant expanse of Sawmill Meadow   Photo by Elizabeth Wenk

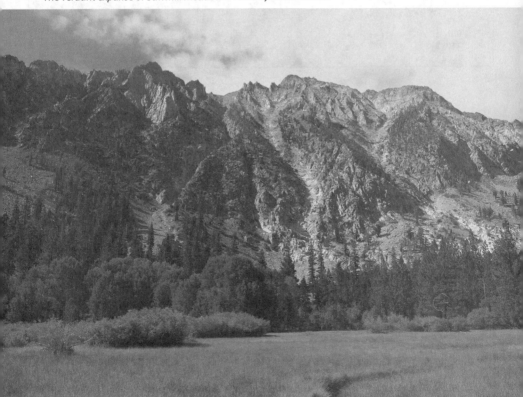

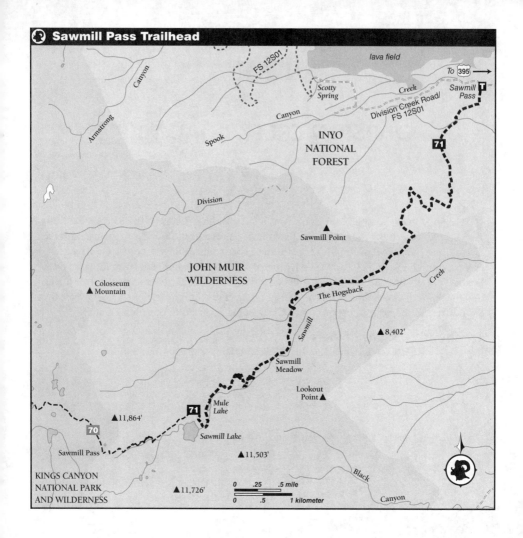

Sawmill Pass Trailhead

INYO NATIONAL FOREST

JOHN MUIR WILDERNESS

KINGS CANYON NATIONAL PARK AND WILDERNESS

lava field

To 395 →

Sawmill Pass

Scotty Spring

FS 12S01

Canyon

Armstrong

Canyon

Spook

Division Creek Road/ FS 12S01

Creek

Canyon

Division

71

Sawmill Point ▲

Creek

Colosseum ▲ Mountain

The Hogsback

Sawmill

▲8,402'

Sawmill Meadow

Lookout Point ▲

71

Mule Lake

▲11,864'

70

Sawmill Lake

▲11,503'

Sawmill Pass

▲11,726'

Black

Canyon

0   .25   .5 mile

0   .5   1 kilometer

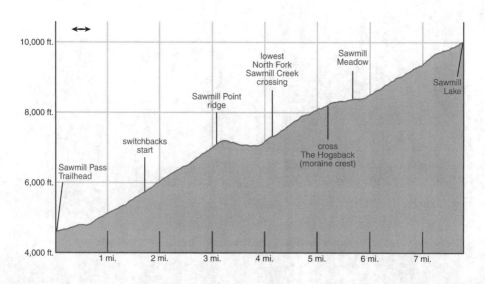

Sawmill Pass Trailhead				4,607'; 36.93891°N, 118.29029°W	
Destination/ GPS Coordinates	Trip Type	Best Season	Pace & Hiking/ Layover Days	Total Mileage	Permit Required
71 Sawmill Lake 36.88671°N 118.34488°W	Out-and-back	Early to late	Strenuous 2/1	15.6	Sawmill Pass
70 Bench Lake and Woods Lake Basin (in reverse of description; see page 370)	Shuttle	Mid to late	Strenuous 5/1	33.4	Sawmill Pass (Taboose Pass as described)

INFORMATION AND PERMITS: This trailhead is in Inyo National Forest. Permits are required for overnight stays and quotas apply. Permits can be reserved up to six months in advance at recreation.gov (60%; $6 permit reservation fee plus $5 per person) or requested in person, first come, first served, a day in advance (40%; free). All permits must be picked up at one of the Inyo National Forest ranger stations, located in Lone Pine (Eastern Sierra Interagency Visitor Center), Bishop, Mammoth Lakes, and Lee Vining (the Mono Basin Scenic Area Visitor Center). If you plan to use a stove or have a campfire while on national forest lands, you must also have a California campfire permit, available from a forest service office or online at preventwildfireca.org/campfire-permit. Campfires are prohibited above 10,400 feet in Inyo National Forest (east of the Sierra Crest). Bear canisters are strongly recommended in this area.

DRIVING DIRECTIONS: From the junction of US 395 and Crocker Street in the center of Big Pine, drive 18.0 miles south to Black Rock Springs Road. This junction is 8.5 miles north of the intersection of US 395 and Market Street in Independence. Turn west onto dirt Black Rock Springs Road. Go west 0.8 mile to a junction with paved Tinemaha Road. Turn right and continue 1.2 miles. Then turn left onto Division Creek Road and follow it 2.0 miles to the trailhead.

trip 71   ## Sawmill Lake

Trip Data: 36.88671°N, 118.34488°W; 15.6 miles; 2/1 days
Topos: *Aberdeen*

HIGHLIGHTS: This extremely strenuous trip climbs steeply from the sweltering Owens Valley at 4,600 feet to a refreshing, beautiful alpine lake at 10,000 feet. After the long, steep, exposed climb, you'll arrive weary but with a mountaineer's "high" from the hard work. Expect solitude here: Few dare tackle this grueling climb. It is a perfect trip to take in late spring, when you're desperate to get high but most trails are still snow-covered.

HEADS UP! *Only strong hikers in top condition should undertake this long, hot slog.*

DAY 1 (Sawmill Pass Trailhead to Sawmill Lake, 7.8 miles): At 4,607 feet, Sawmill Pass Trailhead is the eastern Sierra's lowest trailhead; it is imperative to get an early start, for summer temperatures here regularly surpass 100°F. Your first 0.6 mile traverses a giant alluvial fan, debris carried down Spook Canyon and Division Creek by countless storms. The road downstream of the trailhead gets washed out intermittently by summer thunderstorms. This fan is beautiful in spring, with countless desert shrubs and herbs in bloom, including indigobush, yellow and white buckwheats, and bright blue giant woollystar, but only a few stray flowers usually remain by the time Sawmill Lake is snow-free.

Thereafter the trail begins to gain elevation, climbing briefly across and then above red volcanic cinder cones. With increasing altitude, views of the Big Pine volcanic field appear to the north. The lava field is spotted with reddish cinder cones and black lava flows that erupted from the west side of Owens Valley. The trail makes its first decisive switchback 1.7 miles from the trailhead (5,719'), as it continues up the dry brushy slope, where Mormon tea, sagebrush, rabbitbrush, and cacti continue keeping you company. The shade from trees high on Sawmill Point is still agonizingly far out of reach. At least the sandy tread is pleasant walking and well graded. At 7,088 feet you cross the eastern ridge emanating off Sawmill Point; you've completed the first 3.1 miles of your walk.

Peering one last time to the still-visible trailhead, you cross into the Sawmill Creek drainage and stare at its steep, fractured granite walls, the ends of ridges eroding into triangular faces. The waters of Sawmill Creek appear as a white ribbon 1,000 feet below. The path descends slightly, then contours, and finally climbs along the precipitous north wall of Sawmill Creek's canyon. Looking down you'll see a long triangular rib, the Hogsback. This is a moraine from the most recent glacial maximum, although it has been somewhat reshaped by the two forks of Sawmill Creek that flow down opposite sides of it. You may also notice a more eroded linear feature just north of the trail, the remnants of an older moraine.

As the path nears the sloping ridge of the Hogsback, Jeffrey pine, black oak, and white fir make a most welcome appearance. A careful look at the lower end of the Hogsback may reveal the remains of the Blackrock sawmill and flume (dating from the 1860s), after which Sawmill Creek and Sawmill Pass are named. Above the Hogsback, you can occasionally see stumps, felled trees, and logs used as "gliders" in this long-gone operation to supply Owens Valley miners with lumber.

The trail climbs to meet the sometimes-dry northern fork of Sawmill Creek—the first water you pass on this hot climb. Soon after passing a pleasant shelf above the creek, you cross the channel a second time and then walk past a small basalt flow. The creek corridor through here keeps its color after the surrounding sandy soils are parched, most welcome in midsummer. You continue switchbacking mostly outside the riparian corridor with just scattered Jeffrey pines and occasional black oaks providing shade. You cross the creek a third time in a grove of pleasant white fir and then switchback up to cross the now-less-distinct moraine crest at 8,215 feet.

Now in the true Sawmill Creek catchment, a more gradual ascent across slopes burned in the 2005 Pinyon Complex fire carries you the final 0.5 mile to Sawmill Meadow (8,373'; 36.89784°N, 118.32797°W). Sawmill Meadow is boggy and lush green in early season but dries considerably as the months progress. At the eastern edge of Sawmill Meadow are forest openings with space for many tents in a stand of mostly unburned trees. This makes a good late spring destination when most of the high country is still snow covered and you're itching to get into the backcountry. There are additional campsites as the trail prepares to climb above the meadow, under a mix of burned and surviving conifers.

Leaving Sawmill Meadow, you have a final 1.9 miles and 1,600 feet of elevation gain to Sawmill Lake. The canyon is rugged and stark with stunningly sheer walls. In two straight-line miles, from Sawmill Pass to the meadow, the canyon drops 3,000 feet—and this is just one of tens of equally steep and narrow parallel canyons that descend from the Sierra Crest to the Owens Valley floor. The zigzags continue up the steep gravel-and-sand tread, staying northwest of the creek, sometimes in burned terrain and elsewhere through stands of Jeffrey pine and even red fir, an eastern Sierra rarity. The trail briefly brushes the creek and then passes a sandy, Jeffrey pine-shaded flat, where there are a few poor tent sites.

The remaining distance to Sawmill Lake is a sustained climb, except where it skirts campsiteless and sometimes dry Mule Lake, precariously perched on a small bench high up the canyon. Then the path ascends through a jumbled mass of rocks, home to grass-harvesting pikas. After crossing a side creek, the trail finally arrives at the northeast shore of beautiful Sawmill Lake, where there is fishing for rainbow trout. There are a couple of good campsites under clumps of whitebark pines on the benches east and northeast of the lake (for example, 10,031'; 36.88682°N, 118.34511°W). Above the lake, in all directions you're staring at rocks—cliffs, rounded slabs, and a giant rock glacier to the south—with just a few foxtail pines growing in exposed patches of soil. And in case you wish to continue, it is an additional 1.9 miles to Sawmill Pass (11,327'), from which you can easily access the Woods Lake basin, described in reverse as part of Trip 70. Peak baggers may wish to head to the summit of Colosseum Peak on a layover day, a nontechnical ascent up the sandy southwestern slopes.

DAY 2 (Sawmill Lake to Sawmill Pass Trailhead, 7.8 miles): Retrace your steps.

A mix of metamorphic and granite rock outcrops creates colorful, rugged scenery around Sawmill Lake.   Photo by Elizabeth Wenk

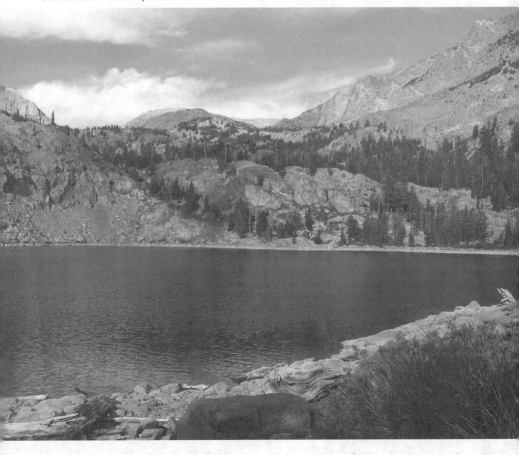

ONION VALLEY ROAD TRIPS

Onion Valley Road leads west from Independence along Independence Creek. This is the least-rugged canyon for many miles north and south, so the road is able to reach an elevation of 9,201 feet. Three trails depart from the end of Onion Valley Road: the Kearsarge Pass Trail, described here, as well as trails to the little-visited Robinson Lakes and Golden Trout Lake. Kearsarge Pass Trail is popular, for it climbs just 2,500 feet to cross the Sierra Crest, just half of the elevation required for any other pass between South Lake and Horseshoe Meadow, and then descends toward the John Muir Trail corridor and Bubbs Creek drainage. A spur off Onion Valley Road, Foothill Road, leads to the Symmes Creek (or Shepherd Pass) Trailhead, located along Symmes Creek at just 6,308 feet. From there, the Shepherd Pass Trail crosses into the Shepherd Creek drainage and climbs to Shepherd Pass on the Sierra Crest by a long, difficult route, then descends Tyndall Creek into the headwaters of the Kern River.

Trailheads: Kearsarge Pass

Symmes Creek (Shepherd Pass)

Gilbert Lake   Photo by Elizabeth Wenk

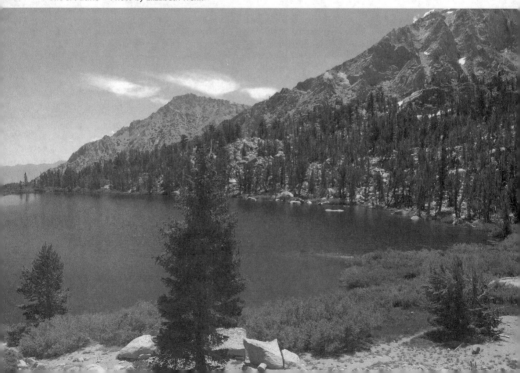

Kearsarge Pass Trailhead			9,201'; 36.77254°N, 118.34107°W		
Destination/ GPS Coordinates	**Trip Type**	**Best Season**	**Pace & Hiking/ Layover Days**	**Total Mileage**	**Permit Required**
72 Flower Lake 36.76909°N 118.35906°W	Out-and-back	Early to late	Leisurely 2/0	5.0	Kearsarge Pass
73 Charlotte, Rae, and Kearsarge Lakes 36.80639°N 118.39794°W (Middle Rae Lake)	Mostly out-and-back, minor semiloop	Mid to late	Moderate 5/1	27.5	Kearsarge Pass
74 Sixty Lake Basin 36.83602°N 118.42125°W (north end Sixty Lake Basin)	Mostly out-and-back, minor semiloop	Mid to late	Moderate 4/2	34.5	Kearsarge Pass

INFORMATION AND PERMITS: This trailhead is in Inyo National Forest. Permits are required for overnight stays and quotas apply. Permits can be reserved up to six months in advance at recreation.gov (60%; $6 permit reservation fee plus $5 per person) or requested in person, first come, first served, a day in advance (40%; free). All permits must be picked up at one of the Inyo National Forest ranger stations, located in Lone Pine (Eastern Sierra Interagency Visitor Center), Bishop, Mammoth Lakes, and Lee Vining (the Mono Basin Scenic Area Visitor Center). If you plan to use a stove or have a campfire while on national forest lands, you must also have a California campfire permit, available from a forest service office or online at preventwildfireca.org/campfire-permit. Campfires are prohibited above 10,000 feet along the Kearsarge Pass Trail and above 10,000 feet in Kings Canyon National Park (west of the Sierra Crest). Bear canisters are required in both Inyo National Forest (east of the Sierra Crest) and Kings Canyon National Park (west of the Sierra Crest) on the hikes that depart from this trailhead.

DRIVING DIRECTIONS: From US 395 in Independence, turn west on Market Street, which becomes Onion Valley Road. Follow this road 13.0 miles to its end in Onion Valley. There are toilets, a campground, a water faucet, and three trailheads here. The Kearsarge Pass Trail, which you want for these trips, is the middle one, to the west of the toilets and just before the campground entrance.

see map on p. 386

trip 72   **Flower Lake**

> **Trip Data:**   36.76909°N, 118.35906 °W; 5.0 miles; 2/0 days
> **Topos:**   *Kearsarge Peak*

HIGHLIGHTS: A short hike on a well-graded trail brings you to the justly popular lakes east of Kearsarge Pass. The angling is good and the scenery grand. This trip also makes an excellent day hike.

DAY 1 (Kearsarge Pass Trailhead to Flower Lake, 2.5 miles): From the trailhead, situated just past the last parking spot and just before you reach the campground, ascend a dry sand-and-gravel slope with sparse shrub cover. After initially trending southwest, the trail turns north, climbing toward the Golden Trout Lake outlet creek. Nearly intersecting the creek, the Kearsarge Pass Trail passes two spurs, at about 0.3 and 0.4 miles, that jog right

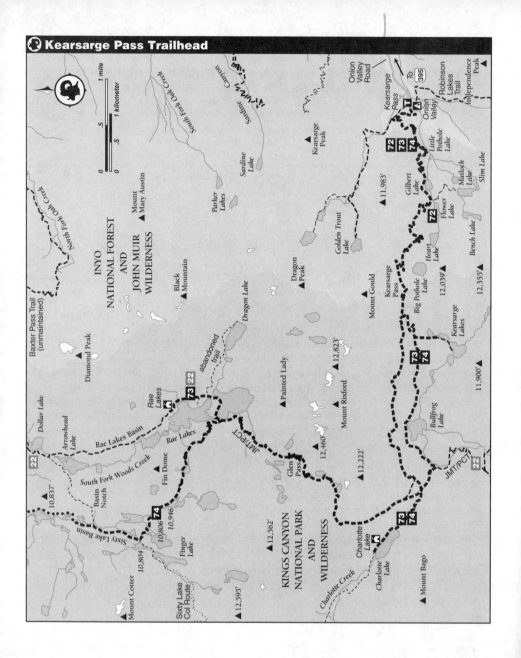

INYO NATIONAL FOREST AND JOHN MUIR WILDERNESS

KINGS CANYON NATIONAL PARK AND WILDERNESS

1 mile
1 kilometer

South Fork Oak Creek

North Fork Oak Creek

Baxter Pass Trail (unmaintained)

Dollar Lake

Arrowhead Lake

Rae Lakes Basin

Rae Lakes

South Fork Woods Creek

Basin Notch

Sixty Lake Basin

Mount Cotter

Sixty Lake Col Route

Finger Lake

Fin Dome

Glen Pass

JMT/PCT

Painted Lady

Saddlerock Canyon

Sardine Lake

Parker Lakes

Mount Mary Austin

Black Mountain

Diamond Peak

Dragon Lake

Dragon Peak

abandoned trail

Kearsarge Peak

Golden Trout Lake

Mount Gould

Kearsarge Pass

Gilbert Lake

Flower Lake

Little Pothole Lake

Matlock Lake

Slim Lake

Bench Lake

Heart Lake

Big Pothole Lake

Kearsarge Lakes

Bullfrog Lake

Charlotte Lake

Charlotte Creek

Mount Rixford

Mount Bago

Orion Valley Road

Kearsarge Pass

To 395

Orion Valley

Robinson Lakes Trail

Independence Peak

▲ 11,983'

▲ 12,039'

▲ 12,355'

▲ 11,900'

▲ 12,823'

▲ 12,460'

▲ 12,222'

▲ 12,562'

▲ 12,595'

▲ 10,837

▲ 10,804

10,806

10,946

JMT/PCT

22 73 74 72 1

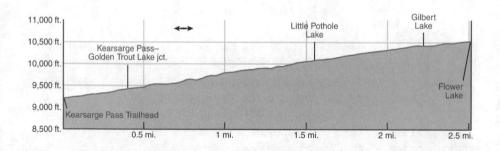

11,000 ft.
10,500 ft.
10,000 ft.
9,500 ft.
9,000 ft.
8,500 ft.

Kearsarge Pass Trailhead

Kearsarge Pass–Golden Trout Lake jct.

Little Pothole Lake

Gilbert Lake

Flower Lake

0.5 mi.   1 mi.   1.5 mi.   2 mi.   2.5 mi.

(northeast) toward the trail to Golden Trout Lake; stay left (northwest) both times. After the second junction, your trail swings south and west again, zigzagging up through sagebrush, mountain mahogany, and greenleaf manzanita, with only a few dry-site flowers like Bridge's penstemon and wavyleaf paintbrush providing dots of color.

By the 0.7-mile mark you are close to the creek draining Flower and Gilbert Lakes, switchbacking steadily up a dry slope well above the creek. Swamp onion and giant red paintbrush provide color as you cross a wetter patch, while magenta mountain pride penstemon emerges from beneath rocks. The trees here alternate between foxtail pine on sandy slopes and whitebark pine on little knobs. Around 1.3 miles from the trailhead the trail is finally close enough to the tumbling creek that only a few steps are needed to reach the wildflower-lined stream bank. At the top of this grade is Little Pothole Lake, with a beautiful pair of cascades dashing into it, although its willow-clad banks don't make it very enticing to visit.

After another set of rocky switchbacks, the trail levels off in a slightly ascending groove across a glacial moraine, then crosses a multicolored talus fan, and arrives at small, round Gilbert Lake (10,425'). Overused campsites dot the shores of this fine swimming lake and fishing for brook trout is good in early season. A final upcanyon traverse beneath some splendid, big foxtail pines leads to the outlet of Flower Lake (10,533'; 36.76909°N, 118.35906°W). There are many highly used campsites under lodgepole and whitebark pine cover along the south and east sides of this shallow lake (for example, 10,541'; 36.76862°N, 118.35909°W; no campfires).

CAMPING FARTHER AFIELD

Slightly less visited and more scenic are two nearby lakes, Matlock and Bench. Reach Matlock Lake by a fairly obvious trail that leads south from the east side of Flower Lake and goes over the ridge south of Flower; it has been plotted on the map on page 386 and heads first southeast, turning southwest and dropping to Matlock Lake once it crosses the shallow ridge separating the two basins. From Matlock Lake, it's a cross-country route west to Bench Lake. Both lakes offer beautiful campsites in sandy flats in the pervasive polished slabs with scattered lodgepole pines and wonderful views, especially south to the steep face of University Peak. These lakes are, however, fishless.

DAY 2 (Flower Lake to Kearsarge Pass Trailhead, 2.5 miles): Retrace your steps.

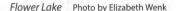

Flower Lake   Photo by Elizabeth Wenk

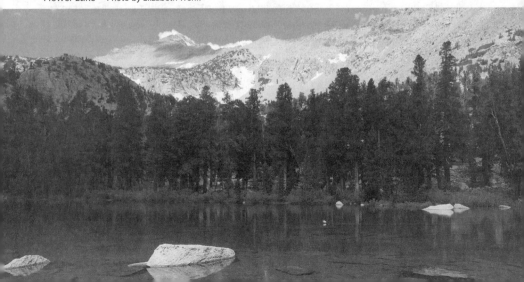

see
map on
p. 386

trip 73 Charlotte, Rae, and Kearsarge Lakes

Trip Data: 36.80639°N, 118.39794°W (Middle Rae Lake);
27.5 miles; 5/1 days

Topos: *Kearsarge Peak, Mount Clarence King*

HIGHLIGHTS: This trip ascends to the alpine moonscape of rugged Kearsarge Pass, descends to the forested shores of bright blue Charlotte Lake, and then joins the John Muir Trail (JMT)/Pacific Crest Trail (PCT) to climb over Glen Pass and visit the rightfully famous—and consequently well-visited— Rae Lakes. It's an exciting mix of grand and varied scenery and good angling.

HEADS UP! *Due to heavy use, camping at Charlotte Lake and the Kearsarge Lakes is limited to a maximum of two nights, and only a single night of camping is permitted at each of the lakes in the Rae Lakes area. If you wish to have a "layover" day in the Rae Lakes area, you must move to a different lake for the second night. Bear canisters are mandatory on this walk.*

DAY 1 (Kearsarge Pass Trailhead to Flower Lake, 2.5 miles): Follow Trip 72, Day 1 to Flower Lake (10,541'; 36.76862°N, 118.35909°W; no campfires). Sturdy hikers may want to continue to Charlotte Lake for the night, as described in Day 2.

DAY 2 (Flower Lake to Charlotte Lake, 6.1 miles): Just barely pausing at Flower Lake, the Kearsarge Pass Trail turns north and resumes a switchbacking ascent through ever sparser forest cover, soon traversing west across the base of a moraine remnant and then following the toe of expansive multihued talus fans. Turning south, the trail crosses a steep rocky slope that holds snow long into July some years, before zigzagging up a whitebark pine–dotted ridge with views to Heart Lake. Eleven exhausting switchbacks later, the trail suddenly rolls over onto an expansive sandy plain sitting atop the cliffband you just surmounted.

Suddenly you can see the trail's route to the summit of Kearsarge Pass, the "pass" sitting high above the ridge's low point. The high elevation limits your pace, but the tread is pleasantly sandy and the trail well graded, allowing good progress. Soon you have views to the nearly perfect blue oval of Big Pothole Lake. The final long switchbacks take you past the uppermost whitebark krummholz, crossing a slope where granitic and metamorphic talus spill together. Finally you reach Kearsarge Pass (11,820'), 2.2 miles beyond Flower Lake. To the west, the impressive view encompasses the Kearsarge Lakes, Bullfrog Lake, and the serrated spires of the Kearsarge Pinnacles. Underfoot are some sky pilot, whose giant spheres of purple flowers rarely grow below 12,000 feet—this is one of the most accessible trailside

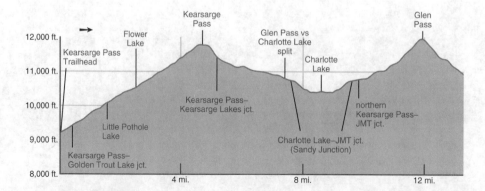

sighting locations in the Sierra. Kearsarge Pass is the easiest Sierra Crest crossing in the southern Sierra. It was an established route used for centuries by American Indian tribes, to cross between Owens Valley to the east and South Fork Kings Valley (Cedar Grove) to the west, for trade and hunting expeditions. It quickly became a well-known route for white pioneers as well, with miners, shepherds, and the first California Geological Survey team to map the southern Sierra, the Brewer Party, all crossing Kearsarge Pass.

On the west side of the pass, your route descends very steeply at first, then more gently, on a traverse high above the basin holding Kearsarge and Bullfrog Lakes. After just over 0.5 mile you pass a spur trail branching left (south) to these lakes, your return route, while now you continue right (west), on the high route, increasingly passing clusters of whitebark pines on your gradual descent. This is a splendid route, cutting across slabs, sandy slopes, and small meadows with unceasing views to the south and west. Ultimately, the trail follows a narrow shelf high above (and below) cliffs; from here you are looking straight down upon Bullfrog Lake and across the canyon to West Vidette, a splendid glacier-carved arête, with Mount Brewer peering out to its right. Rounding a corner, you continue west and gradually down through a dry, sandy landscape with sparse foxtail pine cover. Eventually you reach a trail fork, with both branches leading to the JMT (and PCT). Right (northwest) leads most efficiently to Glen Pass, while left (southwest) is the direct route to Charlotte Lake, so go left, and in just 0.2 mile you reach the JMT at accurately nicknamed "Sandy Junction."

At four-way Sandy Junction, continue straight ahead (west), across the JMT, traversing the sandy flat and then dropping northwest toward Charlotte Lake. As the gradient increases, you suddenly see Charlotte Lake below, in a broad basin with the twin summits of red-hued Mount Bago to the southwest. The dry sandy descent leads to a wet meadow at Charlotte Lake's head and you then follow the northeastern shore to the large lake-end camping area, passing a ranger station shortly before reaching the main collection of tent sites and the often-full bear box (10,436'; 36.77819°N, 118.42831°W; no campfires).

DAY 3 (Charlotte Lake to Middle Rae Lake, 5.8 miles): Retrace your steps 1.3 miles to the junction with the JMT (Sandy Junction) and turn left (north) to begin your climb over Glen Pass. The trail makes a long, steady, rocky ascent, passing the alternate spur to Kearsarge Pass after 0.2 mile, and continuing left (north) up a dry sandy slope that rounds a granite promontory. Here you have fine views of Charlotte Lake, Charlotte Creek's canyon, Charlotte Dome, and the Kings–Kern Divide from Mount Stanford to Thunder Mountain.

The track descends slightly and veers east into a narrow cirque valley, winding between seasonal tarns and then passing a pothole lake with brilliant clear blue water (that occasionally dries out due to its leaky talus dam). Behind the lake is a steep-fronted pile of talus, a

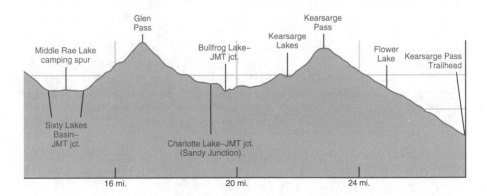

rock glacier. Like an ice glacier, an active rock glacier is slowly moving downslope, pushed along by ice at its core. The well-engineered trail winds up a talus slope and then zigzags tightly up a narrow gully to reach a second lake, this one with a few campsites between timberline whitebark pines. Skirting the lake along its western edge, you pass an area adorned with red mountain heather and Sierra primroses. Staring at the headwall of Glen Pass, it is hard to see where a passable trail could go up the steep slope; the switchbacking trail follows a gravelly gully between cliff bands. Finally at the knife's-edge pass (11,970'), look down on the unnamed glacial lakes immediately north, and to several of the Rae Lakes below. The view south is, however, disappointing, for you can see little beyond the cirque below.

The northern side of the pass is even steeper—both the trail and the slope—and can be snow covered well into July. The trail is routed to avoid the longest-lasting snow banks, but you will likely be following a well-worn and sometimes icy foot trench if you cross in early summer. The rocky zigzags continue all the way to the granite bench holding the clutch of glacial lakes. Passing a few exposed alpine bivy sites, the trail winds across a polished bedrock rib and then drops down a sandy-gravelly slope to a willow-and-grass-covered flat with a small tarn. Notice how there are bands of both black and white rock through here—the rocks here are some of the Sierra's oldest granitic rocks, and subsequent rock formations repeatedly fractured and altered the preexisting rock, creating the beautiful colored stripes crisscrossing the cliff faces. Along the coming miles, keep your eyes open for Sierra Nevada bighorn sheep. A herd of rams is frequently observed on bluffs nearby, one of the best trailside sheep-viewing locales in the Sierra.

After crossing the tarn's outlet stream, the trail resumes its switchbacking descent and steps across a second creeklet three times as it drops down gullies and across slabs to the western shore of Upper Rae Lake. Skirting just above the shore, the trail reaches a junction where left (north) leads to a few small campsites and Sixty Lake Basin (Trip 74), while the JMT leads right (northeast), dropping deeper into the Rae Lakes Basin.

You stay on the JMT, almost immediately crossing the stream connecting the upper and middle lakes (possibly difficult in early season) and then continuing next to the shore of Upper Rae Lake along a narrow isthmus separating the two lakes. The route then swings north, passes the unmarked, unmaintained lateral to Dragon Lake, departing across the sandy strip down the middle of the meadow (Spartan alpine campsites at the lake), and just beyond arrives at a signed spur leading left (west) to the many good but overused campsites near the east shore of Middle Rae Lake (10,570'; 36.80684°N, 118.39941°W, at the bear box above the bay on Middle Rae Lake's east side; no campfires).

Fishing is good for brook trout and some rainbow. Views from these campsites across the beryl-green lake waters to dramatically exfoliating Fin Dome and the King Spur beyond are among the best and longest remembered of the trip, along with morning views of aptly named Painted Lady in the south. A summer ranger is stationed on the northeast shore of the middle lake (10,620'; 36.81093°N, 118.40005°W). Campsites at Middle Rae Lake may be very crowded. There are additional campsites at Lower Rae Lake (0.8 mile farther north) and still-lower Arrowhead Lake (1.5 miles farther north). Having crossed two passes to reach this splendid lakes basin, it is well worth a layover day to enjoy the shores, explore the other lakes in the basin, or perhaps visit Sixty Lake Basin, as described in Trip 74. However, you are only allowed to spend a single night at each lake in the Rae Lakes Basin and therefore must move your campsite to a different lake for the second night.

DAY 4 (Rae Lakes to Kearsarge Lakes, 7.2 miles): Begin by retracing your steps over Glen Pass to Sandy Junction, the junction where right (northwest) leads to Charlotte Lake and

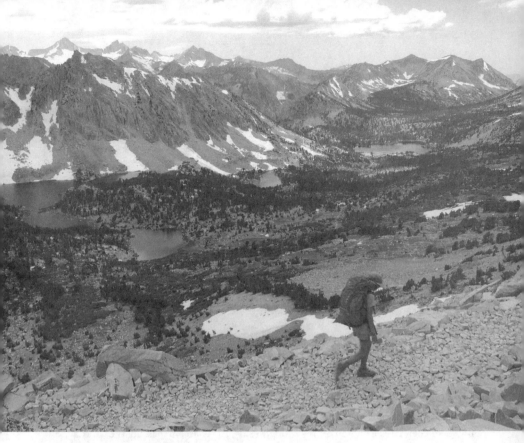

Hiking down the west side of Kearsarge Pass   Photo by Elizabeth Wenk

left (east) to Kearsarge Pass. To take a slightly different return route, continue south on the JMT for an additional 0.4 mile, descending a sandy slope to reach another junction, where the JMT continues right (south), while left (east) leads to Bullfrog Lake and the Kearsarge Lakes. There is a small overused campsite at the junction, but better ones lie ahead. Climbing briefly alongside a small drainage, you pass a pair of splendid tarns and reach meadow-ringed Bullfrog Lake; camping is prohibited within 0.25 mile of Bullfrog Lake. You now wander up this beautiful shallow drainage, increasingly hemmed in to the south by the steep Kearsarge Pinnacles. The trail diverges from the Kearsarge Lakes outlet, climbing alongside a subsidiary creeklet up sandy slopes, across slabs, and past clumps of whitebark pines. Just 1.9 miles beyond the JMT junction, you reach a spur leading right to the popular Kearsarge Lakes (11,039'; 36.77177°N, 118.38586°W). There are other use trails here, but to protect the fragile tundra it is best to wait for the main trail, leading 0.5 mile to the biggest lake (Lake 3,321). The calculated mileage continues just 0.2 mile (to the first lake), but the best campsites are actually before you reach even the first lake, to the west of the trail (10,972'; 36.77030°N, 118.38632°W; no campfires).

DAY 5 (Kearsarge Lakes to Kearsarge Pass Trailhead, 5.9 miles): Retrace your steps up the Kearsarge Lakes spur, then turn right and complete four reasonably steep switchbacks up a sandy whitebark pine–dotted slope to reach the main Kearsarge Pass Trail. Now turn right (east), and retrace your steps 0.5 mile to the summit of the pass and then 4.7 miles down the eastern slopes to the trailhead.

see map on p. 386

trip 74 Sixty Lake Basin

Trip Data: 36.83602°N, 118.42125°W (north end of
Sixty Lake Basin); 34.5 miles; 4/2 days

Topos: *Kearsarge Peak, Mount Clarence King*

HIGHLIGHTS: Sixty Lake Basin is a worthy companion to the nearby Rae Lakes. Its convoluted land-scape leads to generally smaller lakes and a more intimate feel than does the open landscape of the Rae Lakes. Each hollow in the granite holds a pleasant surprise: a meadow, a small campsite, a bub-bling stream, or maybe your own private lake. And, happily, there is no camping limit for backpackers (but stock are not allowed past the uppermost lake).

HEADS UP! *On the way to Sixty Lake Basin, camping is limited to two nights at the Kearsarge Lakes and Charlotte Lake, and to two nights in the Rae Lakes Basin, with just a single night allowed at each lake. Bear canisters are required along this entire hike. And campfires are prohibited in the entire Sixty Lake Basin.*

DAY 1 (Kearsarge Pass Trailhead to Charlotte Lake, 8.6 miles): Follow Trip 72, Day 1 for 2.5 miles to Flower Lake (10,541'; 36.76862°N, 118.35909°W; no campfires). Then follow Trip 73, Day 2 and additional 6.1 miles to Charlotte Lake (10,436'; 36.77819°N, 118.42831°W; no campfires). Some parties may wish to split this hike across two days, spending the first night at Flower Lake.

DAY 2 (Charlotte Lake to northern tip Sixty Lake Basin, 9.3 miles): Retrace your steps 1.3 miles to the junction with the JMT (Sandy Junction) and turn left (north) to begin your climb over Glen Pass. The trail makes a long, steady, rocky ascent, passing the alternate spur to Kearsarge Pass after 0.2 mile and continuing left (north) up a dry sandy slope that rounds a granite promontory. Here you have fine views of Charlotte Lake, Charlotte Creek's canyon, Charlotte Dome, and the Kings–Kern Divide from Mount Stanford to Thunder Mountain.

The track descends slightly and veers east into a narrow cirque valley, winding between seasonal tarns and then passing a pothole lake with brilliant, clear blue water (that occa-sionally dries up due to its leaky talus dam). Behind the lake is a steep-fronted pile of talus, a rock glacier. Like an ice glacier, an active rock glacier is slowly moving downslope, pushed along by ice at its core. The well-engineered trail winds up a talus slope and then zigzags tightly up a narrow gully to reach a second lake, this one with a few campsites between tim-berline whitebark pines. Skirting the lake along its western edge, you pass an area adorned with red mountain heather and Sierra primroses.

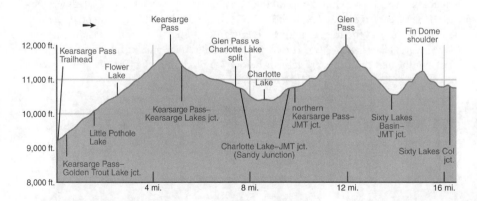

Staring at the headwall of Glen Pass, it is hard to see where a passable trail could go up the steep slope; the switchbacking trail follows a gravelly gully between cliff bands. Finally at the knife's-edge pass (11,970'), look down on the unnamed glacial lakes immediately north, and to several of the Rae Lakes below. The view south is, however, disappointing, for you can see little beyond the cirque below.

The northern side of the pass is even steeper—both the trail and the slope—and can be snow covered well into July. The trail is routed to avoid the longest-lasting snowbanks, but you will likely be following a well-worn and sometimes icy foot trench if you cross in early summer. The rocky zigzags continue all the way to the granite bench holding the clutch of glacial lakes. Passing a few exposed alpine bivy sites, the trail winds across a polished bedrock rib and then drops down a sandy-gravelly slope to a willow-and-grass-covered flat with a small tarn. Notice how there are bands of both black and white rock through here—the rocks here are some of the Sierra's oldest granitic rocks, and subsequent rock formations repeatedly fractured and altered the preexisting rock, creating the beautiful colored stripes crisscrossing the cliff faces. Along the coming miles, keep your eyes open for Sierra Nevada bighorn sheep. A herd of rams is frequently observed on bluffs nearby, one of the best trailside sheep-viewing locales in the Sierra.

After crossing the tarn's outlet stream, the trail resumes its switchbacking descent and steps across a second creeklet three times as it drops down gullies and across slabs to the western shore of Upper Rae Lake. Skirting just above the shore, the trail reaches a junction where the JMT continues right (northeast), heading downcanyon (Trip 73), while you turn left (due north, straight ahead) to cross into Sixty Lake Basin. If you're tired, there are campsites near the junction, on the isthmus between the upper and middle lake, and along the northeastern side of Middle Rae Lake, the latter at a location identified by a signed spur.

Continuing toward Sixty Lake Basin, the trail crosses a marshy area beside a finger of Middle Rae Lake, and then turns west to begin a stiff switchbacking ascent offering superb views of the Rae Lakes and the skyline of steep summits. Winding up a sand-and-slab slope and crossing a delightful flower-rimmed trickle, the route leads west and a little north, crossing the ridge beside a small tarn.

Suddenly you have views to a new mountain wonderland, with the twin pyramids of Mount Cotter and Mount Clarence King rising to the southwest, while equally steep Mount Gardiner peers over Sixty Lake Col. As you sidle north, the lake basin opens up before you—a long chain of island-dotted lakes, becoming shallower to the north. The trail leads steeply down to the shores of Lake 10,946 and then follows its outlet downstream; just before you leave the lake, you'll find small sandy tent sites on a shelf east of the trail,

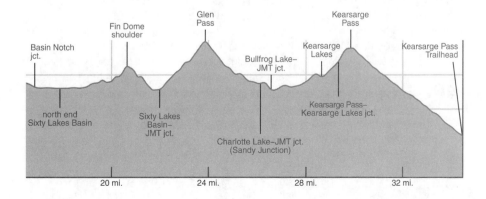

or you can continue farther to a hidden lake just west of Fin Dome. Crossing the inlet and traversing a corridor high above the next lake, look east for an impressive view of Fin Dome, crowning the ridge between Sixty Lake Basin and Rae Lakes Basin. Fin Dome serves as a reference point from most of the high, sparsely forested basin. Bolton Brown saw Fin Dome as part of a massive sea serpent, separating Sixty Lake Basin from the Rae Lakes Basin, assigning the names "The Head" to a knob to the north and "The Tail" to a knob to the south, but only "the Fin" stuck. While other explorers generally named peaks and lakes after famous people, Brown preferred more imaginative or descriptive names; he was the first to map the route over Glen Pass, calling it Blue Flower Pass, probably for the sky pilots.

Climbing slightly, you brush the side of tarns northeast of Lake 10,806 and continue across slabs and through sandy corridors to an unmarked junction, 2.4 miles beyond the JMT (10,816'; 36.81623°N, 118.42586°W). From here a use trail leads to the southwestern lakes, deeper lakes in a yet narrower branch of the basin, and onto Sixty Lake Col and the Gardiner Basin. At all of these lakes you will find small campsites tucked beside whitebark pines, but nothing large.

Stepping across the gushing outlet of Lake 10,804, the trail continues downdrainage. It is a strikingly convoluted basin of polished granite ribs separated by corridors, pocket meadows, creeks, and, in the lowest depressions, the endless lakes. The trail is slow walking as it winds across the landscape to avoid the incessant bluffs and water. Bolton Brown was accurate in calling the northern lakes the "Labyrinth Lakes." After the aforementioned junction there are few campsites until you reach the northern string of lakes. At 0.6 mile past the aforementioned Sixty Lake Col junction (10,636'; 36.82378°N, 118.42338°W), right where a minor side drainage merges from the east, is the route to Basin Notch, a possible easy off-trail route leading to Arrowhead Lake in the Rae Lakes Basin—see sidebar—and a good location to ford the creek. At 0.25 mile later is another good location to cross the drainage and find small, sandy campsites scattered across the pervasive slabs (10,606'; 36.82710°N, 118.42244°W; no campfires). Wherever you stop for the night, the mileage goes to the northernmost lake, for having come so far, you should walk the entire length of the basin and stare north toward the Woods Creek drainage.

SIDE TRIPS FROM SIXTY LAKE BASIN

It's a pleasure simply to explore all the nooks and crannies of Sixty Lake Basin. Or pay a cross-country visit to remote upper Gardiner Basin and its large, alpine lakes by scrambling west over Sixty Lake Col, the low point south of Mount Cotter from the long, slender lake in western Sixty Lake Basin (locally called "Finger Lake"). Stay high around the northern half of Finger Lake's west side and then begin to ramp upward once across the drainage near its midpoint. Crossing Sixty Lake Col at its south end (about 11,656'; 36.80417°N, 118.44145°W) may be easier than at its north end, but let the land tell you where to go; it is Class 2 to easy Class 3 depending on the route you select. Once accessed by a trail from Charlotte Lake over Gardiner Pass, Gardiner Basin is now (mostly) trailless and seldom visited.

From Sixty Lake Col, Mount Cotter is a straightforward, if arduous, ascent, while Mount Clarence King and Mount Gardiner require ropes. These peaks are named for three members of the 1964 Whitney Survey party, and after you have stared at them for several days, you may want to head home to read Clarence King's autobiographical account of his and Richard Cotter's adventures in the Sierra in the 1860s, *Mountaineering in the Sierra Nevada*. It is a thrilling and worthwhile read, though you'll likely concur that King tended to embellish things. Or, perhaps search through archived Sierra Club Bulletins online to read Bolton Brown's account of his two attempts to summit Mount Clarence King, the second, in 1896, successful.

BASIN NOTCH TO RAE LAKES

An easy cross-country pass provides an alternate return route via the Rae Lakes Basin. From the Basin Notch junction (10,636'; 36.82378°N, 118.42338°W) you head 0.2 mile due east past two small tarns and then turn more to the northeast, ascending a broad gully to its head. This leads an easy 0.1 mile to a broad, shallow high point, Basin Notch (10,766'; 36.82523°N, 118.41902°W), a not-so-imaginatively named notch between the two basins. Hopefully you've found the use trail here and can follow it down the steeper terrain on the northeast side. You begin by dropping about 250 feet, to a bit past where the gully broadens, and then you need to begin traversing east (right); avoid dropping too much. Unappealing talus blocks are to your side, but you can walk mostly on sand as you traverse beside them. The key is to aim for a bench with a few scattered trees, not the steep slabs higher up. Then you continue along the base of the cliffs, through lodgepole pine flats and across nearly flat slabs until you land on a beautiful rounded rib overlooking Arrowhead Lake. From here, follow a vegetated gully northeast, soon touching Arrowhead Lake's northwestern shore. You'll find some quiet campsites nearby. Continuing around the lake, you'll shortly intersect the JMT (10,295'; 36.83119°N, 118.40975°W).

Turn right and head upcanyon. There are popular campsites with a bear box at Arrowhead Lake. You then climb up dry slopes far from the river corridor to Lower Rae Lake, with another campsite and bear box. Now in the Rae Lakes Basin proper, the landscape is lush; you step repeatedly over little rills. The Rae Lakes are only a couple of hundred feet lower than the parallel Sixty Lake Basin lakes, but they have a much more open basin. You continue past a spur to the summer-staffed Rae Lakes Ranger Station, Middle Rae Lake (and its large campsite), and then bend right (west) to cross the isthmus separating the upper and middle lakes. Stepping across the connecting stream, you reach the main junction to Sixty Lake Basin, where you complete this optional loop. This alternate route has been 3.8 miles versus 3 miles on the main trail but is considerably slower. If you take this route, you should plan on spending a night at one of the Rae Lakes on the way.

The lowest lake in Sixty Lake Basin   Photo by Douglas Bock

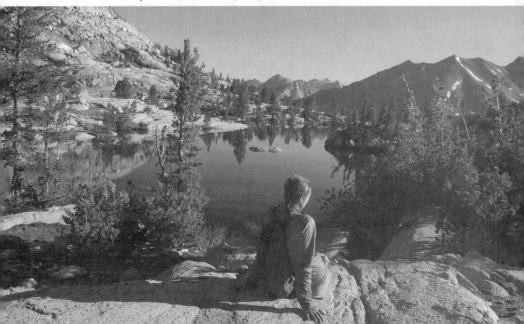

DAY 3 (northern tip of Sixty Lake Basin to Kearsarge Lakes, 10.7 miles): The mileage given is from the northernmost lake in the Sixty Lake Basin. If you are camped there, you may wish to split this day, probably by camping in the Rae Lakes Basin near the junction with the JMT or on the isthmus between the upper and middle lakes. If you are camped farther south in Sixty Lake Basin, reaching the Kearsarge Lakes in a day shouldn't be too difficult; you now have a light pack and are well acclimated.

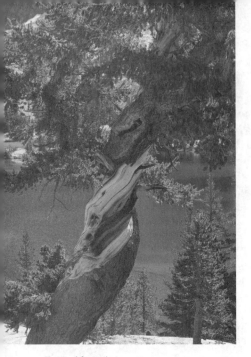

Twisted foxtail pine
Photo by Elizabeth Wenk

Retrace your steps to Rae Lakes Basin and over Glen Pass to Sandy Junction, the junction where left (east) leads over Kearsarge Pass and right (northwest) to Charlotte Lake. To take a slightly different return route, continue south on the JMT for an additional 0.4 mile, descending a sandy slope to reach another junction, where the JMT continues right (south), while left (east) leads to Bullfrog Lake and the Kearsarge Lakes. There is a small overused campsite at the junction, but better ones lie ahead. Climbing briefly alongside a small drainage, you pass a pair of splendid tarns and reach meadow-ringed Bullfrog Lake; camping is prohibited within 0.25 mile of Bullfrog Lake. You now wander up this beautiful shallow drainage, increasingly hemmed in to the south by the steep Kearsarge Pinnacles. The trail diverges from the Kearsarge Lakes outlet, climbing alongside a subsidiary creeklet up sandy slopes, across slabs, and past clumps of whitebark pines. At 1.9 miles beyond the JMT junction you reach a spur leading right to the popular Kearsarge Lakes. There are other use trails leading here, but to protect the fragile tundra it is best to wait for the main trail (11,039'; 36.77177°N, 118.38586°W), leading 0.5 mile to the biggest lake (Lake 3,321). The calculated mileage continues just 0.2 mile (to the first lake), but the best campsites are actually before you reach even the first lake, to the west of the trail (10,972'; 36.77030°N, 118.38632°W; no campfires).

DAY 4 (Kearsarge Lakes to Kearsarge Pass Trailhead, 5.9 miles): Retrace your steps up the Kearsarge Lakes spur, then turn right and complete four reasonably steep switchbacks up a sandy whitebark pine–dotted slope to reach the main Kearsarge Pass Trail. Now turn right (east) and retrace your steps 0.5 mile to the summit of the pass and then 4.7 miles down the eastern slopes to the trailhead.

Symmes Creek (Shepherd Pass) Trailhead
6,308'; 36.72708°N, 118.27888°W

Destination/ GPS Coordinates	Trip Type	Best Season	Pace & Hiking/ Layover Days	Total Mileage	Permit Required
79 Milestone Basin and the Upper Kern *(in reverse of description; see page 427)*	Shuttle	Mid to late	Moderate to Strenuous 7/3	55.6	Shepherd Pass *(Cottonwood Pass as described)*

INFORMATION AND PERMITS: This trailhead is in Inyo National Forest. Permits are required for overnight stays and quotas apply. Permits can be reserved up to six months in advance at recreation.gov (60%; $6 permit reservation fee plus $5 per person) or requested in person, first come, first served, a day in advance (40%; free). All permits must be picked up at one of the Inyo National Forest ranger stations, located in Lone Pine (Eastern Sierra Interagency Visitor Center), Bishop, Mammoth Lakes, and Lee Vining (the Mono Basin Scenic Area Visitor Center). If you plan to use a stove or have a campfire while on national forest lands, you must also have a California campfire permit, available from a forest service office or online at preventwildfireca.org/campfire-permit. Campfires are prohibited above 10,400 in Inyo National Forest (east of the Sierra Crest) and above 10,400 feet in Sequoia National Park (west of the Sierra Crest), as well as at Anvil Camp. Bear canisters are strongly recommended along the Shepherd Pass Trail but required along parts of Trip 79.

DRIVING DIRECTIONS: From Lone Pine, drive 15.7 miles north to Independence. In Independence, turn from US 395 west onto Market Street (Onion Valley Road). Go 4.4 miles to Foothill Road, turn left, and go 1.3 miles to a Y-junction, where you stay right. Continue for an additional 2.0 miles, still on Foothill Road, and then turn right (west) onto Forest Service Road 14S102. Continue another 1.4 miles to the road's end, staying right where two less distinct dirt roads bear south/left.

View from the west side of Shepherd Pass   Photo by Elizabeth Wenk

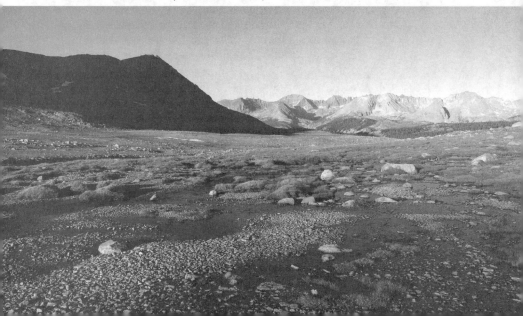

WHITNEY PORTAL ROAD TRIP

Whitney Portal Road leads to Whitney Portal, the start of the famous Mount Whitney Trail to the summit of Mount Whitney. The draw of Mount Whitney led to a road being built high into the Lone Pine Creek canyon. Two trails depart from the road-end parking area, the Mount Whitney Trail, described here, and the Meysan Lakes Trail, a little-used route up the equally steep canyon just to the south, Meysan Creek. The Mount Whitney Trail ascends Lone Pine Creek, crossing the Sierra Crest at Trail Crest, and then connects to the John Muir Trail (JMT), which leads west down Whitney Creek into the Kern River drainage.

Trailhead: Mount Whitney

The summit hut atop Mount Whitney   Photo by Elizabeth Wenk

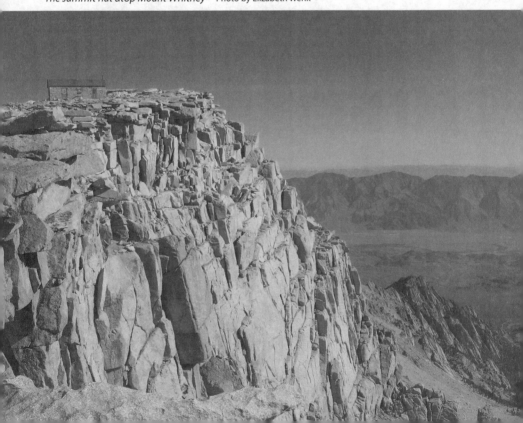

Mount Whitney Trailhead					8,330'; 36.58691°N, 118.24019°W
Destination/ GPS Coordinates	**Trip Type**	**Best Season**	**Pace & Hiking/ Layover Days**	**Total Mileage**	**Permit Required**
75 Mount Whitney Summit 36.57852°N 118.29228°W	Out-and-back	Mid to late	Moderate 4/0	20.8	Mount Whitney Trail
27 High Sierra Trail *(in reverse of description; see page 166)*	Shuttle	Mid to late	Moderate (trans-Sierra) 9/3	68.0	Mount Whitney Trail *(High Sierra Trail issued by Sequoia and Kings Canyon National Parks as described)*
78 Horseshoe Meadow to Mount Whitney *(in reverse of description; see page 420)*	Shuttle	Mid to late	Moderate 6/0	39.5	Mount Whitney Trail *(Cottonwood Pass as described)*

INFORMATION AND PERMITS: This trailhead is in Inyo National Forest. Permits are required for overnight stays and day trips and quotas apply. All permits for Mount Whitney must be picked up at the Eastern Sierra Interagency Visitor Center located 2.0 miles south of the center of Lone Pine, at the southeast corner of the intersection of US 395 and CA 136. The process for obtaining permits for the Mount Whitney Trail is different than for all other Inyo National Forest trailheads—keep reading.

Trailhead quotas are in effect May 1–November 1, with a daily quota of 60 overnight permits and 100 day hike permits. All permits for both day and overnight trips during the quota period are allocated by lottery. Permit requests may be submitted to the lottery between February 1 and March 15, with outcomes being emailed in late March. You may submit up to 15 date choices in a single application. Outside of the quota season, you may simply pick up a first-come, first-served permit at the Eastern Sierra Interagency Visitor Center. To submit a permit request to the lottery, visit tinyurl.com/whitneypermit. There are also additional instructions at this site.

Note that overnight permits must be picked up or confirmed by 10 a.m. on the departure date. Day hike permits must be picked up or confirmed by 1 p.m. the day before the permit date. You may confirm your permit in person or call the Inyo National Forest Wilderness Permit Reservation Office at 760-873-2483. If you wish to pick up your permit after hours, call the number above and have your permit left in the night box, located in a small kiosk along CA 136.

Prior to 2019, last-minute cancellations and no-shows were available for walk-up visitors. In 2019 these permits were available at recreation.gov. It is unclear what the regulations will be post-COVID once visitor centers are open again.

If you plan to use a stove or have a campfire while on national forest lands, you must also have a California campfire permit, available from a forest service office or online at preventwildfireca.org/campfire-permit. Campfires are prohibited along the entire Mount Whitney Trail. Bear canisters are required along the Mount Whitney Trail.

DRIVING DIRECTIONS: From the intersection of US 395 and Whitney Portal Road in the town of Lone Pine—at the town's only traffic light—go 11.8 miles west on Whitney Portal

Road to its end at Whitney Portal. Here you'll find a large parking area with toilets, water, and the Whitney Portal store (including a café).

Mount Whitney Summit

> **Trip Data:** 36.57852°N, 118.29228°W; 20.8 miles; 4/0 days
> **Topos:** *Mount Langley, Mount Whitney*

HIGHLIGHTS: At 14,505 feet, Mount Whitney is the highest peak in the contiguous 48 states. Because of that claim—and the fact that the mountain is accessible and offers unparalleled views over the southern Sierra and the Owens Valley—Whitney is also one of the most sought-after summits in the Sierra. Sixty lucky people receive permits to begin an overnight hike from Whitney Portal each day, the majority hoping to complete this walk. An additional 100 people each day attempt a day hike up Mount Whitney—following the same route described, but in a single day.

HEADS UP! *This walk is written assuming you spend a night at both Outpost Camp (3.8 miles from the trailhead) and Trail Camp (6.1 miles from the trailhead). However, most people will only spend a night at one of these locations, completing the trip in three days. The advantage of splitting your ascent across more days is to acclimatize to the high elevation and increase your chances of successfully summiting Mount Whitney; if you know you are particularly prone to altitude-induced illness—headaches, queasiness, general fatigue— contemplate the described four-day option. Alternatively, spend a few nights camped at a high-elevation car-accessible campground before your trip and then do a three-day hike.*

HEADS UP! *The U.S. Forest Service asks that hikers in the Mount Whitney Zone pack out their solid wastes. Too many people use the trail, and the climate is too unfriendly, for burial and biological degradation to break down your waste. You will receive a human-waste disposal kit for free when you pick up your wilderness permit.*

HEADS UP! *Visit the Facebook page Altitude Acclimatization to find numerous resources on altitude sickness. Many hikers will experience acute mountain sickness (AMS) symptoms ascending Mount Whitney, and it is important to be aware of the symptoms before your hike.*

DAY 1 (Whitney Portal to Outpost Camp, 3.8 miles): The Mount Whitney Trailhead departs from the northern side of the giant Whitney Portal parking area, just east of the Whitney Portal store. You will pass large information plaques and a handy scale to weigh your pack. A couple of quick switchbacks initially direct the sandy trail north. After crossing a small creek, you emerge onto a dry, sandy slope and complete an east-trending switchback, followed by a long, mostly westward traverse along the south side of the canyon. Climbing gently, you cross this open slope, dotted with drought-tolerant shrubs and sporting an understory of colorful flowers in spring and early summer. Along the way, you cross several small trickles, including unofficially named Carillon Creek in a thicket of wild roses and scarlet monkeyflower. Just before you cross the North Fork of Lone Pine Creek, 0.9 mile from the trailhead, a sign points right (northwest) to the use trail that hikers and climbers take to access the east face of Mount Whitney and the Mountaineers Route. You stay left on the main trail, crossing the creek on large boulders (or wet feet at high flows).

After crossing the North Fork of Lone Pine Creek, sidle around to the head of the canyon, and climb a long series of switchbacks. They are well graded, and the trail is sandy with few

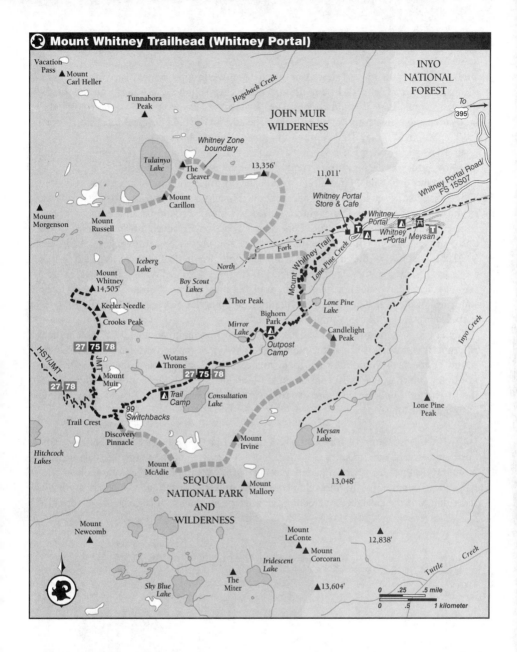

protruding rocks. The slope begins under a tree cover of Jeffrey pine and white fir, then emerges onto a drier slope of chaparral plants, including mountain mahogany, chinquapin, and sagebrush. Higher still, the shrubs slowly become shorter and more intermingled with flowers. This stretch of trail can be scorching by midmorning—begin your hike as early as possible. Breather stops provide a view down the canyon framing the Alabama Hills, the background for hundreds of television shows and movies, especially countless westerns.

Near the end of this climb, the trail veers toward Lone Pine Creek and crosses patches of moister vegetation, where tall corn lilies, lupines, and larkspurs dominate. Just past one open patch with a small meadow and a cluster of lodgepole pines, you reach the Lone Pine Creek crossing. A series of raised logs allows you to traverse the broad crossing easily, although during the highest flows you may get wet while approaching these logs. Beyond the stream, you switchback briefly up through lodgepole pine forest and promptly reach the signed Lone Pine Lake junction (10,041'). Heading left (east) leads to the round lake (and some adequate campsites), perched on the edge of the long drop-off to Whitney Portal. The Mount Whitney Trail continues up to the right (southwest).

In a few steps you reach a sandy flat and pass the sign declaring your entry into the Mount Whitney Zone; permits are required for all hikers beyond this point. To the south is a blocky talus field flanked by tall, steep cliffs, the north face of unofficially named Candlelight Peak. Next, a series of switchbacks takes you in and out of scattered foxtail pine cover as you cross a spur. Dropping slightly, you reach Bighorn Park, a marshy meadow, where you are reunited with meandering Lone Pine Creek. Overhead are towering cliffs. Look upstream, just to your left, and you may see where a spring emerges from exposed bedrock.

At the west end of the meadow is Outpost Camp, the first of the two large campsites along the Mount Whitney Trail (10,374'; 36.57159°N, 118.25886°W; no campfires). There are a few small campsites northeast of the trail, but most people choose to pitch their tents southwest of the trail, beneath tall foxtail pines. South of these campsites, Lone Pine Creek cascades over a cliff face in a tumbling waterfall.

Many people continue on to Trail Camp for their first night, another 1,700 feet higher, although if you aren't well acclimated it might be wise to stop here; you are more likely to suffer the effects of altitude sickness at the higher perch. Some people will day hike straight to Mount Whitney's summit from Outpost Camp—it is a long hike, but for many people the benefit of a good night's sleep in this warmer, less exposed, lower elevation setting outweighs the longer day.

DAY 2 (Outpost Camp to Trail Camp, 2.3 miles): Leaving Outpost Camp, the trail veers north and switchbacks up a dry slope past blossoming creambush, mountain pride penstemon, wavyleaf paintbrush, chinquapin, wax currant, coyote mint, fireweed, and ragwort—to name just a sample. Shortly, the trail intersects the stream drainage and you climb briefly on slabs alongside the creek before crossing the Mirror Lake outlet on large blocks of rock. To

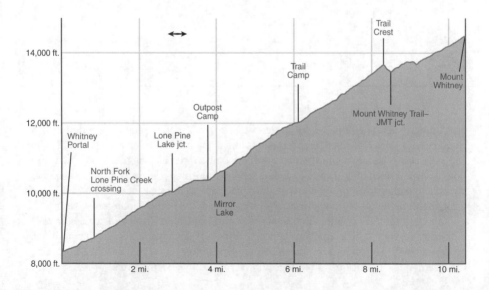

the north is Thor Peak, its steep cliff faces extending all the way to the shores of Mirror Lake (10,686'). Camping is prohibited at Mirror Lake.

Above Mirror Lake, the trail climbs steeply via tight switchbacks that follow sandy ledges up a granite bluff—pay attention to make sure you don't lose the trail here. There are a few small campsites tucked in sandy flats along this climb, but if you choose to use them, you must carry water up from Mirror Lake. You reach the top of a small granite ridge and then turn southwest to rejoin the main Lone Pine Creek drainage. Through this section, the views down to Lone Pine Lake and the Owens Valley are exquisite. To the north are gigantic talus fans spilling down the north flanks of Mount Irvine, and the tall granite walls of the surrounding peaks suddenly feel much closer. You are now walking through a landscape of slabs—in places the trail winds along small sandy passageways, and elsewhere you walk atop the slabs themselves. Here you pass the last trees, mostly foxtail pines, along with a few stunted whitebark and lodgepole pines, and enter the alpine zone. The trail continues along the crest of the granite ridge until it sidles along a sandy bench to Trailside Meadow, an important waypoint: it is almost exactly the halfway point in terms of both distance and elevation from Whitney Portal to the summit of Mount Whitney. The small meadow, covered with shooting stars, is a refreshing place to take a short break, but camping here is prohibited.

Above Trailside Meadow, the trail climbs out of the drainage and back onto slabs. Looking left, you see Lone Pine Creek forking into branches, the southern tributary leading to Consultation Lake and the main creek toward Trail Camp. Shortly you begin a traverse across a steep slope and cross Lone Pine Creek, which is particularly flower-lined at this location, and proceed up more granite slabs toward Trail Camp. Imperceptibly step by step, the trail is becoming rockier; you are increasingly stepping over protruding rocks or walking on cobble and have to pay more attention to your footing. To the south, the skyline from left to right is Mount Irvine, appropriately shaped Arc Pass, Mount McAdie, and Mount Marsh, a small summit just beyond Mount McAdie. Consultation Lake lies below Arc Pass. If you wish to camp at Consultation Lake, there are several small use trails that cross the granite slabs; choose any of them once upstream of Trailside Meadow.

Along the last 0.3 mile to Trail Camp, there are many camping options, with water from Lone Pine Creek just a short distance away. Trail Camp (12,025'; 36.56298°N, 118.27915°W) itself is wonderfully scenic and conveniently located, but also cold, windy, crowded, and utterly lacking in privacy. Your tent site will be a small sandy nook surrounded by slabs, boulders, and other people's tents. There are ample tent sites for everyone, although you can expect to hear the noise of—and see the lights from—other backpackers and day hikers long before first light. Since there are no longer toilets tethering you to this specific location, if you want more privacy, search for alternate campsites a bit farther south, or select one of the campsites before you reach Trail Camp. Beyond Trail Camp the only camping options are a few small bivy sites on the far side of Trail Crest or on the summit of Mount Whitney. The inlet to the Trail Camp tarn is the last reliable water along the trail—fill up before embarking on the summit.

DAY 3 (day hike from Trail Camp to Mount Whitney Summit and back, 8.6 miles): Because of the high elevation and exposure of Mount Whitney's summit, this is not an ordinary day hike. Be sure your day pack includes survival gear like extra food, water, clothing, rain gear, and a map. Allow plenty of time and don't try to hurry.

The next stretch of trail is tough: you are already at 12,000 feet and face a 1,600-foot slope with a relentless set of approximately 99 switchbacks—some short, some long, and, luckily, all well graded. These switchbacks lead up a long talus slope via a route that avoids both cliff

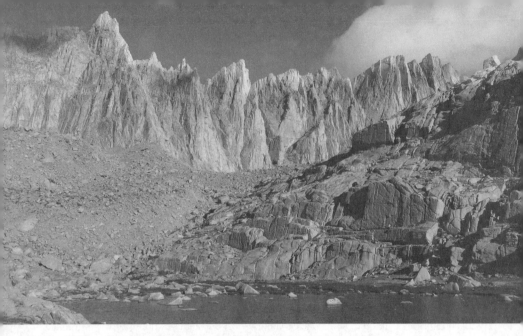

View to Mount Muir and the pinnacles from Trail Camp   Photo by Elizabeth Wenk

bands and a large snowfield that can hug the western side of the slope well into the summer. The trail is well constructed and the footing is mostly straightforward, but like the terrain, the trail becomes increasingly rocky—there are small rocks underfoot, and the tips of embedded boulders must be stepped over. About a third of the way up, you intersect a prominent cliff band where the trail has been blasted into rock. Snow and ice can persist here throughout the summer—a handrail has been installed for safety, but thick snow deposits here effectively block access to the upper switchbacks. If you're hiking in June or early July, ask at the ranger station about this when you pick up your permit because, until the switchbacks are accessible, you must ascend the snowy western bowl, requiring mountaineering skills. Take a moment to gaze down the steep slab of rock extending below the trail and look up at the colorful and jointed rock above the trail. Above this section, the meager vegetation becomes even sparser, but not entirely barren, for, in season, hikers may see a dozen species of flowering plants, climaxed by the blue flower clusters of polemonium—the "sky pilot."

As you take breathers, stop to look at the mountains. The higher you climb, the more peaks come into view. Mount Muir, with a sharp summit and tall, steep east arête, is the peak nearly due west of Trail Camp, and it dominates the view as you ascend the switchbacks. North of Mount Muir is the long ridge of pinnacles ending with the flat-topped Mount Whitney. Mount Whitney is visible from the lowest switchbacks, but then not again until you are nearly at Trail Crest; Keeler Needle, the next summit south, blocks Mount Whitney from your view. Farther north is notably steep Mount Russell, and to its east is the talus field that leads to the summit of Mount Carillon. The last few switchbacks are longer, and after one final westward traverse, you reach Trail Crest (13,600') and cross to the west side of the Sierra Crest, entering Sequoia National Park.

Hikers suddenly have vistas to much of Sequoia, including the Kaweah Peaks Ridge and the entire Great Western Divide. Straight below are the rockbound Hitchcock Lakes. From Trail Crest, you descend briefly but steeply, skirting past a few rock towers and, after 0.15 mile, reaching the junction with the John Muir Trail (JMT). You head right (north), while left (northwest) is the JMT descending to Crabtree Meadow. From this junction to the summit of Mount Whitney, the Mount Whitney Trail, JMT, and High Sierra Trail from the Giant

Forest (Trip 27) follow the same path. You may see backpacks stashed around this junction, as backpackers arriving from the west generally choose to carry only minimal gear to the summit. Beyond the junction, you cross a talus field with a few bivy sites.

At about 13,800 feet, the trail levels off and enters a maze of pinnacles. The slope here has a scalloped appearance due to widespread fractures in the rock, reshaped into avalanche chutes. The sharp ridges of pinnacles mark the boundary between avalanche chutes. Between pinnacles, you have open views to the west; in the distance are the dark, jagged Kaweah peaks, while granite slopes dominate the foreground. You repeatedly pass narrow notches, with jaw-dropping views straight down to the east—watch your footing carefully near there, for the trail is narrow and the drops are very steep.

Leaving the pinnacles behind, you are just 1.0 mile from the summit. Before you is a broad, barren talus field. Large boulders are embedded in sand, with ever smaller numbers of alpine gold and sky pilot growing in sheltered crevices. The trail mimics the surrounding terrain; it is still mostly sandy, but there are also boulders embedded in the trail that require larger steps up—not a welcome proposition at this altitude. Traverse the western face of Crooks Peak (previously named Day Needle) and Keeler Needle, two 14,000-foot points that are too indistinct from Mount Whitney to be considered true peaks.

Beyond Keeler Needle, the trail bends west for a stretch before beginning the final climb to the summit. There are a few halfhearted switchbacks up the last talus field. Nearly everyone heading down will encourage you onward with calls of, "You can't see the summit hut yet, but you're almost there." In fact, because of the summit plateau's very shallow angle, you don't see the summit hut until just minutes before you reach the top. Suddenly, the views open in every direction. A large summit register sits by the entrance to the stone hut. Sign your name, and then head to the giant boulders a short distance east—the true high point—to take a long, well-deserved break (14,505'; 36.57852°N, 118.29228°W).

The peak was named in 1864 for Josiah D. Whitney, California state geologist and chief of the famed "Whitney Survey" of 1860–74. However, European Americans didn't actually climb it until August 18, 1873, when three fishermen from Lone Pine ascended the southwest slope. They named the mountain "Fisherman's Peak," but it was "Mount Whitney" that stuck.

After enjoying the summit, retrace your steps to Trail Camp (or Outpost Camp).

HIGH-ELEVATION HAZARDS

If you see dark clouds approaching, get off the peak quickly! Indeed, do not continue the final 2 miles past Trail Crest if you see storm cells approaching. The summit hut is not considered a safe location to sit out a storm—there have been fatalities in the hut due to its metal roof conducting lightning strikes; the hut has since been retrofitted, but you don't want to be the one to test if it is safe now. And remember, from the summit it will take you more than an hour to get off exposed, high-elevation slopes—don't wait until the rain starts to decide to turn back.

Also, on your return, stay on the trail. It is tempting for hikers to leave the trail at the snowfield on the east side of Trail Crest and glissade (slide in a controlled manner) down. Unfortunately, many who do this are inexperienced and ill equipped. No one should ever glissade down a snowfield without an ice ax and preferably a helmet, as well as the knowledge of how to self-arrest. Even if you are carrying this equipment, be aware that this seemingly innocuous snow patch is often icy partway down, and many people have lost control and gone sliding into the rocks below.

DAY 4 (Trail Camp to Whitney Portal, 6.1 miles): Retrace your steps.

HORSESHOE MEADOWS ROAD TRIPS

Horseshoe Meadows Road leads southwest from Lone Pine to a collection of trailheads that access the Kern Plateau and far southeastern High Sierra. The road climbs impressively up a broad slope to reach the flat upper reaches of Cottonwood Creek, ending just above 10,000 feet. Trips from two trailheads are included in this book: Cottonwood Lakes and Cottonwood Pass Trailheads. The Cottonwood Lakes Trail leads to the Cottonwood Lakes and across to the Rock Creek drainage in Sequoia National Park via New Army Pass. The Cottonwood Pass Trail ascends just 1,000 feet to reach Cottonwood Pass, providing access to the northernmost Kern Plateau and the Pacific Crest Trail (PCT) corridor. Northbound on the PCT is then a delightfully easy way to continue to the Mount Whitney area. Not included in this guide is the trail across Trail Pass, another easy Sierra Crest crossing that leads south onto the Kern Plateau.

Trailheads: Cottonwood Lakes
Cottonwood Pass

South Fork Lakes   Photo by Elizabeth Wenk

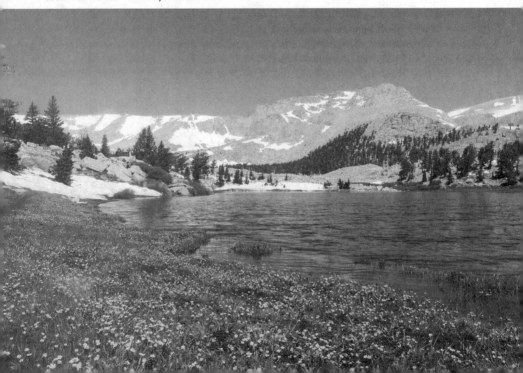

Cottonwood Lakes Trailhead

10,060'; 36.45321°N, 118.17006°W

Destination/ GPS Coordinates	Trip Type	Best Season	Pace & Hiking/ Layover Days	Total Mileage	Permit Required
76 Cottonwood and South Fork Lakes 36.49844°N 118.21981°W (Cottonwood Lake 3)	Semiloop	Early to late	Leisurely 2/2	12.6	Cottonwood Lakes
77 Upper Rock Creek Loop 36.49517°N 118.28407°W (Rock Creek Lake)	Loop	Mid to late	Leisurely 4/2	23.4	Cottonwood Lakes *(Cottonwood Pass in reverse)*

INFORMATION AND PERMITS: This trailhead is in Inyo National Forest. Permits are required for overnight stays and quotas apply. Permits can be reserved up to six months in advance at recreation.gov (60%; $6 permit reservation fee plus $5 per person) or requested in person, first come, first served, a day in advance (40%; free). All permits must be picked up at one of the Inyo National Forest ranger stations, located in Lone Pine (Eastern Sierra Interagency Visitor Center), Bishop, Mammoth Lakes, and Lee Vining (the Mono Basin Scenic Area Visitor Center). If you plan to use a stove or have a campfire while on national forest lands, you must also have a California campfire permit, available from a forest service office or online at preventwildfireca.org/campfire-permit. Campfires are prohibited above 10,400 in Inyo National Forest (east of the Sierra Crest), as well as at Chicken Spring Lake (Trip 77), and above 10,400 feet in Sequoia National Park (west of the Sierra Crest). Bear canisters are required in this area.

DRIVING DIRECTIONS: Turn west from US 395 in Lone Pine onto Whitney Portal Road. Go 3.1 miles and turn left onto Horseshoe Meadows Road. Go straight 19.2 miles and then turn right to the trailhead marked for Cottonwood Lakes and New Army Pass (not Cottonwood Pass). Follow this road 0.5 mile to the trailhead parking. Here you'll also find toilets, water, and a one-night campground.

---

trip 76   ## Cottonwood and South Fork Lakes

see map on p. 408

Trip Data: 36.49844°N, 118.21981°W (Cottonwood Lake 3); 12.6 miles; 2/2 days
Topos: *Cirque Peak, Mount Langley*

HIGHLIGHTS: With relatively little effort, hikers taking this trip can reach a rugged cirque surrounded by peaks up to 14,000 feet and filled with lakes, meadows, and streams—the true High Sierra. The South Fork Lakes, immediately adjacent to the extremely popular Cottonwood Lakes, offer a little more privacy. An easy cross-country section adds adventure to the return route. Layover days are a must to more fully explore this spectacular basin.

HEADS UP! *Due to a trail realignment (many decades back), the first 2.0 miles of trail are not shown on the USGS 7.5' topo, but they are shown on the map in this book.*

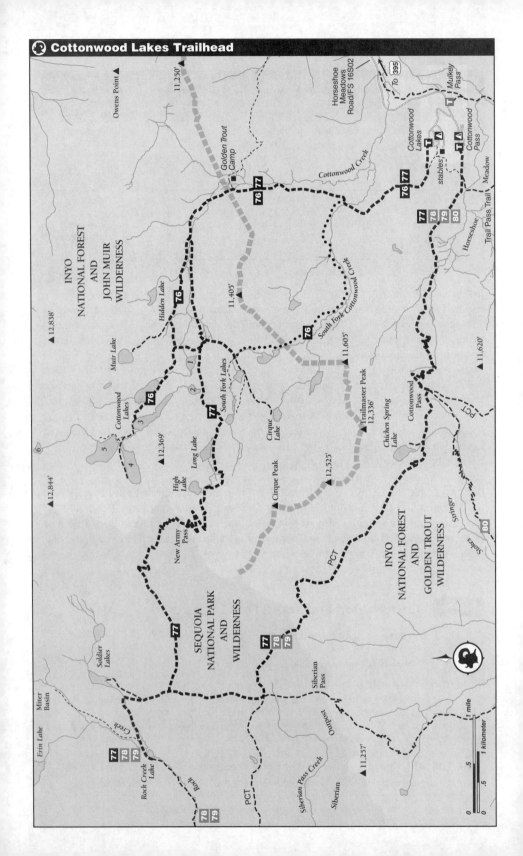

HEADS UP! *Don't expect solitude if you camp at the Cottonwood Lakes: with a trailhead quota of 36, there are often many large groups scattered across the basin. Campfires are prohibited in the Cottonwood Lakes Basin and at the South Fork Lakes.*

DAY 1 (Cottonwood Lakes Trailhead to Cottonwood Lake 3, 5.9 miles): From the trailhead, the trail leads west on a gentle and brief ascent under sparse lodgepole pine cover. The sandy trail passes a spur to the pack station, enters Golden Trout Wilderness, and soon turns north, descending gradually toward South Fork Cottonwood Creek. You'll notice that as soon as the trail is on a slope, foxtail pines replace the lodgepole pines. Then the trail flattens again and crosses South Fork Cottonwood Creek on a flattened log, 1.5 miles from the trailhead. A few steps later an unmarked spur trail departs left (northwest). This is the South Fork use trail on which you will return, but for now stay right (north) on the main trail.

Crossing an insignificant ridge, you sidle into the main Cottonwood Creek corridor, continuing through dry, sandy terrain some distance west of the meandering creek. Skirt the west side of the meadows along Cottonwood Creek and ascend steadily, passing a spur right to the privately operated Golden Trout Camp at the 2.8-mile mark (10,204').

The trail shortly enters John Muir Wilderness and soon crosses Cottonwood Creek on rocks that are submerged at high flow. Beyond the crossing, the trail swings slowly to the west, with the creek and its meadows to the southwest and soon reaches a junction, where right (west-northwest) is the most efficient route to Muir Lake and the upper Cottonwood Lakes, while left (due west) leads more directly to Cottonwood Lakes 1 and 2 and the South Fork Lakes. If you're planning on skipping Cottonwood Lakes 3–5, head left; otherwise, continue right, the route described.

The trail initially follows the meadow edge in lodgepole pine forest and then begins climbing a drier, sandier slope, diverging from Cottonwood Creek. You cross one seasonal tributary and continue upward beneath sparse lodgepole and foxtail pine cover. At the eastern edge of an often-marshy meadow, you reach a junction where you continue left (west) and immediately step across a creek channel, while right (northwest) is a lateral leading 0.6 mile to Muir Lake (and lovely more-secluded campsites). The trail continues west, first skirting a meadow to the south, then a second to the north, before reaching another junction. Here you turn right (west) toward Cottonwood Lakes 3–5, your immediate goal, while left (south) leads to Cottonwood Lake 1 and back to the New Army Pass corridor, your route tomorrow.

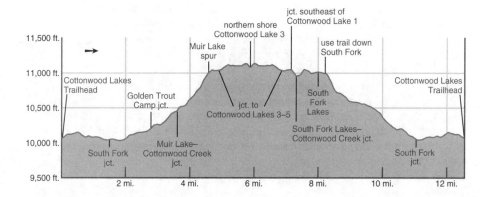

The trail continues west, then northwest to the only unnumbered Cottonwood Lake, a vast, shallow body of water sitting east of the trail. Its lack of a number is because, contrary to its depiction on topo maps, this lake mostly dries out by late summer (or in drought years), becoming a big, shallow puddle. Near the northern end of the lake are a number of lovely, popular campsites in lodgepole and foxtail pine stands.

Curving west leads to the northern tip of elongate Cottonwood Lake 3—and more campsites (11,124'; 36.49844°N, 118.21981°W; no campfires). You're ever closer to the vertical faces of the Sierra Crest, where the sheer, jointed cliffs often erode into triangular profiles. The mileage assumes you stop here, but as described in the sidebar, you can continue up to Cottonwood Lakes 4 and 5—and beyond—but the terrain becomes rockier with notably few campsites.

DAY HIKING AND CAMPING AROUND THE COTTONWOOD LAKES BASIN AND SOUTH FORK LAKES

Cottonwood Lakes 4 and 5 and "Old" Army Pass: Established trails lead to or near all of the Cottonwood Lakes. Peak baggers may want to attempt Mount Langley (14,023'; 36.52342°N, 118.23951°W) from old Army Pass (reached by following an old trail around the northern side of Cottonwood Lake 4 and then up the head of a cirque that holds snow well into summer). The high-altitude meadows around the Cottonwood Lakes are very fragile, especially when wet, so stay on established trail and respect rehabilitation efforts that have blocked off some use trails.

New Army Pass, Long and High Lakes, Cirque Peak: From the junction near the southeastern corner of Cottonwood Lake 1, turn west to continue toward New Army Pass. This trail follows the southern edge of the meadow holding Cottonwood Lakes 1 and 2 (passing several good campsites) and then winds along the northern and then western edges of a truly massive morainal boulder field separating the Cottonwood Lakes and South Fork Lakes. You nearly touch the western South Fork Lake before turning northwest to follow the creek corridor toward Long Lake. This trail passes Long Lake to its south and then heads to High Lake; there's good camping at Long Lake and a little Spartan camping around fragile High Lake. If you continue to New Army Pass (highly recommended and offering great views), from the pass it is a straightforward, 4.0-mile, out-and-back, cross-country route to summit Cirque Peak, which commands panoramic views. From New Army Pass, you follow near the skyline, first southwest and then southeast, looping around to the summit (12,908'; 36.47688°N, 118.23680°W). The route is mostly Class 1, walking on sand, with a short Class 2, easy talus section as you approach the summit.

South Fork Lakes: The trail leads past the eastern side of the easternmost South Fork Lake. From the southeastern corner of the eastern lake, a quasi–use trail leads upstream along the South Fork Lakes. Initially easy, it soon winds onto the interminable, flat talus expanse (moraine deposits) that extends across the South Fork Lakes and north to the Cottonwood Lakes. There will be some talus walking, but it is relatively easy if you follow one of the tree-dotted mini-moraine crests west, only cutting back into the drainage as you approach the westernmost lake. There are some campsites in a patch of lodgepole pines at this lake's inlet. You could return the way you came or cut up to the New Army Pass Trail from here and complete a longer loop through the Cottonwood Lakes Basin past Lakes 1 and 2.

Cirque Lake: From the southeastern corner of the eastern South Fork Lake, a lateral continues 0.5 mile to Cirque Lake, climbing over a shallow spur. There are several lovely campsites at the northeastern corner of the lake. Cirque Lake garners its name from Cirque Peak, but the name doesn't quite fit the lake, which sits in a quite broad, open basin perched above the South Fork Cottonwood Creek drainage.

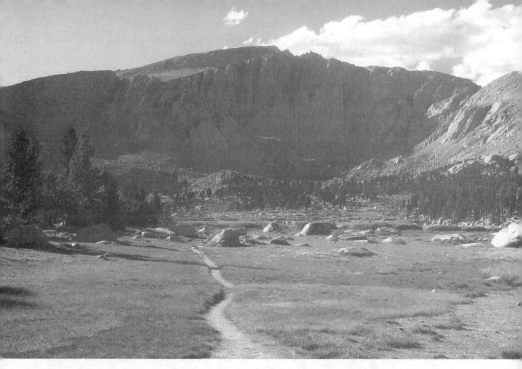

Mount Langley rises above the Cottonwood Lakes Basin.   Photo by Elizabeth Wenk

DAY 2 (Cottonwood Lake 3 to Cottonwood Lakes Trailhead, 6.7 miles, part use trail):
Although official, mapped, maintained trails don't exist for much of this day's route, the
network of use trails pounded out by anglers makes for easy cross-country hiking.

From the northern end of Cottonwood Lake 3, you begin by retracing your steps 1.0
mile south and east to the junction northeast of Cottonwood Lake 1. Now turn south and
cross first Cottonwood Creek (wet in early season) and then a sandy, morainal rib east of
Cottonwood Lake 1. You quickly reach a junction with the New Army Pass Trail, where
you turn left (east) and descend four quick switchbacks to reach a junction where right
(south) is signposted for the South Fork Lakes and left (east) leads back down Cottonwood
Creek—head right for the continued route description or left if you'd like to retrace your
steps to the trailhead along a maintained trail. Turning right, the trail skirts the edge of a
willow-filled slope, crosses a shallow sandy ridge with large, elegant foxtail pines, and drops
to the easternmost South Fork Lake. There are fine campsites nearby (11,016'; 36.48328°N,
118.20902°W; no campfires) and optional excursions to the upper South Fork Lakes or
Cirque Lake, described in the sidebar on page 410.

The official trail ends at this point, but a well-trodden use trail leads down the South
Fork Cottonwood Creek back to the main trail. Your entire route remains on the northeastern bank, never more than 0.1 mile from the drainage, so even if you lose the trail, you're
unlikely to get lost.

Keeping on the north side of the outlet stream, this route descends steeply over heavily
fractured granite past foxtail and lodgepole pines on a slope where the dashing stream cascades and falls from one rocky grotto to the next. Clumps of shooting star, topped by showy
red columbine and orange Kelley's lily, line the stream. The trail levels off in a meadow
and then descends into a larger meadow, where the outlet of Cirque Lake joins South Fork
Cottonwood Creek. In the sandy flats to the northeast are possible campsites, with beautiful views of the long meadow with steep cliffs looming overhead. Following the creek's
course, swing east and descend steeply in lodgepole forest to skirt around another meadow,

this one sufficiently willow-choked that it is hard to reach the creek corridor. Beyond this meadow, the use trail drops again and rounds the base of the moraine between the south fork and the main fork of Cottonwood Creek to reach the main Cottonwood Lakes Trail. Here you turn right (south) to retrace the final 1.5 miles to the trailhead, crossing the South Fork Cottonwood Creek on the flattened log after just 200 feet.

trip 77   # Upper Rock Creek

see map on p. 408

Trip Data: 36.49517°N, 118.28407°W (Rock Creek Lake); 23.4 miles; 4/2 days

Topos: *Cirque Peak, Mount Whitney (just barely), Johnson Peak*

HIGHLIGHTS: One of the finest circuits in the Sierra, this route travels up an elegant cirque past spectacular peaks, visits lonely alpine lakes and meadowed ponds, and climbs past treeline into desolate moonscapes. The scenery and day hiking opportunities are spectacular, while the elevation gain is more moderate than on many trips farther north.

HEADS UP! *Due to a trail realignment (many decades back), the first 2.0 miles of trail are not shown on the USGS 7.5' topo, but they are shown on the map in this book. Campfires are prohibited in the Cottonwood Lakes Basin, at the South Fork Lakes, and within 0.3 mile of Chicken Spring Lake. The top of New Army Pass can have a steep, icy, dangerous snowfield through June; if you are hiking in early season, ask about conditions when you pick up your permit. The Mount Langley topo is helpful if you plan to day hike in the Miter Basin.*

DAY 1 (Cottonwood Lakes Trailhead to Cottonwood Lakes Basin, 6.3 miles): From the trailhead, the trail leads west on a gentle and brief ascent under sparse lodgepole pine cover. The sandy trail passes a spur to the pack station, enters Golden Trout Wilderness, and soon turns north, descending gradually toward South Fork Cottonwood Creek. You'll notice that as soon as the trail is on a slope, foxtail pines replace the lodgepole pines. Then the trail flattens again and crosses the South Fork Cottonwood Creek on a flattened log, 1.5 miles from the trailhead.

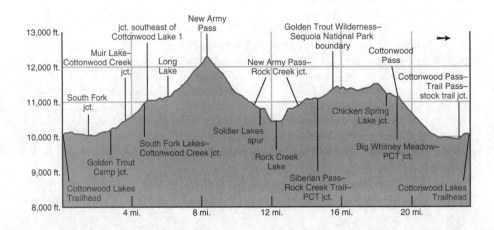

Passing a faint spur up the South Fork (northwest; Trip 76) and then crossing an insignificant ridge, you sidle into the main Cottonwood Creek corridor, continuing through dry, sandy terrain some distance west of the meandering creek. Skirt the west side of the meadows along Cottonwood Creek and ascend steadily, passing a spur right to the privately operated Golden Trout Camp at the 2.8-mile mark (10,204').

The trail shortly enters John Muir Wilderness and soon crosses Cottonwood Creek on rocks that are submerged at high flow. Beyond the crossing, the trail swings slowly to the west, with the creek and its meadows to the southwest, and soon reaches a junction, where you stay left (due west) on a trail that leads most directly to Cottonwood Lakes 1 and 2 and on to New Army Pass, while right (west-northwest) leads to Muir Lake and the upper Cottonwood Lakes (Trip 76).

You immediately cross Cottonwood Creek again (currently on a log) and begin a gentle climb through sandy terrain with sparse lodgepole pine cover. You climb beside the bubbling, willow-choked creek, stopping briefly to admire a small cascade where the creek splits into three forks. The trail continues to the south of these tributaries, climbing more steeply to a junction where left (south) leads to the South Fork Lakes (Trip 76). You continue right (west) and a final four switchbacks carry you up a moraine to the lip of the expansive Cottonwood Lakes Basin, offering sublime views across the basin to Mount Langley.

In a few steps, you meet another junction, where right (north) leads to the upper Cottonwood Lakes (Trip 76), while you stay left (west), skirting the south side of Cottonwood Lake 1. With flat terrain everywhere, campsites are plentiful on the sandy meadow verges—pick your favorite location over the coming mile. Your route continues due west past lakes 1 and 2 and then winds through sandy flats along the northern and then western edges of a truly massive morainal boulder field separating the Cottonwood Lakes and South Fork Lakes. You nearly touch the western South Fork Lake before turning northwest to follow the creek corridor toward Long Lake. (Crossing the creek here leads to a small campsite near the shore of the westernmost South Fork Lake.) On the south bank, about halfway to Long Lake, additional large, sandy areas are suitable for camping and recommended for the views. A final ascent leads to lodgepole pine–ringed Long Lake, lying in a steep-walled cirque. You skirt its southern side, quickly reaching a giant camping area at its head (11,196'; 36.48612°N, 118.22856°W; no campfires).

DAY 2 (Cottonwood Lakes Basin to Rock Creek Lake, 6.0 miles): Climbing again, the trail diagonals up a sandy slope to another flat beside seasonally marshy meadows. Looping south, you pass the most delightful collection of lodgepole pine krummholz—it is a rare treat to see this subalpine tree twisted into ground cover—and continue around the wet willow-filled expanse to the north. Atop the next rise, the trail just touches the southern edge of deep, clear High Lake and its tiny bivy sites, some beneath giant boulders. Here travelers can pause and stare at the upcoming rocky switchbacks.

It is a lengthy 1.4-mile climb from High Lake to New Army Pass, but not a difficult one, as the long zigzags are gently graded and offer amazing bursts of alpine color, especially magenta Sierra primrose in early July and rockfringe in August. The higher the track climbs, the better are the views east to the Cottonwood Creek drainage. Approaching the headwall, the switchbacks become tighter, weaving between blocky, near-vertical outcrops. Although "New" Army Pass was built to replace the original Army Pass because of its long-lasting steep snowfields, New Army can also present problems to early-season hikers when they discover the final 20 feet are near-vertical icy snow. Suddenly the switchbacks end and you are on top of remarkably flat New Army Pass (12,330'). It is a sandy expanse with gigantic embedded boulders, a location that stood above the Pleistocene glaciers, and the boulders have eroded in situ over millions of years. Countless tiny tundra plants cover the ground, their names revealing their stature: dwarf ivesia, pygmy fleabane daisy, dwarf alpine paintbrush, pygmy mountain parsley, and pygmyflower rockjasmine, to name a few.

CLIMBING CIRQUE PEAK

From New Army Pass it is a straightforward, 4.0-mile, out-and-back, cross-country hike to the summit Cirque Peak, which commands panoramic views. You follow near the skyline, first southwest and then southeast, looping around to the summit (12,908'; 36.47688°N, 118.2368°W). The route is mostly Class 1, walking on sand between boulders, with a short Class 2, easy talus section as you approach the summit.

Descending from New Army Pass into Sequoia National Park, the trail crosses a long, barren slope of coarse granite sand sprinkled with granite boulder totems. At 0.8 mile north of the pass, the route passes an unmaintained trail (not shown on the topo map) that branches right to old Army Pass, the original pass built by the army in the 1890s. From old Army Pass a remarkably distinct use trail leads north toward 14,023-foot Mount Langley, one of California's easiest fourteeners to climb. Beyond this junction, the route swings west and descends steeply over rocky tread to level off on a more gentle descent in a barren cirque of talus, cliffs, and sand, including an elongate rock glacier. Slowly the creek corridor becomes greener, and you pass the first straggly, stunted lodgepole pines growing atop lateral moraines. Beyond, the trail crosses to the north side of the unnamed stream and tree cover slowly thickens.

At 2.7 miles from New Army Pass, the trail meets the path that connects the upper Rock Creek drainage to the Pacific Crest Trail (PCT) and Siberian Pass; tomorrow you will take the left (southbound) trail toward the PCT and on to Cottonwood Pass, but for now turn right (north). There are good campsites to either side of the stream at this junction, but better ones ahead at Lower Soldier Lake and Rock Creek Lake.

Heading north, you descend gently across dry sandy and bouldery slopes and then have a nearly flat traverse among lodgepole and a few foxtail pines. Just 0.3 mile later you reach a junction to the Soldier Lakes, unnamed on the USGS 7.5' topos. Heading right (east) along the spur trail leads to a selection of campsites, some on a ledge high above the lower lake after 0.2 mile (10,843'; 36.50020°N, 118.27117°W; no campfires; bear box) and others along its southern shore after 0.5 mile. (*Note:* The current spur trail is along the south side of the Soldier Lakes outlet creek. The old trail along the north side of Lower Soldier Lake has been rehabilitated and does not lead to camping.) Continuing left (north) on the main trail along the western side of the elongate meadow, you soon step across the Soldier Lakes outlet creek on rocks and make a sharp left.

Westbound, the trail now descends steeply alongside a willow-infested tributary of Rock Creek until the rocky slope gives way to a meadow just above the almost heart-shaped lake colloquially known as Rock Creek Lake or Upper Rock Creek Lake (being in Upper Rock Creek) or Lower Rock Creek Lake (being below the Soldier Lakes, which used to be called the Upper Rock Creek Lakes) (10,468'; 36.49517°N, 118.28407°W at the bear box; no campfires). There are fair campsites at the head of this meadow, others at the lake's outlet, and more primitive ones can be found on the south side of the lake. Fishing for golden in the lake and adjoining stream is good. To reach the lakeside campsites take the trail across Rock Creek, a sandy-bottomed wade at higher flows.

DAY HIKING FROM ROCK CREEK LAKE

This marshy-meadowed lake makes a fine base camp for side trips to rugged Miter Basin. A use trail to Miter Basin makes a hard-to-spot exit along the north side of the large campsite at the eastern tip of Rock Creek Lake's meadow (10,455'; 36.49828°N, 118.27912°W). This trail is easy to follow up to the place where Rock Creek cascades out of Miter Basin; from there, it's easy cross-country hiking through meadows and across slabs to a vast wonderland of slab-ringed lakes watched over by steep crests. You can easily spend a day exploring—or may even want to carry your pack upstream.

DAY 3 (Rock Creek Lake to Chicken Spring Lake, 6.3 miles): Begin this hiking day by retracing your steps for 1.25 miles to the meadowed junction with the trail to New Army Pass. Fill your canteens here, for this is the last reliable water source before Chicken Spring Lake. From the junction, continue south (right) and ascend gradually over a moderately to densely forested slope of foxtail and lodgepole pine. The route crosses a barren area, climbs over an easy ridge, and, 1.1 mile south of the last junction, turns left (southeast) onto the PCT at a junction where right (northwest) is the PCT's route down Rock Creek and straight ahead (south) leads to Siberian Pass.

SIBERIAN OUTPOST

Here you are at the head of barren Siberian Outpost, a vast expanse of mounds of sand and seasonally marshy meadows with fascinating soil colors. Spare hours can easily be spent walking the length of Siberian Outpost, possibly even ascending west onto the Boreal Plateau and to Funston Lake, a pothole lake that lacks an outlet. Siberian Outpost also marks the start of the enormous Kern Plateau to the south. In dry periods, all water sources on Siberian Outpost can dry up, so while maps indicate a boggy landscape, it doesn't offer late-summer camping.

Once on the PCT you begin a lengthy traverse south across the base of Cirque Peak's slopes. Siberian Outpost is spread out before you, backdropped, far to the west, by the Kaweah Peaks Ridge rising above the Kern River. Rounding a rocky promontory, a ridge descending off Cirque Peak, you leave Sequoia National Park for Golden Trout Wilderness. The trail now curves into a valley holding two seasonal lakes—do not be fooled by the maps suggesting they are permanent water sources. Looping around a blunt ridge, today's high point at about 11,430 feet, and back onto broad southwest-facing slopes, the sandy trail resumes its southeastward, forever-view-rich course. The trail passes many a twisted, picturesque, wind-battered foxtail pine. For many, small spiraling strips of surviving bark are a testament to their tenacity, as most of the roots, and consequently bark, have died, but the trees eke out a continuing existence. Eventually, the PCT begins a gradual, descending traverse toward the west wall of Chicken Spring Lake's cirque. Follow switchbacks down the wall and reach a spur to the lake (11,219'; 36.45420°N, 118.22510°W at the junction). There's fair camping on its west side and good camping on its east end (11,267'; 36.45541°N, 118.22589°W; no campfires). This foxtail pine–ringed lake is a very popular stop; you're sure to have company.

DAY 4 (Chicken Spring Lake to Cottonwood Lakes Trailhead, 4.8 miles): Leaving Chicken Spring Lake, the trail soon curves east toward Cottonwood Pass, continuing through a delightful foxtail pine forest. Just before the pass, there's a junction where left (east-northeast) leads over Cottonwood Pass to Horseshoe Meadow (your route), right (southwest) leads to

Big Whitney Meadow (Trip 80), and the PCT continues south (straight ahead). You go left and almost immediately summit the 11,167-foot pass. Stealing one last glance at the view west, you turn and look eastward to the Inyo and Panamint ranges.

Moderate switchbacks down a sandy slope with scattered foxtail pines lead to the edge of a small meadow full of willows, which the trail skirts to the west and south, before cutting back across to its northern edge. Continuing through sandy terrain beside the descending water course, another sequence of switchbacks among blocky outcrops leads to a flatter expanse of lodgepole pines. The path presently makes a pair of quick stream crossings, with great red paintbrush, crimson columbine, and monkeyflowers growing along the watercourses.

After a few more steps you see an expanse of meadow opening to your south, Horseshoe Meadow. You skirt the meadow's north side on an increasingly sandy trail. Breaks in the lodgepole and foxtail pine forest permit southward and eastward views of Mulkey Pass, Trail Pass, Trail Peak, and over the shoulder to Cottonwood Pass.

The meadow pinches near its middle, and here, in a gigantic patch of sand, you reach a junction with the trail to Trail Pass (right, south; not shown on USGS 7.5' topos); straight ahead (east) leads to the Cottonwood Pass Trailhead. There is also a track—also not on maps—that leads left (northeast) toward the pack station and will be easily detected by the predominance of hoofprints along it. The pack station is just near the Cottonwood Lakes Trailhead, where your car is parked, so head along this decidedly sandy-sloggy trail. It loops around the west side of the pack station and then turns east to reach the trailhead campground. Then turn left and cut across to the main trailhead parking, the cars visible through the sparse trees.

View to Big Whitney Meadow on the long traverse toward Chicken Spring Lake
Photo by Elizabeth Wenk

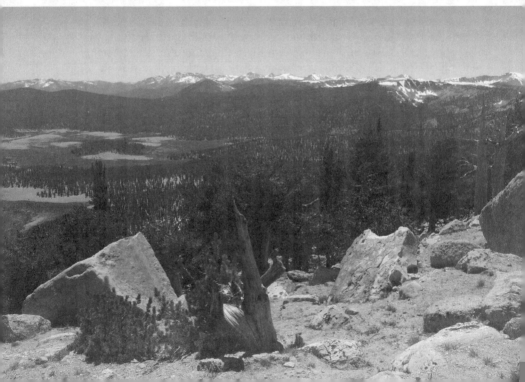

Cottonwood Pass Trailhead   9,949'; 36.44834°N, 118.17070°W

Destination/ GPS Coordinates	Trip Type	Best Season	Pace & Hiking/ Layover Days	Total Mileage	Permit Required
78 Horseshoe Meadow to Mount Whitney 36.57852°N 118.29228°W (Mount Whitney)	Shuttle	Mid to late	Moderate 6/0	39.5	Cottonwood Pass *(Mount Whitney Trail in reverse)*
79 Milestone Basin and Upper Kern 36.64357°N 118.44742°W (Milestone Basin)	Shuttle	Mid to late	Moderate to strenuous 7/3	55.6	Cottonwood Pass *(Shepherd Pass in reverse)*
80 Rocky Basin Lakes 36.44451°N 118.32412°W	Out-and-back	Mid to late	Moderate 4/1	26.8	Cottonwood Pass
77 Upper Rock Creek *(in reverse of description; see page 412)*	Loop	Mid to late	Leisurely 4/2	23.4	Cottonwood Pass *(Cottonwood Lakes as described)*

INFORMATION AND PERMITS: This trailhead is in Inyo National Forest. Permits are required for overnight stays and quotas apply. Permits can be reserved up to six months in advance at recreation.gov (60%; $6 permit reservation fee plus $5 per person) or requested in person, first come, first served, a day in advance (40%; free). Trip 78 exits over Trail Crest, which has an exit quota. When you book your permit at recreation.gov, you must specifically indicate you are exiting via the Whitney Zone; Whitney exit permits are generally available six months plus one week in advance of a particular exit date. These permits are in high demand, so you may have to be flexible with your start (or finish) date. All permits must be picked up at one of the Inyo National Forest ranger stations, located in Lone Pine (Eastern Sierra Interagency Visitor Center), Bishop, Mammoth Lakes, and Lee Vining (the Mono Basin Scenic Area Visitor Center). If you plan to use a stove or have a campfire while on national forest lands, you must also have a California campfire permit, available from a forest service office or online at preventwildfireca.org/campfire-permit. Campfires are prohibited above 10,400 in Inyo National Forest (east of the Sierra Crest) and above 10,400 feet in Sequoia National Park (west of the Sierra Crest), as well as at Chicken Spring Lake (Trips 78 and 79), along the Mount Whitney Trail (Trip 78), at Anvil Camp (Trip 79), and at Rocky Basin Lakes (Trip 80). Bear canisters are required in this area.

DRIVING DIRECTIONS: Turn west from US 395 in Lone Pine onto Whitney Portal Road. Go 3.1 miles and turn left onto Horseshoe Meadows Road. Go straight 19.2 miles, then continue left on the main road at the Cottonwood Lakes Trailhead junction. After an additional 0.2 mile you reach the gigantic parking area, servicing the Cottonwood Pass Trailhead as well as the Trail Pass Trailhead onto the Kern Plateau. There are toilets and water, with a one-night campground nearby at the Cottonwood Lakes Trailhead.

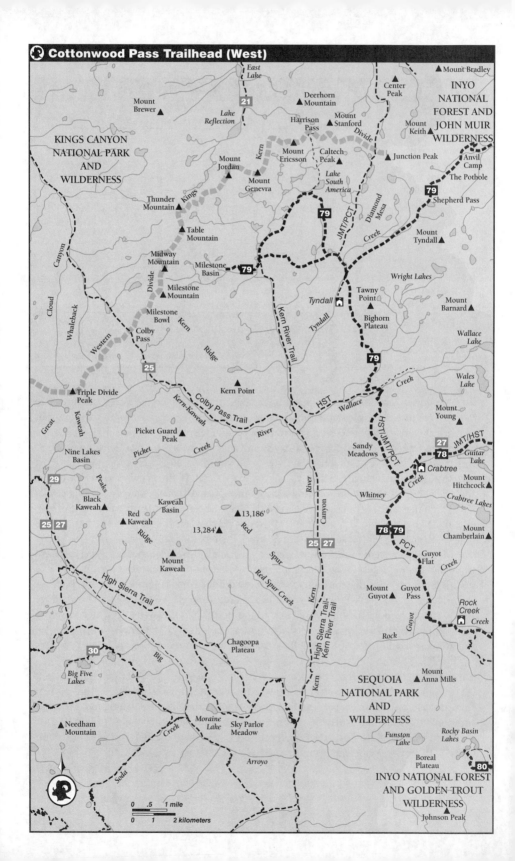

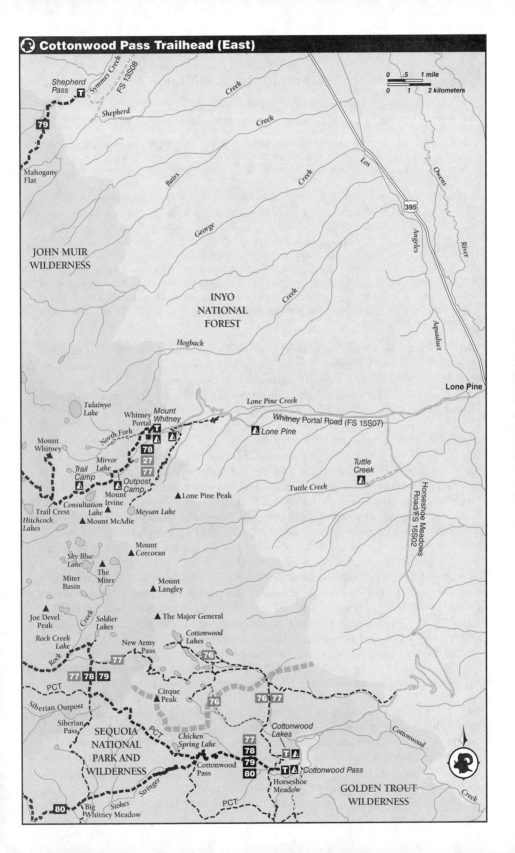

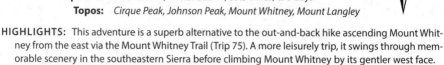

trip 78 Horseshoe Meadow to Mount Whitney

see maps on p. 418–419

Trip Data: 36.57852°N, 118.29228°W; 39.5 miles; 6/0 days
Topos: *Cirque Peak, Johnson Peak, Mount Whitney, Mount Langley*

HIGHLIGHTS: This adventure is a superb alternative to the out-and-back hike ascending Mount Whitney from the east via the Mount Whitney Trail (Trip 75). A more leisurely trip, it swings through memorable scenery in the southeastern Sierra before climbing Mount Whitney by its gentler west face.

HEADS UP! *From Timberline Lake (on the west side) to Lone Pine Lake (on the east side) you need to pack out solid waste—you will receive a human-waste disposal kit for free when you pick up your wilderness permit. Bear canisters are required along the Rock Creek corridor and on the Mount Whitney Trail.*

SHUTTLE DIRECTIONS: From the intersection of US 395 and Whitney Portal Road in the town of Lone Pine—at the town's only traffic light—go 11.8 miles west on Whitney Portal Road to its end at Whitney Portal. Here you'll find a large parking area with toilets, water, and the Whitney Portal store (including a café).

DAY 1 (Cottonwood Pass Trailhead to Chicken Spring Lake, 4.4 miles): The exposed, sandy trail heads west beneath very sparse lodgepole pine shade. After 0.3 mile you reach a junction where left (south) leads across Horseshoe Meadow and onto Trail Pass, while you continue straight ahead (west), along the northern edge of the expansive meadow system. Continued flat, sandy walking takes you northwest and then west to the head of Horseshoe Meadow, where the trail makes a pair of quick stream crossings, with great red paintbrush, crimson columbine, and monkeyflowers growing along the watercourses. After traversing a denser lodgepole pine flat and looping around another seasonally verdant meadow lobe, the trail begins a switchbacking ascent to the north of the willow-clad stream corridor. Winding up among foxtail pines and between small fractured outcrops, the gradient eases briefly where the trail crosses the meadowed river strip.

The trail then carries you north, still alongside a swathe of meadow and willows, before a dozen switchbacks lead west to Cottonwood Pass (11,167'). Views eastward include the Inyo and Panamint Ranges, while to the west you garner glimpses of expansive Big Whitney Meadow and the distant Great Western Divide.

A few feet west of the pass, you come to the famous Pacific Crest Trail (PCT) at a diffuse four-way junction. The PCT leads south–north (left–right), while straight ahead (west) is the trail to Big Whitney Meadow (Trip 80). You turn right, heading northbound on the PCT. Follow the PCT west for an easy 0.6 mile through delightful foxtail pine forest to the outlet of Chicken Spring Lake and a junction (11,219'; 36.4542°N, 118.2251°W). Follow the spur trail upstream toward good campsites east of and fair campsites west of the foxtail pine–rimmed lake (for example, 11,267'; 36.45541°N, 118. 22589°W; no campfires). This is a popular lake, and you're sure to have company here, but by late summer the next water is 5.0 miles ahead.

DAY 2 (Chicken Spring Lake to Rock Creek Lake, 6.4 miles): Leaving Chicken Spring Lake with full water bottles, you climb switchbacks westward, up and away from the lake, crossing a spur and beginning a northwestward traverse across Cirque Peak's extensive southwestern flank. The trail forever passes twisted, picturesque, wind-battered foxtail pines. On many small spiraling strips of surviving bark are a testament of their tenacity, as most of the roots, and consequently bark, have died, with just one branch of the tree eking out a continuing existence. The views west to Big Whitney Meadow and onward to the southern Great Western Divide are continually splendid and the walking is easy—a gentle undulating traverse that descends and then regains about 200 feet over 2.0 miles.

You then turn north and drop just slightly into a tiny valley sculpted into Cirque Peak. Maps show two tempting tarns here, but both can be dry by midsummer; do not depend upon them for water. The walking is rockier as the trail rounds a headwall, turns back to the northwest, and presently enters Sequoia National Park. Here you trade your final views south to Olancha Peak for better ones northwest to the Kaweahs. Still skirting Cirque Peak's western slopes, Siberian Outpost is now spread out before you, a vast expanse of mounds of sand and seasonally marshy meadows with colorful soils. Descending more steeply and then bearing west, you soon reach a junction where you turn right (north) toward the Rock Creek Trail, while the PCT continues straight ahead (west), and left (south) leads to Siberian Pass. Note that continuing along the PCT to the Rock Creek crossing is 0.5 mile shorter, but it's less scenic and you would have to continue nearly 5 miles to water and camping. It is, however, recommended if water levels are high and you want to miss two wet fords of Rock Creek.

Turning right, you drop off an easy ridge, climb very slightly, and then gradually descend a moderately to densely forested slope of foxtail and lodgepole pine. An easy 1.1 miles lead to another junction where right heads up over New Army Pass (Trip 77), while you stay left (north), signposted for the Rock Creek Trail.

Heading north, you descend gently across dry sandy and bouldery slopes and then have a nearly flat traverse beneath open pine cover. Just 0.3 mile later you reach a junction to the Soldier Lakes, unnamed on the USGS 7.5' topos. Heading right (east) along the spur trail leads to a selection of good campsites, some on a ledge high above the lower lake after 0.2 mile (10,843'; 36.50020°N, 118.27117°W; no campfires; bear box) and others along the lake's southern shore after 0.5 mile. (*Note:* The current spur trail is along the slope on the south side of the Soldier Lakes outlet creek. The old trail along the north side of Lower Soldier Lake has been rehabilitated and does not lead to camping.) Continuing left (north) on the main trail along the western side of the elongate meadow holding Lower Soldier Lake, you soon step across the outlet creek on rocks and make a sharp left.

The trail now descends steeply alongside a willow-infested tributary of Rock Creek until the rocky slope gives way to a meadow just above the gleaming blue lake colloquially known as Rock Creek Lake or Upper Rock Creek Lake. There are fair campsites at the head of this meadow, and then following a sandy-bottomed wade of Rock Creek (at high flows) another large area with a bear box near the lake's outlet (10,468'; 36.49517°N, 118.28407°W at the bear box; no campfires). Additional options are to be found on the south side of the lake. Fishing for golden in the lake and adjoining stream is good. If you arrive with hours to spare, Miter Basin, the headwaters of Rock Creek, is well worth exploring.

MITER BASIN

From Rock Creek Lake, a day hike to nearby Miter Basin is always a treat. A use trail to Miter Basin makes a hard-to-spot exit along the north side of the large campsite at the eastern tip of Rock Creek Lake's meadow (10,455'; 36.49828°N, 118.27912°W). This trail is easy to follow to the place where Rock Creek cascades out of the basin; from there, it is easy cross-country hiking through meadows and across bedrock to a vast wonderland of slab-ringed lakes watched over by steep crests. You can easily spend a day exploring the basin.

DAY 3 (Rock Creek Lake to Guyot Creek, 5.0 miles): The coming miles offer relatively few views as you follow the lodgepole pine–shaded Rock Creek corridor west beneath the flanks of massive Joe Devel Peak. Stretches are flatter, with possible campsites, and elsewhere the valley bottom is narrow, steeper, and the river faster flowing. After 1.8 miles you ford Rock Creek (on small logs or a sandy-bottomed wade) and pass a collection of campsites beneath lodgepole pine at the fringe of a meadow through which Rock Creek meanders lazily. Once the meadow pinches closed, a sloping traverse southwest takes you away from the river corridor to a junction where you rejoin the PCT; you turn right (west), signposted for the Lower Rock Creek crossing, while left (southeast) trends back toward Cottonwood Pass.

Switchbacks lead you back toward the now-broad valley bottom, here an expanse of seasonally marshy meadows where Rock Creek, Perrin Creek, and several unnamed tributaries combine. You pass a spur to the summer-staffed Rock Creek Ranger Station (cabin at 9,683'; 36.49541°N, 118.32646°W) and continue past campsites in a lodgepole pine flat, the trail picking a route along raised ribs that mostly avoids walking through the fragile meadow environment. Ahead is a crossing of Rock Creek, often discussed among PCT hikers, as it is notoriously treacherous in early season; hopefully a log will be present and dry for your ford. Just across the creek is a large, overused campsite and a bear box.

On the north side of the ford, the trail begins its long climb northwest and then north to the saddle east of Mount Guyot known as Guyot Pass. You begin with a 700-foot ascent up rocky, bouldery moraine deposits, quickly crossing several small trickles and then increasingly laboring up dry slopes with little shade but lovely views south to Mount Anna Mills and Forgotten Canyon. At about 10,250 feet you reach the moraine crest and continue north across a gently sloping sandy plateau. Beneath sparse foxtail and lodgepole pine cover you shortly reach Guyot Creek and will find many beautiful, low-impact sandy campsites nearby (10,369'; 36.50662°N, 118.34308°W; no campfires). Unseen from the trail, there are meadows both east and west of the trail, with more campsites at their perimeters. This is also your last water source until Whitney Creek in Crabtree Meadow, nearly 5 miles ahead.

DAY 4 (Guyot Creek to Guitar Lake, 8.4 miles): The jumbled, symmetrical crest of Mount Guyot fills the skyline to the west, and highly fractured Joe Devel Peak looms to the east as the PCT begins another steep ascent through lodgepole and foxtail pine. This bouldery climb culminates at Guyot Pass (10,922'), which once rose above the glaciers. The broad, sandy expanse to your north blocks views deep into the Kern Canyon, but you can look across it to the edge of Red Spur and northwest to the Kern–Kaweah River drainage (the

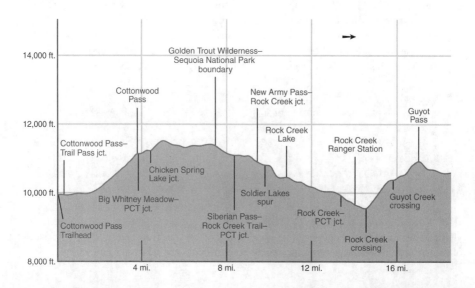

Colby Pass Trail corridor; Trip 25), Kern Point and the evocative Greatest Western Divide peaks ringing Milestone Basin: Milestone, Midway, Table, and Thunder Mountains. From the pass, Mount Guyot is a technically easy, albeit tiring, 1,400-foot ascent mostly up sand and gravel and offers outstanding views of the entire Kern drainage.

The trail descends moderately to the large, sandy basin of Guyot Flat and traverses the open forest east of the flat. It then loops west around a spur emanating off Mount Chamberlain's western summit and climbs just slightly to cross a second sandy ridge. Just thereafter, a barely noticed uphill leads over Whitney Creek's lateral moraine, and you then drop quite steeply down moraine rubble to the stream corridor. The descent into this drainage affords views eastward to Mount Whitney—the long, flat-topped, avalanche-chuted mountain that towers over the nearer, granite-spired shoulder of Mount Hitchcock—and north to the Kings–Kern Divide. The barren, rocky descent leads to beautiful rounded, polished, granite-slab ribs in lower Crabtree Meadow and good campsites with a bear box. The trail then fords Whitney Creek and arrives at a junction. The PCT continues left (north) here, while this trip branches right (northeast) along Whitney Creek's northwest bank on a lateral to the John Muir Trail (JMT), leaving the PCT behind.

Skirting first lower and then upper Crabtree Meadow, an easy 0.7 mile leads to the unsigned, almost invisible old trail heading east to the Crabtree Lakes (golden trout and small campsites). Ahead, Whitney Creek follows a narrow channel and your trail hugs the western bank, curving in tandem with the creek. The trail then fords the creek and climbs to an open area beside a bear box, with many good but busy campsites nearby. If thunderstorms are threatening, or you prefer a forested campsite, pick a location in the vicinity of Crabtree Meadow, but otherwise continue toward Guitar Lake, an additional 2.6 miles, to ease tomorrow's hike. Along a use trail to the right (east) is the summer-staffed Crabtree Ranger Station (10,694'; 36.56465°N, 118.34727°W).

Continuing toward Guitar Lake from the camping area, head north, ford Whitney Creek again, and climb briefly, to arrive at a junction with the JMT. Here you turn right (east), now heading straight toward Mount Whitney, while left (west) is the northbound route of the JMT and also leads back to the PCT. You continue upward, following a river terrace on the north shore of Whitney Creek, passing first through open lodgepole forest (with several campsites) and then increasingly walking across dry, open slopes. A set of switchbacks up

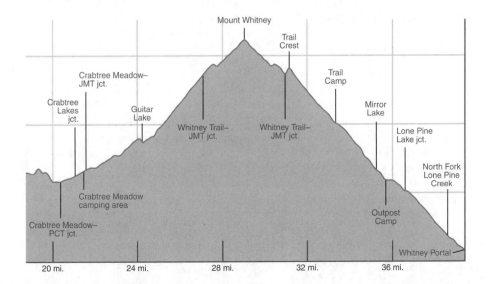

slabs takes you to Timberline Lake (golden trout), where camping and grazing are prohibited, but photographing Mount Whitney mirrored in its still waters is encouraged.

Now passing the final trees, the trail turns northeast, following a trickle past seasonal tarns. The meadow corridor is dotted with alpine flowers, including the August-blooming white Sierra gentians and purple alpine gentians. To your left, Mount Young and Mount Hale, like so many of the peaks in the Whitney region, shed prodigious quantities of coarse gravel and sand. Red mountain heather creeps across the lower-angled slopes, holding the sediment in place. When the trail levels out into a wet-sandy flat, you are nearly at Guitar Lake. Here, you can leave the trail to find campsites above the "guitar's neck." Or, stay on the trail until it approaches Arctic Lake's outlet (11,487'), then follow one of several use trails to additional campsites near Guitar Lake (head south at 11,500'; 36.57230°N, 118.31407°W; no campfires). Cross-country slab-and-sand walking also leads to tarns above the Hitchcock Lakes, offering more privacy; these are best reached by continuing another 0.5 mile along the trail and then striking south. In dry periods this will be your last on-trail water until Trail Camp, so fill all your bottles before continuing.

DAY 5 (Guitar Lake to Trail Camp, 9.1 miles): Get an early start, for even if you were to skip Mount Whitney's summit (saving about 3.9 miles), this is a tough day because you are at high elevation. Leaving Guitar Lake—and crossing Arctic Lake's braided outlet—the route follows a slab bench above Guitar Lake and then skirts a marshy meadow at its head, crossing a broad jumble of rocks that is a debris-flow fan. Mount Whitney's western face is tall and daunting, but beautifully decorated with spires due to joints in the rock. Two switchbacks lead to another shelf, again with a marshy meadow and two small tarns. Then more than a dozen tight zigzags lead up a sometimes-wet corridor to another shelf—from here you could head south toward campsites among tarns above the Hitchcock Lakes.

Leaving these meadow patches you begin barren switchbacks up and up—cutting up talus fans and zigzagging up cliff bands. While the grade is moderate, the increasing altitude leads to frequent rest stops from which the views just get better and better—reward enough for your labor.

SUMMIT PREPARATION

It is a good idea to leave most of your gear at the junction south of Mount Whitney's summit, continuing to the summit with a day pack (or mostly empty overnight pack). Just be sure to lock your food and toiletries in your bear canister to impede the pesky marmots. And do take plenty of food and water, extra warm clothes, and wind- and raingear. Avoid the summit if a storm is brewing—the entire route from here to the summit is exposed in a storm. The summit hut is not a safe shelter; the metal roof conducted fatal electrical jolts to hikers seeking shelter on one occasion, and although it has been retrofitted I wouldn't want to be the one to test it.

Many switchbacks later, the JMT passes a collection of near-crest tent sites, somewhat protected by makeshift rock walls (no water!), and reaches a junction where it turns left (north) to climb to Mount Whitney's summit; the Mount Whitney Trail ascending from Whitney Portal to the east merges from the right (south)—your return route. At about 13,800 feet, the trail levels off and enters a maze of pinnacles. The slope here has a scalloped appearance due to the many avalanche chutes that transect it. The sharp ridges of joint-defined pinnacles mark the boundary between avalanche chutes. Between pinnacles, you have open views to the west; in the distance is the dark, jagged Kaweah Peaks Ridge, while granite slopes dominate the foreground. You repeatedly pass narrow notches, with

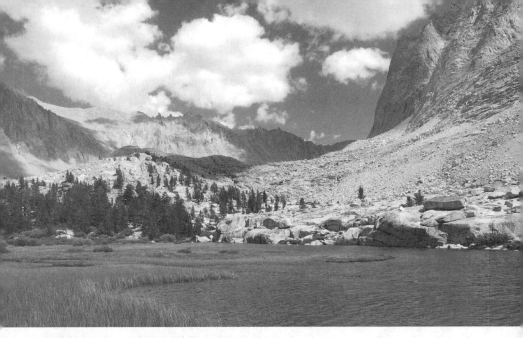

Timberline Lake   Photo by Elizabeth Wenk

jaw-dropping views straight down to the east—watch your footing carefully near there, for the trail is narrow and the drops are very steep.

Leaving the pinnacles behind, you are just 1.0 mile from the summit. Before you is a broad, barren talus field: large boulders surrounded by sand, with ever smaller numbers of alpine gold and sky pilot growing in sheltered crevices. The trail mimics the surrounding terrain; it is still mostly sandy, but there are also boulders embedded in the trail that require larger steps up—not a welcome proposition at this altitude. Traverse the western face of Crooks Peak (previously named Day Needle) and Keeler Needle, two 14,000-foot points that are too indistinct from Mount Whitney to be considered true peaks.

Beyond Keeler Needle, the trail bends west for a stretch before beginning the final climb to the summit. There are a few halfhearted switchbacks up the last talus field. Nearly everyone heading down will encourage you onward with calls of, "You can't see the summit hut yet, but you're almost there." In fact, because of the summit plateau's very shallow angle, you don't see the summit hut until just minutes before you reach the top. Suddenly, the views open in every direction. A large summit register sits by the entrance to the stone hut. Sign your name, and then head to the giant boulders a short distance east—the actual high point—to take a long, well-deserved break.

GEOLOGY AND BOTANY ON THE CLIMB

Particularly striking are the views of the Hitchcock Lakes, gemlike and blue-green in a cirque basin that has changed little since its glacier melted. Notice how the parallel avalanche chutes on the northeast wall of Mount Hitchcock all terminate at the same elevation. This boundary between "steep chute" and "nearly vertical wall" marks the height to which the valley was once filled with ice, known as the *trimline* in the jargon of a geomorphologist. Along the switchbacks, the most prominent flower is the yellow, daisylike alpine gold, whose warm flowers are a magnet for insects. Sky pilot, with its giant purple heads, also manages to grow almost to the peak's summit—but at the very summit temperatures are too cool and winds too strong for either of these species to establish.

Retrace your steps to the junction, bid the JMT farewell, put away the day packs, hoist the backpacks, and follow the Mount Whitney Trail left (southeast). Climbing briefly but steeply, you skirt past a few rock towers, reaching Trail Crest (13,600') after 0.15 mile, crossing into Inyo National Forest and John Muir Wilderness.

You steal one last view west and then stare down the steep eastern escarpment. After a long eastward traverse, the 99 switchbacks begin, leading you 1,600 feet down to Trail Camp. The trail follows a route more or less along a shallow ridge, avoiding most of the long-lasting snowfields, but snow can still persist well into summer. Most notorious is the "cables" section, where the trail cuts through a prominent cliff band and the trail has been blasted into rock. Here water seeps through cracks and snow and ice can persist long after most of the trail is snow-free—a handrail has been installed for safety. The peaks seem taller with each downward step, and soon you are looking up at the Whitney Crest's sawtooth profile from Mount Muir to the Needles; Mount Whitney itself is visible at just the top and bottom of the switchbacks. Mount Irvine looms to the southeast, and rounded Wotans Throne sits to the northeast.

The switchbacks finally cease near Trail Camp, one of the Whitney Trail's two main camping areas (12,025'; 36.56298°N, 118.27915°W; no campfires). Here, tent sites have been created in every flat spot available among the pervasive slabs and boulders—there are many places to camp on both sides of the trail. Since there are no longer toilets tethering you to this specific location, if you want more privacy, search for alternate campsites a bit farther south or a little below Trail Camp. Since you have just completed Mount Whitney and might not wish to be woken by other hikers at 3 a.m., you will particularly appreciate a well-off-trail campsite. The inlet to the Trail Camp tarn is the first reliable water since Guitar Lake.

DAY 6 (Trail Camp to Whitney Portal, 6.1 miles): The Mount Whitney Trail leaves Trail Camp on an eastward descent down sandy passageways on the granite ridge north of Consultation Lake; heading south about 0.4 mile beyond Trail Camp leads to possible campsites closer to this beautiful lake. Winding down to cross nascent Lone Pine Creek, the trail follows a sandy ledge past espaliered rosy-petaled cliffbush and crack-hugging Sierra primrose as it works its way through the tortuous landscape. It curves first away from and then switchbacks back toward Lone Pine Creek, sidling up to the creek in beautiful Trailside Meadow (where camping is prohibited). The trail now follows the crest of a rounded granite ridge. Through this section, the views down to Lone Pine Lake and the Owens Valley are exquisite. Take care not to miss where the trail turns left (north) to begin switchbacking sinuously to Mirror Lake, for straight ahead are steep cliffs. Here you pass your first trees—a few each of lodgepole, whitebark, and foxtail pines—and descend rockily to Mirror Lake (10,686'; no camping), nestled in a steep-walled cirque beneath Thor Peak.

Crossing Mirror Lake's outlet on rocks, the trail descends again, first past a headwall and then down a bouldery-brushy slope among creambush, spiny-fruited chinquapin, wax currant, aromatic coyote mint, and vibrantly magenta mountain pride penstemon—to name just a sample of the many species. The gradient eases in Outpost Camp, a flat of sand and scattered foxtail pines with ample campsites (10,374'; 36.57159°N, 118.25886°W; no campfires). Some of the best are at the south end of the flat, with views to cascading Lone Pine Creek. Beyond, the trail fords the creek on large rock blocks and continues along the south side of Bighorn Park, a marshy meadow with towering cliffs overhead. Look just to your right and you may see where a spring emerges from exposed bedrock. A slight rise leads to a gully south of the main drainage that you descend via elegantly walled switchbacks. In a sandy flat beyond, you exit the Whitney Zone and reach a junction with a spur right (east) to Lone Pine Lake (and your final plausible campsites on this trail).

You continue left, dropping through lodgepole pine cover to another ford of Lone Pine Creek, this one on a series of raised logs. After briefly following the creek corridor, the trail veers north, crosses a patch of moist vegetation, and begins a long series of switchbacks down a dry, exposed slope of chaparral vegetation including mountain mahogany, chinquapin, and sagebrush. Enjoy the view down the canyon framing the Alabama Hills, the background for hundreds of television shows and movies, especially countless westerns. As you begin a long traverse, some Jeffrey pine and white fir finally provide some shade and soon the trail cuts north to cross the North Fork Lone Pine Creek in the thicket of vegetation.

The final 0.9 mile is a descending traverse east, mostly down another sandy slope with scattered shrubs. Bursts of color—and even a little mud—greet you as you cut into the small, informally named Carillon Creek drainage. Finally you switchback west and then turn south for the final descent to Whitney Portal with its parking lot, café, and small store.

trip 79 Milestone Basin and the Upper Kern

see maps on p. 418–419

Trip Data: 36.64357°N, 118.44742°W (Milestone Basin); 55.6 miles; 7/3 days

Topos: *Cirque Peak, Johnson Peak, Mount Whitney, Mount Langley (barely), Mount Williamson, Mount Brewer*

HIGHLIGHTS: Visit some of the most beautiful and sought-after alpine cirques and lakes in the southern Sierra on this multiday adventure that includes famed Milestone Basin and Lake South America. There's no easy way to reach these destinations and as soon as you're off the busy John Muir Trail (JMT)/Pacific Crest Trail (PCT) corridor, you'll find immediate solitude. Having worked so hard to reach these locations, be sure to plan some layover days for exploring the basins.

SHUTTLE DIRECTIONS: From Lone Pine, drive 15.7 miles north to Independence. In Independence, turn from US 395 west onto Market Street (Onion Valley Road). Go 4.4 miles to Foothill Road, turn left, and go 1.3 miles to a Y-junction, where you stay right. Continue for an additional 2.0 miles, still on Foothill Road, and then turn right (west) onto Forest Service Road 14S102. Continue another 1.4 miles to the road's end, staying right where two less distinct dirt roads bear south/left (6,308'; 36.72708°N, 118.27888°W).

DAY 1 (Cottonwood Pass Trailhead to Lower Soldier Lake, 9.8 miles): Follow Trip 78, Day 1 for 4.4 miles across Cottonwood Pass to Chicken Spring Lake. If you wish to have a shorter first day, follow the outlet upstream toward good campsites east of the foxtail pine–rimmed lake (11,267'; 36.45541°N, 118. 22589°W; no campfires). By late summer, the next water is 5.0 miles ahead, so fill your water bottles here. Continuing your day, follow Trip 78, Day 2 for the first 5.4 miles to the Soldier Lakes junction (10,800'; 36.49759°N, 118.27294°W).

Heading right leads to a selection of good campsites, some on a ledge high above the lake after 0.2 mile (10,843'; 36.50020°N, 118.27117°W; no campfires; bear box) and others along the lower lake's southern shore after 0.5 mile. (*Note:* The current spur trail is along the slope on the south side of the Soldier Lakes outlet creek.) There are many additional campsites 1.0 mile ahead at Rock Creek Lake.

DAY 2 (Lower Soldier Lake to Lower Crabtree Meadows, 10.6 miles): Continue following Trip 78, Day 2 for 1.0 mile to Rock Creek Lake. Then follow Trip 78, Day 3 for 5.0 miles to Guyot Creek. Fill up on water, for this is your last water source until Whitney Creek in Crabtree Meadow, nearly 5 miles ahead.

The jumbled, symmetrical crest of Mount Guyot fills the skyline to the west, and highly fractured Joe Devel Peak looms to the east as the PCT begins another steep ascent through lodgepole and foxtail pine. This bouldery climb culminates at Guyot Pass (10,922'), which once rose above the glaciers. The broad sandy expanse to your north blocks views deep into the Kern Canyon, but you can look across it to the edge of Red Spur and northwest to the Kern–Kaweah River drainage (the Colby Pass Trail corridor; Trip 25), Kern Point and the evocative Greatest Western Divide peaks ringing Milestone Basin. You will camp beneath Milestone, Midway, and Table Mountains in a few days' time. From the pass, Mount Guyot is a technically easy, albeit tiring, 1,400-foot ascent mostly up sand and gravel and offers outstanding views of the entire Kern drainage.

The trail descends moderately to the large, sandy basin of Guyot Flat and traverses the open forest east of the flat. It then loops west around a spur emanating off Mount Chamberlain's western summit and climbs just slightly to cross a second sandy ridge. Just thereafter, a barely noticed uphill leads over Whitney Creek's lateral moraine and you then drop quite steeply down moraine rubble to the stream corridor. The descent into this drainage affords views eastward to Mount Whitney—the long, flat-topped, avalanche-chuted mountain that towers over the nearer, granite-spired shoulder of Mount Hitchcock—and north to the Kings–Kern Divide. The barren, rocky descent leads to beautiful rounded, polished, granite-slab ribs in lower Crabtree Meadow and good campsites with a bear box (10,347'; 36.55189°N, 118.35836°W; no campfires).

DAY 3 (Lower Crabtree Meadow to Tyndall Frog Ponds, 8.0 miles): Beyond the campsites, the trail fords Whitney Creek and arrives at a junction, where the PCT continues straight ahead (north), while right (northeast) is a cutoff connector leading up Whitney Creek to the Crabtree Ranger Station, main Crabtree Meadow camping area, and Mount Whitney (Trip 78). Staying left on the PCT, you very gently ascend an open sandy slope, skirt the head of a pocket meadow, and climb more steeply through a foxtail pine forest. This foxtail forest, with its dead snags, fallen trees, and lack of ground cover has an otherworldly quality—a moonscape with statues. Enjoying views to Mounts Hitchcock, Pickering,

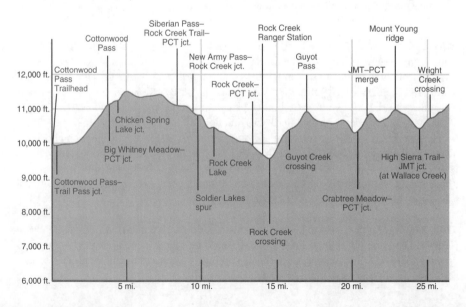

Chamberlain, and Whitney, you shortly reach a junction where the PCT is joined from the right by the JMT, coming east from Mount Whitney. This is also the route of the High Sierra Trail from Crescent Meadow (in the west) to Mount Whitney (Trip 27).

Continue left (north) on the now-busier trail corridor, the trail flattening as it summits a broad rib. It then descends to cross a seasonal creeklet at the head of one of Sandy Meadow's many tentacles and proceeds across the top of this seasonally verdant expanse, covered with orange sneezeweed and corn lilies by midsummer, while diminutive primrose monkeyflower decorates the banks of the creeklets. There are a handful of small campsites in the forest upslope, but note that these drainages can run dry. Following the northernmost stringer meadow upstream, you climb to the apex of a sandy shoulder that once stood above the glaciers, the most prominent ridge extending west of Mount Young (10,990′).

From this saddle, the route descends gently on a sandy trail, leveling off as it crosses onto a bouldery lateral moraine. The trail winds among the massive boulders that comprise the moraine, and then drops back onto sloping polished slabs, sandy strips, and suddenly lodgepole pine stands. Here you have fine views of Mount Ericsson, Tawny Point, Junction Peak, the flank of Mount Tyndall, Mount Versteeg, Mount Williamson, and, farthest right, massive Mount Barnard.

After fording a tributary of Wallace Creek, the descent steepens, and the trail switchbacks a half mile down to campsites (and a bear box) on the south side of the Wallace Creek ford. This crossing is broad, rocky, and can be very difficult during peak flows; it is likely to result in wet shoes through much of the summer. Once across Wallace Creek, the High Sierra Trail turns left (west; Trip 27) toward Giant Forest while the JMT/PCT continues ahead (north). Heading east (right) from the junction, you'll discover a good use trail that leads up Wallace Creek to the sublime Wallace and Wales Lakes, each sitting in broad granite slab basins above which rise vertical, fractured summits. This basin and the Wright Creek drainage (the next basin north) are each well worth a day's exploration (or more) if you have spare days.

You continue north along the JMT/PCT for a circuitous 0.7 mile, as you climb a moraine crest and then drop modestly to the ford of Wright Creek (also can be difficult in early season but is generally an easier wade). There are campsites to either side of the crossing and more as you follow the drainage upstream. Ascending gradually, the trail now crosses

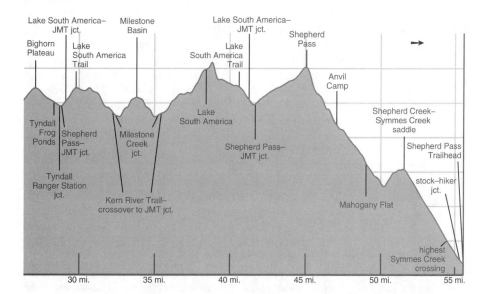

the multiple stringer meadows that coalesce into Wright Creek, traverses minor bedrock ridges, and walks through endless piles of sand transported from the rubbly granite slopes to the east. The trail levels as it reaches Bighorn Plateau. A delightfully round, mostly groundwater-fed tarn sits in its center, with ample campsites once you're outside its grassy fringe. Tawny Point, to the east, is a straightforward ascent that yields panoramic views, although walking to the western edge of Bighorn Plateau suffices for a spectacular vista that begins with Red Spur in the southwest and sweeps north along the Great Western Divide, then east along the Kings–Kern Divide to Junction Peak. In addition, you can see, to the southeast, Mount Whitney, Mount Young, and Mount Russell.

From Bighorn Plateau a gradual descent on a rocky trail through a sparse foxtail cover leads to good campsites at the so-called Tyndall Frog Ponds, a chain of tarns strung along the base of Tawny Point, dammed by Tyndall Creek's lateral moraine. The lakes offer good swimming, and there are fine campsites near where the trail crosses the outlet creek (10,978', 36.64299°N, 118.38767°W; no campfires).

DAY 4 (Tyndall Frog Ponds to Milestone Basin, 5.5 miles): Continue north along the JMT/PCT toward Tyndall Creek. As you approach its banks you reach a junction with a spur trail that leads 0.6 mile downstream (left; southwest) to the sometimes-staffed Tyndall Creek Ranger Station (ranger station at 10,692'; 36.63256°N, 118.39196°W). A little-used trail, the John Dean Cutoff, continues downstream to the Kern. Another 0.1 mile north on the JMT leads to a junction with the Shepherd Pass Trail (right; northeast), your exit route in some days' time. (*Note:* The USGS 7.5' topo incorrectly shows these two junctions in the opposite order.) Continuing straight ahead (left; north) along the JMT, you drop to ford Tyndall Creek, a very difficult ford in early season: the flows are significant, the gradient here is not flat, the base is rocky, and the water is frigid—take care. Just beyond is a collection of campsites with a bear box. Then, less than 0.2 mile beyond the campsites, you reach another junction, where the JMT/PCT is the right-hand (north) option, bound for Forester Pass, while you turn left (northwest), toward Lake South America and the Kern River.

After a brief ascent up sandy slopes, you pass a tarn and begin a delightful romp through an unmatched expanse of alpine tundra. With an occasional wind-blasted foxtail pine for foreground, unforgettable views extend in all directions as you walk east across the alpine fellfields. Soon you reach the next junction, where left (straight ahead; west) leads most directly to Milestone Basin, your route now, while the described route returns via the longer Lake South America loop, the right-hand (north) choice. Continuing due west, you wander on and on through this wonderland, hopefully on a day without storms brewing. Enjoy the views in all directions, especially those to Mounts Milestone, Midway, Table, and Thunder along the Great Western Divide, for their profiles will vanish as you drop down.

You step across the outlet stream of Lake 3,490 (golden trout), pass a small tarn, and eventually begin a rocky descent across the quite-steep front of a gigantic flat-topped talus pile, a moonscape of undulating boulder ribs that is a moraine from an early Pleistocene glaciation; this slope was last under ice 180,000 years ago, not 15,000 years like the surrounding valleys. You then traverse past tall foxtail pines—and many dead snags—to reach an unnamed creeklet whose drainage you follow west beneath a sparse cover of foxtail and whitebark pines. The trail crosses to the north side of the drainage as it arrives at a picture-book lake that is fast (geologically speaking) turning to meadow—the natural fate of all these lakes. After climbing slightly, your route begins the last, very steep descent to the Kern River, where it meets the Kern River Trail at an unnamed lake (10,662'; about 3,250 meters on the *Mount Brewer* topo; golden and rainbow-golden hybrids).

You turn left (south) on the Kern River Trail, while right leads to the headwaters of the Kern, your return route. If there is a safe logjam at this lake's outlet you should cross to the west side of the river, for you will follow the Kern River downstream for less than 0.2 mile before turning west toward Milestone Basin. At the actual (unmarked) trail junction, the crossing is usually a wade and can be difficult in early season. If you continue down the east side of the creek, the junction with the spur trail to Milestone Basin is marked only by a small cairn (10,632'; 36.64573°N, 118.43325°W); you know you've missed it when the Kern River Trail starts to trend left, away from the riverbank.

Once on the west side of the Kern River, the trail is more obvious. It heads to the southwest, dropping a token amount of elevation as it contours across lodgepole pine flats into the Milestone Creek drainage. Staying on the north side of the river, the trail then begins a zigzagging ascent up fractured, polished slabs. Walking across the sandy tops of the slabs, you are again next to the creek, now in a small meadow, beside which there are ample campsites. The next stretch of trail is less distinct—where the gradient increases, the trail veers northwest through lodgepole pine forest, diverging from the creek, before turning west beneath a headwall and following a sandy corridor. Continuing west, you soon reach some idyllic campsites atop sandy knobs with brilliant views both east to the Sierra Crest from Mount Tyndall to Mount Whitney and west to the wonderful profiles of Milestone, Midway, and Table Mountains; one large site is located at 11,119'; 36.64357°N, 118.44742°W; no campfires. Fishing in Milestone Creek is good for rainbow trout.

Just past this campsite, you reach a many-tentacled meadow enveloped by slabs where the two main forks of Milestone Creek merge. The trail diagonals up the slope toward the unnamed northern branch and soon vanishes in the endless slab. The trip's mileage likewise ends here, but opportunities for exploring have just begun. There are sandy nooks for one or two tents throughout the basin, some closer to lakes and others atop rocky ribs. Or you can set up a base camp in the relative shelter of the location described and explore without the weight of an overnight pack.

EXPLORING MILESTONE BASIN

The westernmost part of Milestone Basin is what makes the area famous: expansive polished slabs backdropped by near-vertical peaks. To reach it, ascend the shallow slab rib between the main Milestone Creek and its northern tributary; you might cross the occasional strip of sand with footprints, but there is no consistent use trail. Passing a boomerang-shaped lakelet set beneath a steep wall, you find yourself back along the main creek near where it bends to the north. From here you can walk up to the large lake at 11,920 feet or simply while away the hours atop a smooth, polished slab. Peak baggers are advised to seek out detailed route descriptions from other sources, but briefly, Milestone Mountain is a straightforward Class 3; you head up a Class 3 gully just north of the summit, drop 50 feet down the west side, follow a ramp left onto the west face, and then climb Class 2 and 3 slabs to the summit. Midday Mountain is Class 2 talus from the northeast. Table Mountain is Class 3 via a route that undulates across its steep southeast face to the table but requires excellent route-finding to avoid trickier terrain. Meanwhile, the cluster of lakes in the northwestern corner of Milestone Basin is tucked away in a steep, awkward landscape—navigating to them is cumbersome and not as rewarding as the western basin.

DAY 5 (Milestone Basin to Lake South America, 4.6 miles): If you've spent so many days exploring Milestone Basin that you now need to beeline for the trailhead, you should retrace your steps to the Shepherd Pass junction on the JMT, shaving 2.8 miles off the described distance. However, the headwaters of the Kern are as enchanting as Milestone Basin and you are within a couple hours' walk of it, so that is where you are directed next.

First retrace your steps down to the Kern River Trail, ford the Kern River, and turn left (north) to ascend the river drainage. As before, either cross at the official junction or

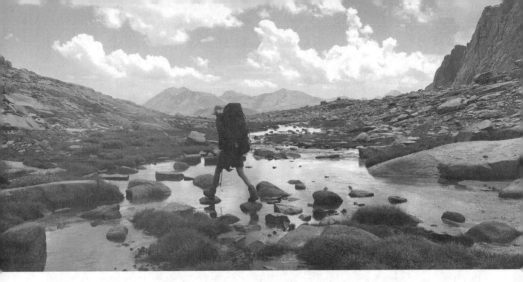

Walking through upper Milestone Basin   Photo by Elizabeth Wenk

upstream on the log jam. At the junction that cuts east (right) to the JMT (your previous route), continue straight ahead (left; north). Continuing up broken slabs beside the bubbling river, you pass a second lake (10,767') and then proceed northeast across a landscape of broken slab and ever sparser lodgepole and then whitebark pines. Marshy meadows are speckled with tundra aster and alpine shooting stars. You pass a trio of amoeba-shaped lakelets at about 11,270 feet (with decent campsites) and then turn farther to the east, away from the main Kern. If you haven't yet done so, turn around now and stare down the straight, narrow Kern drainage. Upstream, cross-country travel leads easily to the true headwaters of the Kern; see the sidebar "Headwaters of the Kern River" below.

The trail toward Lake South America winds upward, near a small creeklet. You are first on its southeastern side and then, above a small meadow, cross to the northern bank. Onward, you follow passageways and benches positioned along fractures and weaknesses in the bedrock. Ultimately turning to the east again and bidding the final krummholz farewell, a gentler gradient leads across barren terrain to a junction (11,973'; 36.67489°N, 118.40592°W), where right (southeast) leads back to the JMT, while left (north) leads 0.2 mile north past a tarn to Lake South America (11,829'; 36.67791°N, 118.40479°W). There are ample sandy, exposed campsites in the area with perfect sunrise views of the Great Western Divide.

HEADWATERS OF THE KERN RIVER

Broad, open, mostly sandy or grassy, low-angle slopes make the Kern River's headwaters easy to explore without a trail. The eastern branch leads from Lake South America north to Harrison Pass. A trail is marked on the USGS 7.5' topos, but only token sections of it exist on the ground; no need to worry, for a trail is superfluous for the easy 2-mile jaunt to Harrison Pass. You cross meadows, sand, and almost no talus to surmount the Kings–Kern Divide. However, as you stare down the steep, bouldery northern side of Harrison Pass, you'll be glad you get to retrace your steps to Lake South America.

Alternatively, if you were to leave the trail well below Lake South America, at the lakes around 11,300 feet (near 36.66932°N, 118.41629°W), you could walk an equally straightforward 2.5 miles up past lakes and tarns to Lucys Foot Pass, the true headwaters of the Kern. Here you would stare down an even steeper, rockier escarpment. Peak baggers will be particularly enamored by the view down the Kern from atop Mount Genevra (Class 2 from the southeast), but Mount Ericsson (Class 2 from the west) is also a wonderful summit.

DAY 6 (Lake South America to Anvil Camp, 8.6 miles): Retrace your steps to the junction by the tarn, just south of Lake South America, and turn left (southeast), heading across alpine fellfields to the summit of a broad saddle west of Caltech Peak's southern summit. A steep but pleasantly sandy trail snakes its way south, soon reaching a spring-fed marshland where flowers are prolific all summer. Skirting the edge of the meadows, you continue past a tarn, reveling in the easy walking and expanding views south. Crossing a shallow ridge, you reach a junction from a few days ago, where right (west) was the route you took to Milestone Basin, while left (east) leads back to the JMT corridor; turn left. Now retrace your steps 0.7 mile to the JMT, turn right (south), and continue 0.4 mile south along the JMT, crossing Tyndall Creek to reach the Shepherd Pass Trail junction. Turn left (east) onto the Shepherd Pass Trail.

The Shepherd Pass Trail winds up moraine deposits, slowly diverging from Tyndall Creek. A couple of switchbacks carry you into an isolated stand of lodgepole pine before you embark on a barren ascent toward Shepherd Pass. The trail is carefully routed to follow sand-and-rock ribs, but much of the broad shallow basin is covered in seasonal trickles and meadow patches. Admire the colorful streamside flowers where you cross tributaries and elsewhere stare closely at the gray sands to discern the tiny alpine tundra species. Turning around, you have views of the now-familiar skyline around Milestone Basin, the vista now evoking personal memories of a difficult-to-reach beautiful corner of the High Sierra. To your right (south) rises the broad northern flank of Mount Tyndall, while to the south stands aptly named Diamond Mesa, an unglaciated landform. Just before Shepherd Pass is a large lake (12,209') that can remain half frozen into summer. It offers chilly, windy campsites popular with climbers seeking the summit of Mount Williamson, California's second highest summit.

MOUNT TYNDALL'S FIRST ASCENT

The traveler who has read the incredible first chapter of Clarence King's *Mountaineering in the Sierra Nevada* may speculate on where King and Richard Cotter crossed the Kings–Kern Divide in July 1864 (the experts still do), but it is known that they traversed the west side of Shepherd Pass on their way to ascending Mount Tyndall. They had left the main Brewer survey party in hopes of summiting Mount Whitney, which they would have seen when they summited Mount Brewer a few days earlier. King did not document in his journal why they selected a lesser summit as their destination. Maybe it was their frightening crossing of the Kings–Kern Divide or slower-than-expected progress across this unmapped landscape that made them opt for a closer goal. Certainly they found the ascent up Mount Tyndall's north face to be legend worthy and the view from the summit worth a long description.

The view from Shepherd Pass (12,052') down to the Owens Valley, 8,000 feet below, is intimidating, and unless you welcome a steep talus descent, the coming half mile isn't much fun. In early summer you must first inch across a quite steep snow slope, hopeful that others have etched out a foot trench you can follow. Beyond are rough switchbacks down a steep slope; this trail is infrequently maintained, and small rockslides commonly remove parts of the tread. Weaving down between imposing cliff faces, you eventually reach a lower angle jumble of huge boulders, an amalgamation of rock glaciers and moraines. The trail follows a welcome strip of sand between two talus ribs, where wax currants have successfully established. Here the trail is in good condition, an amazing sandy passage between the rock piles. You cross a broad shallow creek and then wind down a gravelly rib with whitebark pine krummholz, passing the first plausible campsites. Crossing a second drainage among willows, you reach the Pothole and some more small campsites. With steep walls (or talus piles) rising on three sides, this indeed feels like a pothole, but the name would have been even more fitting for hikers completing the JMT before the trail over Forester Pass was built. Between 1916 and 1931, hikers wishing to cross the Kings–Kern Divide between Bubbs Creek and Tyndall Creek crossed Junction Pass, high to your north, and had to drop to the Pothole, before ascending Shepherd Pass. To them, it must have been a most unwelcome 1,200-foot-deep pothole—but at least they had a stock-passable route.

Rounding the front on an inactive rock glacier, the trail winds easily down. Whitebark pine cover increases, and you pass more small campsites before sidling back up to the creek corridor and soon crossing Shepherd Creek. Just beyond is Anvil Camp, a broad collection of good campsites under foxtail and whitebark pine cover on the north side of Shepherd Creek (10,349'; 36.68949°N, 118.32964°W; no campfires). *Note:* Anvil Camp is 0.2 mile southwest of where it is marked on the USGS 7.5' topo.)

DAY 7 (Anvil Camp to Symmes Creek [Shepherd Pass] Trailhead, 8.5 miles): Leaving Anvil Camp, descend on a good trail through talus. Most noteworthy over the coming mile are the repeated debris flow channels that bisect the talus fans. At the most prominent one, the trail has recently been rerouted, and now completes a pair of ascending switchbacks to enter the debris flow channel. In late July 2013, the runoff from a severe thunderstorm sculpted a channel that was in places more than 20 feet deep, with giant jagged boulders embedded in the vertical dirt walls—not a route stock or most hikers could confidently use. Once you're across this unmapped drainage, the foxtail pines abruptly end and the path begins a long series of gentle switchbacks through dry eastside terrain—mountain mahogany and sagebrush are now the dominant shrubs—to reach Mahogany Flat. There are several campsites here and water if you leave the trail and descend to the creek (9,240'; 36.69309°N, 118.31877°W; well north of the words *Mahogany Flat* on the 7.5' Mount Williamson quad).

Continuing the switchbacking descent, ford a year-round Shepherd Creek tributary after 0.7 mile and then cross onto a more open slope, still recovering from a fire decades ago. A final stream crossing after an additional 1.1 miles (at 8,550' and often dry by midsummer) marks the beginning of a discouraging 500-foot ascent. The first steep section of climbing carries you to a small ridge radiating off Mount Keith; there is a dry campsite with views that make up for the absence of water. Shepherd Creek has carved a steep canyon to the south, capped by towering Mount Williamson, the only 14,000-foot peak in the Sierra not on the crestline. Sidling in and out of two other drainages, across sloggy, sandy slopes so steep they seem to exceed the angle of repose, and over two small ridges, you are finally on the divide separating Shepherd Creek's canyon from Symmes Creek's (9,090'). You are most pleased to trade the mountain mahogany and pinyon pine cover of the south-facing Shepherd Creek slope for limber pines on the Symmes Creek side. There are ample campsites set in trees on this waterless saddle.

From this saddle, the trail begins a relatively gradual switchbacking descent, dropping the 2,100 feet to Symmes Creek over 2.9 miles. The trail as marked on the USGS 7.5' topo shows just 22 switchbacks, but a rerouting in the late 1970s decreased the gradient and increased the zigzags to the current count of 30. With continued descent, white firs join the pinyon and limber pines, the firs preferring the sheltered draws and deeper soil farther west in the gully, while the pinyon pines thrive on the rockier, drier slopes on the eastern edge of the slope. Finally you drop to the riparian thicket fringing Symmes Creek (6,971') and reach your first water in 4.8 miles.

With just 1.1 miles remaining to the car, the trail now winds down this steep, narrow canyon. You must ford Symmes Creek four times over this distance—easy in a dry year or in late summer, but sure to wet feet and threaten footing in early summer. If water levels are particularly onerous, you can remain on the north bank between the second and third crossings, working your way across talus and through scrub. In places, the trail has also been reworked here following the 2013 debris flows. Alders, willows, and interior rose grow thickly along the banks, with black cottonwood appearing as the canyon mouth opens. At the mouth, there is a fork, where the stock trail trends to the left and fords the creek again, while hikers go right (east) a final 0.2 mile to the Symmes Creek Trailhead (6,308'; 36.72708°N, 118.27888°W).

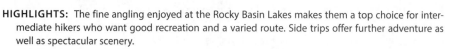

trip 80   **Rocky Basin Lakes**

see maps on p. 418–419

Trip Data: 36.44451°N, 118.32412°W; 26.8 miles; 4/1 days
Topos: *Cirque Peak, Johnson Peak*

HIGHLIGHTS: The fine angling enjoyed at the Rocky Basin Lakes makes them a top choice for intermediate hikers who want good recreation and a varied route. Side trips offer further adventure as well as spectacular scenery.

HEADS UP! *Wood fires are not allowed at the Rocky Basin Lakes.*

DAY 1 (Cottonwood Pass Trailhead to Big Whitney Meadow, 7.8 miles): The exposed, sandy trail heads west beneath very sparse lodgepole pine shade. After 0.3 mile you reach a junction where left (south) leads across Horseshoe Meadow and onto Trail Pass, while you continue straight ahead (right; west), along the northern edge of the expansive meadow system. Continued flat, sandy walking takes you northwest and then west to the head of Horseshoe Meadow, where the trail makes a pair of quick stream crossings, with great red paintbrush, crimson columbine, and monkeyflowers growing along the watercourses. After traversing a denser lodgepole pine flat and looping around another seasonally verdant meadow lobe, the trail begins a switchbacking ascent to the north of the willow-clad stream corridor. Winding up among foxtail pines and between small fractured outcrops, the gradient eases briefly where the trail crosses the meadowed river strip.

The trail then carries you north, still alongside a swathe of meadow and willows, before a dozen switchbacks lead west to Cottonwood Pass (11,167'). Views eastward include the Inyo and Panamint Ranges, while to the west you garner glimpses of expansive Big Whitney Meadow and the distant Great Western Divide. A few feet west of the pass, you come to the famous Pacific Crest Trail (PCT) at a diffuse four-way junction. The PCT leads south–north (left–right), while your route, the trail to Big Whitney Meadow, is straight ahead (west). The trail descends alongside the headwaters of one of the branches of Stokes Stringer through a "meadow" of sagebrush. About 0.4 mile past the junction, where the trail cuts to the north side of the creek, the sandy slopes to the north offers campsites beneath foxtail and lodgepole pines as long as there is still water in the creek.

Soon the terrain steepens and the trail begins switchbacking beside the now-willow-choked creek, soon crossing the fork of Stokes Stringer that drains Chicken Spring Lake. Eighteen well-graded switchbacks then lead down a steep sandy slope of foxtail pine to another ford of Stokes Stringer after exactly 1.0 mile, this time crossed on logs. Another dozen, very gentle zigzags, now in a mixed foxtail and lodgepole pine forest, lead to the eastern precincts of Big Whitney Meadow.

The sandy trail skirts the edge of the meadow, sometimes across sand flats and elsewhere beneath stands of lodgepole pines. The meadow's periphery is sagebrush, while a verdant meadow stripe winds down its middle. Eventually, the trail cuts across the meadow, cross-ing Stokes Stringer on large rocks, traversing a huge sandy flat, and then crossing a forested ridge to the true start of Big Whitney Meadow. Multiple stringers coalesce in this expansive meadow-and-sand basin, eventually exiting the meadow as Golden Trout Creek.

You soon drop to cross one of Big Whitney Meadow's seasonally marshy lobes, this one draining lands to the northeast; the two channels within it are broad and must often be waded. Beyond, you arrive at a large island of sand and lodgepole pines in the middle of the meadow and walk along the meadow-sand boundary. This lump of sand, like others found in the Kern Plateau's expansive meadows are likely dunes, created soon after glaciers retreated. The recently deglaciated landscape would have been covered by a blanket of fine sediment, easily whipped into dunes by strong winds. Near here is a good place to end your first day, with water available nearby and expansive views (9,724'; 36.43866°N, 118.26187°W).

DAY 2 (Big Whitney Meadow to Rocky Basin Lakes, 5.6 miles): The trail continues west along the northern perimeter of the sandy island. Mountain bluebirds and killdeer are both common on the Kern Plateau's vast meadows; so, too, are coyotes, and you were hopefully treated to their chorus last night. The endless sandy flat eventually leads to a jump-across crossing of the stringer flowing south from Siberian Pass, your last reliable water before Rocky Basin Lakes. Now at the western edge of Big Whitney Meadow, the track continues through sloggy sand to the signed junction with the trail north (right) to Siberian Pass; you continue due west (straight ahead). Just 450 feet later you reach a second junction, where straight ahead (right; southwest) leads to Rocky Basin Lakes, while left (south) is signposted for Tunnel Meadow.

Onward toward the Rocky Basin Lakes, you climb gently up a shallow spur through open lodgepole pine forest, big rectangular feldspar crystals decorating the sandy ground. After dropping just slightly, you proceed up alongside a small creek, step across it, and then trend straight up a sandy slope. Continued ascent, including a cluster of tight, easy switch-backs, leads to a broad shallow saddle, from which a short descent takes you to a cryptic, but signed, trail junction (10,111'; 36.42734°N, 118.30204°W): right (north) leads to the Rocky Basin Lakes, straight ahead to Little Whitney Meadow (on a mostly abandoned trail), and left to Golden Trout Creek (on a mostly abandoned trail). Turn right.

The trail ascends through lodgepole pine forest alongside Barigan Stringer, the Rocky Basin Lakes outlet. It is a decent trail, ascending gently to moderately through forest flats and alongside meadow strips, but becoming rockier with increasing elevation. After just under 1 mile, where the trail turns to cross Barigan Stringer, hikers may see a sign that indi-cates FOOT TRAIL (right, northwest) and HORSE TRAIL (left, west)—and a reminder that no campfires are allowed (10,359'; 36.43732°N, 118.30718°W). The indistinct, unmapped foot trail offers a shorter but steeper scramble over a rocky, foxtail-clad ridge above Barigan

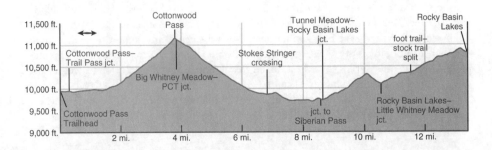

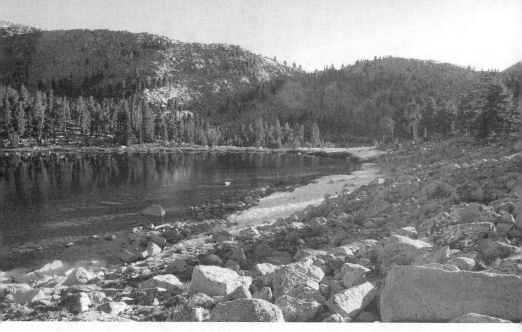

Rocky Basin Lakes   Photo by Elizabeth Wenk

Stringer, past a wedge-shaped seasonal lakelet, to the largest Rocky Basin lake, and then across talus bands to the western lakes.

The distinct, longer horse trail, the route shown on the USGS 7.5' topo map and described here, hops across the creek and zigzags up an open bouldery foxtail pine slope to a small tarn. The trail skirts its southern shore and climbs northwest up broken slab to the next step, a pocket meadow, before continuing mostly west as it winds around a knob and thereafter north as it climbs up an unmapped seasonal drainage. Passing a small ephemeral tarn, the trail turns north-northeast, winding up a bouldery trough with scattered foxtail pines. The trail flattens atop a broad saddle and drops gently to the westernmost Rocky Basin lake, where it ends.

The best campsites are at the northeastern corner of this lake, in sandy flats beneath whitebark pines (10,828'; 36.44451°N, 118.32412°W; no campfires), although there are additional small tent sites on the rib separating the middle and easternmost lakes. The Rocky Basin Lakes feel quite unique among high Sierran lakes. First of all, they are leaky, and in drought years their water levels drop significantly—quite different to the standard bedrock-dammed lakes whose water levels drop only slightly. Moreover, they lie in one of the Sierra's southernmost glaciated basins, but the glacier here wasn't terribly thick or erosive, and although the granite slabs are polished, mostly it is just a basin of rubble, set not far beneath the broad, flat, unglaciated Boreal Plateau—it is astoundingly stark and desolate, even by Sierran standards. Nearby Johnson Peak and the Boreal Plateau with Funston Lake offer adventurous cross-country goals for a layover day. Johnson Peak is a straightforward climb up its northwestern ridge and offers an outstanding view of the Kern Plateau. Heading west and then north leads to the Boreal Plateau and Funston Lake. A confident cross-country traveler could return to the trailhead via the Boreal Plateau, Siberian Outpost, and then the PCT, but note that the only guaranteed water is at Funston Lake and Chicken Spring Lake, so be prepared for a long, waterless hike to the car.

DAYS 3–4 (Rocky Basin Lakes to Cottonwood Pass Trailhead, 13.4 miles): Retrace your steps, perhaps selecting a different campsite to break the return trek.

Useful Books

BACKPACKING AND MOUNTAINEERING

Aksamit, Inga. *The Hungry Spork: A Long Distance Hiker's Guide to Meal Planning*. Pacific Adventures Press, 2017.

Aksamit, Inga, Kenny Meyer, and Leslie Rozier. *An Unofficial Acclimatization Guideline: Your High-Altitude Guideline for the John Muir Trail*, 2020.

Beck, Steve. *Yosemite Trout Fishing Guide*. Portland, OR: Frank Amato Publications, 1996.

Beffort, Brian. *Joy of Backpacking: Your Complete Guide to Attaining Pure Happiness in the Outdoors*. Berkeley, CA: Wilderness Press, 2007.

Berger, Karen. *Hiking Light Handbook: Carry Less, Enjoy More*. Seattle, WA: Mountaineers Books, 2004.

Clelland, Mike. *Ultralight Backpackin' Tips: 153 Amazing & Inexpensive Tips for Extremely Lightweight Camping*. Lanham, MD: Rowman & Littlefield, 2011.

Forgey, M. D. William W. *Wilderness Medicine: Beyond First Aid*. 7th ed. Guilford, CT: Falcon Guides, 2017.

Ghiglieri, Michael Patrick, and Charles R. Farabee. *Off the Wall: Death in Yosemite: Gripping Accounts of All Known Fatal Mishaps in America's First Protected Land of Scenic Wonders*. Flagstaff, AZ: Puma Press, 2007.

Ladigin, Don. *Lighten Up!: A Complete Handbook for Light and Ultralight Backpacking*. Lanham, MD: Rowman & Littlefield, 2005.

Wilkerson, James A. *Medicine for Mountaineering & Other Wilderness Activities*. 6th ed. Seattle, WA: The Mountaineers Books, 2010.

GUIDEBOOKS

Roper, Steve. *The Sierra High Route: Traversing Timberline Country*. Seattle, WA: The Mountaineers Books, 1997.

Secor, R. J. *The High Sierra: Peaks, Passes, Trails*. Seattle, WA: The Mountaineers Books, 2009.

Wenk, Elizabeth. *John Muir Trail: The Essential Guide to Hiking America's Most Famous Trail*. 5th ed. Birmingham, AL: Wilderness Press, 2014

———. *One Best Hike: Mount Whitney*. 2nd ed. Birmingham, AL: Wilderness Press, 2017

White, Mike. *Sequoia & Kings Canyon National Parks: Your Complete Hiking Guide*. Birmingham, AL: Wilderness Press, 2012.

———. *Top Trails: Sequoia and Kings Canyon National Parks: 50 Must-Do Hikes for Everyone*. 2nd ed. Birmingham, AL: Wilderness Press, 2016.

HISTORY AND LITERATURE

Aksamit, Inga. *Highs and Lows on the John Muir Trail*. San Bernardino, CA: Pacific Adventures Press, 2015.

Alsup, William. *Missing in the Minarets: The Search for Walter A. Starr, Jr. Illustrated Edition*. El Portal, CA: Yosemite Conservancy, 2005.

Arnold, Daniel. *Early Days in the Range of Light: Encounters with Legendary Mountaineers*. Berkeley, CA: Counterpoint Press, 2011.

Blehm, Eric. *The Last Season*. New York: HarperCollins, 2009.

Brewer, William H. *Up and Down California in 1860–1864: The Journal of William H. Brewer*. Berkeley, CA: University of California Press, 2003.

Brewer, William Henry, William H. Alsup, and Yosemite Association. *Such a Landscape!: A Narrative of the 1864 California Geological Survey Exploration of Yosemite, Sequoia & Kings Canyon from the Diary, Field Notes, Letters & Reports of William Henry Brewer*. El Portal, CA: Yosemite Association, 1999.

Brown, Bolton Coit. "Another Paradise." Sierra Club Bulletin 3 (1900): 135–49.

———. "Wanderings in the High Sierra Between Mt. King and Mt. Williamson." Sierra Club Bulletin 2 (1897): 17–28.

Browning, Peter. *Sierra Nevada Place Names.* 3rd ed. Lafayette, CA: Great West Books, 2011.

———. *Splendid Mountains.* Lafayette, CA: Great West Books, 2007.

Farquhar, Francis Peloubet. *History of the Sierra Nevada.* Berkeley, CA: University of California Press, 2007.

Jackson, Louise A. *Mineral King: The Story of Beulah.* Sequoia, 2006.

———. *The Sierra Nevada Before History: Ancient Landscapes, Early Peoples.* Mountain Press Publishing Company, Incorporated, 2010.

Johnson, Shelton. *Gloryland: A Novel.* Berkeley, CA: Counterpoint Press, 2010.

King, Clarence. *Mountaineering in the Sierra Nevada.* Lincoln, NE: University of Nebraska Press, 1997.

Le Conte, Joseph N. "The High Mountain Route Between Yosemite and the King's River Canon." Sierra Club Bulletin 7, no. 1 (1909): 1–22.

Muir, John. *The Mountains of California.* Berkeley, CA: Ten Speed Press, 1894 (1977).

———. *My First Summer in the Sierra.* San Francisco, CA: Sierra Club, 1911 (1990).

Roberts, Suzanne. *Almost Somewhere: Twenty-Eight Days on the John Muir Trail.* Lincoln, NE: University of Nebraska Press, 2012.

Rose, Gene. *High Odyssey: The First Solo Winter Assault of Mount Whitney and the Muir Trail Area, from the Diary of Orland Bartholomew and Photographs Taken by Him.* Panorama West Books, 1987.

———. *Kings Canyon, America's Premier National Park: A History.* Three Rivers, CA: Sequoia Natural History Association, 2012.

Roth, Hal. *Pathway in the Sky.* Howell-North Books, 1965.

Sargent, Shirley. *Solomons of the Sierra: The Pioneer of the John Muir Trail.* Flying Spur Press, 1989.

Strong, Douglas Hillman. *From Pioneers to Preservationists: A Brief History of Sequoia and Kings Canyon National Parks.* Three Rivers, CA: Sequoia Natural History Association, 2000.

Tweed, William. *Kaweah Remembered: The Story of the Kaweah Colony and the Founding of Sequoia National Park.* Three Rivers, CA: Sequoia Natural History Association, 1986.

———. *Shorty Lovelace, Kings Canyon Fur Trapper.* Three Rivers, CA: Sequoia Natural History Association, 2012.

Tweed, William C., and Lary M. Dilsaver. *Challenge of the Big Trees: The Updated History of Sequoia and Kings Canyon National Parks. Illustrated Edition.* Staunton, VA: George F. Thompson Publishing, 2017.

GEOLOGY

Glazner, Allen F., and Greg M. Stock. *Geology Underfoot in Yosemite National Park.* Missoula, MT: Mountain Press, 2010.

Guyton, Bill. *Glaciers of California: Modern Glaciers, Ice Age Glaciers, Origin of Yosemite Valley, and a Glacier Tour in the Sierra Nevada.* Berkeley, CA: University of California Press, 2001.

Huber, N. King, and Wymond W. Eckhardt. *Devils Postpile Story.* Three Rivers, CA: Sequoia Natural History Association, 2001.

Moore, James Gregory. *Exploring the Highest Sierra.* Palo Alto, CA: Stanford University Press, 2000.

BIOLOGY

Anderson, M. Kat. *Tending the Wild: Native American Knowledge and the Management of California's Natural Resources.* Berkeley, CA: University of California Press, 2013.

Beedy, Edward C., and Edward R. Pandolfino. *Birds of the Sierra Nevada: Their Natural History, Status, and Distribution.* Berkeley, CA: University of California Press, 2013.

Gaines, David. *Birds of Yosemite and the East Slope.* Lee Vining, CA: Artemisia Press, 1992.

Johnston, V. R. *Sierra Nevada: The Naturalist's Companion.* Berkeley, CA: University of California Press, 2000.

Laws, John Muir. *The Laws Field Guide to the Sierra Nevada.* Berkeley, CA: Heyday, 2007.

Sibley, David. *The Sibley Field Guide to Birds of Western North America.* New York: Knopf, 2003.

Storer, Tracy I., Robert L. Usinger, and David Lukas. *Sierra Nevada Natural History.* Berkeley, CA: University of California Press, 2004.

Weeden, Norman F. *A Sierra Nevada Flora.* Berkeley, CA: Wilderness Press, 1996.

Wenk, Elizabeth. *Wildflowers of the High Sierra and John Muir Trail.* Birmingham, AL: Wilderness Press, 2015.

Wiese, Karen. *Sierra Nevada Wildflowers.* 2nd ed. Lanham, MD: Rowman & Littlefield, 2013.

Willard, Dwight. *A Guide to the Sequoia Groves of California.* El Portal, CA: Yosemite Association, 2000.

Guides to the Sierra Nevada from Wilderness Press

AFOOT & AFIELD: TAHOE-RENO *by Mike White*
The completely updated second edition of this comprehensive guide features more than 175 trips in a diverse range of terrain around Lake Tahoe and the communities of Reno, Sparks, Carson City, and Minden-Gardnerville. These trips are tailored for every type of hiker, and many are suited for mountain bikers.

JOHN MUIR TRAIL: THE ESSENTIAL GUIDE TO HIKING AMERICA'S MOST FAMOUS TRAIL
by Elizabeth Wenk
This is the best guide to the legendary trail that runs from Yosemite Valley to Mt. Whitney. Written for both northbound and southbound hikers, it includes updated two-color maps.

SEQUOIA & KINGS CANYON NATIONAL PARKS *by Mike White*
This information-packed guide to the peaks and gorges of the majestic apex of the Sierra Nevada includes detailed maps, comprehensive trail descriptions, and enlightening background chapters.

SIERRA NORTH *by Elizabeth Wenk and Mike White*
This completely revised and updated classic—the companion to *Sierra South*—showcases new trips and old favorites. With trips organized around major highway sections, using this guide is easier than ever.

TOP TRAILS: LAKE TAHOE *by Mike White*
This indispensable guide features the 50 best hikes in the Tahoe area, including the north side's splendid backcountry; the lake's sedate western side; the picturesque and popular areas south of the lake, including Desolation Wilderness and D. L. Bliss and Emerald Bay State Parks; and the relatively undeveloped eastern side.

TOP TRAILS: SEQUOIA AND KINGS CANYON NATIONAL PARKS *by Mike White*
The southern High Sierra, including Sequoia and Kings Canyon National Parks and the surrounding John Muir, Jennie Lakes, and Monarch Wildernesses, is one of the most magnificent natural areas in the world. This guide presents the best curated selection of trips suitable for varied skill levels to explore this wonderland.

TOP TRAILS: YOSEMITE *by Elizabeth Wenk and Jeffrey P. Schaffer*
Now in full color, the second edition of *Top Trails Yosemite* helps you sort through the amazing number of choice hiking destinations in Yosemite National Park. Whether you're looking for a scenic stroll, a full-day adventure, or a spectacular backpacking trip, you'll find it here.

YOSEMITE NATIONAL PARK *by Elizabeth Wenk and Jeffrey P. Schaffer*
Called the Cadillac of Yosemite books by the National Park Service, the completely revised sixth edition of this guide details more than 90 trips, from day hikes to extended backpacks, and now includes a map specific to each trip.

Index

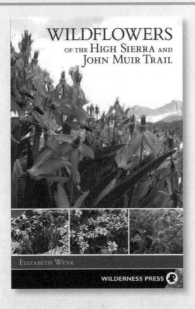
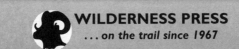
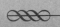

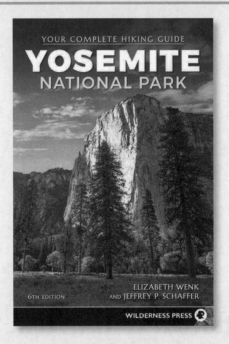
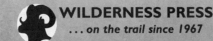

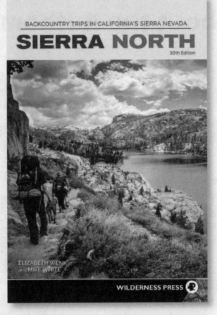
 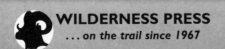

About the Authors

Elizabeth Wenk has hiked and climbed in the Sierra Nevada since childhood and continues the tradition with her husband, Douglas Bock, and daughters, Eleanor and Sophia. As she obtained a PhD in Sierran alpine plant ecology from the University of California, Berkeley, her love of the mountain range morphed into a profession. Writing guidebooks has become her way to share her love and knowledge of the Sierra Nevada with others. Lizzy continues to obsessively explore every bit of the Sierra, spending summers hiking on- and off-trail throughout the range, but she currently lives in Sydney, Australia, during the "off-season." Other Wilderness Press titles she has authored include *John Muir Trail, Top Trails Yosemite, One Best Hike: Mount Whitney, One Best Hike: Grand Canyon, Backpacking California, Sierra South, 50 Best Short Hikes: Yosemite,* and *Wildflowers of the High Sierra and John Muir Trail,* the latter a perfect companion book for all naturalists. Lizzy is also a board member of the John Muir Trail Wilderness Conservancy, a foundation dedicated to the preservation of the JMT corridor and surrounding High Sierra lands.

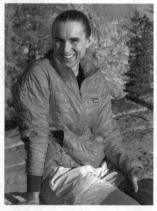

Photo by Douglas Bock

Mike White was born and raised in Portland, Oregon. He learned to hike, backpack, and climb in the Cascade Mountains, and he honed his outdoor skills further while obtaining a bachelor's degree from Seattle Pacific University. After college, Mike and his wife, Robin, relocated to the Nevada desert, where he was drawn to the majesty of the High Sierra. In the early 1990s, Mike began writing about the outdoors, expanding the third edition of Luther Linkhart's *The Trinity Alps* for Wilderness Press. His first solo title was *Nevada Wilderness Areas and Great Basin National Park.* Many more books for Wilderness followed, including the Snowshoe Trails series; books about Sequoia, Kings Canyon, and Lassen Volcanic National Parks; *Backpacking Nevada; Top Trails: Northern California's Redwood Coast; Best Backpacking Trips in California and Nevada; Best Backpacking Trips in Utah, Arizona, and New Mexico; 50 of the Best Strolls, Walks, and Hikes Around Reno;* and *Afoot & Afield: Tahoe-Reno.* Mike has also contributed to the Wilderness classic, *Backpacking California.* Two of his books, *Top Trails: Lake Tahoe* and *50 Classic Hikes in Nevada,* have won national awards.

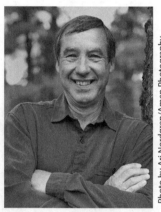

Photo by Ari Nordgren/Amen Photography

A former community college instructor, Mike is a featured speaker for outdoor groups. He and Robin live in Reno; his two sons, David and Stephen, live in the area as well.